Hari's
Essentials of
Clinical Medicine

Hari's Essentials of Clinical Medicine

Third Edition

P Baburaj MD
Professor
Department of Medicine
Jubilee Mission Medical College and Research Institute
Thrissur, Kerala, India

Formerly, Professor and Head
Department of Medicine
Government Medical College
Thrissur, Kerala, India

Shankara BV DNB (Med)
Assistant Professor
Department of Medicine
Jubilee Mission Medical College and Research Institute
Thrissur, Kerala, India

Foreword
MV Muraleedharan

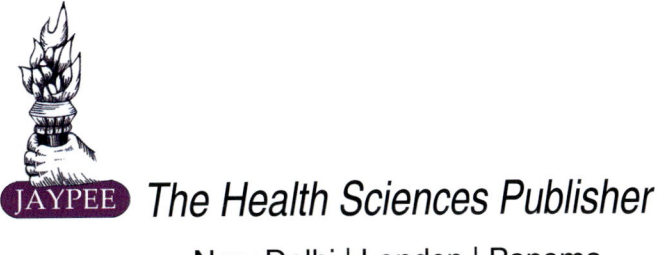

JAYPEE *The Health Sciences Publisher*
New Delhi | London | Panama

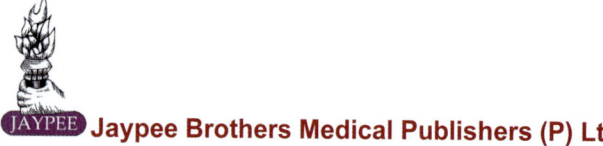

Jaypee Brothers Medical Publishers (P) Ltd

Headquarters
Jaypee Brothers Medical Publishers (P) Ltd
4838/24, Ansari Road, Daryaganj
New Delhi 110 002, India
Phone: +91-11-43574357
Fax: +91-11-43574314
Email: jaypee@jaypeebrothers.com

Overseas Offices

J.P. Medical Ltd
83 Victoria Street, London
SW1H 0HW (UK)
Phone: +44 20 3170 8910
Fax: +44 (0)20 3008 6180
Email: info@jpmedpub.com

Jaypee Brothers Medical Publishers (P) Ltd
17/1-B Babar Road, Block-B, Shaymoli
Mohammadpur, Dhaka-1207
Bangladesh
Mobile: +08801912003485
Email: jaypeedhaka@gmail.com

Jaypee-Highlights Medical Publishers Inc
City of Knowledge, Bld. 235, 2nd Floor, Clayton
Panama City, Panama
Phone: +1 507-301-0496
Fax: +1 507-301-0499
Email: cservice@jphmedical.com

Jaypee Brothers Medical Publishers (P) Ltd
Bhotahity, Kathmandu
Nepal
Phone: +977-9741283608
Email: kathmandu@jaypeebrothers.com

Website: www.jaypeebrothers.com
Website: www.jaypeedigital.com

© 2019, Jaypee Brothers Medical Publishers

The views and opinions expressed in this book are solely those of the original contributor(s)/author(s) and do not necessarily represent those of editor(s) of the book.

All rights reserved. No part of this publication may be reproduced, stored or transmitted in any form or by any means, electronic, mechanical, photocopying, recording or otherwise, without the prior permission in writing of the publishers.

All brand names and product names used in this book are trade names, service marks, trademarks or registered trademarks of their respective owners. The publisher is not associated with any product or vendor mentioned in this book.

Medical knowledge and practice change constantly. This book is designed to provide accurate, authoritative information about the subject matter in question. However, readers are advised to check the most current information available on procedures included and check information from the manufacturer of each product to be administered, to verify the recommended dose, formula, method and duration of administration, adverse effects and contraindications. It is the responsibility of the practitioner to take all appropriate safety precautions. Neither the publisher nor the author(s)/editor(s) assume any liability for any injury and/or damage to persons or property arising from or related to use of material in this book.

This book is sold on the understanding that the publisher is not engaged in providing professional medical services. If such advice or services are required, the services of a competent medical professional should be sought.

Every effort has been made where necessary to contact holders of copyright to obtain permission to reproduce copyright material. If any have been inadvertently overlooked, the publisher will be pleased to make the necessary arrangements at the first opportunity. The **CD/DVD-ROM** (if any) provided in the sealed envelope with this book is complimentary and free of cost. **Not meant for sale.**

Inquiries for bulk sales may be solicited at: jaypee@jaypeebrothers.com

Hari's Essentials of Clinical Medicine

First Edition: 2008
Second Edition: 2017
Third Edition: **2019**
ISBN: 978-93-5270-534-4
Printed at: Samrat Offset Pvt. Ltd.

Dedicated to

My Father

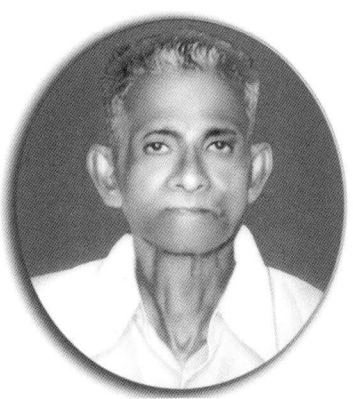

Sh K Parameswaran

and

My Beloved Teachers

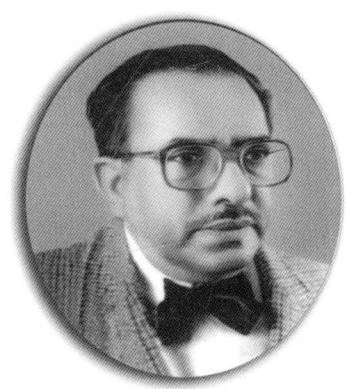

Prof MG Sahadevan

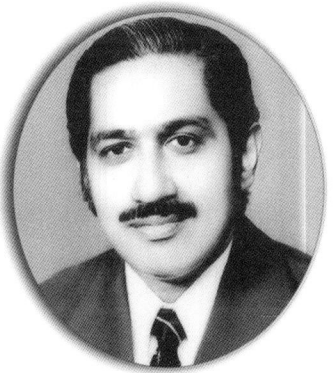

Prof VC Mathew Roy

Foreword to the Third Edition

As a medical teacher for almost 45 years, I look with great pleasure the launching of the third edition of *Hari's Essentials of Clinical Medicine* by Professor P Baburaj and Dr Shankara BV. In the era of rapid advances in the field of medicine, textbook needs a lot of efforts and determination which makes the third edition of this book a reality.

Clinical medicine is a challenging field. Our teachers have shown us the way to practise clinical methods as advanced investigations of today were not existing. It is founded on scientific principles of history taking and physical examination which is done with utmost commitment in a systemic manner, even in this era of investigative medicine, clinical medicine has great importance in a country, where investigations are not within the reach of average patient. Dr P Baburaj and Dr Shankara BV have written this book fully understanding the reality. It is heartening to note that new chapter of relevance and new photographs are added. The following topics are revised in the third edition—general examination findings, speech disorders, common disorders in cardiovascular system, systemic lupus erythematosus, nephrology. In the present format, this book will be a ready-reckoner to the basic students and also for specialists and subspecialists practicing medicine. I take this opportunity to wish Dr P Baburaj and Dr Shankara BV, the very best in their new endeavor.

MV Muraleedharan MD DM MRCP (UK)
Retired Professor and Head
Department of Medicine and Endocrinology
Jubilee Mission Medical College and Research Institute
Thrissur, Kerala, India

Foreword to the First Edition

Clinical medicine is an ever-interesting science and provides satisfaction to the practitioners and comfort to his patients. It is founded on the well-defined principles of history taking and physical examination done in a methodical manner.

The art of history taking and examination is the theme of a number of books and manuals. Each author views these skills from his/her point of view.

This book titled *Hari's Essentials of Clinical Medicine* written by Professor P Baburaj will be a useful addition to the large number of titles already existing in this field. In this publication, Dr P Baburaj has incorporated his vast skills and knowledge as a teacher and practitioner which span over three decades. During his educational career, he qualified as the best student in medicine in his batch with gold medal to his credit and he proved his consistency by being honored with the best teacher award.

Many believe that technical advances in the field of medicine would replace the art and science of clinical medicine. On the contrary, one has to view the data obtained from such investigations on the background of the data obtained by the clinician during his interview with the patient. Professor P Baburaj has fully taken this point when writing this book and, hence, it would be an excellent source of information for the medical students, practicing doctors and postgraduate students preparing for the examination. It will be a useful ready reference for the subspecialists in the discipline of internal medicine.

I wish Professor P Baburaj every success in his endeavor.

MV Muraleedharan MD DM
Professor and Head
Department of Medicine
Jubilee Mission Medical College and Research Institute
Thrissur, Kerala, India

Preface to the Third Edition

We feel great pleasure in presenting the third edition of *Hari's Essentials of Clinical Medicine*. Various suggestions from the students, teachers and professors of medicine are included. Some of the chapters in cardiology and locomotor system are revised and certain topics regarding the spinal cord are rewritten. New topics, like "Diseases of the Peripheral Nerve" are included. New photographs are added for easy appreciation. The following topics are revised in the third edition—general examination findings, speech disorders, common disorders in cardiovascular system (CVS), systemic lupus erythematosus (SLE), nephrology.

The book is a ready-reckoner for preparing clinical discussion and clinical examination for both undergraduates and postgraduates.

P Baburaj
Shankara BV

Preface to the First Edition

It gives me great pleasure to present this book *Hari's Essentials of Clinical Medicine* before the medical fraternity.

Examination of a patient at the bedside to elicit the signs and symptoms of the disease to arrive at a diagnosis forms the basis of clinical medicine. It is on this basis that investigations are planned to confirm the clinical diagnosis and treatment plans are evolved. Skill in eliciting history and art of clinical examination establishes rapport between the patient and clinician. This rapport is important for the patient to develop confidence on his/her doctor. Even with availability of advanced and accurate investigations, clinical examination is important in arriving a logical diagnosis.

This book on Essentials of Clinical Medicine incorporates the fundamentals of clinical examinations like eliciting history and physical findings. The knowledge derived thus forms the essential tool for the student preparing for his/her examination at undergraduate and postgraduate levels. It is equally important when he/she starts practising the profession later.

The chapters on major systems like Neurology, Cardiology, Alimentary System and Pulmonology are given in detail and aim at the undergraduate and postgraduate students preparing for the examination. Chapters on Rheumatology, Renal Medicine, Hematology and Endocrinology give enough information for the examination and to practise medicine.

Common disorders of each system are highlighted. This would help the students as rapid reference before the examination.

This book will also give directions for the junior teachers preparing for clinical teaching sessions.

I have immense pleasure in placing on record my gratitude and appreciation to Professor MV Muraleedharan, my teacher, for being kind enough to write a foreword for this book. I also thank M/s Jaypee Brothers Medical Publishers (P) Ltd, New Delhi, India, for their wholehearted help and cooperation extended to me in bringing out this book in an elegant manner.

P Baburaj

Acknowledgments

We are deeply indebted to the following members, for helping us in preparing the various chapters of the third edition *Hari's Essentials of Clinical Medicine,* bringing out in a good shape.

- Dr BL Harikrishnan MD (Assistant Professor, Department of Medicine)
- Prof MV Muraleedharan MD DM (Professor, Department of Medicine and Endocrinology)
- Prof KB Mohan MD (Professor, Department of Medicine)
- Prof MA Andrews MD DM (Professor, Department of Medicine and Neurology)
- Prof CV Radha (Professor, Department of Ophthalmology)
- Prof R Krishnan MD (Professor, Department of Medicine)
- Dr PM Jayaraj MD DM (Senior Nephrologist)
- Dr Dinesh Prabhu MD DTCD (Professor, Department of Pulomonology)
- Dr Karunadas MD DM (Assistant Professor, Department of Cardiology)
- Dr Premalatha MD DM (Assistant Professor, Department of Gastroenterology)
- Dr Rajkrishna MD
- Dr CV Lakshmy MBBS
- Dr Swapna MD
- Dr KG Gopakumar
- Dr BL Lakshmi
- Dr Lalitha kumari MBBS DGO

Abbreviations

AGN	Acute glomerulonephritis	LSB	Left sternal border
AION	Anterior ischemic optic neuritis	LVE	Left ventricular enlargement
AKI	Acute kidney injury	LVF	Left ventricular failure
ALL	Acute lymphatic leukemia	MCTD	Mixed connective tissue disease
ARDS	Acute respiratory distress syndrome	MI	Myocardial infarction
AVM	Arteriovenous malformation	MND	Motor neuron disease
B/L	Bilateral	MS	Multiple sclerosis
BIH	Benign intracranial hypertension	NHL	Non-Hodgkin's lymphoma
CHD	Congenital heart disease	NSAIDs	Nonsteroidal anti-inflammatory drugs
CHF	Congestive heart failure	OCP	Oral contraceptive pill
CJ disease	Cruetzfeld Jacob disease	OP	Organophosphorus
CKD	Chronic kidney disease	PAN	Polyarteritis nodosa
CLL	Chronic lymphoid leukemia	PCOD	Polycystic ovarian disease
CML	Chronic myeloid leukemia	PDA	Patent ductus arteriosus
CMV	Cytomegalovirus	PND	Paroxysmal nocturnal dyspnea
COPD	Chronic obstructive pulmonary disease	PNS	Paranasal sinus
CRF	Chronic renal failure	PSS	Progressive systemic sclerosis
DIP	Distal interphalangeal joint	PTA	Persistent ductus arteriosus
DPH	Diphenyl hydantoin	PUO	Pyrexia of unknown origin
DVT	Deep vein thrombosis	RICS	Right intercostal space
ECF	Extracellular fluid	RSOV	Rupture of sinus of Valsalva
EPS	Extrapyramidal system	RS_3PE	Remitting symmetrical seronegative synovitis with pitting edema
GBS	Guillain-Barré syndrome		
HBV	Hepatitis B virus	RTI	Respiratory tract infection
HL	Hodgkin's lymphoma	SCLE	Subacute cutaneous lupus erythematosus
IBD	Inflammatory bowel disease	SDH	Subdural hematoma
ICP	Intracranial pressure	SLE	Systemic lupus erythematosus
ICSOL	Intracranial space-occupying lesion	SMA	Spinal muscular atrophy
ILD	Interstitial lung disease	SSPE	Subacute sclerosing pan-encephalitis
IMN	Infectious mononucleosis	TAPVC	Total anomalous pulmonary venous connection
IVC	Inferior vena cava		
LGV	Lymphogranuloma venereum	U/L	Unilateral
LICS	Left intercostals space	UMN	Upper motor neuron
LMN	Lower motor neuron	UTI	Urinary tract infection

Contents

1. **History Taking**   1
   - General Principles of History Taking   *1*
   - History Taking Sequence   *1*

2. **Physical Examination**   4
   General Examination   *4*
   - Appearance of the Patient   *4*
   - Consciousness and Cooperation   *4*
   - Apparent Age   *4*
   - Build and Nourishment   *4*
   - Anemia   *5*
   - Polycythemia   *6*
   - Jaundice   *6*
   - Cyanosis   *7*
   - Edema   *8*
   - Dyspnea   *9*
   - Posture of the Patient   *10*
   - Hydration   *11*
   - Examination of Nail   *11*
   - Skin   *12*
   - Hair   *17*
   - Thyroid Gland   *17*
   - Examination of Lymph Nodes   *17*
   - Hand and Systemic Diseases   *19*
   - Diagnostic Facies   *19*
   - Vital Signs   *20*
   - Usual Features of Fever   *21*

3. **Examination of Nervous System**   23
   Review of Neuroanatomy and Physiology   *23*
   - Motor System   *23*
   - Sensory System   *24*
   - Extrapyramidal System   *26*
   - Cerebellum   *26*
   - Spinal Cord   *26*
   - Cerebral Cortex   *27*
   - Blood Supply of Brain and Spinal Cord   *27*
   - Symptomatology in Disorders of Nervous System   *29*
   - History Taking in Nervous System Disorder   *31*
   - General Examination in Nervous System Disorder   *31*
   - Examination of Nervous System   *32*
   - Examination of Higher Functions   *33*

   Examination of Cranial Nerves   *37*
   - Olfactory Nerve   *37*
   - Optic Nerve   *38*
   - Ocular Motor Nerves   *42*
   - Ocular Muscles   *44*
   - Ptosis   *47*

- Pupil and Light Reflex 48
- Other Abnormal Movements of Eye 50
- Clinical Approach to Ophthalmoplegia 51
- Trigeminal Nerve 56
- Facial Nerve 59
- Vestibulocochlear Nerve 64
- Glossopharyngeal and Vagus Nerve 65
- Accessory Nerve 67
- Hypoglossal Nerve 68
- Examination of Motor System 69
- Bulk of Muscle 69
- Power of Muscle 73
- Reflexes 78
- Coordination of Movement 86
- Gait 87
- Involuntary Movements 88
- Examination of Sensory System 90
- Examination of Cerebellar Signs 96
- Signs of Meningeal Irritation 98
- Skull and Spine Examination 98
- Spine 98
- Examination of Unconscious Patient 99
- Clinical Evaluation of Hemiplegia 100
- Neurovascular Syndromes 102
- Clinical Assessment of Diseases of Spinal Cord 103
- Peripheral Neuropathy 106

4. **Examination of Cardiovascular System** 109
   - Symptomatology 109
   - History in Cardiovascular Disorders 111
   - General Examination in Cardiovascular System 111
   - Pulse 113
   - Jugular Venous Pressure and Pulsation 117
   - Examination of Precordium 120
   - Clinical Features of Common Cardiovascular Disorders 129
   - Mitral Regurgitation 131
   - Mitral Valve Prolapse 132
   - Aortic Stenosis 133
   - Aortic Regurgitation 134
   - Tricuspid Valvular Disease 136
   - Pulmonary Valvular Disease 136
   - Common Congenital Heart Diseases 137
   - Atrial Septal Defect 138
   - Ventricular Septal Defect 139
   - Patent Ductus Arteriosus 140
   - Eisenmenger Syndrome 141
   - Tetralogy of Fallot 142
   - Coarctation of Aorta 143
   - Pulmonary Hypertension 144
   - Pericardial Diseases 145
   - Infective Endocarditis 146
   - Clinical Evaluation of Heart Failure 148

5. Examination of Respiratory System — 151
- Functional Anatomy *151*
- Pleura *152*
- Symptomatology *152*
- History Taking in Respiratory Diseases *154*
- General Examination in Respiratory System *155*
- Examination of Respiratory System *155*
- Examination of Chest *156*
- Clinical Features of Common Respiratory Diseases *165*

6. Examination of Alimentary System — 180
- Symptomatology *180*
- Upper GI Symptoms *180*
- Lower GI Symptoms *185*
- General Symptoms *187*
- History Taking in Alimentary System *189*
- General Examination in Alimentary System *190*
- Alimentary System Examination *191*
- Examination of Esophagus *194*
- Examination of Abdomen *194*
- Inspection of Abdomen *195*
- Palpation of the Abdomen *197*
- Percussion of Abdomen *201*
- Auscultation of Abdomen *202*
- Examination of Groins *203*
- Examination of Anus and Rectum *204*
- Examination of Acute Abdomen *204*
- Other System Examinations in Alimentary Disorders *205*
- Differential Diagnosis of Common Clinical Signs of Abdomen *205*
- Clinical Evaluation of Ascites *207*
- Malabsorption Syndrome *210*
- Inflammatory Bowel Disease *211*
- Clinical Evaluation of Jaundice *213*
- Differentiating Features of Various Types of Jaundice *215*
- Viral Hepatitis *215*
- Chronic Hepatitis *216*
- Cirrhosis Liver *217*
- Portal Hypertension *220*
- Upper GI Bleed *222*
- Hepatic Encephalopathy *223*

7. Examination of Musculoskeletal System — 226
- Commonly Used Terms in Rheumatology *226*
- Symptomatology *226*
- History Taking *227*
- Examination *227*
- Differential Diagnosis of Arthritis *232*
- Common Rheumatological Disorders *234*
- Rheumatoid Arthritis *234*
- Systemic Lupus Erythematosus *238*
- Seronegative Spondyloarthropathy *241*
- Diagnostic Criterias of Rheumatological Disorders *241*

8. Examination of Endocrine System — 245
- Symptomatology 245
- History Taking in Endocrine Disorders 248
- Examination of Endocrine System 249
- Examination of a Diabetic Patient 251
- Examination of a Hypertensive Patient 253

Common Clinical Disorders of Endocrine System 254
- Acromegaly 254
- Hypopituitarism 256
- Hypothyroidism 257
- Thyrotoxicosis 260
- Graves' Disease (Basedow's Disease) 260
- Cushing's Syndrome 263
- Hypoadrenalism 264
- Disorders of Calcium Homeostasis 266

9. Examination of the Kidneys and the Urinary System — 269
- Symptomatology 269
- History Taking in Renal Disorders 272
- Examination of the Kidneys and Urinary System 272
- Systemic Examination 273
- Normal Urine 273
- Clinical Presentation of Renal Diseases 273
- Primary Glomerular Diseases 274
- Nephrotic Syndrome 276
- Acute Renal Failure 278
- Chronic Renal Failure 280
- Common Electrolyte Disturbances 283
- Hyponatremic Disorders 284

10. Examination of Hemopoietic System — 286
- Symptomatology 286
- History Taking 287
- Examination of Hemopoietic System 287

Common Disorders of Hemopoietic System 290
- Anemia 290
- Hemorrhagic Disorders 296
- Plasma Cell Proliferative Disorders 299
- Hematological Values 301

Index 303

CHAPTER 1

History Taking

Clinical examination of patient consists of history taking and physical examination. This will lead on to clinical diagnosis which is further confirmed by the appropriate investigation. There are three pillars for the diagnosis—history taking, physical examination and investigation.

To quote Sir William Osler's words (Father of Clinical Medicine)—"Clinical Medicine is learned by the bedside than in the classroom (Fig. 1.1)."

GENERAL PRINCIPLES OF HISTORY TAKING

Interrogation with the patient is the first step for making a diagnosis. Accurate history is the most valuable for bringing a correct diagnosis and of course it is the least expensive of all investigations. Careful medical history should precede both examination and treatment. History taking is the beginning of doctor-patient relationship.

It is important to try to put the patient at ease, encourage the patient to talk freely, thus have a good rapport with the patient. Patient's first impression of a doctor's professional manners will have a lasting effect on him. Each doctor should learn this difficult part of the examination by their own method and guided by the clinical teacher. Try to call the patient by name and start the interrogation by a non-committal remark like "What help can I do for you?". In case the patient's consciousness is disturbed or he is extremely ill, information may be collected from a near relative. In spite of advanced modern diagnostic tests, history taking and physical examination still remain the essential skills.

HISTORY TAKING SEQUENCE

1. Biodata
2. Presenting complaint
3. History of present illness
4. History of past illness
5. Family history
6. Personal history
7. Treatment history
8. Menstrual history
9. Occupational history
10. Socioeconomic Status
11. System review

Biodata

Name, age, address, gender.

Presenting Complaint

The symptoms with which the patient present to the doctor. Some patients have more than one complaint, record these complaints in the words of the patient, in chronological order with duration. Leading questions can be asked in the next step of the history of present illness.

History of Present Illness

Each of the presenting complaints has to be dealt in detail. In general a number of facts has to be uncovered about each complaint:

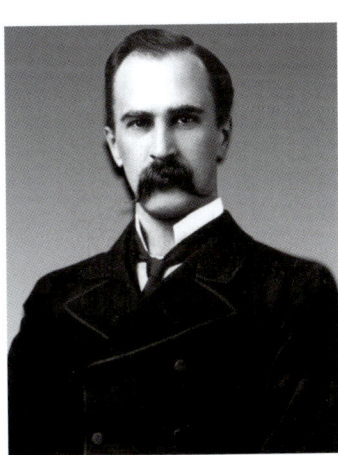

Fig. 1.1: Sir William Osler.

- Mode of onset—acute, subacute or insidious
- Duration
- Site and radiation—especially of pain
- Character
- Severity
- Relieving and aggravating factors
- Associated symptoms
- Course of the illness, from the first symptoms to the time of presentation.

Onset of Symptom

- Acute—within hours/abrupt, e.g. vascular lesion
- Subacute—within days/weeks to develop the full symptoms, e.g. infection, inflammation
- Insidious—slow in onset, patient cannot remember the exact date of onset, e.g. neurodegenerative disease, neoplasms.

Course of illness may be:
- Progressive
- Static
- With remissions and relapse.

Leading questions to be asked depend on the symptoms of each system. Patients who insist on talking with medical terms like rheumatism, anxiety should be gently discouraged and tell them to discuss in their own words.

Symptoms referable to other systems should also be enquired as in review of other systems. A negative data is also equally important like absence of cough in respiratory diseases, breathlessness in cardiovascular illness and paralysis in nervous system disorders. Enquire whether the patient is harboring other common diseases on the top of which present illness started-like systemic hypertension, diabetes mellitus, coronary artery disease (CAD), etc. Specific symptoms of each systems are detailed in the subsequent chapters on each system.

History of Past Illness

Include the following points in the history of past illness:
- All the illness in the past from infancy onward and list in chronological order
- Similar illness in the past, especially for diseases with recurring nature-like seizure disorder, migraine, duodenal ulcer
- Past history of certain specific diseases which lead to the present illness, e.g.
  - Rheumatic fever → valvular heart diseases
  - Viral hepatitis → cirrhosis liver
  - Childhood respiratory disease → suppurative lung disease (bronchiectasis)
  - Sexually transmitted diseases → neurosyphilis/cardio-vascular syphilis
  - Recent loss of consciousness as in alcoholism, seizure
  - General anesthesia → aspiration pneumonia and lung abscess
- History of travel abroad or residence abroad → malaria, kala azar, tropical sprue, etc.

Family History

- Note the health status of other members of the family—grandparents, spouse, children, parents and siblings.
- History of consanguinity for the possibility of autosomal recessive inheritance.
- History of similar illness in the family.
- Diseases with specific pattern of inheritance
  - Metabolic diseases
  - Bleeding diathesis
  - Congenital anomalies
- Diseases with multifactorial inheritance, like:
  - Diabetes mellitus
  - Coronary artery disease
  - Hypertension
  - Dyslipidemia
- Communicable diseases, like:
  - Measles
  - Mumps
  - Chickenpox
  - Enteric fever
  - Tuberculosis

Attempt to construct the family tree showing the pattern of inheritance.

Personal History

- Habit of smoking—substance used, amount and duration relevant for:
  - Coronary artery disease
  - Chronic obstructive pulmonary disease (COPD)
  - Bronchogenic carcinoma
- Alcoholism—amount, duration, nature of alcohol
  - Acute and chronic liver disease
  - Neuropathy
- Chewing tobacco—duration and substance used
  - Carcinoma cheek
  - Leukoplakia
- Drug abuse—susceptible for HIV, infective endocarditis, psychiatric problems
- Dietetic history—nutritional disorders
  - Deficiency disease—protein calorie malnutrition, megaloblastic anemia, iron deficiency anemia
  - Parasitic infestation
  - Obesity/overweight
- Sleep—quality of sleep, duration, sleep rhythm
  - Any specific sleep disorders-like narcolepsy/sleep palsy
  - Other nocturnal symptoms-like PND, headache, cough
  - Use of any sedatives
- Appetite—good, anorexia, bulimia, distorted by the illness
- Bowel and bladder habits—any alteration by the illness
- Domestic and marital relationship
  - Feelings toward other members of the family
  - Hobbies, lifestyle and pets.

Treatment History

- Details of the drugs used for the present illness
  - For the correct dose and duration of treatment
  - To ascertain any drug resistance
- Allergy or other side effects of the drug
- Any regular use of drugs for DM, hypertension, epilepsy, psychiatric illness, oral contraceptives
- Use of analgesics and NSAIDs
- Anesthesia and surgery
- Immunization
- Self medication.

Menstrual and Obstetric History

Note the following things: Age of menarche, details of menstrual cycle, age of menopause.

Importance

- Endocrine disorders affecting the menstrual cycle
  - Turner's syndrome—primary amenorrhea
  - Polycystic ovarian disease—irregular menstruation/secondary amenorrhea
  - Thyroid disorders—irregular menstruation, menorrhagia, oligomenorrhea
- History of intrapartum and postpartum hemorrhage—hypopituitarism—Sheehan's syndrome
- Menorrhagia-blood loss → Anemia
- Peripartum cardiomyopathy
- Premenstrual tension and edema
- Postmenopausal symptoms and osteoporosis
- Oral contraceptives → seizure and headache-cortical venous thrombosis.

Occupational History

- Enquires about:
  - Present and previous occupation
  - Exposure to dust and chemicals
  - High altitude work
  - Business affairs
- Importance:
  - Occupational respiratory disease
    - Pneumoconiosis
    - Nasobronchial allergy
    - Fibrosing alveolitis
  - Leptospirosis—paddy field workers, pineapple farmers
  - Veterinary workers—anthrax, brucellosis
  - Communicable diseases from workmates.

Socioeconomic Status

- Poverty and illiteracy
  - Under nutrition
  - Increase the incidence of infection and infestation
  - No immunization coverage
- Problems of affluent society
  - Over eating, sedentary life
  - Obesity, hypertension, dyslipidemia, etc.
- Socioeconomic status will tell the affordability of investigations, drug treatment and other modalities of treatment.

System Review

Enquire about the symptoms of major systems other than the presenting complaints

- Cardiovascular system—dyspnea, palpitation, chest pain, edema
- Respiratory system—cough and expectoration, hemoptysis, dyspnea, wheeze
- Nervous system—headache, seizure, cranial nerve symptoms, paralysis, sensory symptoms, bladder symptoms
- Alimentary system—abdominal pain, distention of abdomen, vomiting, dysphagia, diarrhea, constipation, jaundice.

CHAPTER 2

Physical Examination

It can be considered under two headings—general examination and systemic examination.

Physical examination is the second tool for diagnosis. Diagnosis is a crucial process that labels the illness, propels specific treatment and decides the prognosis. Diagnosis should always precede treatment.

Ancestor's word to be remembered—"More mistakes are made from want of proper examination than for any other reason. Doctors know more but see less. Doctors should have kite's eye for keen observation, lady's finger for good perception by touch and palpation and lion's heart for courage to face any emergency situation".

GENERAL EXAMINATION

Look for:
- Appearance
- Consciousness and cooperation
- Apparent age
- Build and nourishment
- Anemia
- Polycythemia
- Jaundice
- Cyanosis
- Edema
- Dyspnea/posture
- Nails—clubbing/koilonychia
- Lymph node enlargement
- Thyroid
- Skin and hair
- Hand
- Body habits
- Hydration
- Vital signs
  - Temperature
  - Pulse
  - Blood pressure
  - Respiratory rate.

APPEARANCE OF THE PATIENT

Normal, not in distress, looks ill, very ill.

CONSCIOUSNESS AND COOPERATION

Whether the patient is fully conscious and cooperative in giving information and allowing examination.

APPARENT AGE

Looks of his age
- Looks young
  - Physiological variations
  - Pathological variations—infantile appearance in endocrine disorders
- Premature aging
  - Physiological
  - Pathological—various systemic illness, progeria, etc.

BUILD AND NOURISHMENT

It is considered as the skeletal structure in relation to age, sex as compared to a normal person.
- Observation
  - Normal
  - Abnormal—somatotypes
  - Asthenia—poor built, thin long, flat chest, slender fingers
  - Normosthenia—normal built
  - Sthenia—broad, stout, short neck, muscular chest, stumpy finger.

Anthropometry: Measurements of height, weight, arm span, upper-lower segment ratio.
- *Anthropometry types are:*
  - Endomorphy—soft rounded body, digestive viscera dominate
  - Mesomorphy—muscles, bones and connective tissue derived from the embryonic mesoderm dominate

- Ectomorphy—fragile, thin built with linearity or angularity.
- Normal
  - Upper segment (US), Lower segment (LS) ratio is 1:1 (1.8:1 at birth, become 1:1 at 11–12 years)
- Infantile body proportions
  - US > LS
  - Height > arm span
- Eunuchoid and Marfan syndrome
  - LS > US
  - Arm span > height.

Marfan's index
- Arm span 7.5 cm > height
- Lower segment, 5 cm > upper segment.

Common causes for tall stature
- Marfan's syndrome
- Gigantism
- Klinefelter's syndrome
- Eunuchoidism
- Familial
- Homocystinuria.

Common causes of Dwarfism (Fig. 2.1)
- Proportionate
- Disproportionate
  - Familial
  - Endocrine—cretinism, panhypopituitarism, Juvenile Cushing's syndrome
  - Racial
  - Musculoskeletal—achondroplasia, rickets
  - Mongolism
  - Nutritional—Protein-calorie malnutrition (PCM)
  - Major organ disease in childhood.

Nourishment: State of nutrition—distribution of adipose tissue in the body

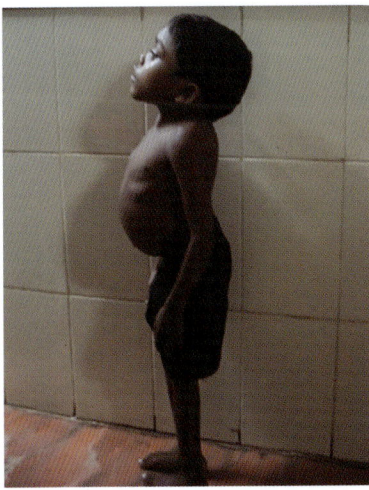

Fig. 2.1: Dwarfism, short neck in a patient with mucopolysaccharidosis

- Normal
- Under weight
- Overweight
- Obese.

Body Mass Index (BMI)

$$BMI = \frac{Weight\ (kg)}{[Height\ (meters)]^2}$$

- Male → 20–25
- Female → 18–23

Grades of obesity
- 25–30 → overweight
- 30–40 → obese
- >40 → very obese

Ideal body weight (IBW)
- Males = $22.5 \times [Height\ (meters)]^2$
- Females = $0.94 \times 22.5 \times [Height\ (meters)]^2$

Types of obesity: Generalized obesity
- Android obesity: Excessive fat deposition at waist
- Gynoid obesity: Excessive fat deposition at hip or thigh
- Truncal obesity: Excessive fat deposition on face, neck and upper body.

Waist-hip ratio: The *waist* is measured by taking a circumference that gives narrowest measurement between the ribcage and the iliac crest.

The *hip measurement* is taken by measuring at a level that gives maximum measurement of the hip over the buttocks.
- </= 0.8—pear-shaped obesity
- >/= 0.9—apple-shaped obesity: more risk.

Under weight: BMI <18—cachexia

Causes of cachexia:
- Malnutrition, diabetes mellitus
- Anorexia nervosa, tuberculosis
- Internal malignancy, Addison's disease
- Malabsorption, thyrotoxicosis, acquired immune deficiency syndrome (AIDS).

ANEMIA (TABLE 2.1)

Mucous membranes and nailbed are normally pink, depending on the amount of hemoglobin (Hb) in the circulating blood.

Clinically, anemia means pallor of the conjunctiva (Fig. 2.2), oral mucosa, tongue, palm and nailbed. Best site for examining the pallor of anemia is palmar creases and mucosa of the palate.
- Pallor > anemia is seen in CRF, hypopituitarism, etc.
- Facial pallor is seen in shock and low cardiac output state.
- Pale complexion is seen in people without anemia also.

Table 2.1: Laboratory criteria to define anemia.			
	Males	Females	Children
Hb	<13 g%	<12 g%	6 months–6 years : <11 g% 6 years – 14 years : <12 g%
PCV	<42%	<36%	
RBC count	<4.5 million/mm³	<4 million/mm³	

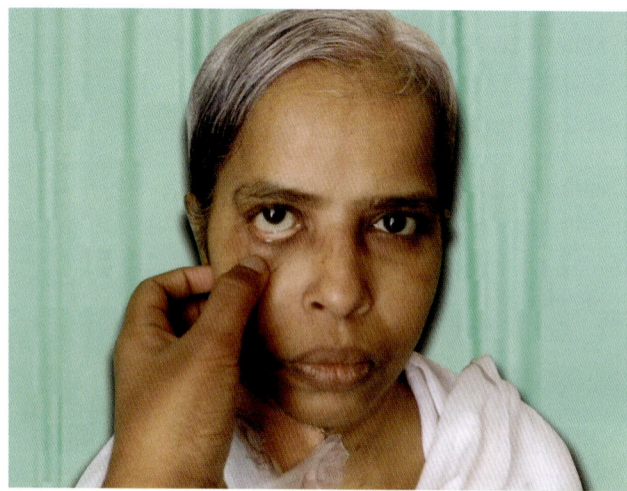

Fig. 2.2: Pale appearance of conjunctiva shows sign of anemia.

- Usually pallor appears when the Hb < 10 mg%
- Pale palmar creases are seen when Hb < 8 g%.

POLYCYTHEMIA

Excessive amount of RBC mass leads to redness of conjunctiva, mucous membrane, skin and nailbed.

This is often accompanied by central cyanosis and clubbing as in congenital cyanotic heart disease and interstitial lung disease called secondary polycythemia.

Primary proliferative polycythemia is the malignant counterpart.

Anoxia or excess erythropoietin → secondary polycythemia.

To produce polycythemia:
- In males
  - RBC mass is > 36 mL/kg
  - PCV >55%
- In females
  - RBC mass >32 mL/kg
  - PCV >47%.

JAUNDICE

Yellowish discoloration of skin, sclera, mucous membrane and nailbed due to excess amount of serum bilirubin of >2 mg/dL.

Serum bilirubin 1–2 mg/dL is subclinical jaundice. Normal being < 1 mg/dL.

Sclera is rich in elastic fibers. Serum bilirubin has affinity to elastic fibers. Periphery of the sclera being thick, early staining by bilirubin will occur at the periphery. In marked hyperbilirubinemia, all tissues except the brain is stained by bilirubin, the blood–brain barrier will block the bilirubin staining of the brain.

Mechanism

Three basic mechanisms of jaundice:
1. Hemolytic anemia—lemon yellow jaundice, pallor, splenomegaly without bilirubinuria—acholuric jaundice
2. Hepatocellular jaundice—jaundice, bilirubinuria with other stigmas of hepatocellular damage and features of primary liver disease
3. Obstructive jaundice—greenish dark yellow jaundice, pruritus, pale stool, palpable gallbladder ±. It can be either intra- or extrahepatic cholestasis.

Carotenemia (Fig. 2.3) is characterized by yellowish discoloration of skin (carotenoderma) sparing the sclera.

"While examining for jaundice, elevate the upper eyelid, ask the patient to look down and then look at the periphery of the sclera in bright natural day light" (Figs. 2.4 and 2.5).

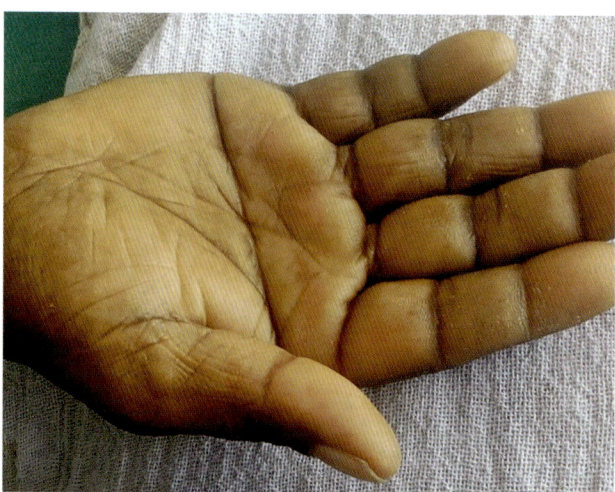

Fig. 2.3: Carotenemia.

Physical Examination

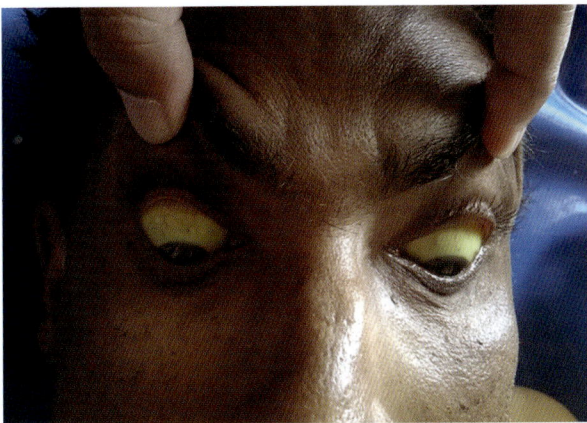

Fig. 2.4: Yellowish discoloration of sclera—jaundice.

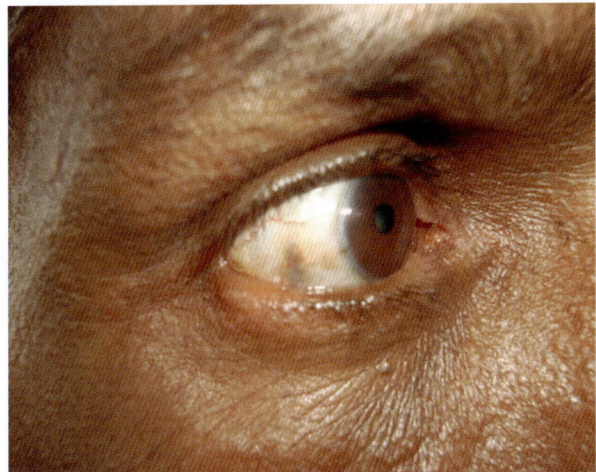

Fig. 2.5: Pigmented lesion over the eye— Osler's sign in alkaptonuria.

CYANOSIS

Bluish discoloration of oral mucosa, tongue, skin or nailbed due to excess amount of reduced Hb >5 g/dL.

Early cyanosis is observed as bluish tinge at the surface of the tongue and fingertip (tuft cyanosis). Anemia may mask the cyanosis even if hypoxemia is present, but in primary polycythemia, cyanosis is present without hypoxemia—red cyanosis.
- Cyanosis with hypoxemia—when reduced Hb >5 g/dL
- Hypoxemia without cyanosis—moderate-to-severe anemia
- Cyanosis without hypoxemia—primary polycythemia.

Clinical Types of Cyanosis
- Central
- Peripheral
- Mixed
- Differential

Central Cyanosis

Warm and cold areas are affected, bluish discoloration of tongue, oral mucosa, skin and nailbed, extremities are warm.
Etiopathogenesis
1. *Defect in heart:* Cardiac cyanosis
   - Cyanotic congenital: heart disease, right → left shunts as in TOF—mixing of venous and oxygenated blood
2. *Defect in lung:* Pulmonary cyanosis
   - Either ventilatory defect as in COPD or
   - Diffusion defect as in interstitial lung disease
3. *Defects in Hb:*
   - Excess Hb—primary polycythemia
   - Abnormal Hb:
     - Methemoglobinemia—met Hb >1.5 g% → cyanosis
     - Congenital—Hb M, enzyme glutathione deficiency
     - Acquired—drugs like phenacetin and sulpha
     - Sulfhemoglobinemia—Sulf Hb >0.5 g% → cyanosis
   - Drugs (sulphone)
   - Chief complaint—constipation—sulfur absorbed from intestine.
4. *Defect in atmospheric oxygen content:* High altitude, atmospheric oxygen content is less → alveolar oxygen content → central cyanosis.

Rarely, central cyanosis is seen as chief complaint in liver diseases (cirrhosis liver) because of pulmonary AV shunting, portopulmonary connection and ↓ in tidal volume due to associated ascites.

Exercise may increase right → left shunts—cardiac cyanosis ↑.

Oxygen inhalation may reduce the pulmonary cyanosis.

Central cyanosis is added with secondary polycythemia and clubbing in cyanotic CHD and ILD.

Peripheral Cyanosis

Bluish discoloration of the cold areas of the body like nailbed, fingers, toes, tip of nose, ear lobes, sparing warm areas-like oral mucosa and tongue where there is no vasoconstriction. Extremities are cold.

Etiopathogenesis: Peripheral cyanosis is due to microcirculation defect, more extraction of oxygen by tissues leading to increase amount of reduced Hb.

Types:
- Generalized—cold weather—cyanosis of lips and finger tips; shock, low cardiac output; severe right heart failure and severe PAH.
- Localized—major vein occlusion like SVC, IVC and femoral vein.

Pigmentation of tongue and oral mucosa may resemble cyanosis; press with a glass slide (diascopy), no change occurs with pigmentation and blanching occurs in cyanosis.

Mixed Cyanosis

Features of both central and peripheral cyanosis, in situations like acute pulmonary edema with shock producing diffusion defect and defect in microcirculation as in acute MI. Clinically, it is characterized by signs of peripheral cyanosis and cyanosis of warm areas.

Differential Cyanosis

Evidence of central cyanosis and clubbing, either in both lower extremities or in both the upper extremities, including conjunctiva, oral mucosa, and tongue, e.g.
- PDA with reversal of shunt—cyanosis and clubbing of toes in both lower extremities
- TGA with PDA—cyanosis with clubbing of fingers in both upper extremities.

Note: Cyanosis is a grave sign inviting good care of the patient.

EDEMA

Excessive collection of ECF is called edema. More than 6 liters of excess fluid in extracellular compartment is needed to produce clinical edema. If it is less, it is called subclinical edema.

Factors Responsible for Edema Formation (Fig. 2.6)

- Hydrostatic pressure of the capillary
- Osmotic pressure of the plasma protein
- Permeability of the capillary
- Lymphatic obstruction.

Clinical Demonstration

Sites of edema
- Ambulant—pedal edema
- Bed ridden—sacral edema.

Procedure

Press over the bony areas like shin of tibia, sacrum or medial malleolus for a few seconds (10-15 seconds), pitting means presence of edema.

Types of Edema
- Soft pitting—recent edema
- Hard pitting—long-standing edema with secondary tissue changes
- Nonpitting—filarial edema (Fig. 2.7), myxedema.

Causes of Edema

Generalized Edema
- Cardiac edema, renal edema, hepatic edema and hypoalbuminemia
- Hypothyroidism, premenstrual edema, wet beriberi
- Idiopathic cyclical edema (childbearing age—multiple factors responsible)
- Drugs—NSAIDs, steroids, insulin (Na-H_2O retention).

Localized Edema
- Venous obstruction—DVT, varicose veins, venous obstruction by tumors and lymph node
- Lymphatic obstruction—filariasis, congenital Milroy's edema
- Inflammatory edema.

Mechanism of Edema

1. *Cardiac edema:* Sign of right heart failure, clinically dependent pitting edema
   Mechanism
   - ↑ hydrostatic pressure of the capillary
   - ↓ renal perfusion in CHF → ↑ renin → secondary hyperaldosteronism → ↑ Na and H_2O retention
   - ↑ sympathetic activity as compensation in CHF → ↑ renin → ↑ Na and H_2O retention
   - ↑ capillary permeability.
2. *Renal edema:*
   - Clinically, puffiness of face, then spread of edema to other parts
   - ↓ GFR → ↑ Na and H_2O as in acute glomerulonephritis
   - Proteinuria → hypoalbuminemia as in nephrotic syndrome

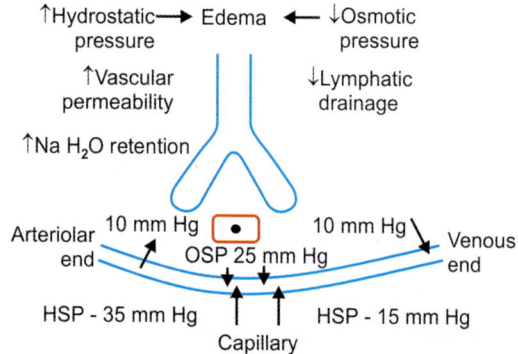

Fig. 2.6: Pathogenesis of edema.
(HSP—hydrostatic pressure; OSP—osmotic pressure)

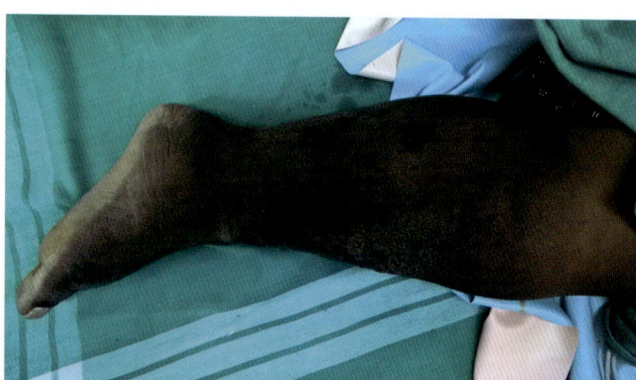

Fig. 2.7: Nonpitting edema—elephantiasis.

- ↑ renin → ↑ Na and H_2O as in renovascular lesion
- More than one above factors.
3. *Hepatic edema*
   - Clinically ascites, abdominal edema spreading to periphery
   - *Mechanisms*
     - Hypoalbuminemia
     - Secondary hyperaldosteronism—↑ Na and H_2O retention
     - For ascites, besides the above two mechanisms—portal hypertension and peritoneal lymphatic obstruction also.
4. *Hypoalbuminemia:* As in malnutrition, malabsorption, protein losing enteropathy will produce pitting edema
   Mechanism—hypoalbuminemia and decreased osmotic pressure.
5. *Idiopathic cyclical edema:* Seen in females of childbearing age group due to multiple factors, including hormonal imbalance, diagnosed by process of exclusion.
6. *Anemia and edema* (Fig. 2.8)
   - Anemia → CHF
   - Anemia with hypoproteinemia
   - Hb is inhibitory to N_2O formation
   - Anemia → ↑ nitric oxide → ↑ vasodilation and permeability → edema.

Pedal Edema

- *Bilateral*—as in:
  - Congestive heart failure
  - Renal disease
  - Hepatic disease
  - Other causes of hypoalbuminemia
  - Beriberi
  - IVC obstruction
  - Hypothyroidism

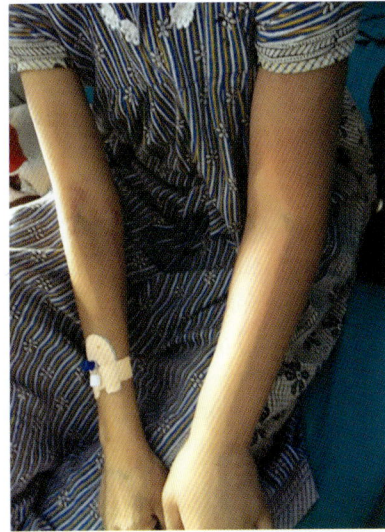

Fig. 2.9: Unilateral edema—left upper limb.

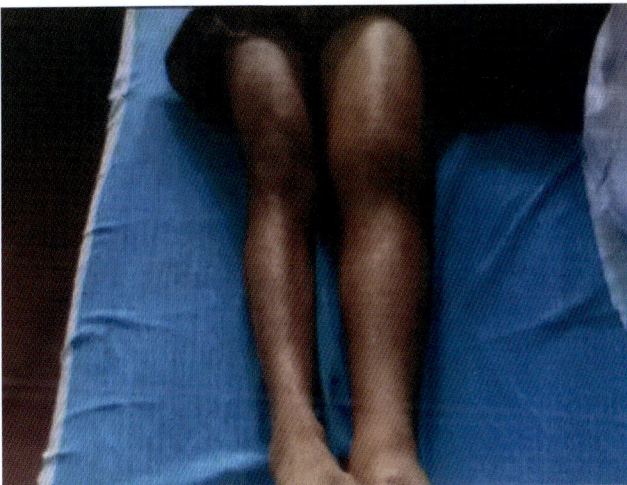

Fig. 2.10: Unilateral edema—left lower limb.

- Drug induced
- Idiopathic cyclical edema
- *Unilateral* (Figs. 2.9 and 2.10)
  - *Venous:* DVT, c/c venous insufficiency in varicose veins, obstruction by tumor or enlarged lymph node
  - *Lymphatic:* Infection—filariasis, congenital: Milroy's edema, tumor invasion of lymph node and surgical removal of lymph node as in block dissection
  - Inflammatory—cellulitis.

DYSPNEA

Unpleasant awareness of one's own breathing. Dyspnea can be a sign as well as symptom. Dyspneic patient requires emergency care and full evaluation for the cause.

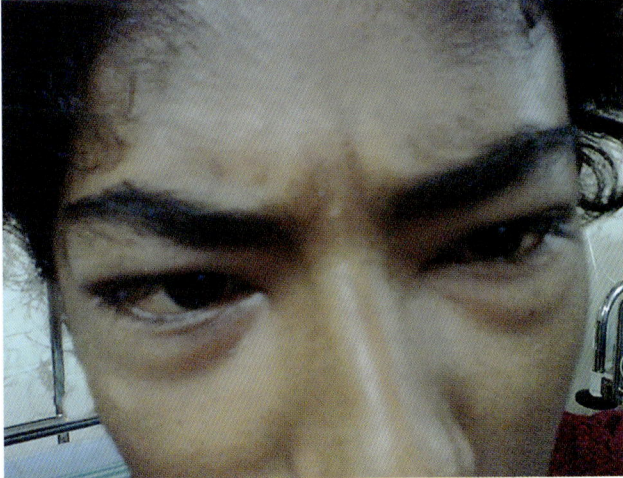

Fig. 2.8: Periorbital edema in capillary leak syndrome in a case of snake bite.

Factors responsible are:
- Pulmonary capillary congestion ↓ compliance of the lung as in LVF ← interstitial and alveolar edema.
- Ventilation and perfusion abnormality in the lung as in COPD, ILD, ARDS.
- Chest wall abnormality—impeding the movement of the chest wall as in obesity, thick chest wall, kyphoscoliosis.
- Neuromuscular diseases affecting the respiratory muscles as in muscular dystrophy, myasthenia, GBS, OP poisoning.
- Defective O_2 carrying capacity of blood as in anemia.

Clinical detection—Patient in distress
- Rate of respiration is more (> 22/min—tachypnea).
- Visible action of accessory muscles of respiration like sternocleidomastoid, scalene and serratus anterior.

Clinical Types

Exertional dyspnea: The most common symptom of left heart disease and pulmonary disease.

Mechanism: Exercise → ↑ venous return → ↑ blood flow to lung → pulmonary capillary congestion around each alveoli, when the left side of heart is damaged → ↓ compliance of lung → exertional dyspnea.

Grading of Exertional Dyspnea by New York Heart Association (NYHA)

- Grade I—Dyspnea on competitive exercise
- Grade II—Dyspnea while walking on level ground and climbing stairs
- Grade III—Dyspnea on day-to-day activity—combing hair, dressing, etc.
- Grade IV—Dyspnea at rest.

 Individual variation in tolerance of dyspnea—dyspnea threshold.

 Change in dyspnea grade indicates progression or regression of disease.

Orthopnea

Dyspnea on lying flat—upright breathing.

Mechanism

- ↑ venous return to the pulmonary vascular system on lying flat → pulmonary congestion → ↓ compliance of the lung.
- Mechanical disadvantage of diaphragmatic movement due to viscera in lying position.
- The part of the lung lying below the level of heart is more in lying position—thus more area of lung congestion.

 These changes will be reversed in upright position; orthopnea is an important feature of left heart failure and also observed in acute asthma, COPD and diaphragmatic paralysis.

Paroxysmal Nocturnal Dyspnea

Paroxysm of dyspnea occurring during sleep.

Mechanism

- All the factors mentioned in orthopnea will come to play in the lying position.
- ECF shift to intravascular compartment due to ↓ vascular tone, this further ↑ the venous return-vascular volume expansion.
- Compensatory sympathetic over activity in failing heart is less during night.
- Thus the pulmonary capillary pressure exceeds to produce interstitial edema → stiffness of lung, making the patient to get up due to discomfort of breathing.
- While adopting sitting or standing position, the hemodynamic burden on pulmonary capillary vessel will reverse, producing relief of dyspnea. PND also produces nocturnal cough. PND is a symptom of decompensation of left heart.

Acute Dyspnea

Severe dyspnea at rest is seen in patients with
- Acute LVF
- ARDS
- Acute exacerbation of asthma, COPD
- Tension pneumothorax
- Massive pleural effusion
- URT obstruction due to laryngeal edema/angiedema
- Massive pulmonary embolism
- Foreign body in respiratory tract, irritant gas inhalation.

 Inspiratory dyspnea occurring with upper airway obstruction should be identified promptly for the immediate relief of obstruction; otherwise, it may endanger the life, as in angioedema, Ludwig's angina, laryngeal diphtheria, foreign body, etc.

 Hyperventilation means deep rapid breathing as in acidosis, upper brainstem lesion, hypoxia and hysterical salicylism.

 Tachypnea is RR >22/min
 Bradypnea is RR <10/min.

POSTURE OF THE PATIENT

Patient may adopt certain posture, depending on the disease to get some relief of discomfort.
- Propped up position—LVF, acute asthma
- Opisthotonus—tetanus, acute meningitis
- Curled position—acute meningitis
- Pleuritic pain and pleural effusion—lying on the affected side for relief of pain and dyspnea
- Flexed attitude of the whole body—parkinsonism

- Hippocratic facies with immobile distended abdomen—acute peritonitis
- Deviation of head and eyes—cerebellar hemorrhage.

HYDRATION

To assess the hydration of the patient—look for:
- Dryness of oral mucosa and tongue
- Sunken eyes
- ↓ skin turgor—pinch the skin, on releasing, normal skin returns within 2 seconds (except old age and infancy)
- Postural fall of BP >10 mm Hg/postural dizziness
- Oliguria
- Invisible jugular venous column in lying position.

Signs of Dehydration

- ECF loss
  - Dryness of oral mucosa and tongue
  - Sunken eyes
  - ↓ skin turgor
- IVF loss
  - postural fall of BP >10 mm Hg/postural dizziness
  - Oliguria—↑ specific gravity of urine >1.025
  - Tachycardia
  - Prerenal azotemia
  - ↑ PCV
- ICF loss
  - Altered sensorium
  - Encephalopathy
  - Seizure
  - ± features of shock.

EXAMINATION OF NAIL

A lot of clinical signs are reflected in the nails as a marker of various systemic diseases.

Clubbing (Fig. 2.11)

Normal angle between the skin and nailbed is 160° (Lovibond angle).

More than this, is an early sign of clubbing, also have increase in the soft tissue of distal part of fingers and toes leading to biconvexity of the nail and bulbous distal portion. In normal nails, when the thumb nails are placed in opposition, there is lozenge shaped gap, whereas in clubbing, this gap is decreased, called Schamroth's window test or sign.

Pathogenesis: Arterial hypoxia and neurohumoral stimuli → hypervascularity and opening of anastomotic channels in the nailbed → overgrowth of soft tissues, is the basic mechanism of clubbing.

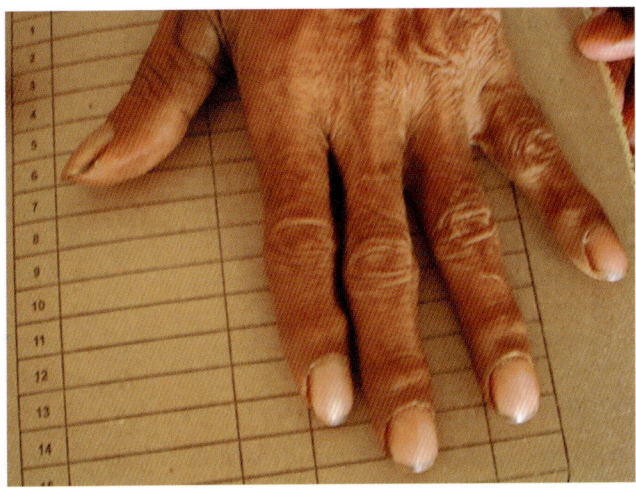

Fig. 2.11: Clubbing of the fingers.

Grades of Clubbing

- Increased fluctuation of nailbed—↑ looseness of base of nail
- Obliteration of nailbed angle and exceeding ≥ 180°. It can be demonstrated by keeping the finger in profile view—called profile sign
- Parrot beaking—biconvexity of nail
- Drumstick clubbing—bulbous terminal segment of fingers and toes
- Hypertrophic osteoarthropathy—with the above changes, thickening of periosteum, distal arthropathy, periosteal tenderness and heaviness of hands.

Causes of Clubbing

- CVS
  - Infective endocarditis
  - Cyanotic CHD
  - Myxoma of atria
  - Aneurysm of major vessels—aorta, subclavian, etc.
- GIT
  - Malabsorption
  - IBD—Crohn's, ulcerative colitis
  - Cirrhosis liver especially in primary biliary cirrhosis.

Respiratory system: Bronchogenic carcinoma
- Suppurative lung disease
- Interstitial lung disease (ILD)
- Empyema
- In pulmonary TB, it denotes
  - Post-TB bronchiectasis
  - Diffuse bilateral lung fibrosis
  - TB empyema.

Unilateral Clubbing

- Subclavian aneurysm
- Aortic aneurysm
- Arteriovenous malformation of limb
- Pancoast's tumor.

Others:
- Congenital—pachydermoperiostosis
- Thyrotoxicosis—thyroid acropachy
- Acromegaly
- Unidigital—sarcoidosis, trauma, gout.

Koilonychia

Dry brittle spoon-shaped nail, early stage there is flattening of nail. This is usually observed in iron deficiency anemia.

Splinter hemorrhage: Linear subungual hemorrhage in IE (vertical) and trichinosis (horizontal).

Beau's lines: Transverse furrow in nail plate due to temporary arrest of nail growth.

Mee's lines: White transverse band in nailplate—arsenic poisoning. Septicemia.

Half-half nail (Lindsay nail): Proximal dull white portion and distal pink or brown portion with well-demarcated line of separation, seen in chronic renal disease.

Leukonychia: White nail/Terry's nail—seen in hypoalbuminemia, in cirrhosis and nephrotic syndrome.

Blue nail: Azure lunula—bluish discoloration of lunula of nail—Wilson's disease.

Yellow nail syndrome: Combination of yellow nail, bronchiectasis and nephropathy.

Plummer's nail: Brittle nail with longitudinal ridges and distal onycholysis in hypothyroidism—onychopathy in myxedema.

Glassy nail: Cirrhosis liver.

Nailbed infarct: Vasculitis—SLE, PAN.

Nailfold telangiectasis: Periungual telangiectasis, PSS, SLE, dermatomyositis.

Subungual fibroma: Tuberous sclerosis.

Pitting of nail: Psoriasis.

Onychomyosis: Fungal infection of nail.

Nail growth is distorted in ectodermal dysplasia, chondroectodermal ectoplasia, and nail-patella syndrome.

Discoloration of nail is produced by drugs like busulfan, zidovudine, phenothiazine, antimalarials and antibiotics.

SKIN

Skin is a mirror of systemic disease. Examination of skin will reveal specific sign of systemic disease.

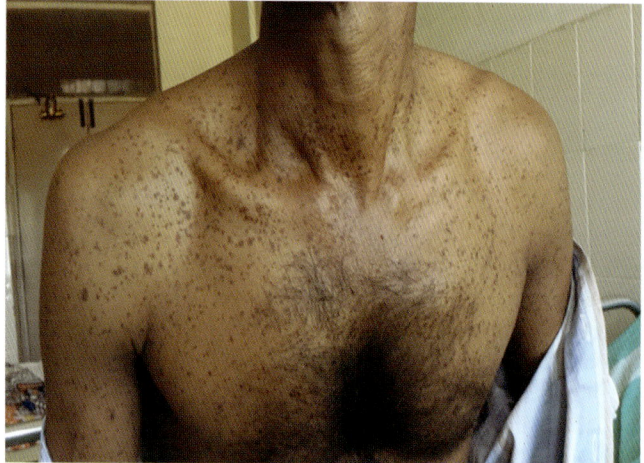

Fig. 2.12: Multiple black macules seen over chest and upper limbs—lentigines.

Primary skin lesions:
- Macules (flat lesions <1 cm) (Fig. 2.12)
- Papules (palpable solid elevation <1 cm)
- Maculopapular (both macule and papule)
- Vesicles (lesions <1 cm fluid filled epidermal elevations) (Figs. 2.13 to 2.15)
- Bullae (>1 cm fluid filled elevation) (Fig. 2.16)
- Pustules (epidermal elevations <1 cm containing pus) (Fig. 2.17)
- Patch (large macule >2 cm size)
- Plaque (papular lesions >1 cm).

Secondary skin lesions:
- Cutis laxa—in Ehlers-Danlos syndrome (Fig. 2.18)
- Scar—replacement by fibrous tissue (Fig. 2.19)
- Excoriation—loss of skin substance produced by scratching
- Fissure—any linear slit or discontinuity of skin

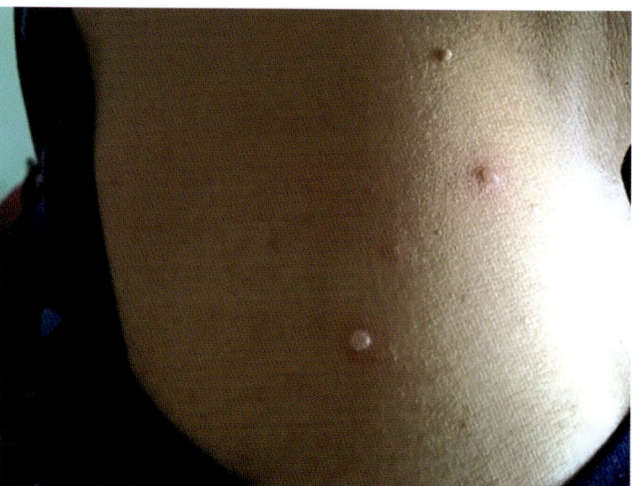

Fig. 2.13: Vesicles of chickenpox.

Physical Examination

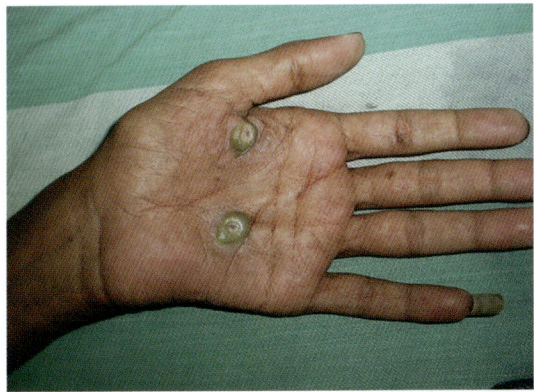

Fig. 2.14: Vesicular lesion on palm of hand—cowpox.

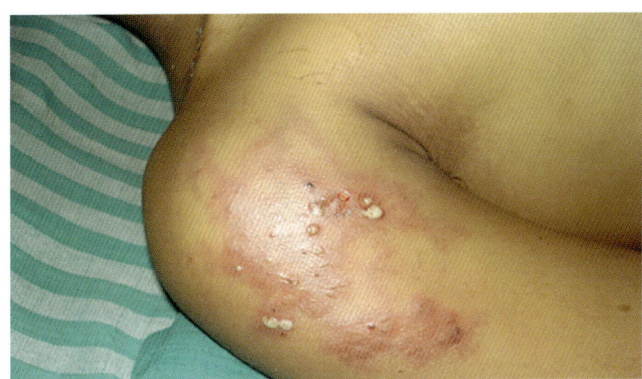

Fig. 2.17: Staphylococcal skin lesion showing pustules and redness—cellulitis.

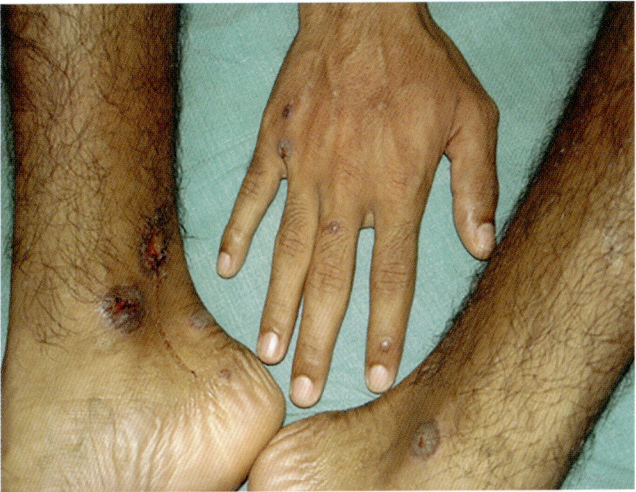

Fig. 2.15: Vesicular lesion of the hand and foot in a patient with hand-foot- mouth disease.

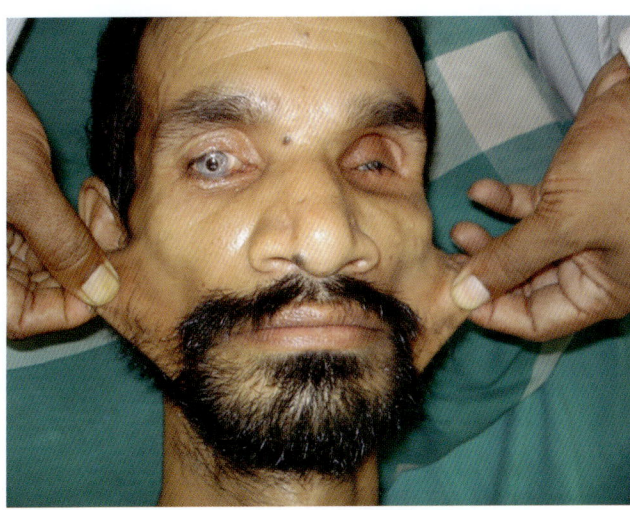

Fig. 2.18: Cutis laxa in a patient with Ehlers-Danlos syndrome.

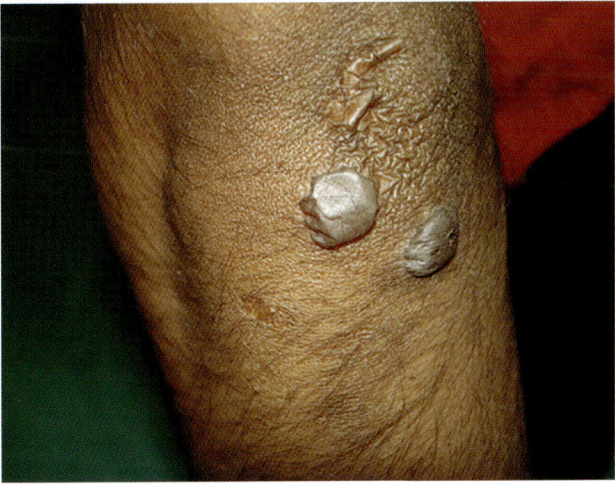

Fig. 2.16: Bullous lesion of the skin in a patient with hand-foot- mouth disease.

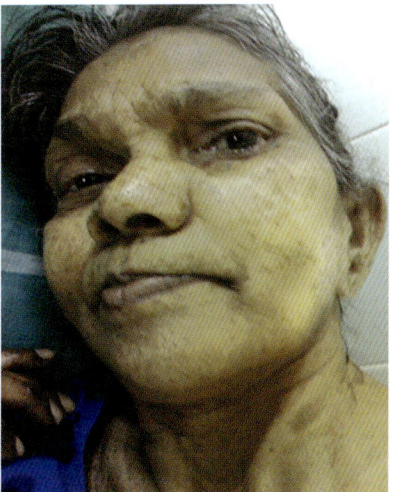

Fig. 2.19: Pitted scar–healed smallpox.

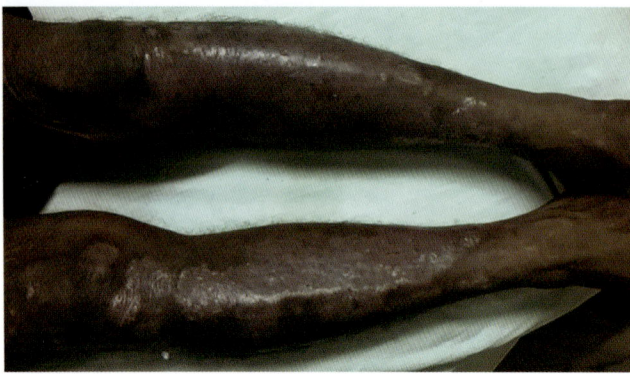

Fig. 2.20: Psoriasis.

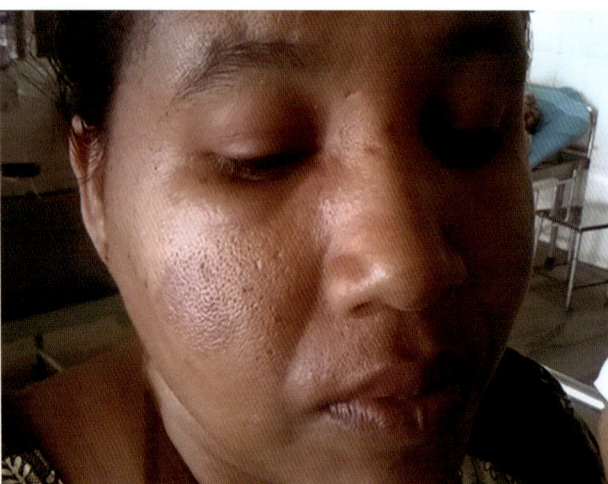

Fig. 2.21: Angioedema of face and lips.

- Scales—desquamated epithelium (Fig. 2.20)
- Ulcers—loss of epidermis, dermis and often with loss of underlying tissue (Fig. 2.21)
- Crust—dried up exudates.

Color of Skin

- Pallor—anemia, hypopituitarism, CRF
- Bluish discoloration—cyanosis
- Yellowish—jaundice
- Hyperpigmentation
  - Megaloblastic anemia—hands and face
  - Addison's disease
  - Nelson's syndrome—post adrenalectomy
  - Chronic liver disease
  - Arsenic poisoning
  - Internal malignancy
  - Hemochromatosis

  Acanthosis nigricans—pigmented velvety thickness of skin.

Benign:
- Obesity
- Cushing's syndrome.

Drugs:
- OCP
- Nicotinic acid
- Protease inhibitors.

Malignant: Internal malignancy.

Flushing of Skin

- Alcoholism
- Antabuse therapy
- Carcinoid syndrome
- Polycythemia vera
- Diabetes mellitus—rubeosis faciei.

Vitiligo (Fig. 2.22)

- Idiopathic
- Autoimmune disease
  - Thyroid disease
  - Pernicious anemia.

Hypopigmented Lesions

- Early vitiligo
- Leukoderma
- Tinea versicolor
- Pityriasis alba
- Hansen's disease
- Nevus anemicus
- Leafy macules—tuberous sclerosis.

Skin Markers in Collagen Vascular Disease

- Systemic lupus erythematosus
  - Butterfly rash
  - Telangiectasia
- Pan and antiphospholipid syndrome
  - Livedo reticularis
  - Purpura

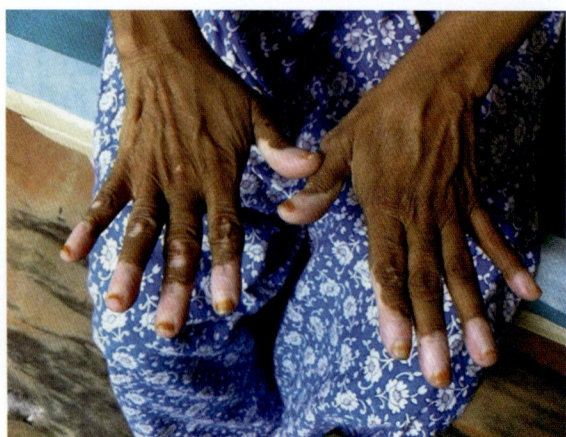

Fig. 2.22: Vitiligo.

- Progressive systemic sclerosis (PSS)
    - Acrosclerosis
    - Ulcers
    - Calcinosis
- Dermatomyositis
    - Heliotrope rash
    - Periorbital edema
    - Gottron's papules.

Skin Changes in Diabetes Mellitus

- Necrobiosis diabeticorum—popular/nodular—brownish yellow with waxy surface and telangiectasia → ulceration → scar formation due to microangiopathy
- Diabetic rubeosis—flushed skin over the face
- Diabetic dermopathy—pigmented pretibial dermatosis/shin spots/spotted leg syndrome—pigmented macules and dull red flat topped papules—microangiopathic lesion
- Scleredema diabeticorum—diffuse waxy nonpitting induration of skin—on the back of the neck and upper trunk
- Ear lobe crease—diagonal ear lobe crease
- Skin infection—bacterial and fungal infection.

Skin Markers in GIT Diseases

- Pigmentation—perioral, lips and hand—Peutz-Jeghers syndrome
- Dermal cyst—Gardener's syndrome
- Pyoderma gangrenosum—ulcerative colitis
- Dermatitis herpetiform—gluten sensitive enteropathy
- Vesiculobullous lesion of acral parts—acrodermatitis enteropathica
- Cirrhosis liver—dry skin, pruritus, palmar erythema, purpura and jaundice
- Migratory thrombophlebitis—carcinoma head of pancreas—Trousseau syndrome
- Palmar tylosis—Ca esophagus
- Acute necrolytic migratory erythema—glucagonoma
- Flushing of skin—carcinoid syndromes
- Dermatomyositis—GI malignancy
- Pityriasis rotunda—hepatocellular carcinoma, hyperpigmented scaly lesions of trunk and thighs.

Skin in CVS Diseases

- Infective endocarditis—Osler's nodes
    - Janeway lesions
- Rheumatic fever
    - Erythema marginatum
    - Erythema nodosum
    - Subcutaneous nodules.

Skin Markers in Endocrine Diseases

- Cushing's syndrome—striae, acne, hirsutism, purpura, acanthosis nigricans
- Acromegaly—thick hyperpigmented skin on acral parts of the body—acanthosis nigricans
- Addison's disease—hyperpigmentation of skin of axillae, groin, areola of nipple and palmar creases
- Hyperthyroidism—warm moist skin; pretibial myxedema
- Myxedema—dry cold skin; nonpitting edema
- Hypopituitarism—pale complexion
- Dyslipidemia—xanthoma—yellowish orange papule or nodule of skin due to lipid loaded cells
    - Xanthelasma
    - Xanthoma tuberosum
    - Xanthoma tendinosum
    - Eruptive xanthoma.

Neurocutaneous Diseases

- Tuberous sclerosis
    - Angiofibroma of face—adenoma sebaceum
    - Subungual fibroma
    - Shagreen patch
    - Leafy macule
- von Recklinghausen's disease
    - Multiple cutaneous and subcutaneous neurofibroma
    - Café-au-lait spots > 6 in no: >1.5 cm in size
    - Axillary freckles
- Sturge-Weber syndrome—capillary hemangioma in trigeminal nerve distribution
- Hereditary hemorrhagic telangiectasia—multiple telangiectasia of skin, mucosa, and pulmonary AVM.

Skin Markers in Internal Malignancy

- Acanthosis nigricans—adenocarcinoma of stomach (patchydermatoglyphy—diffuse yellowish palmoplantar keratoderma is a feature of malignant accanthosis nigricans)
- Palmoplantar keratoderma—Tylosis—Ca esophagus, Bronchogenic Ca (thick hard hyperkeratotic skin)
- Migratory thrombophlebitis—Ca pancreas
- Pellagra like skin lesions—carcinoid syndrome
- Pruritus—lymphoma, polycythemia vera
- Lesser-Trelat sign—multiple intensely pruritic seborrheic keratosis
- Dermatomyositis—GI malignancy.

Umbilicated papules and nodular lesions—malignant melanoma (Fig. 2.23).

Systemic Diseases with Pruritus

- Obstructive jaundice
- CRF
- Carcinoid syndrome
- Diabetes mellitus

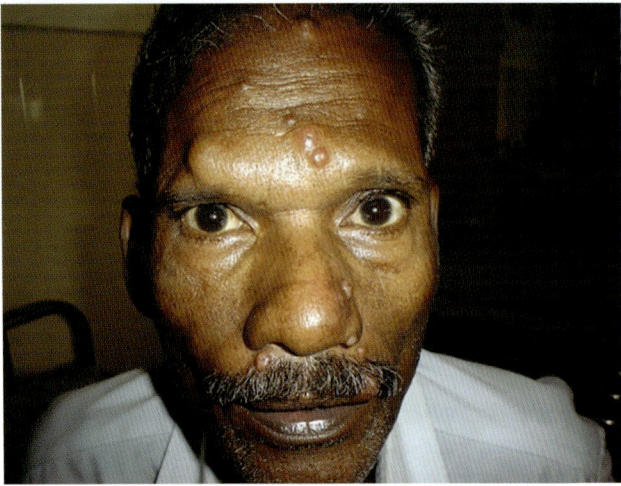

Fig. 2.23: Multiple umbilicated papules and nodular lesions in a patient with malignant melanoma.

- Hypothyroidism
- Hyperthyroidism
- Psychosis
- Polycythemia vera
- Int: malignancy—lymphoma, myeloma
- Drugs

Skin in Hematological Diseases

- Hyperpigmentation—megaloblastic anemia
- Urticaria—hot water bath and palmar erythema—polycythemia vera
- Painful ecchymosis—at the site of minor trauma—autoerythrocyte sensitization syndrome (sensitization to extravasated RBCs)
- Cutaneous bleeds—
  - Patechiae < 2 mm size
  - Purpura 2–5 mm size
  - Ecchymosis > 5 mm size.

Exanthematous Fever and Skin

- Time of appearance of rash is specific for exanthematous fevers
- 1st day rash—covered area of the body—*chickenpox*
- 2nd day rash—*German measles*
- 3rd day rash—centripetal distribution—*smallpox*
- 4th day rash—*scarlet fever*
- 5th day rash—*measles*
- End of 1st week—*typhoid*.

Life-threatening infection with skin rash
- Meningococcemia
- Dengue hemorrhagic fever (Fig. 2.24)
- Mountain spotted fever
- Septicemia—*Pseudomonas* → Ecthyma (Figs 2.25 and 2.26).

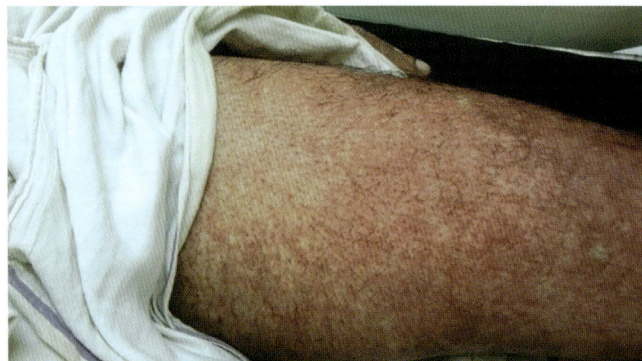

Fig. 2.24: Dengue rash with islands of non-erythematous area.

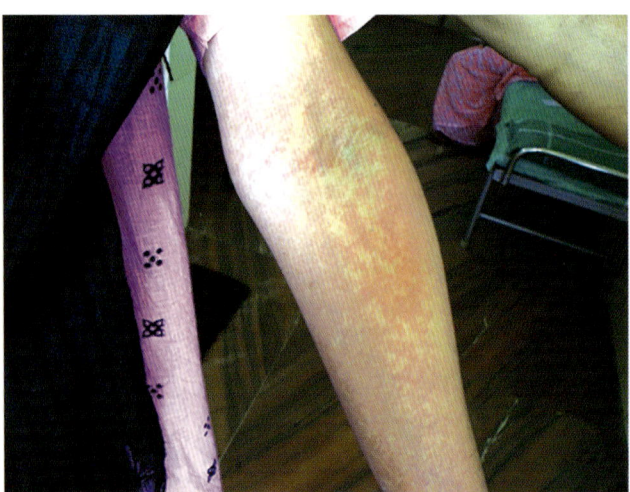

Fig. 2.25: Drug-induced rash—Dapsone.

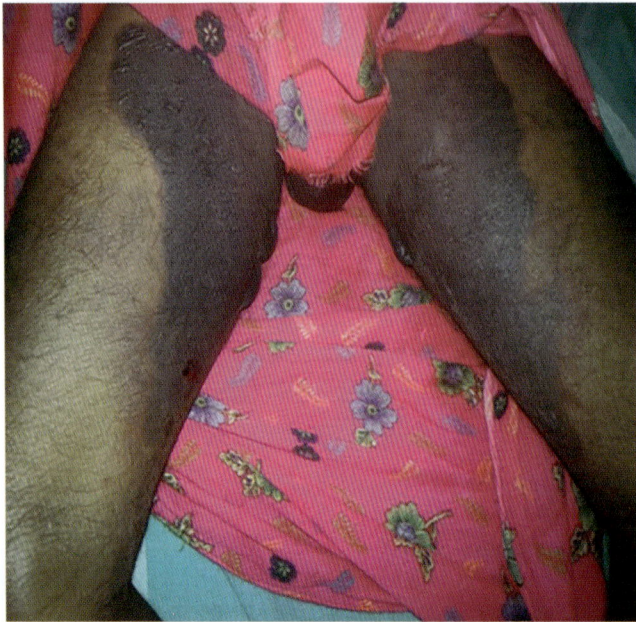

Fig. 2.26: Fixed drug eruption.

HAIR

Examination of hair consists of:
- Distribution—normal or abnormal
- Color of hair
- Alopecia
- Hypertrichosis
- Hirsutism.

Alopecia: Loss of hair from skin. It is of 2 types:
- Cicatricial—due to primary dermatological conditions
- Noncicatricial.

Systemic diseases with alopecia: Noncicatricial
- Physiological—male pattern of alopecia
- SLE (Fig. 2.27)
- Hypothyroidism
- Cirrhosis liver
- Postpartum alopecia
- Enteric fever
- Cytotoxic drugs—cyclophosphamide
- Alopecia in females—virilizing tumor of ovary or adrenal.

Hypertrichosis: Excessive growth of hairs in a generalized or localized pattern but not of male pattern distribution.
- Congenital—porphyria cutanea tarda, Hurler's syndrome, giant pigmented nevus (bathing suit nevus)
- Acquired—malignancy—bronchogenic carcinoma; drugs—phenytoin, steroids, minoxidil, diazoxide, streptomycin.

Hirsutism: ↑ growth of terminal hair in women similar to male secondary sexual pattern.

Causes
- Idiopathic
- Virilization in adrenal and ovarian tumors
- PCOD
- Corticosteroid therapy.

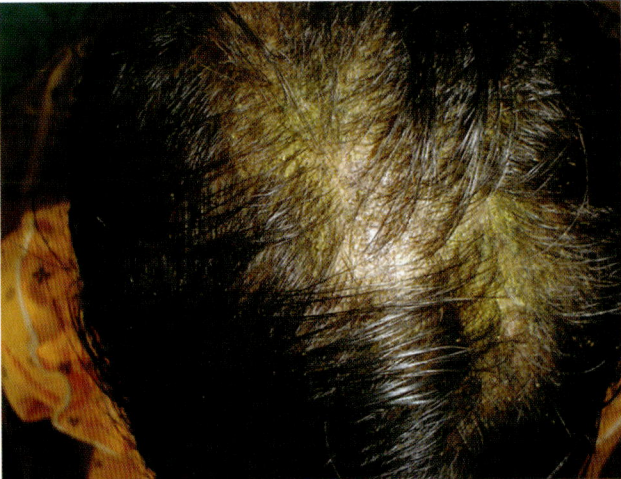

Fig. 2.27: Alopecia in SLE.

Graying of hair:
- Aging process
- Age >20—white
- Age >30—black
  Poliosis means gray hair in a circumscribed pattern.

Premature graying:
- Megalobastic anemia
- Diabetes mellitus
- Hyperthyroidism
- Dystrophia myotonica
- Rare syndromes like Werner's syndrome, Vogt-Koyanagi syndrome, Waardenburg syndrome, Chediak-Higashi syndrome.

THYROID GLAND

Clinical examination of thyroid gland is also included in general examination. Observe the gland for any generalized or local enlargement, inspect its movement during swallowing. Stand behind the seated patient and palpate the gland with one hand on each side of the neck. Assess the thyroid enlargement—whether it is uniform, nodular—single or multiple; soft, firm or hard. Mild enlargement is better seen than felt, auscultation for bruit is important in hyperthyroidism.

Causes for thyromegaly are:
- Goiter (iodine deficiency)
  - Diffuse
  - Nodular—
    - Single
    - Multiple
- Autoimmunity
- Thyroiditis
- Neoplasm
  - Benign
  - Malignant.

EXAMINATION OF LYMPH NODES

Following features are to be noted while examining lymph nodes:
- Site
- Size
- Number
- Consistency—soft, firm or hard
- Tenderness
- Mobility
- Matted/discrete
- Fixity to skin
- Condition of overlying skin
- Lesions in the area of drainage.

Important groups are normal adults have 400–450 lymph nodes:
1. *Cervical group*
   - Vertical
   - Anterior cervical—along anterior jugular—infrahyoid, prelaryngeal and pretracheal

- Superficial cervical—along external jugular
- Deep cervical—along internal jugular—upper - jugulo-digastric- lower - jugulo-omohyoid
- Circular—upper
  - Occipital, posterior auricular, preauricular
  - Buccal, submandibular and submental
- Circular—lower
  - Supraclavicular—Virchow's node—left supraclavicular node (Troisier's sign enlarged Virchow's node)
  - Scalene node—in relation to scaleneus anterior deep to sternocleidomastoid right scalene LN—drains whole of right lung and left lower lobe left Scalene LN—drains left upper lobe.
2. *Axillary group*—apical, medial, lateral, anterior—pectoral and posterior—subcapular
3. *Epitrochlear*
4. *Deltopectoral*—infraclavicular
5. *Inguinal*
   - Superficial
     - Upper group—in relation to inguinal ligament
     - Lower group—in relation to the saphenous vein
   - Deep
     - Vertical—in relation to femoral vein
     - Horizontal—in relation to inguinal ligament
6. *Mediastinal group*
7. *Abdominal group.*

Method of Examination

Cervical Group (Figs. 2.28A and B)

Cervical lymph nodes should be examined by standing behind the patient. Slightly flex the neck of the patient, start palpating from submental onward both circular and vertical groups. Care must be taken to palpate scalene LN on both sides and Virchow's node on the left side.

Axillary Group

Axillary lymph nodes are palpated by raising the patient's arm using right hand of the examiner for the left axilla and vice versa; push the fingers as high as possible in the axilla. Patient's arm is then brought to rest on the examiner's forearm.

Inguinal Group

In the supine position palpate with the palm of the hand.

Abdominal Group

Method of palpation like any other abdominal mass, lymph node enlargement is felt as nodular discrete or matted mass.

Mediastinal Group

Mediastinal group enlargement is detected by percussion or looking for pressure effect on the neighboring structures.

Causes of Lymph Node Enlargement

Generalized Lymphadenopathy

- ***Infections***
  - Viral—IMN, CMV, AIDS, HBV
  - Bacterial—syphilis (secondary stage), TB, brucellosis, Hansen's disease in reaction, melioidosis
  - Parasitic—toxoplasmosis, kala azar, trypanosomiasis
  - Rickettsiae—scrub typhus, rickettsial pox
  - Fungal—histoplasmosis, coccidioidomycosis
- ***Non-infections***
  - Neoplasms-lymphomas—HL and NHL; leukemias—ALL, CLL, CML with blast crisis
  - Others
    - Drugs—phenytoin (pseudolymphoma)
    - SLE, rheumatoid arthritis—Still's disease
    - Serum sickness
    - Generalized skin diseases

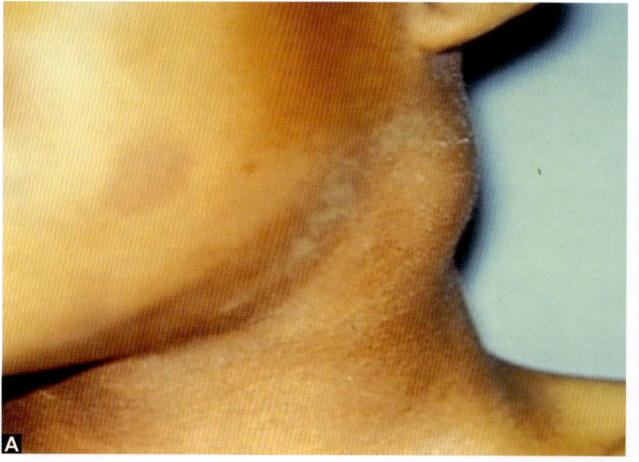 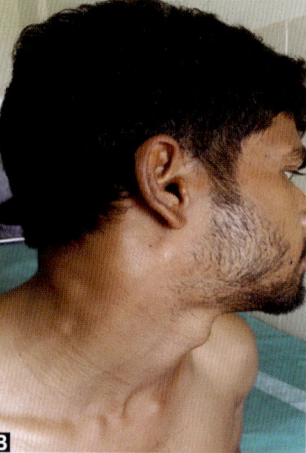

Figs. 2.28A and B: Cervical lymphadenopathy.

- Exfoliative dermatitis, pyoderma
- Sarcoidosis
- Hyperthyroidism, primary biliary cirrhosis
- *Rare conditions:*
  - Angioimmunoblastic lymphadenopathy
  - Kikuchi's disease—histiocytic necrotizing lymphadenitis
  - Castleman's disease—giant LN hyperplasia—mediastinal
  - Sinus histiocytosis with massive lymphadenopathy—Rosai-Dorfman syndrome.

Localized Lymphadenopathy

- *Infections*—Rubella, TB, bubonic plague, LGV, granuloma inguinale, filariasis, infection in drainage area
- *Non-infections*
  - Secondary LN—scalene (lung malignancy)
  - Virchow's LN—upper GIT malignancy and testicular tumors
  - Hodgkin's disease.

HAND AND SYSTEMIC DISEASES

Examination of hand reveals specific features of systemic diseases.
- Cold clammy hand with peripheral cyanosis—shock
- Cold moist hand—anxiety state
- Cold dry hand—myxedema
- Warm moist hand—thyrotoxicosis
- Pallor of palmar crease—anemia
- Hypertrophic osteoarthropathy—bronchogenic Ca
- Wasting and fasciculation of hand muscles—MND, syringomyelia
- Myotonic disorders—slow relaxation on shaking hand
- Cyanosis and clubbing together—cyanotic CHD, ILD
- Nailfold infarct and telangiectasia—vasculitis, SLE, PAN, PSS
- Osler's node—splinter stage, Janeway lesion—IE
- Pigmentation—Addison's disease, megaloblastic anemia
- Arachnodactyly—Marfan's syndrome
- Deformed hand—rheumatoid arthritis
- Sclerodactyly—PSS, MCTD
- Heberden's node—osteoarthritis
- Involuntary movement—chorea, athetosis, tremor
- Clawing of hand—T_1 segment lesion or both ulnar and median nerve lesion
- Dupuytren's contracture—alcoholic liver disease, trauma
- Gottron's papule—dermatomyositis
- Large spade hand—acromegaly
- Short 4th metacarpal
  - Pseudohypoparathyroidism
  - Reverse Marfan's syndrome (Weill-Marchesani syndrome)
  - Turner's syndrome (Fig. 2.29)
- Long thumb—fingerization—Holt-Oram syndrome

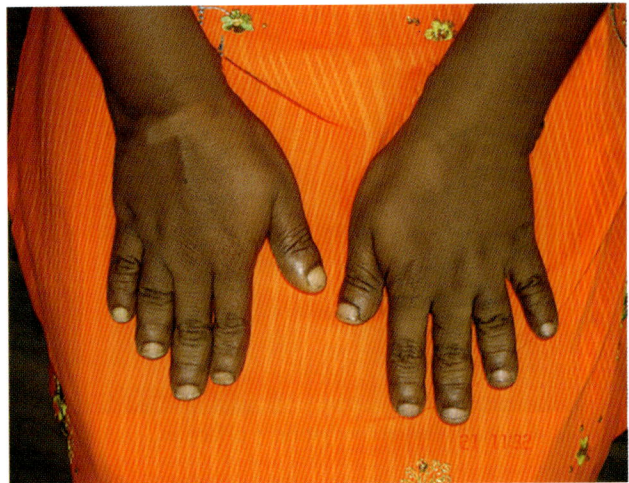

Fig. 2.29: Short 4th metacarpal seen in Turner's syndrome.

DIAGNOSTIC FACIES

Specific diagnostic facies can be made from facial appearances.
- Acromegaly—coarse features, prominent lower jaw, large nose, lips and ears, prominent cheek bone and forehead, wide spread teeth
- Cushing's syndrome—moon face with plethoric appearance
- Hypothyroidism—puffy pale face, swollen eyelids, dull expression and loss of hair of eyebrows
- Cretinism—pale face, broad and flattened face, thick lips and large protruding tongue
- Hyperthyroidism—anxious look with bilateral ptosis and infrequent blinking of eyes, visibility of sclera all around the cornea
- Hippocratic facies—sunken eyes and cheeks, dry lips, looks severely ill
- Leonine facies—thickening of skin and earlobes, with a flattened nose, loss of hair over the lateral part of eyebrows (madarosis)
- Myasthenic facies—bilateral ptosis, wrinkling of forehead and partially opened mouth with vertical smile—myasthenic snarl
- Dystrophia myotonica—bilateral ptosis, frontal baldness, wasting of sternocleidomastoid, temporalis and masseter, transverse smile—hatchet face and swan neck (Fig. 2.30)
- Parkinsonism—fixed expressionless face, with infrequent blinking and reptilian stare
- Tabetic facies—bilateral partial ptosis with miosis, compensatory partial wrinkling of forehead and anhidrosis—bilateral Horner's syndrome
- Chip munk facies—frontomaxillary prominence due to marrow expansion—hemolytic facies in hemolytic anemias
- Mucopolysaccharidosis (Hurler's)—coarse features of face, hypertrichosis, large tongue and corneal haziness
- Tetanus—characteristic risus sardonicus—blepharospasm and spasm of facial muscles

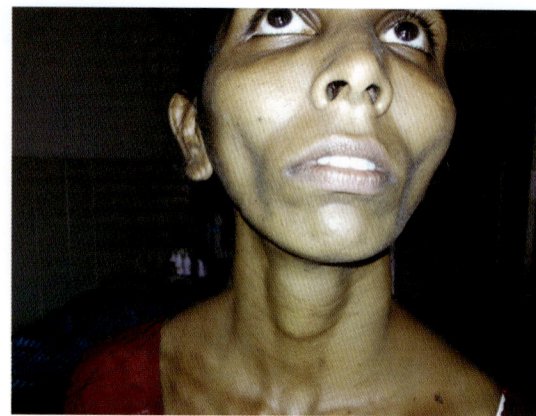

Fig. 2.30: Partial lipodystrophy of face and neck.

- Elfin facies—William's syndrome—wide mouth with wide pouty lips, widely spaced teeth and eyes
- Face in scleroderma—shiny taut skin over the face, microstomia with wrinkles around the mouth, pinched nose
- Face in SLE—butterfly rash—nasal bride and upper face
- Cirrhotic facies—sunken eyes and cheeks, bilateral enlargement of parotid especially in alcoholic cirrhosis.

Body Habitus

First impression of a patient's appearance will lead to diagnosis, but one should substantiate by seeking for other signs on proper examination—may be labeled as spotters.
- Acromegaly—characteristic facies with acral enlargement
- Gigantism—tall stature, bilateral acral enlargement and prognathism
- Thyrotoxicosis—anxious look, bilateral ptosis, restlessness, thin built body, tremor of hands
- Myxedema—characteristic facies, dull expression and edema of legs
- Cretinism—characteristic facies, dwarfism and protruding tongue
- Addison's disease—hyperpigmentation, asthenia and thinning of body
- Cushing's syndrome—moon face, plethoric face, striae, obesity—truncal obesity and buffalo hump
- Pseudohypoparathyroidism—short stature, moon face and brachydactyly
- Rickets—dwarfism, frontoparietal bossing, rachitic rosary, bowing of legs, delayed dentition
- Marfan's syndrome—tall stature, long thin extremities and arachnodactyly
- Klinefelter's syndrome—tall stature, absence of secondary sexual characters, alopecia ± gynecomastia
- Turner syndrome—short stature, cunbitus valgus, webbing of neck and widely spaced nipple
- Achondroplasia—dwarfism, normal trunk size, short limbs especially proximal parts, macrocephaly, saddle nose, increased lumbar lordosis

- Mongolism—characteristic facies—mongoloid slant of eyes, protruded tongue with open mouth, hypotonic muscles, single transverse crease of hand
- Mucopolysaccharidosis—short stature, characteristic facies, joint stiffness, kyphoscoliosis
- SLE—characteristic facies
- PSS—characteristic facies—vitiligo—pepper and salt appearance, sclerodactyly, hyperpigmentation, digits—telangiectasia, ulcers, pitted scars
- Ankylosing spondylitis—posture of patient due to spine involvement, loss of lumbar lordosis, increased dorsal kyphosis and forward stoop of neck, flexion of hip and knee joints, limitation of spine movement
- Dystrophia myotonica—baldness with characteristic facies
- Abnormal movement—chorea, athetosis, dyskinesia, tics, hemifacial spasm
- Charcot-Marie-Tooth disease—peroneal muscular atrophy, inverted champagne bottle appearance of legs.

VITAL SIGNS

Temperature

Temperature should always be recorded as a part of initial clinical examination. Oral temperature is measured by placing the clinical thermometer under the tongue with mouth closed for a period of 1 minute. Prior to measurement no oral feeds for 15 minutes, wash the thermometer with antiseptic solution, mercury in the thermometer is gently shaken down.

Oral temperature is less than rectal temperature by 0.2-0.5°C, axillary temperature is less than oral by 0.5°C. Diurnal variation of body temperature is lowest in the morning and reaches a peak between 6 and 10 pm.

	Degree Celsius	Degree Fahrenheit
Normal temperature	36.6–37.2	98–99
Febrile	>37.2	>99
Hyperpyrexia	>41.6	>107
Subnormal	<36.6	<98
Hypothermia	<95	<35

Types of Fever

- *Continuous fever:* Fluctuation of temperature <1°C, does not touch baseline, e.g. lobar pneumonia, upper UTI, rheumatic fever.
- *Remittent fever:* Fluctuation of temperature >2°C, does not touch the baseline, e.g. invasive phase of enteric fever—stepladder pattern of temperature.
- *Intermittent fever:* Temperature touches normal at least once in 24 hours, e.g. malaria.

Types of Intermittent Fever

- Quotidian—every day
- Tertian—every 48 hours

- Quartan—once in every 72 hours.
Note: All types *of intermittent fever* seen in malaria.

Relapsing Fever

Temperature remains normal, for days, before rising again as in Hodgkin's lymphoma—"Pel-Ebstein's fever".

Pattern of rise and fall of temperature in various diseases:
- Abrupt rise of temperature is seen in lobar pneumonia, upper UTI
- Step ladder type of fever is seen in—enteric fever
- High temperature in fever touches normal within days—lysis of fever—enteric fever
- High temperature in fever touches normal within hours—crisis of fever—lobar pneumonia and malaria
- Short febrile illness <7 days—viral fever
- Prolonged fever >7 days—RTI, UTI, etc.
- **PUO**—Pyrexia of unknown origin
- Fever lasting >3 weeks where no cause is found despite clinical examination and basic investigation
  - Infections—IMN, HIV, TB, c/c malaria, kala azar, toxoplasmosis, brucellosis, occult abscess anywhere
  - Collagen vascular disease
  - Internal malignancy—lymphoma, renal cell carcinoma, hepatoma.

Hyperpyrexia

- Lobar pneumonia
- Septicemia
- Acute pyogenic meningitis
- Cerebral malaria
- Pontine hemorrhage
- Neuroleptic malignant syndrome
- Heat stroke

Hypothermia

- Myxedema coma
- Phenobarbitone poisoning
- Exposure to cold—frost bite
- Alcohol intoxication
- Hypoglycemia.

USUAL FEATURES OF FEVER

- CVS-tachycardia—rise of HR by 10° F above 100° F
- Relative bradycardia—rise <10° F—viral fever, enteric fever, meningitis
- Relative tachycardia
  - Rise > 10° F—rheumatic fever
  - High volume pulse and wide pulse pressure—because of vasodilatation
- Respiratory system
  - Rise in respiratory rate by 4° F rise above 100° F
  - Tachypnea especially in pneumonia

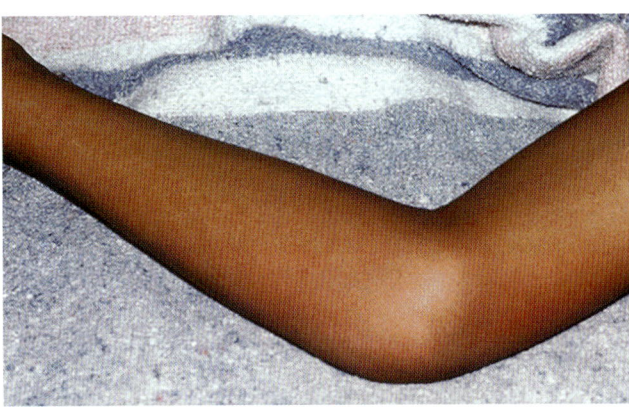

Fig. 2.31: Macular rash in a patient with dengue fever.

- CNS—headache due to vasodilatation
  - Febrile convulsion, especially in children
  - Acute confused state and delirium—toxic encephalopathy
- GIT—anorexia, constipation, herpes labialis—especially in pneumonia and malaria (rare in enteric fever), furring of tongue
- Skin—miliaria—Sweat retention rash in exanthematous fevers (refer examination of skin) (Fig. 2.31).
- Dehydration—increased sweating, vomiting and decreased fluid intake.

Pulse

Count the pulse for a full minute while patient is at rest. Details of the method of palpation of pulse and clinical abnormalities are detailed in the CVS chapter. Normal pulse can be expressed as 72/minute, regular in rhythm, volume and character normal, condition of the vessel wall normal, all peripheral pulses felt equally, no radial femoral delay.

Blood Pressure

Blood pressure recording is essential to assess the patient's blood pressure, to know whether the patient is having normal blood pressure, hypertension or hypotension. Sphygmomanometer was discovered by Riva Rocci. Mercury type of manometer is the most reliable standard instrument. Rubber cuff has a width of 12.5 cm and length of 25 cm. in obese people cuff width is 15 cm. For measuring lower limb, BP cuff width is 18 cm.

Procedure

- BP should be first recorded by palpation and then by auscultatory method.
- Rubber cuff should cover 80% of arm.
- Lower border of cuff is not <2 cm from the cubital fossa.
- No smoking or coffee for 30 minutes prior to BP recording.
- Recording should be done after 5 minutes of rest.

- Patient should be seated in a chair or in supine position.
- Inflate the cuff while palpating the radial pulse to 30 mm Hg above the level at which the radial pulse is not felt.
- Keep the stethoscope lightly over the brachial artery and deflate at a rate of 5 mm/sec until the first sound of the Korotkoff is heard (phase 1). This is taken as the systolic BP, continue to lower the pressure in the cuff until the sounds disappear (phase V), this indicates the diastolic BP.

"Nikolai Korotkoff described these sounds in 1905". At times the Korotkoff's sounds disappear between auscultations, this is called the 'auscultatory gap' or the 'silent gap'. Three BP measurements done, 2 minutes apart if the value difference is >5 mm Hg between the first two measurements, then the average is taken. BP difference between the right and left arm is 10 mm Hg. Arm and leg difference is 20 mm Hg. On standing systolic BP falls and diastolic BP rises. Fall of systolic BP >10 mm Hg while standing for 3 minutes or more is indicative of postural hypotension.

Lower limb BP is recorded if coarctation of aorta, aorto-arteritis and aortic regurgitation (Hill's sign) are present. Before labeling a person hypertensive, 2 or more BP recording at each visit for 3 or more occasions at an interval of 2–3 weeks is a must.

Classification of blood pressure for adults—JNC 7 report.		
Category	SBP	DBP
Normal	<120	<80
Pre-HTN	120–139	80–89
Stage I HTN	140–159	90–99
Stage II HTN	≥160	≥100

JNC—Joint National Committee on Prevention, Detection, and Evaluation of High Blood Pressure

BP Goal: According to JNC 8.	
Age	BP goal
≥ 60 years No DM/CKD	<150/90
<60 years or ≥60 years with DM/CKD	<140/90

- *Isolated systolic hypertension*
  - SBP >140 mm Hg
  - DBP <90 mm Hg
- *Accelerated hypertension*—recent increase in BP over the previous BP value with evidence of vascular changes in the optic fundi without papilledema.
- *Malignant hypertension*—is a triad of
  - High BP of 200/140
  - Papilledema and
  - Renal dysfunction.
- *Hypertensive emergency*—is a marked elevation of BP with evidence of end organ damage, demanding prompt control of BP.
- *White coat hypertension*—high BP recording in individuals at physician's office or hospital, otherwise normal BP.

Sphygmomanometer is used
- To measure the BP
- To measure the difference in BP in limbs in occlusive arterial diseases
- To demonstrate postural hypotension
- To demonstrate Hill's sign in AR
- To demonstrate pulses alternans
- To demonstrate pulses paradoxus
- To determine IVY method of bleeding time
- To look for Hess' test
- To elicit latent tetany—Trousseau's sign.

Respiratory Rate

Rate, rhythm and type of respiration should be noted. Respiratory rate is counted by placing the hand over the abdomen, feel for the anterior movement of the anterior abdominal wall with each respiration and count the number of forward movements for one full minute.

Normal respiratory rate is 18/min (16–22) >22 is called tachypnea.

Types of respiration—male—abdominothoracic: female—thoracoabdominal.

Changes in the Rhythm of Respiration

- Upper airway obstruction—inspiratory stridor—noisy respiration with indrawing of suprasternal, supraclavicular and intercostal spaces.
- Whoop—inspiratory noise after a bout of cough in whooping cough
- Wheeze—in COPD/asthma high pitched ronchi heard during expiration
- Rattling noise—severe pulmonary edema, both in cardiogenic and non-cardiogenic (death rattle)
- Cheyne-Stoke's breathing—periods of apnea alternate with hyperpnea, delay in the chemoreceptor response to blood gas changes as in CHF and upper brainstem damage
- Biot's breathing—breathing irregular in time and depth as in brainstem damage
- Kussmaul's breathing—acidotic breathing—deep rapid breathing.

CHAPTER 3

Examination of Nervous System

REVIEW OF NEUROANATOMY AND PHYSIOLOGY

MOTOR SYSTEM

Upper Motor Neurons

Pyramidal system: Corticospinal and corticonuclear fibers.

Extrapyramidal tracts: Vestibulospinal, rubrospinal, olivospinal and tectospinal fibers.

Pyramidal System

Pyramidal system consists of 10 lakhs fibers arising from Betz cells situated in the 5th layer of cerebral cortex—precentral gyrus, parietal lobes, area 6 and 8 of frontal lobes and other parts of brain. Number of Betz cells are 25,000–35,000. Pyramidal fibers pass down through corona radiata into the genu and anterior 2/3rd of posterior limb of internal capsule. A part of fibers are also present in the posterior 1/3rd of anterior limb of internal capsule (Fig. 3.1).

Body Representation at the Motor Cortex and Internal Capsule

- *In the motor cortex*: Center for the larynx and pharynx are at the lowermost part of precentral gyrus, in the ascending order—center for palate, jaw, tongue, mouth and face, forehead, neck, thumb, fingers, wrist, elbow, shoulder, thorax and abdomen, lower limbs and sacral region are represented on the medial surface of the hemisphere. Areas for the tongue, face and digits are large.
- *In the internal capsule*: Those to the face is anterior, followed posteriorly by upper limbs, trunk and lower limbs.
- *In the midbrain*: Pyramidal fibers lie in the intermediate 3/5 of cerebral peduncle.
- *In the pons:* Basilar part of pons, separated by transverse fibers.
- *In the medulla*: Pyramidal fibers are on the ventral aspect (Fig. 3.1).

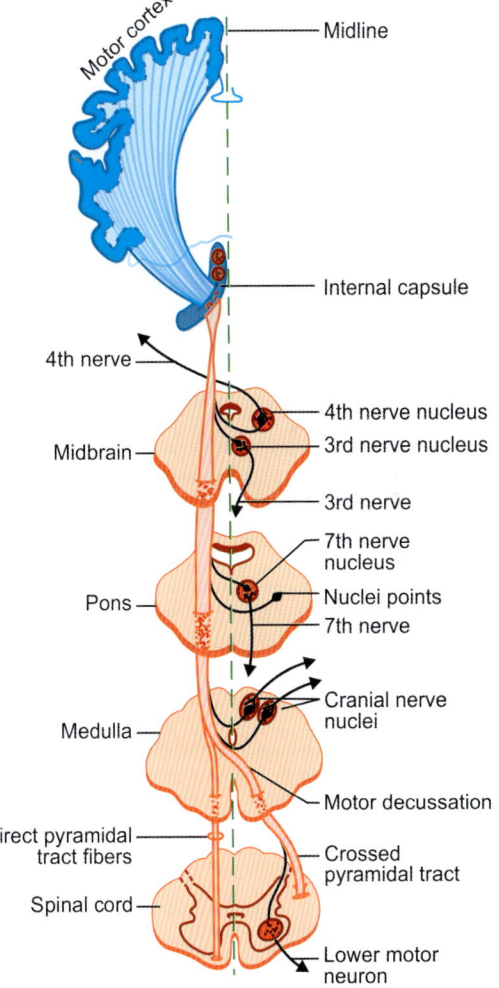

Fig. 3.1: Pyramidal tract.

Corticonuclear fibers cross before synapsing with the cranial nerve nuclei of opposite side. Brainstem nuclei are innervated by both crossed and uncrossed fibers. Pyramidal fibers to spinal cord descend as corticospinal fibers at the caudal part of medulla. The 80–90% decussate and

descend through the lateral column of spinal cord as lateral corticospinal pathway and synapse with anterior horn cells.
- Fifty percent of lateral corticospinal fibers terminate at cervical region.
- Twenty percent of lateral corticospinal fibers terminate at thoracic region.
- Thirty percent of lateral corticospinal fibers terminate at lumbosacral region.

Small anterior corticospinal fibers descend uncrossed in ipsilateral anterior column of spinal cord not beyond mid thoracic region, these fibers also cross before termination. One pyramidal fiber may supply more than one neuron of spinal cord.

Pyramidal system is concerned with voluntary skilled, fine movement of limbs especially distal portion which is more for the extensors and external rotators in the upper limb, flexors and internal rotators in the lower limb.

Extrapyramidal system tracts consists of vestibulospinal, reticulospinal, rubrospinal, olivospinal and tectospinal. Cortical center influencing the extrapyramidal fibers is area 6 of premotor region of frontal lobe.

Lesion of pyramidal system alone will produce flaccidity of muscles, but lesion of both pyramidal and extrapyramidal tracts will result in spasticity at the early. Lamination in the corticospinal tract from lateral to medial is sacral, lumbar, dorsal and cervical.

Lower Motor Neurons

It is the connecting link between the CNS and skeletal muscle.
- Anterior horn cell/brainstem motor nuclei of cranial nerve
- Anterior root ± plexus
- Peripheral nerve to the muscle.

Features of UMN Lesion

- Loss of power
- Hypertonia-spasticity (clasp knife)
- Exaggerated DTR ± clonus
- Loss of superficial reflexes and extensor plantar.

Features of LMN Lesion

- Loss of power, wasting and fasciculation
- Hypotonia-flaccidity
- Hyporeflexia/areflexia
- Superficial reflexes—normal, plantar flexor (except in situation of lesion of reflex arc).

Acute Phase of UMN Lesion

- Loss of:
  - Power
  - Tone
  - Reflexes: Both deep and superficial
- On recovery: Reflex recovers first, then tone, lastly power, proximal earlier than distal.

SENSORY SYSTEM

Sensory input to the brain is usually through three orders of neurons from the receptors.

Receptors:
- Pain: free nerve endings
- Touch: free nerve endings, Meissner's corpuscles and Merkel's disc
- Thermal: Cold-Krause's end bulb, free nerve endings
- Warm: Free nerve endings, Ruffini's corpuscle
- Pressure: Pacinian corpuscle
- Proprioception: Muscle spindle, Golgi tendon organ.

Pathways of Pain and Thermal Sensation

Receptor → 1st order of neuron → peripheral nerve ± plexus → posterior root → substantia gelatinosa of Rolando at the posterior horn of spinal cord.

Second order of neuron → from SGR to the opposite lateral column and ascend as lateral spinothalamic tract in the spinal cord, spinal lemniscus in the brain-stem terminate at the ventral posterolateral nucleus of thalamus.

Third order of neuron → from thalamus to the sensory cortex as thalamoparietal fibers (Fig. 3.2).

Pathway of Touch Sensation

Dual pathway:
- *Fine touch through posterior column*
- *Crude touch through anterior spinothalamic tract → spinal lemniscus in brainstem → thalamus → sensory cortex.*

Pathway of Proprioception and Fine Touch

- *First order: Receptor → peripheral nerve ± plexus → central axons of posterior root ganglion → posterior column in the spinal cord (tract of Goll and Burdach) → nucleus of Gracilis and Cuneatus*
- *Second order: From nucleus of gracilis and cuneatus-cross to opposite side → medial lemniscus in brainstem → thalamic chief sensory nucleus*
- *Third order: From the chief sensory nucleus of thalamus → sensory cortex as thalamoparietal projection.*

Sensory Cortex

It is the post central gyrus of the parietal lobe (Area 3, 1, 2 of Brodmann).

Representation of body appears upside down; foot occupies the medial part of gyrus, face on the lower lateral part of gyrus.

Applied Anatomy of Sensory Pathways

Lamination of fibers in spinothalamic tract: From lateral to medial: Sacral, Lumbar, thoracic and cervical.

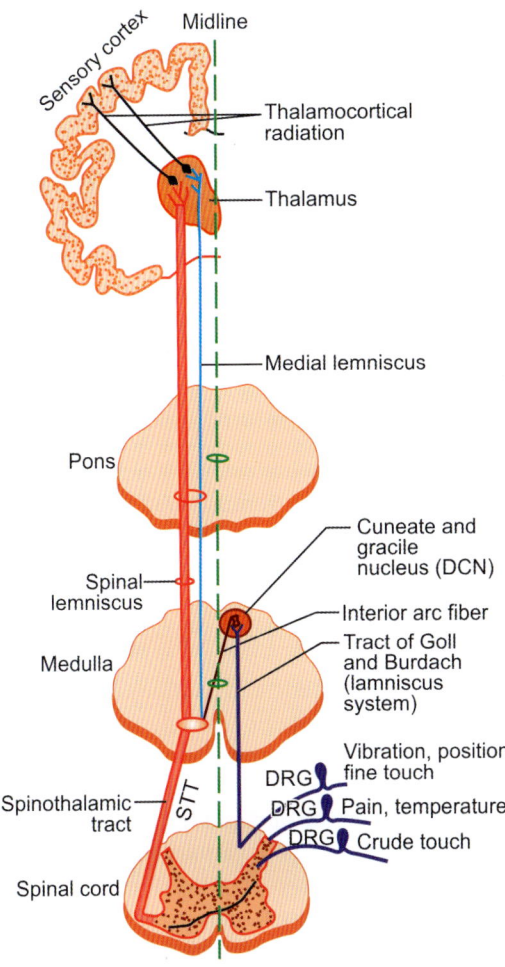

Fig. 3.2: Important sensory pathways.

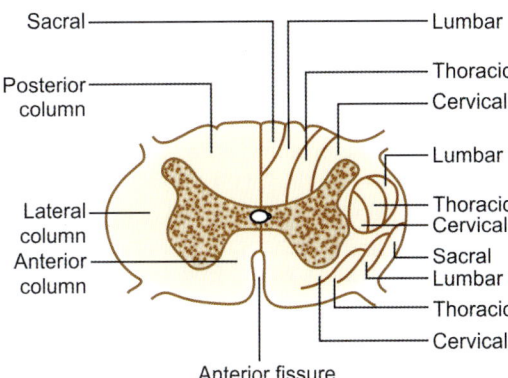

Fig. 3.3: Lamination of fibers of pathways of spinal cord.

Lamination of fibers in posterior column: From lateral to medial cervical, thoracic, lumbar and sacral.

Peripheral lesion of spinothalamic tract: Fibers from lower part of the body (sacral and lumbar) are 1st affected sensory loss at a lower level—opposite side.

Central lesion of spinothalamic tract: Fibers from upper part of the body (cervical and thoracic) are 1st affected with sparing of sacral sensory fibers (Fig. 3.3).
- Second order of neurons becoming spinothalamic tract may ascend a few segments in the same side before crossing, thus lesion of spinothalamic tract produce loss of sensation at the opposite side at a lower level.
- Fibers carrying pain and thermal sensation while crossing to the opposite side are lying close to the central canal of spinal cord, dilatation of this, as in syringomyelia, will damage these fibers early, producing dissociated sensory loss.
- Primary modalities of sensation like touch, pain, and thermal sensation are appreciated at the thalamic level, thus lesion of 1st and 2nd order neurons can produce total loss of primary modalities of sensation, lesion of 3rd order of neuron will produce no total loss of sensation, but dulling of primary modalities of sensation.
- Loss of proprioception can be due to lesion anywhere from peripheral nerve to sensory cortex.

Terms for Description

- *Mononeuropathy/mononeuritis:* Neural pattern of involvement of single peripheral nerve.
- *Mononeuritis cranialis:* Involvement of single cranial nerve.
- *Polyneuropathy:* More than one nerve is involved.
- *Mononeuritis multiplex:* Asymmetrical involvement of multiple nerves.
- *Polyneuritis cranialis:* Lesions affecting multiple cranial nerves.
- *Peripheral neuropathy:* Distal symmetrical involvement of peripheral nerves (glove and stocking pattern).
- *Radiculopathy:* Lesions of nerve root
  - *Anterior:* segmental motor defect.
  - *Posterior:* segmental or dermatome pattern of sensory loss and reflex loss.
- *Radicular pain:* Shooting type of pain radiating to a dermatome, increased by straining like cough and movement of spine.
- Bilateral radicular pain in the trunk is called girdle pain.
- Sclerotome and myotome pain, deep pain arising from connective tissue and muscles of a segment in posterior root lesion.
- *Tract pain:* Lesion of spinothalamic tract produce non-localized, diffuse, burning type of pain below the level of tract lesion.

Important Dermatomes to Remember

It is easier to remember the dermatomes with the following facts:
- C1 gives no supply to skin—occiput supplied by C2
- C5 supplies shoulder region—deltoid region
- C7 supplies middle finger area
- D2/D3 supplies axilla

- D7, D10 and D12 supplies epigastrium, umbilicus and pubic symphysis
- L3 at the knee, L5—outer aspect of leg
- S1–lateral aspect of sole (walking on S1)
- S3, S4, S5—around the anus (sitting on S3, S4, S5)
- At sternal angle—junction of C4–D2/D3
- Upper medial side of thigh—junction of L2 and S2.

EXTRAPYRAMIDAL SYSTEM

It consists of basal ganglia, subthalamic nucleus, substantia nigra, red nucleus and other structures in the brainstem. It controls the LMN through rubrospinal, reticulospinal, vestibulospinal and olivospinal tract. Extrapyramidal system is in close relation with motor system and influence the proper motor activity like posture, initiation of movement, and movements affecting the postural mechanism like sitting, standing and turning.

Lesions of EPS affect:
- The tone of muscle—rigidity
- Impaired initiation and poverty of movement
- Abnormal movements
- Retained muscle power
- Postural instability.

CEREBELLUM

It forms 10% weight of cerebrum. Cerebellum receives sensory inputs from spinal cord, vestibular system and cerebral cortex.

Functions

- Control of equilibrium
- Coordination of movement, rate, range and force of movement acting on agonist, antagonist, fixators and synergists.
- Facilitatory action on tone and reflex activity.
- Visceral functions—BP, heart rate and bladder function.

Three circuits for the input of impulses to cerebellum from vestibular system, spinal cord and cerebral cortex.
  A. *Input from vestibular system:*
  Labyrinth → vestibular nerve → medial and superior vestibular nucleus → vestibulocerebellar tract → flocculonodular lobe of cerebellum → fastigial nucleus → lateral vestibular nucleus → vestibulospinal tract → anterior horn cell.
  Function: Control of equilibrium.
  B. *Input from the spinal cord:*
  Spinocerebellar tracts—dorsal and ventral → superior and inferior cerebellar peduncle → paleocerebellum → N. globosus and emboliformis → opposite red nucleus; recrosses (double decussation) → rubrospinal tract → anterior horn cell.
  Function: Control and coordination of voluntary movement, control of visceral activity.
  C. *Input from cerebral cortex:*
  Cerebral cortex—motor area and premotor areas (4 and 6) → Fronto-ponto-cerebellar tract → middle cerebellar peduncle → ansiform lobe of neocerebellum → dentate nucleus → Dentatorubrothalamocortical fibers and dentatothalamocortical fibers to cerebral cortex (Area 4 and 6)

Cerebellar lesions → asthenia, ataxia, atonia—Luciani's triad.
Cerebellum controls the same side of the body because of recrossing (double decussation) of rubrospinal fibers to the same side of cerebellar hemisphere and descends to reach the anterior horn cell.

Localization of Cerebellar Lesion

- Hemispheric lesion → limb ataxia of same side
- Anterior lobe and upper vermis lesion → gait ataxia
- Lower vermis lesion → truncal ataxia—inability to sit and stand (astasia abasia).

Sites of Lesion Producing Cerebellar Signs

- *Cerebellum:* Hemispheric and midline vermis lesion
- *Cerebellar peduncle:* Superior, middle and inferior
- *Frontal lobe lesion:* Via frontopontocerebellar fibers to cerebellum as in ataxic hemiparesis (both cerebellar and pyramidal signs on the same side)
- *Brainstem lesion:* Fibers of various circuit of input going through brainstem.
- *Posterior radicular lesion at spinal level:* Fibers intending to become spinocerebellar tracts are selectively damaged by demyelination as in Miller Fisher variant of GBS.

SPINAL CORD

Spinal cord extends from foramen magnum to the level between 1st and 2nd lumbar vertebra, and ends at a conical structure called conus medullaris. Spinal cord has anterior median fissure and posterior median sulcus. Anterior root exits at anterolateral sulcus carrying efferent impulse from spinal cord. Posterior root enters at the posterolateral sulcus carrying afferent impulse to spinal cord. Anterior and posterior roots join to form the peripheral nerve. Nerve roots emerge through the intervertebral foramen. The fissure, sulci and root zones divide the spinal cord into anterior, posterior and lateral column.

Ascending Pathways

- Lateral spinothalamic tract
- Ventral spinothalamic tract
- Dorsal and ventral spinocerebellar tracts
- Spino-olivary, spinotectal and spinovestibular tract
- Posterior column (fasciculus gracilis and cuneatus).

Descending Pathways

- Lateral corticospinal tract
- Ventral corticospinal tract
- Reticulospinal tract
- Olivospinal tract
- Vestibulospinal tract
- Tectospinal tract
- Rubrospinal tract
- 31 pair of spinal nerves: 8 cervical, 12 thoracic, 5 lumbar, 5 sacral, and 1 coccyx. Length of the spinal cord is less than the length of the spinal canal of the spine.

Spinal Segments Corresponding to Vertebrae

Vertebral Body Level Spinal Segment

Cervical vertebrae	Add 1
Dorsal vertebrae 1–6	Add 2
Dorsal vertebrae 7–9	Add 3
D 10	L1 and L2 segment
D 11	L3 and L4 segment
D 12	L5 segment
L1	Sacral and coccyx segment

- *Conus medullaris*: Lower most part of spinal cord consisting of S3, S4, S5 and coccyx 1 segment.
- *Epiconus*: It consists of L4, L5 and S1, S2 segments.
- *Cauda equina:* L2 nerve root down, descends to escape through respective intervertebral foramen. This group of nerve roots on either side is called cauda equina.

Important Spinal Segments to Remember

- C5—Abduction of shoulder
- C6—Flexion of elbow
- C7—Extension of elbow
- C8—Wrist flexion and extension
- T1—Small muscles of hand
- L1—Flexion of hip
- L2—Adduction of hip
- L3—Extension of knee
- L4—Dorsiflexion of ankle and inversion of foot
- L5—Eversion of foot
- S1—Plantar flexion of ankle
- S2,3—Small muscles of foot
- L4–L5—Abduction of hip
- L5, S1—Extension of hip and flexion of knee.

CEREBRAL CORTEX

Important cortical areas
- **Frontal lobe:**
  - Area 4—Motor area precentral gyrus
  - Area 6—Premotor area—cortical origin of EPS
  - Area 8—Frontal eye field
    - Superior frontal gyrus
    - Lateral gaze center
  - Area 44—Broca's area—posterior part of inferior frontal gyrus
- **Parietal lobe:**
  - Area 3, 1, 2—Chief sensory area—posterior central gyrus
  - Area 5, 7—Sensory association area
  - Area 43—Taste center—lower part of posterior central gyrus
- **Temporal lobe:**
  - Area 41—Primary auditory area—superior temporal gyrus
  - Area 42—Auditory association area
  - Area 39, 40—Wernicke's area—posterior part of superior temporal gyrus
- **Occipital lobe:**
  - Area 17—Primary visual area
  - Area 18, 19—Visual association area.

BLOOD SUPPLY OF BRAIN AND SPINAL CORD

- Brain receives 700–800 mL of blood/minute (55 mL/100 g/min)
- Less than 30 mL/100 g/minute will lead to ischemia
- 80% of blood to the gray matter and 20% to white matter (Figs. 3.4 and 3.5).

Blood Supply to Brain

- Carotid system—Two internal carotid arteries
- Vertebrobasilar system—Two vertebral arteries.

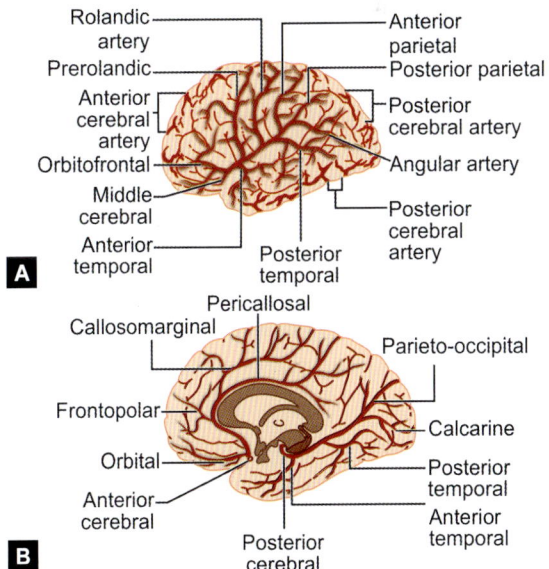

Figs. 3.4A and B: Blood supply of the cerebral cortex. (A) Lateral surface of the brain; (B) Medial surface of the brain.

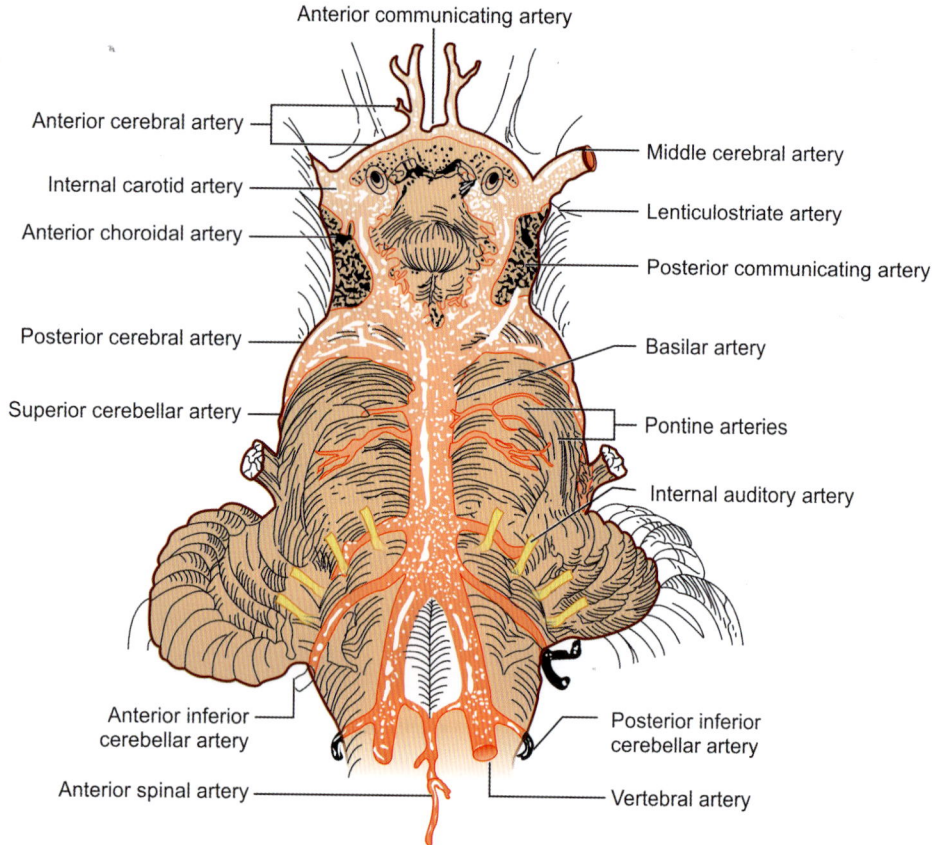

Fig. 3.5: Circle of Willis and principal arteries of the brain.

Internal carotid has four portions:
- Cervical
- Petrous
- Cavernous
- Cerebral

Branches of cerebral portion of internal carotid artery
- Ophthalmic → central retinal artery
- Posterior communicating artery
- Anterior choroidal artery
- Anterior cerebral artery
- Middle cerebral artery.

Main branches: Divided into:
A. Cortical
B. Central (penetrating branches).

Cortical branches: Supply the frontal, parietal, lateral aspect of temporal lobe.

Central branches: Supply the basal ganglia and internal capsule.

They are of two groups:
- *Medial striate:* Lenticulo-optic
- *Lateral striate:* Lenticulostriate (Charcot's artery of cerebral hemorrhage).

Vertebrobasilar System

Branches
- Vertebral artery:
  - Posterior inferior cerebellar artery—supplies lateral medulla
  - Anterior spinal artery—supplies medial medulla
- *Basilar artery:*
  - Paramedian branches—medial portion of pons
    Short circumferential—lateral portion of pons
    Long circumferential:
    - Anterior inferior cerebellar artery
    - Internal auditory artery
    - Superior cerebellar artery
- *Posterior cerebral artery:*
  Supply: Brainstem, thalamus, inferior portion of temporal lobe and occipital lobe.
  Carotid system and vertebrobasilar system anastomose at the base of the skull to form circle of Willis.
- *Middle cerebral artery:*
  - Cortical branches:
    - Upper and lower → Islands of speech area
    - Lateral surface of hemisphere
    - Lateral orbitofrontal surface

- *Central branches:* Medial and lateral striate → basal ganglia → upper half of internal capsule
- *Anterior cerebral artery:*
  - Cortical branches →
    Medial orbitofrontal surface
    Medial surface of brain from frontal pole to parieto occipital sulcus
    Strip of lateral surface; superomedial area
  - Central branches →
    Heubner's artery (recurrent branch of anterior cerebral artery) supply → inferior half of anterior limb of internal capsule
    Part of caudate nucleus
- *Posterior cerebral artery:*
  - Cortical branches →
    Inferior surface of temporal lobe
    Occipital lobe
  - Central (deep) branches →
    Midbrain, thalamosubthalamic region, hypothalamus, mammillary body, medial and lateral geniculate body.

Blood Supply of Internal Capsule

MCA ↓	MCA ↓
Anterior limb— superior half	Posterior limb— superior half
Inferior half	Inferior half

Huebner's artery of ACA anterior, 1/3rd
    Posterior communicating artery
    Posterior 2/3rd—anterior choroidal artery

Venous Drainage of Brain

Sinuses and Veins

Sinuses →
- *Paired:*
  - Cavernous sinus
  - Superior petrosal sinus
  - Inferior petrosal sinus
  - Transverse sinus
  - Sigmoid sinus
- *Unpaired:*
  - Superior sagittal sinus
  - Inferior sagittal sinus
  - Straight sinus
  - Anterior intercavernous
  - Posterior intercavernous

Veins →
- Superficial:
  - Superior → superior sagittal sinus
  - Inferior → transverse sinus and sigmoid sinus
- Deep: From choroid plexus of lateral and 3rd ventricle arises 2 internal cerebral veins which join to form great cerebral vein of Galen and drains to straight sinus.

Blood Supply of Spinal Cord

Spinal cord blood supply is by anterior spinal artery and two posterior spinal arteries. Anterior spinal artery is formed by the union of the branch arising from two vertebral arteries which is reinforced by lateral spinal artery which divides into anterior and posterior radicular branches.
- Lateral spinal artery arises
- Cervical region: superior cervical artery
- Thoracic region: intercostal artery
- Lumbosacral region:
  - Lumbar
  - Iliolumbar
  - Lateral sacral

Two important reinforcing arteries:
- Lower cervical region
- Lower lumbar region: artery of Adamkiewicz.

Watershed areas: Lower cervical and upper dorsal, C8 T1 segment, lower thoracic region.

Anterior spinal artery supplies anterior 2/3rd of spinal cord sparing posterior column.

Posterior spinal artery supplies → posterior 1/3rd of spinal cord mainly posterior column.

Peripheral part of spinal cord is supplied by the arterial vasocorona plexus formed by the branches of anterior and posterior spinal arteries.

Venous Drainage of Spinal Cord

By the spinal veins emerging through the intervertebral foramen into the epidural venous plexus and external vertebral venous plexus to the thoracic, abdominal and pelvic veins. Direction of blood flow is from the vertebral venous plexus upward into the intracranial venous sinuses. This is the reason for the xanthochromia and high CSF protein in Froin's syndrome due to extramedullary compressive myelopathy.

SYMPTOMATOLOGY IN DISORDERS OF NERVOUS SYSTEM

Symptoms can be grouped as:
- Headache
- Symptoms due to higher function disorder
- Symptoms of cranial nerves disorder (refer cranial nerves)
- Symptoms of motor system disorder
- Symptoms of cerebellum and extrapyramidal system disorder
- Symptoms of sensory system disorder
- Symptoms of bowel and bladder
- Symptoms of autonomic nevrous system
- Symptoms pertaining to other systems.

Headache

Intracranial pain sensitive structures are blood vessel, meninges, sensory neurons.

Mechanism

- ***Intracranial:***
  - Vascular
  - Meningeal
  - Neuralgic pain—trigeminal, ciliary, glossopharyngeal
  - Increased intracranial pressure—ICSOL
- ***Extracranial:***
  - Paranasal sinus origin
  - Ocular cause
  - Dental cause
  - Psychogenic origin

Vascular headache—characterized by throbbing nature, occurs:
- *Migraine:*
  - Classical
  - Common
  - Tension vascular headache (TVH)
- *Complicated migraine:* With focal neurological defect
  - Facioplegic, ophthalmoplegic, hemiplegic
  - Vertebrobasilar migraine, meningitic
- *Symptomatic migraine:* Intracranial aneurysm
  - Angiomatous malformation
  - ICSOL
  - Systemic hypertension
  - Pheochromocytoma

Other causes:
- Drugs—nitrates
- Hypercapnia
- Vasodilatation in fever.

Symptoms due to Higher Function Disorder

- Altered level of consciousness
- Loss of memory
- Speech abnormality
- Seizure—
  - Focal/generalized
  - Convulsive
  - Nonconvulsive
  - Sensory
  - Autonomic
- Behavior abnormality
- Hallucinations, illusion and delusion.

Symptoms of Motor System Disorder

- Paralysis
- Onset
  - Acute, subacute or insidious
  - Progressive, regressing or static
    Precipitating event like febrile illness, vaccination, trauma.
- Onset:
  - Acute (abrupt):
    - Traumatic
    - Vascular
  - Subacute (days):
    - Infection
    - Demyelination
  - Insidious (slow, progressive)
    - Degenerative
    - Nutritional
    - Neoplastic
  - Recurrent episode
    - Demyelination
    - Vascular
    - Diabetes mellitus
- *Wasting*: Loss of muscle mass (refer motor system examination)
- *Fasciculation*
- *Stiffness of muscle* as in parkinsonism
- *Involuntary movement* (refer motor system examination).

Symptoms of Disorder of Cerebellum

- Incoordination of voluntary movement
- Gait ataxia
- Speech abnormality—ataxic dysarthria
- Tendency to fall
- Tremor while reaching for objects
- Weakness due to hypotonia.

Symptoms of Extrapyramidal System Disorder

- Poverty of movement
- Stiffness of muscle—rigidity
- Frequent fall
- Involuntary movements.

Symptoms of Sensory System Disorder

- Hyperesthesia, paresthesia, hypoesthesia and anesthesia—progressive damage of sensory neuron will produce these symptoms
- Altered pain sensation—increased, decreased or loss of pain sensation
- Ataxia of gait with diurnal variation
- Trophic changes, ulcers
- Sensory seizure or aura
- Enquire the pattern of sensory symptom—whether neural pattern, radicular dermatome pattern, one half of body, part of trunk and both lower limbs, all limbs and trunk.

Bowel and Bladder Symptoms

- Constipation and incontinence of motion
- Urgency, precipitancy, hesitancy of micturition
- Retention, incontinence of urine (refer Neurogenic bladder).

Autonomic Nervous System Symptoms

- Abnormality of sweating, impotence, postural syncope
- Diarrhea, constipation, retention of urine.

Symptoms Pertaining to Other Systems

- *CVS:* Embolic stroke, syncopal attack, systemic hypertension, Stokes-Adams seizure
- *Respiratory symptoms*
  - Respiratory failure → altered sensorium
  - Bronchogenic carcinoma → Secondaries brain with seizure and focal neurological deficit
  - Lung abscess, lobar pneumonia → CNS infection
  - Altered rhythm of breathing in brainstem damage.
- *GIT:*
  - Liver disease → encephalopathy
  - Projectile vomiting—increased ICP
  - Constipation and incontinence of motion—spinal cord problem
  - Abdominal pain in tabes dorsalis, porphyria, radicular pain radiating to abdomen, herpetic neuralgia
  - Malabsorption syndrome—nutritional neuropathy-B_{12} neuropathy.
- *Hematological disorders* like bleeding disorders, thrombophilic state, hematological malignancies, megaloblastic anemia, sickle cell anemia.
- *Neuroendocrine*: Hypothalamo-pituitary tumors, hypothyroidism, Cushing's syndrome, thyrotoxicosis, hypocalcemia → tetany and seizure, hypercalcemia → altered sensorium.
- *Renal disease*: Chronic renal failure → encephalopathy, neuropathy, flap, myoclonus, restless leg syndrome, acute glomerulonephritis → hypertensive encephalopathy.

HISTORY TAKING IN NERVOUS SYSTEM DISORDER

- *Presenting symptoms:*
  In chronological order
- *History of present illness:*
  Detailing of each symptom:
  - Onset
  - Course
  - Recurrence
  - Aggravating and relieving factors
- *Past history*
  History of CNS infection—encephalitis or meningitis → sequelae
  History of head/spinal injury
  History of similar illness—seizure, migraine headache, demyelinating disorders, periodic paralysis
  History of recent febrile illness—post infectious demyelination
  History of otitis or PNS infection → CNS infection
  History of birth injury, anoxic injury, antenatal infection like rubella
  History of any major illness of other system.
- *Personal history*
  - Alcoholism
    - Various neurological manifestations
    - Head injury → subdural hematoma
    - Wernicke's encephalopathy
  - Smoking-ischemic vascular episode
  - Drug abuse/drug usage
  - Overseas travel
- *Family history*
  H/o similar illness
  - Heredofamilial diseases
  - Metabolic disorders
  - Degenerative disorders
  - Muscular dystrophy, myotonia
  History of consanguinity
  History of communicable diseases—tuberculosis, viral illness.
  Mental health of other members.
- *Treatment history*
  Antiepileptics, drugs for parkinsonism
  Antipsychotic
  Oral contraceptives, antihypertensives, antidiabetics, corticosteroids.

GENERAL EXAMINATION IN NERVOUS SYSTEM DISORDER

- *Pallor*
  - Megaloblastic anemia—B_{12} neuropathy
  - CRF—neuropathy, asterixis, encephalopathy, restless leg syndrome
  - Hypothyroidism, entrapment neuropathy, myopathy (Hoffman's syndrome).
- *Cyanosis*
  - Cyanotic congenital heart disease—cerebral abscess, paradoxical embolism, thrombotic stroke, secondary polycythemia
  - Respiratory failure—carbon dioxide narcosis
  - Hypoxic encephalopathy, seizures.

- *Clubbing:*
  - Cyanotic congenital heart disease, infective endocarditis → embolic stroke
  - Bronchogenic carcinoma → cerebral metastasis
  - Cirrhosis liver → encephalopathy.
- *Azure lunula:* Bluish discoloration of base of nail—Wilson's disease or hepatolenticular degeneration—cerebellar and EPS.
- *Jaundice:* Hepatic encephalopathy, TTP, septicemia
- *Edema:* Cirrhosis liver, renal disease, hypothyroidism, beriberi
- *Lymphadenopathy:* Tuberculosis, HIV, lymph node metastasis, lymphoma
- *Skin:*
  - Vesicles—herpes zoster, herpes encephalitis-HSV1
  - Rash—exanthematous fever → chickenpox encephalitis, IMN → GBS like syndrome
  - Neurocutaneous syndrome:
    - Adenoma sebaceum—tuberous sclerosis (Fig. 3.6)
    - Angioma—trigeminal area—Sturge-Weber syndrome
    - Multiple neurofibromatosis—von Recklinghausen's disease
  - Pigmentation—megaloblastic anemia—B_{12} neuropathy (Fig. 3.7)
  - Telangiectasia, purpura, cutaneous infarct—collagen vascular disease
  - Trophic changes—syringomyelia, autonomic neuropathy.
- *Hair:*
  - Premature graying—megaloblastic anemia, hypothyroidism, Vogt-Koyanagi-Harada syndrome
  - Baldness—dystrophia myotonica
  - Tuft of hair in lumbosacral region—Satyre's tail—congenital spinal anomaly
- *Facies:* In neurological disease (refer facies)
- *Eyes:*
  - KF ring—Wilson's disease
  - Arcus senilis

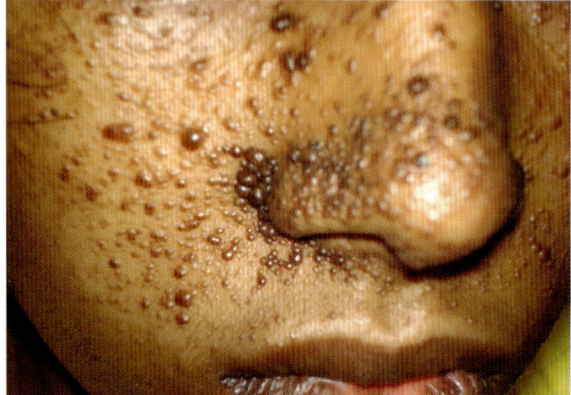

Fig. 3.6: Adenoma sabaceum in tuberous sclerosis.

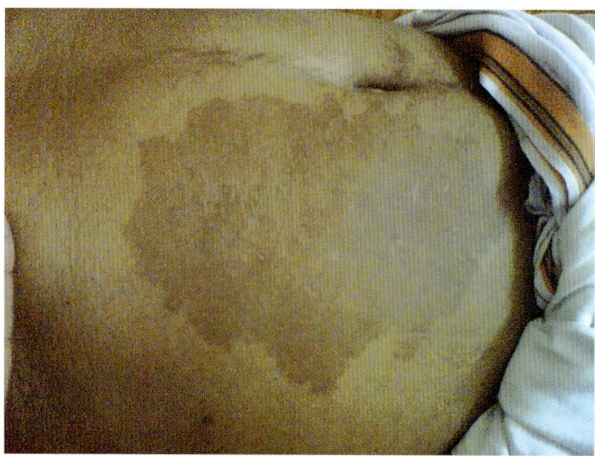

Fig. 3.7: Café-au-lait spot.

  - Proptosis—hyperthyroidism, multiple neurofibromatosis, caroticocavernous fistula
- *Ear:*
  - Otitis media—CNS infection, sigmoid sinus thrombosis, facial palsy
  - Ear bleeding—fracture petrous, glomus jugulare—multiple cranial nerve palsy
- *Mouth:* Gum hypertrophy—dilantin toxicity
- *Thyroid:* Hypo- and hyperthyroidism with neurological disorders
- *Pulse:*
  - Absent—occlusive arterial disease
  - Arrhythmia—embolism
  - Bradycardia—increased intracranial pressure
- *Blood pressure:* Hypertension—stroke (ischemic and hemorrhagic), hypertensive encephalopathy, pseudobulbar palsy, increased ICP
- *Temperature:*
  - Fever
    - CNS infection—meningitis, encephalitis and brain abscess
    - Delerium and toxic encephalopathy
    - Meningism
    - Febrile convulsions
    - Parainfectious demyelination
  - Hypothermia—myxedema coma.

EXAMINATION OF NERVOUS SYSTEM

Examination of nervous system consists of examination of the following:
- Higher functions
- Cranial nerves
- Motor system
- Sensory system
- Cerebellar signs
- Signs of meningeal irritation
- Skull and spine
- Peripheral nerves.

EXAMINATION OF HIGHER FUNCTIONS

- Handedness
- Level of consciousness
- Orientation in time, place and person
- Appearance and behavior
- Emotional state
- Hallucination, illusion, delusion
- Memory
- Intelligence
- Speech.

Handedness

Shake the patient's hand and ask whether he is right or left handed. About 94% of the people are right handed and 50% of the left handed people have dominant hemisphere on left side. Dominant hemisphere controls language and mathematical functions.

Level of Consciousness

Consciousness is maintained by reticular activating system—ill-defined neuronal mass extending throughout the brainstem and projected to both hemispheres.

- *Fully conscious:* Means awareness of oneself and surroundings with appropriate response to external stimuli.
- *Confusional state:* Disorientation in time, place, person and lack of awareness of surroundings.
- *Delirium:* Acute confusional state with excitement, increased motor activity ± hallucinations and tremulousness.
- *Drowsiness:* Resembling normal sleep, can be aroused by stimuli like verbal stimuli, to complete wakefulness and co-operation for examination.
- *Stuporous:* Person can be aroused by stimuli like pain, but slip into sleep once the stimuli ceases.
- *Coma:* Deeply unconscious, no response to any external stimuli, even to painful stimuli.
- *Deep coma:* No response to any external stimuli, no elemental reflex activity like cough.
- *Assess the patient's altered sensorium:*
  - Asking the patient for time, place and person
  - The type of external stimuli required to arouse the patient.
  - Unresponsiveness to any external stimuli
  - Elemental protective reflex activity.

Orientation in Time, Place and Person

- *Time:* Ask the patient about the time, day and month of the year, etc.
- *Place:* Ask the patient where he is at home or hospital.
- *Person:* Ask the patient who he is? What is his work and occupation?

Appearance and Behavior

- Look for attitude, conduct and reaction
- Tidy, neat, clean and good appearance
- Condition of hair and dress
- Free and alert in his reaction
- Anxious, tense, agitated and hostile.
- Communication—silent/over talkative.

Emotional State

- Normal emotional display—be calm, quiescent and composed
- Manic state—cheerful, playful, euphoric and silly
- Depressed state—despondent, despairing and hopeless.

Organic diseases like
- Multiple sclerosis →
  - Euphoria
  - Lack of insights
  - Emotionally labile
- Frontal lobe lesion
  - Lack of inhibition, silly
  - Inappropriate joking
  - Alternation between dullness and excitement
- Pseudobulbar palsy
  - Emotional incontinence
  - Precipitant cry and laughter
- Hypothyroidism
  - Depressive illness.

Delusion, Hallucination and Illusion

- *Delusion:* False beliefs which cannot be corrected with real facts
- *Hallucination:* False perception through a special sense (visual, auditory, olfactory, gustatory) without a stimuli
- *Illusion:* False interpretation through a special sense with a stimulus.

Disorders like:
- *Temporal lobe epilepsy (TLE):* Auditory or olfactory hallucination.
- *Delirium tremens:* Visual, tactile hallucination (insect crawling).
- *Migraine:* Visual aura—scintillating scotoma or teichopsia
- *Occipital lobe lesion:* Visual aura.
- *General paralysis of insane (GPI):* Delusion, hallucination and illusion.

Memory

Components of memory are *perception, registration, retention* and *recall.*
Clinically 3 forms of memory are tested:

1. *Remote memory:* Ask for memorable events in the past, like place of birth, date of birth, beginning of school, date of marriage, history of severe illness in the past.
2. *Recent memory*
   - Date and time of admission to hospital
   - What he had in the recent meals
   - Events in the previous day.
3. *Immediate recall*
   - Digit span test—recites a series of digits at the rate of 1/sec, ask to repeat, normal person is able to repeat 7–8 digits forward and 6 digits in the backward order.
   - Ask him to remember the name of three unrelated objects like red, pen, and apple given at the early part of examination and recall it later.

Disorders like
- Impaired immediate recall and remote memory intact—organic dementia
- Recent memory impaired and remote memory intact
   - Wernicke-Korsakoff syndrome
   - Post-traumatic amnesia
   - Toxic encephalopathy

Intelligence

An appreciation of patient's intellectual capacity may be extremely important in nervous system examination. Consideration regarding his educational and professional capacity, vocabulary and choice of words, general knowledge, calculation judgment, etc. is noted.

Intelligent Quotient

An arbitrary statement of intellectual capacity is obtained by dividing the mental age by the chronological age.
- Intelligence quotient:
   - 90–110—normal
   - 80–90—subnormal—average intelligence
   - <50—Imbecile
   - <25—Idiocy
   - 110–120—super intelligent
   - 120–140—very intelligent
   - >140—near genius

Amnesia

Disorder of memory with impaired ability to remember past events and to learn new information despite normal consciousness and attention.
- Retrograde amnesia—memory disturbance for events that occurred before the time of injury
- Anterograde amnesia—impairment of learning new materials which follows after the time of injury (post-traumatic amnesia).

Dementia

It is a syndrome of acquired global impairment of cognitive function with decline in intellect, memory and personality in the presence of normal consciousness.
- *Causes of dementia*
   - Primary
   - Secondary

Primary causes
- Alzheimer's disease
- Pick's disease.

Secondary causes
- Chronic infection
  Syphilis—GPI
- Slow viral disease SSPE, CJ disease HIV, papovavirus
- Vascular dementia
  Multi-infarct dementia
  Carotid stenosis, cerebral arteriovenous malformation
- Condition with increased intracranial pressure ICSOL hydrocephalus, chronic SDH
- Degenerative disorders
  Huntington's chorea, Steele-Richardson syndrome, Cerebrocerebellar degeneration in hereditary ataxia
- Diffuse cerebral damage
  Anoxic encephalopathy
  Encephalitis
  Head injury
- Endocrine disorders
  Hypothyroidism
  Hypo- and hyperparathyroidism
  Addison's and Cushing's syndrome
- Vitamin deficiency
  B_{12} deficiency
  Thiamine deficiency
  Pellagra
- Others
  Chronic alcoholism
  Dialysis dementia
  Wilson's disease
- Presenile dementia—occurring <65 years—Alzheimer and Pick disease
- Senile dementia—occurring >65 years
- Reversible dementia:
   - Endocrine disorders → Dementia
   - Vitamin deficiency → Dementia
   - SDH, ICSOL → Dementia
   - Chronic alcoholism
   - Dialysis dementia
   - Chronic infection—syphilis and TB.

Speech

- Speech—symbolic expression of ideas
- Language—audible articulate human speech produced by the actions of tongue and vocal cord

- Components of speech—comprehension, formulation, and expression.

Abnormality of Speech

- *Dysphasia:* "This word was coined by Trousseau in 1862" central defect. Decline in already acquired faculty of speech due to lesion in cortical center and its communications producing disturbance of structure and organization of language.
- *Dysarthria:* Peripheral defect. It is a defect in articulation leading to imperfect utterance and formulation of words with normal phonation.

Anatomy of Speech Areas

- *Broca's area:* Area 44—posterior part of inferior frontal gyrus, motor speech area for fluency and expression of speech.
- *Wernicke's area:* Area 39-40, posterior part of superior temporal gyrus, sensory speech area for comprehension of speech.
- *Writing:* Exner's writing center—anterosuperior to Broca's area, near the motor area for hand.
- *Reading area:* Medial aspect of left occipital cortex.

These islands of speech areas are inter connected, sensory and motor areas are connected by the arcuate fibers through the angular gyrus. These islands of speech areas are supplied by the middle cerebral artery—upper and lower division lying in the lateral sulcus.

Examination of Speech Function

- **Look for:**
  - Fluency
  - Comprehension
  - Repetition
  - Naming ability
  - Reading and writing ability.
- **Fluency of speech:**
  - Function of Broca's area
  - Assess the spontaneous speech
  - Selection and sequence of words
  - Misusing words—paraphasia
  - Using words not in vocabulary—neologism
  - Involuntary repetition of words—perseveration
  - Average word output is 100–150/minute
- **Comprehension of speech:**
  Spoken and written language
  - Observe answers to ordinary conversation like age, name and address.
  - Understanding simple comments—
    Ask the patient to show teeth and close eyes.
  - Understanding complex comments
    Lift your right hand with eyes closed
  - Skill in reading and understanding written comments.
- **Repetition:**
  - Presence of repetition means intactness of arcuate fibers
  - Ask the patient to repeat a simple sentence which is clear to the patient
  - Verify that the patient heard and understood the sentence. Later use complex sentences or digits to repeat as in digit span test.
- **Naming ability:**
  - Show familiar objects like pen, key to identify and name it. Sometimes the patient may identify and tell the use of the object without naming, on helping him with three or four names, including the name of the object in question, patient will pick up the name from them.
  - Naming ability is the first one to lose among the components of speech faculty and is the weakest link in speech.

  Impaired naming ability is called amnesic aphasia or nominal aphasia.
- **Reading test:**
  - Check that no visual impairment
  - Visual comprehension of written language
  - Test the skill in reading silently and obey the written comments like "close your eyes".
  - *Reading loud*—testing both visual comprehension of written language and spoken speech.
- **Writing test:**
  - Verify that there is no weakness or in coordination of muscle for the act of writing.
  - Written reply for a verbal command like name, address, occupation and dictation.
  - Copying newspaper, assessing both writing ability, comprehension of written language.

Clinical Types of Aphasia

Considering the functions like:
- Fluency
- Comprehension
- Repetition
- Naming ability

Aphasia without repetition: Global aphasia, motor aphasia, sensory aphasia, conduction aphasia.

Aphasia with repetition: Transcortical (motor and sensory) aphasia, nominal aphasia and echolalia.

Type of aphasia	Fluency	Comprehension	Repetition	Naming ability	Site of lesion
Global aphasia	↓	↓	↓	↓	Both motor and sensory speech area
Broca's aphasia (motor aphasia)	↓	N	↓	↓	Broca's area
Wernicke's aphasia (sensory aphasia)	N	↓	↓	↓	Wernicke's area
Nominal aphasia	N	N	N	↓	No localization value
Transcortical motor aphasia	↓	N	N	↓	Lesion separating Broca's area from its association area
Transcortical sensory aphasia	N	↓	N	↓	Lesion separating Wernicke's area from its association area
Conduction aphasia	N	N	↓	↓	Lesion of arcuate fibers

Isolation of speech →areas from rest of brain
Progressive narrowing of MCA→ Echolalia → Preservation only

Other terms related with aphasia		
Term	Feature	Lesion
Pure alexia (word blindness)	Inability to read	Left occipital medial part or its connection with angular gyrus
Agraphia	Inability to write	Left angular gyrus lesion
Alexia with agraphia	Inability to read and write	Left angular gyrus lesion
Pure word deafness	Inability to comprehend spoken language Comprehension of written language is normal Repetition–normal	Lesion Heschl's Gyrus or its connection
Semantic aphasia	Impaired comprehension of both written and spoken language Repetition-normal	Lesion-parieto temporal border zone. Angular gyrus and its connection with temporal cortex
Jargon aphasia	Severe form of sensory aphasia with neologism and paraphasia	Left superior temporal gyrus
Pure word dumbness	Apraxia of muscles of articulation	Widespread lesion of left hemisphere

Dysarthria

Normal requisites for production of syllables
- Muscles of articulation → labial, lingual and palatal muscles
- Phonation → Larynx
- Resonance → Nasopharynx
- Normal respiration

1. **Spastic dysarthria:** Strained, slurred, slow impressive syllables
   Lesion—bilateral UMN lesion of muscles of articulation, e.g. pseudobulbar palsy and MND
2. **Flaccid dysarthria:**
   Bulbar dysarthria: Strangulated speech with hypernasality, impaired phonation, stridor, low voice
   Lesion—bilateral LMN lesion, e.g. progressive bulbar palsy—MND
   Multiple cranial palsy as in brainstem stroke—myasthenia gravis.
3. **Ataxic dysarthria:**
   Two types:
   1. Scanning speech
      – Undue separation of syllables, monosyllable speech
      – Make the patient to say Thiruvananthapuram, Artillery
   2. Staccato speech
      – Explosive type of speech, undue emphasis on syllables
      – Make the patient to say—Kattachakonam
      – Lesion—cerebellar diseases with incordination of muscles of speech.
4. **Hypokinetic dysarthria**
   Slow, low voice, monotonous, monopitch speech with inappropriate silence.
   Lesion—retardation of motor activity as in Parkinsonism.
5. **Hyperkinetic dysarthria**
   Distorted speech, continuous change in (consonants and vowel) syllable articulation.
   Lesion—dyskinesia of articulation as in chorea, athetosis orofacio lingual dyskinesia.

- Other related terms
  Mutism—Unable to speak or make sound
  Aphonia—Unable to produce sound
  Aphemia—loss of speech.

Apraxia and Agnosia

Apraxia

Failure to carry out well organized voluntary movement, despite normal motor, sensory and coordination function.

Clinically Four Types
1. *Ideomotor apraxia*: Automatic movement is normal, unable to do it on command like blowing nose, pushing back hair, etc.

2. *Ideational apraxia*: Carrying out the whole of complex movement is defective, execution of different parts of movement is normal. Lighting a cigarette—not possible but its different parts of movement is normal like taking a matchbox, holding it correctly and opening it, taking the match, cigarette from cigarette box, etc.
3. *Constructional apraxia*:
   - Failure to make design
   - Draw pictures like star
   - Kohs block – This is a series of blocks with colors occupying the whole half of one side, persons with construction apraxia is unable to make the simplest design.
4. *Dressing apraxia*: Putting the cloth in the wrong way, unable to start the motion for dressing.

Lesion in Apraxia
- Lesion in the interruption of connection of dominant parietal cortex and the ipsilateral motor cortex area and opposite motor cortex corpus callosum—disconnection syndrome.
- Lesion of dominant supramarginal gyrus → bilateral apraxia.
- Lesion of connection of dominant supramarginal gyrus to the left motor cortex → right-sided apraxia.
- Lesion of connection of dominant supramarginal gyrus to the right motor cortex through corpus callosum → left-sided apraxia.
- Lesion of nondominant parietal lobe → constructional apraxia.

Agnosia

Failure to recognize the nature of sensory input when the sense organ by which it is normally recognized remain intact.
- *Visual agnosia of object, color and space:* Lesion of occipital cortex of dominant hemisphere.
- *Tactile agnosia*: Inability to identify the size, shape and naming of object—lesion of left supramarginal gyrus of parietal lobe.
- *Auditory agnosia*: Inability to identify familiar sounds, sound of striking match, tearing cloth, etc. lesion—posterior part of dominant temporal lobe.

EXAMINATION OF CRANIAL NERVES

OLFACTORY NERVE

- *Neuroanatomy:* Central process of sensory cells of olfactory epithelium → 20 unmyelinated fibers → olfactory nerve which passes through the cribriform plate of ethmoid, synapse with olfactory bulb—neurons form the olfactory tract which lies in the olfactory sulcus of frontal lobe → olfactory trigone dividing into medial and lateral striae. Some fibers of the medial join with the opposite side → medial striate terminates in the medial surface of cerebral hemisphere—subcallosal and cingulate gyrus, lateral striae ends in piriform lobe of hippocampus, amygdaloid nucleus and hypothalamus.
- *Function*: To carry smell sensation from nasal mucosa to olfactory bulb.
- *Related terms:*
  - Anosmia—loss of smell sensation
  - Hyposmia—decreased acuity of smell
  - Parosmia—perversion of appreciation of smell
  - Cacosmia—unpleasant odor
  - Hyperosmia—increased acuity of smell
- *Method of testing:* Substance with familiar odor like asafoetida, coffee powder and almond are used. Verify whether local lesions like rhinitis, nasal block are present. Test odor is placed under one nostril while the other is compressed. Asked to have two sniffs, test is repeated in the other nostril. The test is usually done with two or more substances, familiar to the patient.
- *Interpretation:*
  i. Detection, recognition and naming
  ii. Detection, recognition and not naming
  iii. Detection, but no recognition and naming
  All the above three conditions can be considered for the normal olfactory function.
  - Detection—means neural pathway is intact
  - Recognition and naming—cortical function
  - Unilateral cortical lesion—no loss of olfactory function since bilateral representation.
- **Clinical disorders of olfactory nerve**
  - Anosmia or hyposmia
    - Rule out acute or chronic inflammatory lesion of nasal mucosa
    - Head injury—cribriform plate of ethmoid bone closed head injury
    - Basal meningitis
    - Anterior communicating artery aneurysm
    - Intracranial space-occupying lesions—olfactory groove meningioma, sphenoid ridge meningioma, frontal lobe tumor or abscess, parasellar tumor, osteoma of frontal and ethmoid bone. Foster-Kennedy syndrome—subfrontal tumors—ipsilateral optic atrophy, anosmia and contralateral papilledema
    - Familial—anosmia with hypogonadism. Kallmann's syndrome—male. De Morsier's syndrome in either sex
    - Rarely in pernicious anemia, Korsakoff's psychosis, zinc and vitamin A deficiency
    - Olfactory hallucination—uncinate fits aura—complex partial seizure (CPS)
  - Parosmia and cacosmia: Hysteria, head injury or depressive illness.
  - Hyperosmia: Migraine, hyperemesis gravidarum.

OPTIC NERVE

- **Neuroanatomy:** Optic nerve is formed from the axons of ganglion layer of retina, course to optic disc to form the optic nerve, which is 5 cm long, has 4 parts: intraocular 0.7 mm, intraorbital 2.5-3 cm, intracanalicular 1 cm and intracranial 1 cm. Fibers are unmyelinated in the retina and myelinated beyond the lamina cribrosa. Optic nerve leads to optic chiasma where the lower retinal fibers are situated at the inferior portion of chiasma. Nasal fibers cross at the chiasma with uncrossed temporal fibers to form the optic tract. Ratio of crossed and uncrossed fibers is 2:1. Crossed fibers loop into the opposite optic nerves called Wilbrand's knee. Optic tract reaches the lateral geniculate body (LGB). From LGB, the geniculocalcarine fibers—optic radiation → passes through the posterior limb of internal capsule, splay out through the subparietal and subtemporal region—the part encircling the lateral ventricle—Meyer's loop and reaches the striate cortex of occipital lobe area 17. Area 17 is connected with parastriate area 18 and peristriate area 19 for visual perception and spatial orientation.
- **Function:** To carry visual impulses from retina to optic chiasma. Afferent pathway for pupillary light reflex (Fig. 3.8).
- **Light reflex pathway:** Afferent impulses through optic nerve → optic chiasma → optic tract → pretectal nucleus of midbrain at superior colliculus before reaching LGB → to Edinger-Westphal nucleus of both sides → third nerve and ciliary ganglion → short ciliary nerves → constrictor pupillae and ciliary body.
- **Accommodation reflex pathway:** Afferent visual pathway to occipital lobe → frontal lobe → frontal eye fields → corticomesencephalic fibers through internal capsule → 3rd cranial nerve nucleus—medial rectus nucleus and Edinger-Westphal nucleus.
- **Clinical examination of optic nerve**
  Consists of:
  - Acuity of vision
  - Field of vision
  - Color vision
  - Optic fundi

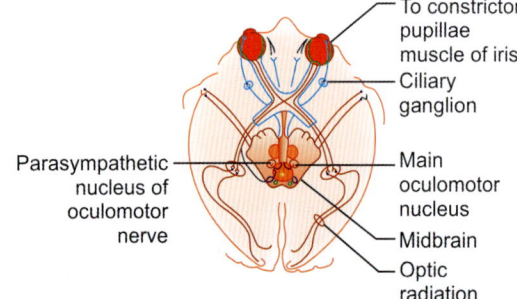

Fig. 3.8: The optic pathways and visual reflexes.

Acuity of Vision

Distant Vision

Assessed by using Snellen's chart kept at a distance of 6 m or using a mirror and 3 m chart with reversible letters, each eye is tested separately. Normal visual acuity is when the line marked 6 can be read correctly with each eye— 6/6 Snellen. If the patient cannot read the largest letter of the chart, acuity of vision is <6/60, then ask for finger counting, perception of hand movement. Failing these, light perception is tested. In total blindness, perception of light is also absent.

Near Vision

Tested by asking the patient to read the letters of different sizes printed on a reading card, e.g. Jaeger's test chart. The reading card is held at 30 cm away from the patient's eye. The near vision is recorded as the smallest type which the patient can comfortably read.

At bedside, rough assessment is done by making the patient to read bed number at a distance of approximately 6 m, if it fails, go for other measures as above. Near vision can be tested by asking the patient to read ordinary newspaper or similar printed material.

Loss of visual acuity: Diseases of cornea, lens, retina, optic nerve or the visual pathway.

- **Bilateral blindness of rapid onset:**
  - Ischemia of occipital lobe ischemic stroke of posterior circulation, vasospasm—migraine, hypertensive encephalopathy, subarachnoid hemorrhage
  - Occipital lobe trauma
  - Hemorrhagic stroke of occipital lobe
  - Bilateral optic nerve damage in methyl alcohol poisoning, pituitary apoplexy
  - Hysteria
- **Unilateral blindness of rapid onset:**
  - Central retinal artery occlusion
  - Central retinal vein occlusion
  - Optic neuritis—papillitis/retrobulbar neuritis
  - Anterior ischemic optic neuritis (AION)—ciliary vessel involvement
  - Retinal detachment
  - Traumatic lesion of eye
- **Bilateral blindness of gradual onset:**
  - Cataract, glaucoma
  - Diabetic retinopathy, macular degeneration
  - Retinitis pigmentosa
  - Bilateral optic nerve or chiasmal compression
  - Bilateral optic atrophy
  - Toxic and nutritional amblyopia

Field of Vision

Confrontation method: Patient and examiner face each other with a distance of one meter between them (one arm distance). For testing the left eye of the patient, examiner covers his left eye and patient covers his right eye, either with a shield or palm. Examiner moves the finger or red tip pin in a plane, midway between the patient and examiner, inwards in each of the four quadrants from just outside the limit of his own field. Patient must say as he sees the movement of finger or the object. It can be compared with the examiner's normal field of vision. To avoid missing quadrantanopia, finger can be moved in all the four quadrants in oblique direction also.

Central field of vision: A red tip pin is used to map out central scotoma or blind spot. Examine as described above, ask for the disappearance of pin around the center of the field of each eye, only gross enlargement may be detectable.

When the field of examination is completed, both eyes are uncovered, examiner hold both hands in the outer part of field, moving one hand or other hand and both together, ask the patient to point to the hand moved. This will detect the visual inattention in parietal lobe lesion.

Perimetry: Visual fields can be mapped out accurately by perimetry. The output of the average field of vision is 100° laterally, 60° superiorly and medially and 75° inferiorly.

Bjerrum's screen: Presenting objects against wall mounted black screen (Bjerrum's screen) at a distance of 1 or 2 meter from the patient. By this method, blind spot and scotoma can be detected precisely.

Localization of Lesion in the Visual Pathway (Fig. 3.9)

a. Enlarged blind spot—papilledema.
b. Central and centrocecal scotoma
   - Intrinsic lesion of optic nerve and chiasma
   - Demyelination as in multiple sclerosis
   - Methyl alcohol poisoning
   - Nutritional amblyopia
   - Glioma of optic nerve.
c. Total unilateral loss of vision
   - Optic nerve lesion
   - Papillitis
   - Retrobulbar neuritis
   - Optic nerve compression
   - Optic atrophy
d. Total unilateral loss of vision with temporal field of vision on opposite side
   - Optic nerve lesion close to chiasma involving Wilbrand's knee.
e. Monocular, temporal field hemianopia
   - Ischemic lesion of optic nerve involving nasal fibers alone.
f. Altitudinal hemianopia
   - Unilateral
     - Partial central retinal artery occlusion
     - Retinal detachment
     - Optic neuritis—early anterior ischemic optic neuritis

- Bilateral
  - Ischemic lesion of retina and optic nerve
  - Occipital lobe lesion
- *Chiasmal lesion*
  - **Anterior chiasmal lesion**—junctional syndrome
    - Unilateral optic nerve defect and temporal field loss on opposite side.
  - **Middle chiasmal lesion**
    - Suprachiasmatic
      - Craniopharyngioma   } Bilateral
      - 3rd ventricular dilatation } Temporal
    - Infrachiasmatic   } Hemianopia
      - Pituitary tumor
      - Meningioma of sella
    - Perichiasmatic
      - Bilateral ICA aneurysm   } Binasal
      - Meningitis   } Hemianopia
      - Opto chiasmatic
      - Arachnoiditis
  - **Posterior chiasmatic lesion**
    - Bilateral temporal scotoma
    - Pituitary tumor
    - Craniopharyngioma.
- *Homonymous hemianopia*

  Lesion at
  - Optic tract
  - Lateral geniculate body
  - Optic radiation
  - Occipital lobe
  - *Optic tract:* Homonymous hemianopia incongruous, pupillary reflex absent, no macular sparing
  - *Lateral geniculate body:* Homonymous hemianopia incongruous, sparing, pupillary reflex and macular sparing of horizontal sector between the upper and lower quadrants. LGB—supplied by anterior choroidal artery. Middle of LGB—supplied by lateral choroidal artery.
  - *Optic radiation:* Homonymous hemianopia congruous—sparing of pupillary reflex and no macular sparing.
  - *Occipital lobe*: Homonymous hemianopia congruous—sparing of pupillary reflex and macula.
- *Upper quadrant homonymous defect*
  - Subtemporal lobe lesion—damage of inferior fibers of optic radiation.
  - Inferior lip of calcarine fissure—lingual gyrus
    Causes are:
    - HSV encephalitis
    - Tumor
    - Vascular lesion.
- *Lower quadrant homonymous defect*
  - Subparietal lobe lesion—superior fibers of optic radiation as in vascular lesion
  - Superior lip of calcarine fissure—cuneus gyrus

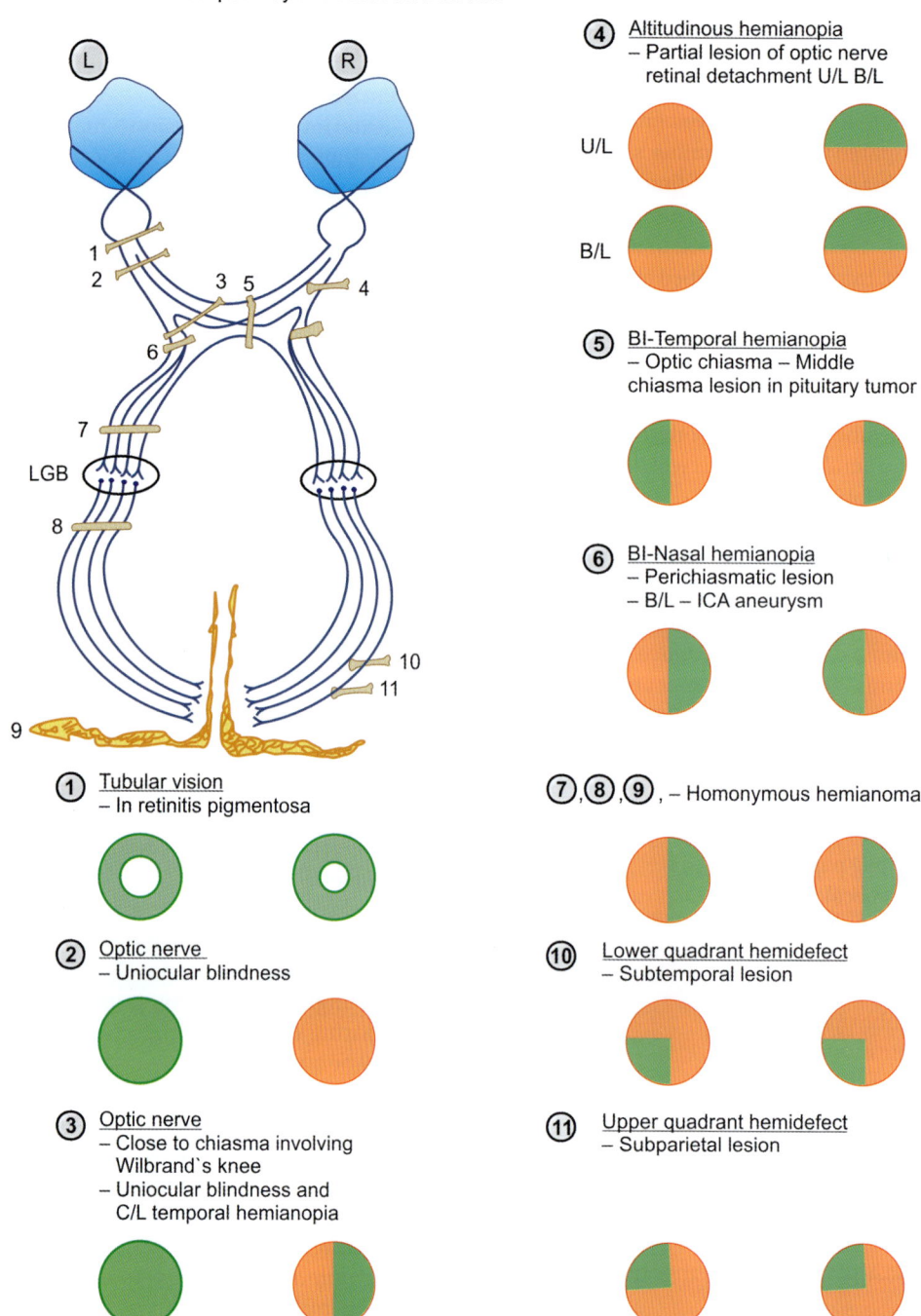

Fig. 3.9: Visual pathway and associated defects. (*Abbreviations*: B/L, bilateral; U/L, unilateral; ICA, internal carotid artery).

In bilateral occipital lobe lesion, in addition to cortical blindness, denial of visual defect is present—known as Anton's syndrome.

Charcot-Wilbrand syndrome—loss of ability to recall visual images and to draw or construct from memory—striate cortex lesion in occipital lobe.

- **Tubular vision:** Concentric narrowing of field of vision *Causes:* Glaucoma, retinitis pigmentosa, quinine amblyopia, CRA occlusion with presence of cilioretinal artery which supplies the macula.
- **Cortical blindness:** Double hemianopia—bilateral hemianopia

- Anoxic encephalopathy
- Vasospasm of posterior cerebral artery
  - Hypertensive encephalopathy
  - Migraine
  - Subarachnoid hemorrhage
- Tentorial herniation.

Color Vision

Primary colors are red, blue and green.

Each eye is tested separately by showing objects of different colors. More sensitive test is Ishihara's pseudoisochromatic plates consisting of multicolored dots. Patient with defective color vision will make mistake in correct identification of colors.

Color Vision Anomaly

- Red green anomaly—X-linked recessive
- Total color blindness—rare
- Retinal disease—loss of blue color vision first, green last.
- Optic nerve lesion—loss of red and green color first.

Optic Fundus Examination

By examination of optic fundus, direct visualization of optic disc and retina is possible. Optic fundus examination is a part of routine examination irrespective of patient complaint.

Method of Examination

Requirement
Good ophthalmoscope
- Dilated pupil
- Still face

Darken the illumination of the room, instruct the patient to fix the gaze at a distant object. Examiner's right eye is used for the visualization of patient's right eye. Hold the ophthalmoscope in the right hand, vice versa for the left eye. To get the proper view of the media, start with +10 lens for cornea, lens and vitreous, and then gradually reduce the strength of the lens, for the retina start with 0 lens.

Features to be Noted

- Optic disc
- Retinal vessels, macula
- Periphery of retina.

Optic Disc

- Can be visualized by following the vessels to the side of convergence.
- Color—normally pink, temporal pallor present.
- Clarity of edge—mild nasal blurring is normal.

- Cup depression in disc where arteries and veins pass through it.
- Cribrosa—lamina cribrosa—Sieve like structure at the center of the cup where pearly white nerve fibers are arranged in a sieve like fashion.
- Circulation—note the vein, artery, its size, color, AV crossing
  - Retinal vessels radiating from the disc
  - Arteries are narrower than veins and bright red.
  - Veins are large, dark red, pulsatile
  - Normal A:V ratio is 2:3
  - Artery crosses the vein.

Macula

Posterior part of retina containing xanthophilic pigment at the temporal side of the disc. Center of macula lutea fovea (5 mm size) which is devoid of vessels.
- Increased cup size in glaucoma
- Pale, white clear edge of disc—primary optic atrophy
- Pale, white blurred margin—secondary optic atrophy as in posterior papilledema optic atrophy
- Red color—hyperemic disc—papilledema
- Blurring of margins in papilledema and papilitis.

Rest of retina: For other retinal diseases like chorioretinitis, retinitis pigmentosa, retinal tear.
- *Retinal hemorrhage*—4 types
  1. Flame shaped streaky hemorrhage related to vessel
  2. Large hemorrhage—obliterating vessels
  3. Deep hemorrhage—dot like rounded
  4. Subhyaloid hemorrhage—in subarachnoid hemorrhage.
- *Microaneurysm*—in diabetes mellitus
- *Exudates*
  - Soft fluffy cotton wool patch in papilledema, systemic hypertension and CRF
  - Hard crystalline streaks—arteriosclerosis, CRF, diabetes mellitus.
    - *Tubercle:* Rounded pale yellowish at the center, pink margin half the size of disc.
    - *Phakoma:* Collection of neuroglial cells, large bluish white plaque half to 2/3rd size of disc.
    - *Pigmentation*: Chorioretinitis, toxoplasmosis, syphilis spidery black pigment—retinitis pigmentosa.
    - *Opaque nerve fibers*: Myelinated nerve fibers in retina—white foam like spread from disc—differential diagnosis of exudates.
- *Papilledema*
  - *Appearance:* Hyperemic disc, margin blurred, veins dilated with no pulsation. Exudates, hemorrhages and macular star present. Loss of visual acuity is less, enlargement of blind spot, usually bilateral.
  - *Causes*
    - Increase in ICP as in ICSOL, benign intracranial hypertension, hydrocephalus

- Malignant hypertension, hypercapnia, hypoparathyroidism.
    - GBS—due to raised cerebrospinal fluid (CSF) protein.
- *Increased ICP without papilledema*—optochiasmatic arachnoiditis previous optic atrophy severe myopia.
- **Optic neuritis:**
  Papillitis—inflammation of nerve head
  Retrobulbar neuritis—inflammation of retrobulbar portion of optic nerve.
- Papillitis
  Appearance
  - Red disc—margins blurred veins less dilated, pulsations normal.
  - Acuity of vision is markedly decreased.
  - Usually unilateral, acute and painful.
  Causes
  - Multiple sclerosis, AION
  - Toxins and drugs—methyl alcohol, tobacco, ethambutol
  - Infection—infectious mononucleosis, mumps
  - Idiopathic.

Optic atrophy
- *Primary:* Pale white, clear edge of disc, number of capillaries crossing the disc margin is less than 7. Normal is 10—Kestenbaum sign.
- *Secondary:* Pale disc with indistinct margin—optic atrophy following papilledema.
- *Consecutive:* Primary retinal disease leading to optic atrophy as in retinitis pigmentosa and chorioretinitis.

Causes
- Papilledema, optic neuritis, AION, CRA occlusion
- Compression of optic nerve as in Foster-Kennedy syndrome
- Methyl alcohol, ethambutol
- Retinal disease—retinitis pigmentosa, chorioretinitis
- Familial Leber's optic atrophy.

Retinitis pigmentosa: Spidery black pigmentation
Causes
- Congenital
- Laurence-Moon-Biedl syndrome
- Refsum's syndrome
- Abetalipoproteinemia (Bassen-Kornzweig syndrome)
- Olivopontocerebellar atrophy (OPCA).

OCULAR MOTOR NERVES

Third—oculomotor nerve
Fourth—trochlear
Sixth—abducent nerve.

Oculomotor Nerve: Neuroanatomy

Nuclear complex situated 5 mm ventral to aqueduct-one unpaired, 4 paired column of nuclei.

Unpaired nuclear column—rostral part—Edinger-Westphal nuclei which supply constrictor pupillae and ciliary muscle, caudally subnucleus of levator palpebrae superioris of both sides.

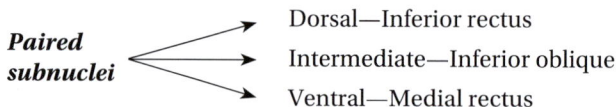

Paired subnuclei
- Dorsal—Inferior rectus
- Intermediate—Inferior oblique
- Ventral—Medial rectus

Subnucleus of superior rectus crosses to opposite side, traverse through the subnuclei of the opposite side and supply the opposite superior rectus.

Complete lesion of the nucleus can produce: Ipsilateral inferior rectus (IR), inferior oblique (IO), medial rectus (MR) palsy (Fig. 3.10).
- Bilateral SR palsy
- Bilateral ptosis
- Mydriasis.

Incomplete lesion can spare levator palpebrae superioris (LPS) muscles and pupil.

Course

Following distinct sites to be remembered for localization of infranuclear lesion.
a. *Brainstem:* fascicular portion traverse through the red nucleus, emerges ventrally to the medial part of cerebral peduncle.
b. *Subarachnoid space/posterior cranial fossa:* Passes between superior cerebellar and posterior cerebral artery—medial to uncus of temporal lobe, closely related to posterior communicating artery.
c. *Cavernous portion:* Pierces the dura at lateral aspect of posterior clinoid process, enters the lateral wall of cavernous sinus in relation to 4th, 5th and 6th cranial nerves.

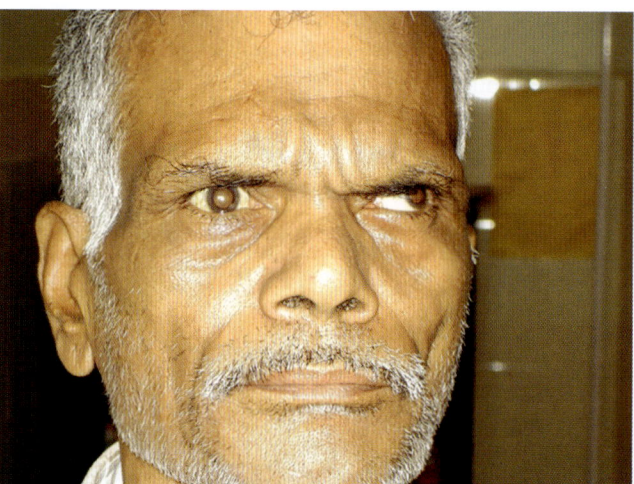

Fig. 3.10: Right medial rectus palsy in right 3rd nerve palsy.

d. *Superior orbital fissure:* 3rd nerve divides into superior and inferior division, lies inside the tendinous ring.
e. *Intraorbital portion:* Superior division—supplies superior rectus and levator palpebrae superioris (LPS).
Inferior division—supplies
   1. Parasympathetic, ciliary ganglion, short ciliary nerves, constrictor pupillae and ciliary muscle
   2. Medial rectus (MR), inferior rectus (IR), inferior oblique (IO)

Parasympathetic fibers lie at the peripheral part of trunk, dorsomedial aspect, dual blood supply to peripheral part of nerve trunk via vasa nervosum and sheath vessel.

Developmentally subnucleus for levator palpebrae superioris and superior rectus are from the same nuclear mass.

Congenital ptosis—superior rectus also involved.

Pressure lesion—pupil is early involved, if it can resist (pressure resistant pupillomotor fibers) pressure, pupil may escape.

Ischemic lesion—pupil is spared, since the center of the nerve is affected early.

Trochlear Nerve: Neuroanatomy

- Nucleus at the level of inferior colliculus—midbrain
- Nerve fascicle—course posteromedially to decussate in the dorsal midbrain, emerge at dorsal part of brainstem below inferior colliculi
- Cisternal segment of nerve traverse around the brainstem, passes anteriorly encircling the surface of tentorium cerebelli edge → pierce the dura → cavernous sinus–lateral wall→ superior orbital fissure → orbit to supply the superior oblique.
- Nuclear lesion—contralateral superior oblique palsy, infranuclear after decussation → ipsilateral superior oblique palsy.

Abducent Nerve: Neuroanatomy

Nuclei situated at the dorsal part of the tegmentum of the pons posterior to facial nucleus, facial fibers surround the nuclei—facial colliculi, 6th nerve escape at pontomedullary junction, ascends between base of pons and clivus in the prepontine cisterns, enters the Dorello's canal beneath the petroclinoid ligament—Gruba's ligament, then pierces the duramater → cavernous sinus, lie close to internal carotid artery → superior orbital fissure → orbit supplies the lateral rectus. It has the longest intracranial course.

Cortical Centers for Gaze Movement

a. *Lateral gaze center:* Frontal eye field. Area 8—fibers descend through the internal capsule, crosses to opposite side upper brainstem → parabducent nucleus of pons → abducent nerve→lateral rectus-opposite side. From parabducent nerve (pontine lateral gaze center) → MLF → medial rectus nerve of same side. Stimulation of frontal eye field (FEF) → conjugate gaze to opposite side. Paralytic or destructive lesion of frontal eye field (FEF) → lateral gaze palsy to opposite side. Both eyes turn to same side.

Frontal eye field also controls saccadic movement to opposite side.

Both eye fields control vertical saccadic movement.

Also has regulatory effects on LPS. Stimulation → contraction of LPS → opening of eye and dilatation of pupil

b. *Occipital gaze center*
   - Area 18-19 → corticofugal fibers → optic radiation → posterior limb of internal capsule → cerebral peduncle → 3rd nuclei and medial longitudinal fasciculus (MLF).
   - Control the pursuit movement - occipital gaze center of one side
   - Control pursuit movement to the opposite side and same side.
   - Both occipital gaze centers together control vertical pursuit movement.
c. *Interstitial nucleus of Cajal:* Level of superior colliculus—control the vertical gaze.
d. *Central nucleus of Perlia:* In the mid brain—center for convergence.
e. *Pontine lateral gaze center:* Close to 6th cranial nerve nuclei, send impulses to ipsilateral lateral rectus nuclei and contralateral medial rectus nuclei through MLF.
Stimulation → lateral gaze to same side
Destruction → lateral gaze to opposite side.

Ocular Sympathetic

Sympathetic fibers—1st order of neurons descend from hypothalamus → brainstem → spinal cord intermediolateral horn at C8 T1 ± T2 ciliospinal center, 2nd order neurons preganglionic fibers → superior sympathetic ganglion—3rd order of neurons—posterior ganglionic fibers around carotid artery → ophthalmic division of 5th nerve → nasociliary → long ciliary → oculopupillary fibers → dialator pupillae and smooth muscles of eyelids (Muller's muscle).

Horner's Syndrome

Lesion can be-
   a. Descending sympathetic fibers from brainstem to spinal cord—1st order
   b. Cervical sympathetic-preganglionic fibers—2nd order
   c. Posterior ganglionic fibers around the carotid artery—3rd order.

Difference of Preganglionic and Postganglionic

Postganglionic
- Incomplete Horner's—secretomotor fibers to sweat gland go through the external carotid artery.
- Hypersensitivity to epinephrine → dilation of pupil.

Preganglionic
- Complete Horner's syndrome, no hypersensitivity to epinephrine.

OCULAR MUSCLES

Physiology of Ocular Movement

There are 3 planes of movement of eyeball **(Table 3.1):**
1. Vertical plane
   - Adduction—medial rectus
   - Abduction—lateral rectus
2. Horizontal plane
   - Elevation—superior rectus and inferior oblique
   - Depression—inferior rectus and superior oblique
3. Diagonal plane
   - Intorsion—superior rectus and superior oblique
   - Extorsion—inferior rectus and inferior oblique.

Agonist	Synergist	Antagonist
MR	SR/IR	LR, SO/IO
LR	SO/IO	MR, SR/IR
SR	IO/MR	IR/SO
IR	SO/MR	SR/IO
SO	LR/IR	IO/SR
IO	SR/LR	SO/IR

Abbreviations: MR: medial rectus; LR: lateral rectus; SR: superior rectus; IR: inferior rectus; SO: superior oblique; IO: inferior oblique

Normal range of eye movement:
- Abduction—60°
- Adduction—50°
- Depression—50°
- Elevation—30°

Types of ocular movement
- Saccadic movement—Jerky voluntary movement from an object to another
- Pursuit movement—Smooth follow movement
- Fixation movement—Move the head while the gaze is fixed
- Reflex movement—Oculocephalic, oculovestibular movement.

Table 3.1: Action of extraocular muscles.

Muscle	Primary	Secondary	Tertiary
Medial rectus	Adductor	–	–
Lateral rectus	Abductor	–	–
Inferior rectus	Depression (in abduction)	Extorsion (in adduction)	Adduction
Superior rectus	Elevation (in abduction)	Intorsion (in adduction)	Adduction
Superior oblique	Intorsion (in abduction)	Depression (in adduction)	Abduction
Inferior oblique	Extorsion (in abduction)	Elevation (in adduction)	Abduction

Symptoms of ocular motor system: Diplopia, squint, ptosis, defective vision, dizziness (ocular vertigo).

Clinical Examination
- Testing ocular movement of each muscle (Fig. 3.11)
- Testing LPS and ptosis
- Pupil and light reflex
- Nystagmus and other involuntary movement of eye.

Testing Ocular Movement

Aim: To detect failure of eye movement and assess diplopia.

Ask the patient to look at the examiner's finger or red topped hat pin which is kept at 60 cm away from the patient's face, assess the movement of both eyes, make the patient look voluntarily to right, right up, right down, left, left up, and left down and also upward, and downward movement from primary position. In each direction, look for any lag of movement and diplopia (Figs. 3.12 to 3.14).

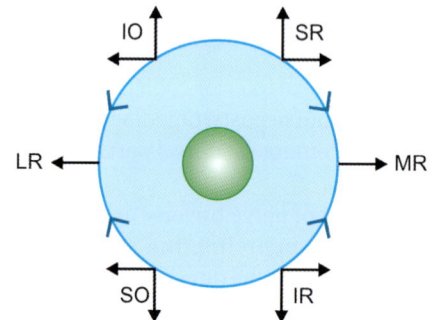

Fig. 3.11: Physiological action of individual muscles.

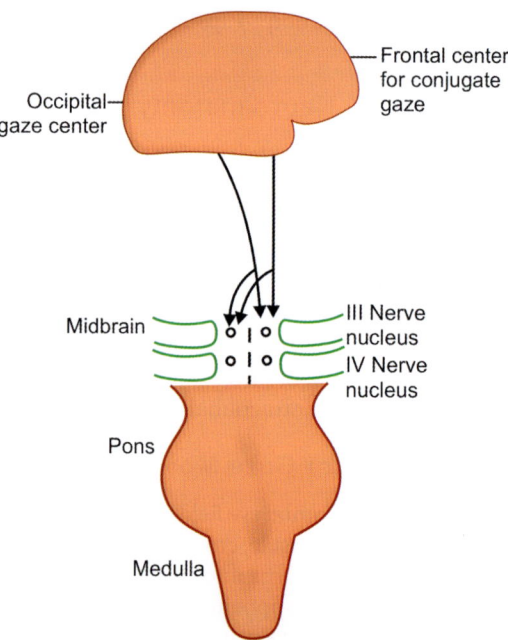

Fig. 3.12: Vertical eye movements.

Examination of Nervous System

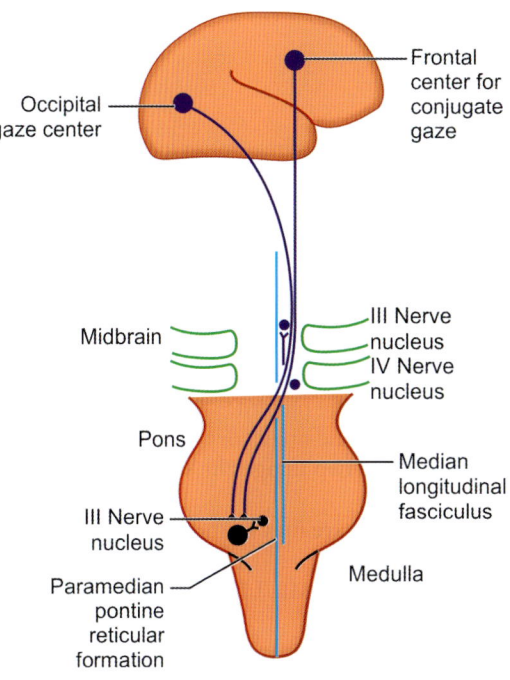

Fig. 3.13: Horizontal eye movements.

Testing Individual Muscles

By an 'H' pattern of movement all muscles can be tested (Fig. 3.15).

Abnormal eye movement are due to:

- Lesion of ocular motor nerves (3, 4, 6 cranial nerves)
- Gaze palsies
- Involuntary movement of eyeball.

Clinical Signs of 3rd Nerve Lesion

- Ptosis, complete or incomplete.
- Divergent squint—eye—abduction and depression
- Mydriasis—unreactive to light reflex—direct and consensual unreactive to accommodation

Clinical Signs of 4th Nerve Lesion

- Weakness of superior oblique, defective downward movement in adducted position, difficulty in descending stairs, head tilted to the shoulder of involved side, eye position—elevation and adduction
- Nuclear lesion → contralateral superior oblique weakness
- Nerve lesion → ipsilateral superior oblique weakness.

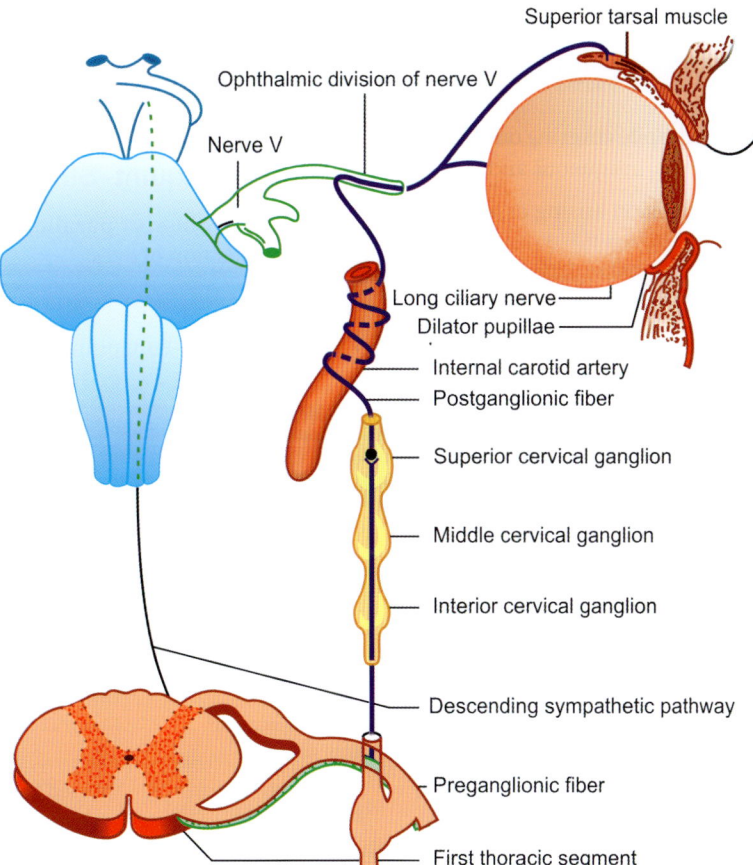

Fig. 3.14: The cervical portion of the sympathetic division of the autonomic nervous system.

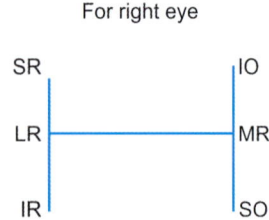

Fig. 3.15: Testis of an 'H' pattern muscle movement

Lateral rectus—abductor	Medial rectus —Adductor
Superior rectus—elevator in Abduction	Inferior rectus —Depression in abduction
Inferior oblique— elevation in adduction	Superior oblique —Depression in adduction

Clinical Signs of 6th Nerve Lesion

- Defective abduction in horizontal plane
- Eye is directed inward with horizontal squint
- Face is turned to affected side.

Clinical signs of individual muscle weakness are described in Table 3.2.

Diplopia Analysis

It can occur even before evidence of muscular weakness, light rays fail to fall on exactly corresponding parts of two retinae. False image formed is indistinct in eye with defective muscle movement.

Mono-ocular diplopia: Persisting despite covering one eye as in cataract, retinal disease, foreign body in aqueous and vitreous.

Binocular diplopia: It is a double vision arising as a result of strabismus.

Rules of Diplopia

- Displacement of false image:
  - Horizontal
    - Higher
    - Lower
  - Vertical
- Separation of images is maximum in the direction of action of weak muscle.
- The false image is displaced farthest in the direction in which the weak muscle should move the eye.

Method of Test for Diplopia

Cover one of the patient's eye with a transparent red shield. Move a point of light in the direction of action of each muscle. In each position ask the patient.

- Whether he sees one object or two
- If double, do the two images lie side by side or one above the other
- In which position are they farthest
- Which is red image.

Image side by side—MR/LR, one above the other—SR/IR, SO/IO (Fig. 3.16).

Assess the muscle pair involved and in which the image is double, e.g. both eyes moving to right and up (testing right SR and left IO). Image is double. Red glass over the right eye. Red image is farthest means superior rectus, white image is farthest means IO.

Superior rectus, white image is farthest means IO.

Various charts are used for representing diplopia diagrammatically, of which the Hess chart is used usually.

Analysis of Squint–Strabismus

Squint means loss of parallelism of eyeball resulting in abnormal position of eyes.

Squint
- Paralytic
- Nonparalytic—concomitant

Table 3.2: Clinical signs of individual muscle weakness.				
Muscle	Action	Movement Affected	Squint (paralytic position)	Diplopia (position of false image)
Lateral rectus	Abduction	Abduction	Convergent squint	Uncrossed, maximum looking laterally
Medial rectus	Adduction	Adduction	Divergent squint	Crossed, maximum looking medially
Superior oblique	Intorsion and depression in adduction	Downward movement in adduction	Elevation, convergence and extorsion	Uncrossed, vertical and lower level. Maximum on looking down and medially
Inferior oblique	Extorsion and elevation in adduction	Upward movement in adduction	Depression, convergence and intorsion	Uncrossed, vertical at a higher level. Maximum on looking up and medially
Superior rectus	Elevation in abduction, intorsion	Upward movement in abduction	Depression, divergence and extorsion	Crossed, vertical, higher level. Maximum on looking up and laterally
Inferior rectus	Depression in adduction and extorsion	Downward movement in abduction	Elevation divergence and intorsion	Crossed, vertical, lower level. Maximum on looking laterally and down

Examination of Nervous System

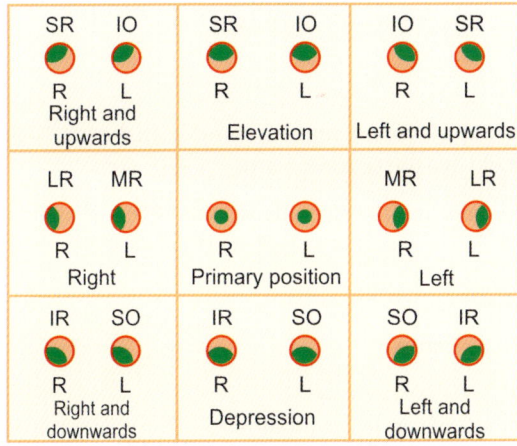

Fig. 3.16: Nine diagnostic positions of gaze.

Deviation of paralytic eye is primary, deviation of sound eye is secondary.

Cover test: To assess the primary and secondary deviation, ask the patient to fix his gaze on an object, cover the fixing eye, watch the deviation of uncovered eye (primary deviation). Then note the deviation of the covered eye. Normal eye—secondary deviation. Note the degree of primary and secondary deviation.

In paralytic squint—secondary deviation > primary deviation.

Nonparalytic squint—primary deviation = secondary deviation.

Nonparalytic squint is characterized by:
- Starts early in childhood
- Ocular movement is full in all directions
- No diplopia
- Primary and secondary deviation are same
- Deviating eye has defective vision.

Testing Levator Palpebrae Superioris

Function: Voluntary elevation of upper eyelid. Frontal belly of occipitofrontalis also help in the action.

Press over the eyebrows to nullify the action of frontal belly of occipitofrontalis and ask the patient to elevate the upper eyelid. Normally upper eyelid will cover 0.5–1 mm of the cornea. Lower eyelid comes to lower border of cornea in neutral position.

Levator function—maximum elevation of eyelid from down gaze to upward gaze is 10–12 mm, 8 mm or more is good levator function, <5 mm is poor.

PTOSIS

a. Neurogenic:
   - Supranuclear—frontal lobe lesion—opposite side ptosis.
   - 3rd nerve—mydriasis and squint, ptosis due to LPS weakness (Figs. 3.17A and B).
   - Sympathetic—Horner's syndrome—ptosis, miosis, LPS—N elevation of lower eyelid also present.
b. Neuromuscular: Myasthenic—fatigability present, which can be demonstrated by asking the patient to look up for 30–45 sec, progressive ptosis will occur. Pupil normal, usually bilateral, diplopia present (unequal muscle weakness of paired group), neostigmine test positive.
c. Myogenic—ocular myopathy—usually bilateral, pupil normal, no fatigability, no diplopia (equal weakness of paired group of muscles): Disease of LPS—no diplopia, tendon damage, sarcoidosis of LPS, disinsertion of LPS—occur in old age—involutional ptosis.
d. Disease of eyelid: Pseudoptosis—mechanical impairment of upward eyelid movement, orbital inflammation, edema of eyelid, orbital tumor.

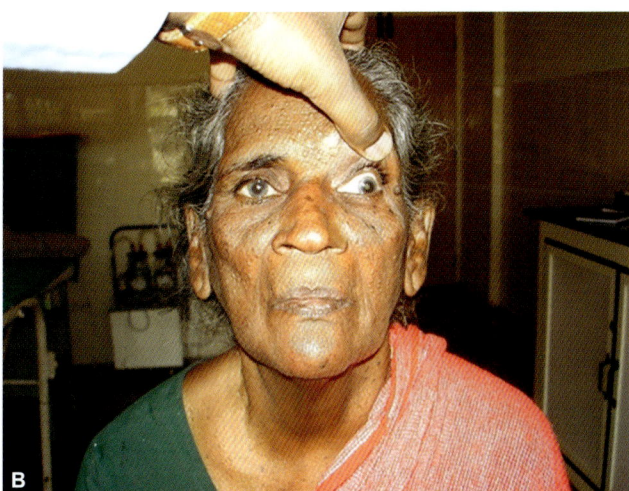

Figs. 3.17A and B: Complete ptosis of left eye with abducted eyeball—left 3rd nerve palsy.

Bilateral Ptosis (Fig. 3.18)

Causes
- Congenital
- Bilateral 3rd nerve lesion—as in brainstem stroke, GBS and basal meningitis
- Bilateral Horner's syndrome—as in tabes dorsalis due to degeneration of descending sympathetic
- Myasthemia gravis
- Ocular myopathy, dystrophia myotonica
- Marcus Gunn phenomenon.

Narrow palpebral fissure
- Ptosis, pseudoptosis
- Blepharospasm
- Enophthalmos
- Apraxia of eyelid opening as in Huntington's chorea, Steele-Richardson disease (progressive supranuclear palsy).

Retraction of upper eyelid
- Thyrotoxicosis, pheochromocytoma
- Marcus Gunn phenomenon
- Aberrant regeneration following 3rd nerve palsy
- Irritation of ocular sympathetic—Claude Bernard syndrome
- Opposite to the side of ptosis due to myasthenia
- Scar of upper eyelid
- Large eye globe
- Collier's sign in upper midbrain lesion
- Short LPS tendon.

Retraction of lower eyelid
- Early stage of facial palsy
- Myasthenia, ocular myopathy
- Proptosis
- Ectropion
- Claude Bernard syndrome.

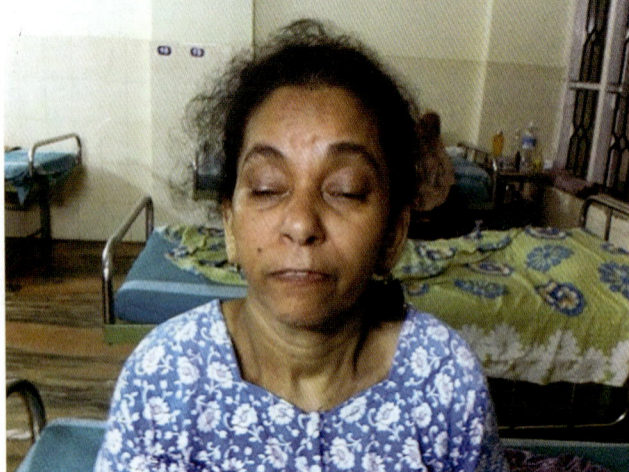

Fig. 3.18: Bilateral ptosis.

PUPIL AND LIGHT REFLEX

Pupil

Normal pupil is round, regular, centered in the iris, 3–4 mm in size. In old age the size is < 3 mm.

Examination: Look for size, shape, whether equal on both sides and position of pupil.

Miosis

Pupil size < 2 mm.

Causes:
- Paralysis of cervical sympathetic—Horner's syndrome
- Irritation of parasympathetic
- Drugs—morphine, organophosphate poisoning, levodopa
- Deep coma, increased ICP, pontine hemorrhage
- Rowland Payne syndrome—consists of Horner's syndrome, phrenic nerve and recurrent laryngeal nerve involvement. It is caused by metastatic tumor at neck from malignancy like carcinoma breast, also in bronchogenic carcinoma.

Mydriasis

Pupil size > 5 mm

Causes:
- 3rd nerve paralysis
- Irritation of sympathetic nerve—Claude Bernard syndrome
- Anxiety, fear
- Cerebral anoxia, death
- Optic atrophy, optic tract lesion
- Drugs—atropine, mysoline
- Myopia.

Hippus

Alternating dilatation and constriction of pupil.

Causes:
- Autonomic imbalance
- Recovering 3rd nerve lesion
- Chorea
  No significant localizing value.

Anisocoria

- Ask the patient to gaze at lighted window or at some other distant light source so as to see the pupil size.
- Look for unequal pupil, associated ptosis, squint, reaction to light, to detect which side is normal.
- *Causes:* Unilateral sympathetic paralysis or irritation unilateral 3rd nerve lesion as in:
  - Brainstem damage
  - Transtentorial herniation
  - Pressure effect on 3rd nerve in tumor, aneurysm.

Horner's Syndrome (Fig. 3.19)

a. Central Horner's syndrome (1st order of neuron). Hypothalamic lesion, tumor, hemorrhage, brainstem stroke, lateral medullary syndrome, syringomyelia
   Cervical sympathetic—preganglionic (2nd order of neuron)
   Bronchogenic carcinoma—Pancoast's tumor
   Metastatic carcinoma of neck—Rowland Payne syndrome
   T1 radiculopathy
b. Postganglionic—carotid artery disease (aneurysm) at cavernous sinus
   - Reader's paratrigeminal syndrome (painful Horner's syndrome)—due to compression of 5th cranial nerve by ICA aneurysm.
   - Parkinson's syndrome—6th N lesion + Horner's syndrome (HS)

   Others:
   - HS + 2nd N lesion—ICA disease
   - HS + 3rd N lesion—Intracavernous ICA aneurysm
   - HS + 4th N lesion—ipsilateral HS + contralateral 4th N palsy as it winds around brainstem
   - HS + 5th N lesion—reader's paratrigeminal syndrome
   - HS + 6th N lesion—intracavernous lesion of ICA.

Light Reflex

Afferent through the optic nerve and efferent through the 3rd nerve.
   Center—midbrain.

Direct light reflex: Bright beam of light is shown to one eye from the side of the eye and then to the other eye (showing light in front of eye produces convergence). Pupil constricts briskly and compare the reaction.
   Observe the reaction—brisk/sluggish/absent

Indirect light reflex (consensual): Throw light from the side of one eye, watch the reaction of the pupil of the other eye, repeat the same in the other eye. To visualize the pupil for consensual reaction, while throwing the light on the contralateral side with another torch, light can be thrown on the anterior chamber of I/L eye, so as to see the reaction of pupil.

Accommodation Reflex

It is a triad of responses:
- Miosis
- Convergence
- Increased convexity of lens.

Ask the patient to look at a distance, then suddenly focus the eyes on an object, such as finger kept 15 cm in front of bridge of nose. Normally, bilateral convergence and constriction of pupil is seen. If near object is very close to the eye, there will be lowering of eyelids. This will obscure the observance of reflex.

Clinical Abnormalities of Light and Accommodation Reflex

1. Afferent lesion—optic nerve—ipsilateral direct light reflex and contralateral consensual reflex lost. I/L consensual present.
2. Efferent lesion—3rd nerve—ipsilateral direct and consensual absent. Contralateral consensual and direct present.
3. Marcus Gunn pupil—in afferent lesion—(optic nerve lesion), affected pupil will dialate paradoxically after a short time, when the light is moved from normal eye to affected eye. This is due to the relaxation after the consensual response in the affected eye which may have poor response to direct light.
4. Argyll Robertson pupil (ARP) (Reflex iridoplegia): Pupil are small, constricted, <3 mm, do not react to light reflex, but react to accommodation reflex, the lesion is in pretectal region of midbrain, where the light reflex pathway and descending sympathetic are affected not impeding accommodation reflex pathway. ARP is seen in neurosyphilis, multiple sclerosis, syringobulbia, autonomic neuropathy.
5. Holmes-Adie's syndrome—tonic pupil—it can be unilateral or bilateral. Delayed pupillary constriction to light or accommodation reflex, once constricted, dilatation is also slow. It is associated with ipsilateral loss of deep tendon reflex (DTR)—ankle jerk. Holmes-Adie's syndrome with segmental hypohydrosis is Ross syndrome. It is supposed to be due to parasympathetic denervation.
6. Horner's syndrome.

Nystagmus

Involuntary rhythmic oscillatory movement of eyeball without affecting the voluntary movement.

Clinically 2 types
1. *Pendular nystagmus:* To and fro movement are equal. Ocular cause—defective vision as in albinism, macular defect, infantile myopia, Miner's nystagmus.

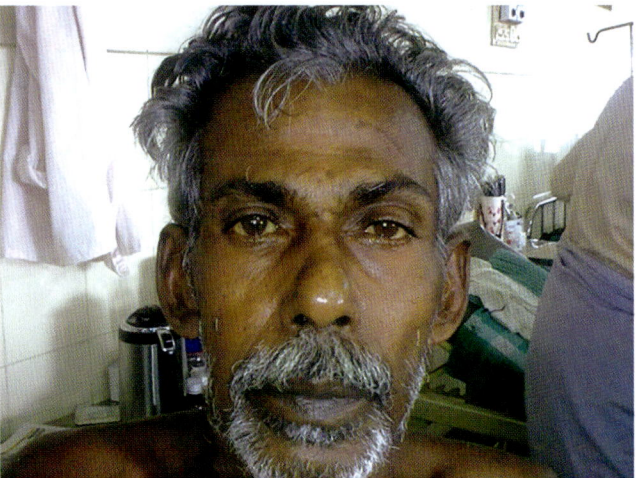

Fig. 3.19: Horner's syndrome left side—partial ptosis of the left eye.

2. *Phasic nystagmus:* Jerk nystagmus—slow and fast component. Direction of nystagmus is named by its fast phase.

Phasic Nystagmus

- Horizontal
- Vertical
- Rotatory—nystagmus in more than in one plane.

Testing Nystagmus

- Fix the head of the patient with the left hand of the examiner.
- Ask the patient to look at the examiner's finger kept at 60 cm away from the patient. The finger should be in the field of binocular vision, means not >30° from primary position or the medial limbus of the opposite eye should not cross the punctum of the eyelid on that side.
- Keep it for 5 seconds to detect latent nystagmus
- Note the following while testing—type, rate, amplitude, grade, direction of fast movement, plane of movement.
  - Slow nystagmus 10-40 movement/minute
  - Medium nystagmus 40-100 movement/minute
  - Fast nystagmus > 100 movement/minute
  - Fine nystagmus—oscillation < 1 mm
  - Coarse nystagmus—oscillation > 3 mm.

Causes of Phasic Nystagmus

- *Vestibular (peripheral) lesion:* Fast phase away from the side of lesion.
- *Cerebellar:* Fast phase to the point of fixation—lateral gaze dependent. Amplitude of oscillation is greater towards the side of lesion.
- *Rotatory nystagmus:* Brainstem lesion involving vestibular nucleus.
- *Ataxic nystagmus:* In internuclear ophthalmoplegia—abducting eye has nystagmus.
- *See saw nystagmus:* Spontaneous nystagmus—one eye is moving up while the other is moving down—in suprasellar lesion.
- *Convergent divergent nystagmus:* Spontaneous convergent divergent movement—lesion at superior collicular level, Parinaud's syndrome.
- *Down beating nystagmus:* Fast downward movement and slow upward movement, increased on lateral gaze—in foramen magnum lesion—CV junction anomaly—Arnold-Chiari malformation.
- *Up-beating nystagmus:* Fast upward movement and slow downward movement increased on upward gaze—lesion of vermis of cerebellum.
- *Optokinetic nystagmus:* Eyes fix at a moving object and then reflex to primary position by a fast movement in the opposite direction, slow movement in the direction of movement of object, fast movement in the opposite direction—railway tract nystagmus.

Slow phase controlled by—occipital lobe
Fast phase controlled by—premotor area of frontal lobe.
Optokinetic nystagmus is demonstrated by using a drum painted with black and white vertical strips
  - Right to left or left to right → horizontal OKN
  - Above downward movement → vertical OKN.

Clinical Use of OKN

- Parietal lobe lesion—no OKN in the direction toward the side of lesion.
- Slow phase absent—occipitoparietal pathway.
- Fast phase absent—frontopontopathway.
- Assess hysterical blindness, testing visual acuity in children when conventional methods are defective.
- Evaluating gaze palsy, saccadic movement, etc.

Positional nystagmus

- Benign paroxysmal positional nystagmus—lesion of utricle and saccule—developing in a particular position of head, later disappear, habituation present.
- Malignant paroxysmal positional nystagmus—lesion is peduncular tumor of ventricle—Brun's syndrome. Nystagmus present in a particular position but no habituation.
- Positional nystagmus can be elicited by placing the patient lying in supine position with the head of the patient outside the edge of the cot and 45° below horizontal, patient's head is held by the examiner, slightly extended and turned to one side at about 45° whereas the patient is asked to look straight at the roof called Hallpike maneuver.
- Oscillopsia—visual symptoms of nystagmus—objects are shaky.

OTHER ABNORMAL MOVEMENTS OF EYE

- *Oculogyric crisis:* Involuntary conjugate upward deviation of the eyeballs which can be transient or lasting for hours. *Cause:* Postencephalitic syndrome, familial parkinsonism, phenothiazine toxicity, 3rd ventricular tumor.
- *Skew deviation of eye:* Ipsilateral eye down and medial, contralateral eye up and lateral, acute cerebellar lesion and posterior fossae lesion.
- *Spasm of upward gaze:* Petit mal epilepsy
- *Adversive seizure:* Focal discharge from area 8, head and eyes will turn away from side of focal discharge.
- *Ocular dysmetria:* Over shooting of the eyes—on attempted rapid fixation of gaze towards either side—in cerebellar lesion.
- *Ocular myoclonus:* Rapid involuntary conjugate saccadic movement of eyes in posterior encephalitic syndrome and neuroblastoma.
- *Ocular bobbing:* Periodic brisk downward movement of both eyes and slow drift upward to the primary position—due to pontine lesion.

- *Ocular flutter:* Episodes of pendular horizontal movement on fixing gaze on an object in cerebellar lesion.
- *Opsoclonus:* Coarse irregular nonrhythmic oscillations of eyeball in both vertical and horizontal planes, persist for a long period of time seen in encephalitis, cerebellar lesion, brainstem damage and metabolic disorders.
- *Ocular apraxia*: Impaired ability to initiate saccades on command, reflex mediated saccades like optokinetic and vestibular stimulation are retained.
- *Oscillopsia*: Illusionary perception of object movement—shaky objects in nystagmus.
- *Superior oblique myokymia*: Uniocular, rapid, small amplitude, intermittent phasic contraction of superior oblique muscle—causing oscillopsia.
- *Slow ocular movement:* In Wadia syndrome, parkinsonism, pseudobulbar palsy.

CLINICAL APPROACH TO OPHTHALMOPLEGIA

Terms to remember:
a. *Internal ophthalmoplegia:* Paralysis of constrictor pupillae and ciliary muscle.
b. *External ophthalmoplegia:* Paralysis of extraocular muscles.
c. *Total ophthalmoplegia:* Both internal and external ophthalmoplegia.

Depends on site of lesion
a. Supranuclear
b. Internuclear
c. Nuclear and infranuclear.

Causes of 3rd Nerve Palsy (Table 3.3)

- Congenital
- Vascular: Brainstem stroke, ICA aneurysm, cavernous sinus thrombosis. Idiopathic granulomatous inflammation of anterior part of cavernous sinus—Tolosa-Hunt syndrome.
- Meningitis, demyelination—Miller-Fisher syndrome, nonspecific mononeuritis.
- Diabetes mellitus, superior orbital fissuritis—Tolosa-Hunt syndrome.
- Pituitary apoplexy, parasellar meningioma.

Causes of Trochlear Nerve Palsy (Table 3.4)

- Isolated lesion—rare
- Upper brainstem stroke, meningitis
- Cavernous sinus, superior orbital fissure, intraorbital lesion as in 3rd nerve palsy.

Causes of 6th Cranial Nerve Palsy (Table 3.5)

- Brainstem stroke, diabetes mellitus, herpes zoster
- Meningitis, CP angle lesion, Gradenigo syndrome
- Increased ICP, cavernous sinus, superior orbital fissure and orbital lesion (refer to 3rd N) *Parkinson's syndrome.*

Table 3.3: Localization of lesion of third nerve.

Site	Structures involved	Clinical features
Brainstem	a. *Nucleus*: complete lesion—uncommon; partial lesion—subnucleus—common b. *Fascicle:* 1. Partial and complete lesion 2. Fascicle + red nucleus 3. Fascicle + superior cerebellar peduncle 4. Fascicle + cerebral peduncle 5. Fascicle + pyramidal cerebellar peduncle + red nucleus	Ipsilateral total ophthalmoplegia, contralateral ptosis ± superior rectus palsy Isolated muscle weakness and isolated ptosis Partial or complete ophthalmoplegia ± pupil Benedickt's syndrome- ipsilateral ophthalmoplegia + contralateral tremor Nothnagel syndrome—ipsilateral ophthalmoplegia + contralateral ataxia Weber's syndrome—ipsilateral ophthalmoplegia + contralateral hemiplegia Claude's syndrome—combination of above syndromes in complete or incomplete form
Subarachnoid space/posterior cranial fossa	Nerve trunk	Complete unilateral or bilateral ophthalmoplegia Pupil + in pressure lesion Sparing pupil—in ischemic lesion.
Cavernous sinus	3rd N trunk ± 4th, 6th N, 5th—ophthalmic and maxillary, pericarotid sympathetic fibers	Partial ophthalmoplegia ± Horner's syndrome ± proptosis, chemosis, papilledema
Superior orbital fissure/anterior cavernous	3rd N upper and lower divisions, 4th, 6th and 5th ophthalmic	Painful ophthalmoplegia
Orbit	3rd N superior and inferior division, optic N, 4th, 6th,5th—ophthalmic, other orbital structures	Branch palsy of 3rd N ± 4th, 5th, 6th—loss of vision, chemosis, proptosis, lid edema

Table 3.4: Localization of lesion of fourth nerve.

Site	Structures involved	Clinical features
Brainstem	Nucleus and fascicle ± Superior cerebellar peduncle ± descending sympathetic at anterior medullary velum (decussating site)	Contralateral superior oblique palsy Ipsilateral cerebellar ataxia Ipsilateral Horner's syndrome Bilateral superior oblique palsy
Subarachnoid space	Nerve ± Superior cerebellar peduncle ± cerebral peduncle	Ipsilateral superior oblique palsy Ipsilateral ataxia Contralateral hemiplegia
Cavernous sinus and superior orbital fissure	4th N + 3rd, 6th, 5th—ophthalmic ± maxillary	Ipsilateral painful ophthalmoplegia
Orbit	4th + 3rd + 6th + 5th—ophthalmic, optic N, Superior oblique tendon mechanical restriction	Partial or complete ophthalmoplegia, loss of vision, chemosis, proptosis, etc. Brown's superior oblique tendon sheath syndrome → ↓ mobility of superior oblique muscle

Abducent Nerve

Table 3.5: Localization of lesion of sixth nerve.

Site	Structures involved	Clinical features
Brainstem	Nucleus/fascicle + pyramidal + 7th cranial nerve ± Pontine lateral gaze center Agenesis of nucleus Agenesis of 6th, 7th nuclei ± 8th cranial nerve	*Raymond syndrome:* Ipsilateral lateral rectus + contralateral hemiplegia *Millard Gubler syndrome:* Ipsilateral 6th and 7th cranial nerve lesion + contralateral hemiplegia *Foville syndrome:* Ipsilateral 6th, 7th + gaze palsy ± ipsilateral Horner's (anterior inferior cerebellar artery lesion) *Duane's retractor phenomenon:* Restriction of abduction, retraction of eye on abduction, narrowing of palpebral fissure *Moebius syndrome:* Oculofacial diplegia
CP angle	6th N + 8th + 5th + 7th cerebellum	Corneal reflex absent, cerebellar ataxia, tinnitus, deafness, LMN facial palsy, lateral rectus palsy
Petrous apex, Dorello's canal	6th CN + 5th—ophthalmic ± 8th	*Gradenigo's syndrome:* Apical petrositis—lateral rectus palsy + sensory features of 5th—ophthalmic *Pseudo-Gradenigo's syndrome/Citelli's syndrome:* Secondary in petrous apex, arising from nasopharyngeal carcinoma intracranial extension through foramen lacerum
Cavernous sinus, Superior orbital fissure, orbit	Refer—3rd cranial nerve	

Etiology of Ophthalmoplegia (3rd, 4th, 6th)

a. *Congenital*
   - Agenesis of nucleus—ptosis
   - Oculofacial diplegia—Moebius syndrome
   - Duane's retractor phenomenon.
b. *Traumatic*
   - 3rd nerve palsy—anatomically 3rd N is fixed at the brainstem and at the site of piercing the duramater
     - Head trauma with shaking movement of brain can produce stretch in 3rd N → neuropraxia
   - Brainstem injury
   - Subdural hematoma with pressure effect
c. *Vascular disorders*
   - Brainstem stroke, aneurysm of ICA, posterior communicating artery.
   - Ophthalmoplegic migraine—Moebius disease.
   - Cavernous sinus thrombosis, caroticocavernous fistula, atheroma of ICA.
d. *Demyelinating disorders*
   - Miller Fisher variant of GBS, disseminated sclerosis
   - Nonspecific neuritis—polyneuritis cranialis

e. *Infections*
   - Brainstem encephalitis, Bickerstaff encephalitis
   - Meningitis—tubercular meningitis, neurosyphilis.
   - Infection with exotoxin producing bacteria—tetanus, botulism, diphtheria
   - Apical petrositis—Gradenigo's syndrome
   - Orbital cellulitis, mucormycosis
f. *Metabolic disorders*
   - Diabetes mellitus and Wernicke's encephalopathy
g. *Entrapment*
   - Superior orbital fissuritis and orbital apex syndrome
h. *C/c Neurological diseases*
   - Hereditary ataxia
   - Progressive bulbar palsy
   - Syringobulbia
i. *Neuromuscular disorders*
   - Myasthenia gravis
   - Botulism
   - Snake venom
j. *Myopathy:*
   - Ocular, oculopharyngeal, mitochondrial myopathy
   - Ragged red fiber syndrome—Kearns-Sayre syndrome
k. *Tumors*
   - Pituitary macroadenoma with apoplexy
   - Brainstem glioma
   - Clivus meningioma
   - False localizing sign in ICSOL.

Depends on Duration of Ophthalmoplegia

- Acute ophthalmoplegia—traumatic and vascular
- Subacute ophthalmoplegia—infection, demyelination, entrapment, metabolic
- Chronic ophthalmoplegia—congenital, degenerative disease, neuromuscular, myopathy and tumors
- Recurrent ophthalmoplegia—disseminated sclerosis, diabetes mellitus, ophthalmoplegic migraine.

Ophthalmoplegia with sparing of pupil
- Diabetes mellitus
- Myopathy
- Myasthenia gravis
- Partial 3rd N palsy.

Ophthalmoplegia with pupil involvement
- Total 3rd N palsy
- Pressure lesion—aneurysm and tumors.

Painful Ophthalmoplegia

Causes: Cavernous sinus thrombosis, superior orbital fissuritis, pituitary apoplexy, caroticocavernous fistula, ophthalmoplegic migraine, orbital apex syndrome, orbital myositis and cellulitis.

Aberrant regeneration of 3rd nerve on recovery from paralysis.
a. Fibers for medial rectus
   Supply levator palpebrae also:
   Abduction → Ptosis (inhibition of medial rectus and levator palpebrae superioris)
   Adduction → elevation of eyelid (inverse Duane's retraction).
b. Fibers for inferior rectus
   Supply levator palpebrae also:
   Downward movement → retraction of eyelid—pseudo-Graffe's syndrome
c. Fibers for medial rectus
   Supply constrictor pupillae—adduction → miosis also, Pseudo-ARP.

Gaze Palsy (Supranuclear Ophthalmoplegia)

Lateral Gaze Palsy

1. *Frontal eye field:* Destructive lesion of area 8 produces loss of lateral gaze to opposite side. Unbalanced action of opposite lateral gaze center. Both eyes turn to the side of lesion–looking towards the side of lesion—vulpian sign. Irritative lesion of area 8 → both eyes turn to opposite side.
2. *Pontine lateral gaze center*
   Destructive lesion → loss of lateral gaze to the same side
   Irritative lesion → lateral gaze to the same side

Vertical Gaze Palsy

Upward gaze palsy
- Lesion—upper midbrain at superior collicular level involving nucleus of Cajal—upward gaze center—as in Parinaud's syndrome, pinealoma, vascular lesion, encephalitis.
- Progressive supranuclear ophthalmoplegia-Steele-Richardson syndrome—affect the vertical saccades
- Wernicke's encephalopathy
- Forced downward gaze—hydrocephalus
  Thalamic hemorrhage—retraction of eyelids also—setting sun appearance
- Parkinsonism
- Posterior 3rd ventricular tumor.

Downward gaze palsy
- Progressive supranuclear ophthalmoplegia
- Olivopontocerebellar ataxia (OPCA)
- Huntington's chorea
- Parkinsonism
- Niemann-Pick disease
- Levy body disease
- DAF syndrome—downward gaze palsy, ataxia/athetosis and foam cells—sea blue hystiocytosis syndrome.

Combined upward and downward gaze palsy
- Bilateral frontal lobe lesion
- Progressive supranuclear ophthalmoplegia
- Parkinsonism

- Huntington's chorea
- Midline—midbrain lesion—vascular and tumor.

Difference between gaze palsy and LMN ophthalmoplegia (Table 3.6).

Table 3.6: Difference between gaze palsy and LMN ophthalmoplegia.

	Gaze palsy	LMN ophthalmoplegia
Movement affected	Gaze movement	Single and multiple muscle action
Pupil	N	±
Diplopia	Absent	+
Squint	Absent	+
Reflex movement (vesitbulo-ocular reflex)	+	absent

Abbreviation: LMN, lower motor neuron.

Internuclear Ophthalmoplegia—Dysconjugate Gaze Palsy (Fig. 3.20)

a. **Superior internuclear ophthalmoplegia**—*Lhermitte's syndrome:* In MLF lesion, on lateral gaze, impulses are not reaching the ipsilateral medial rectus → ipsilateral loss of adduction. Presence of contralateral abduction of eye with nystagmus of abducting eye. But medial rectus will act on convergence.
   Causes:
   - Unilateral—vascular lesion of brainstem
   - Bilateral—disseminated sclerosis, tumor, paraneoplastic encephalomyelitis.

b. **Inferior internuclear ophthalmoplegia**—*Lutz Internuclear ophthalmoplegia:* Lesion is at the connecting link of pontine lateral gaze center to abducent nucleus. On lateral gaze, absence of ipsilateral abduction of eye and presence of contralateral eye adduction. Contralateral adducting eye will have nystagmus, ipsilateral abduction will be present for reflex movement.

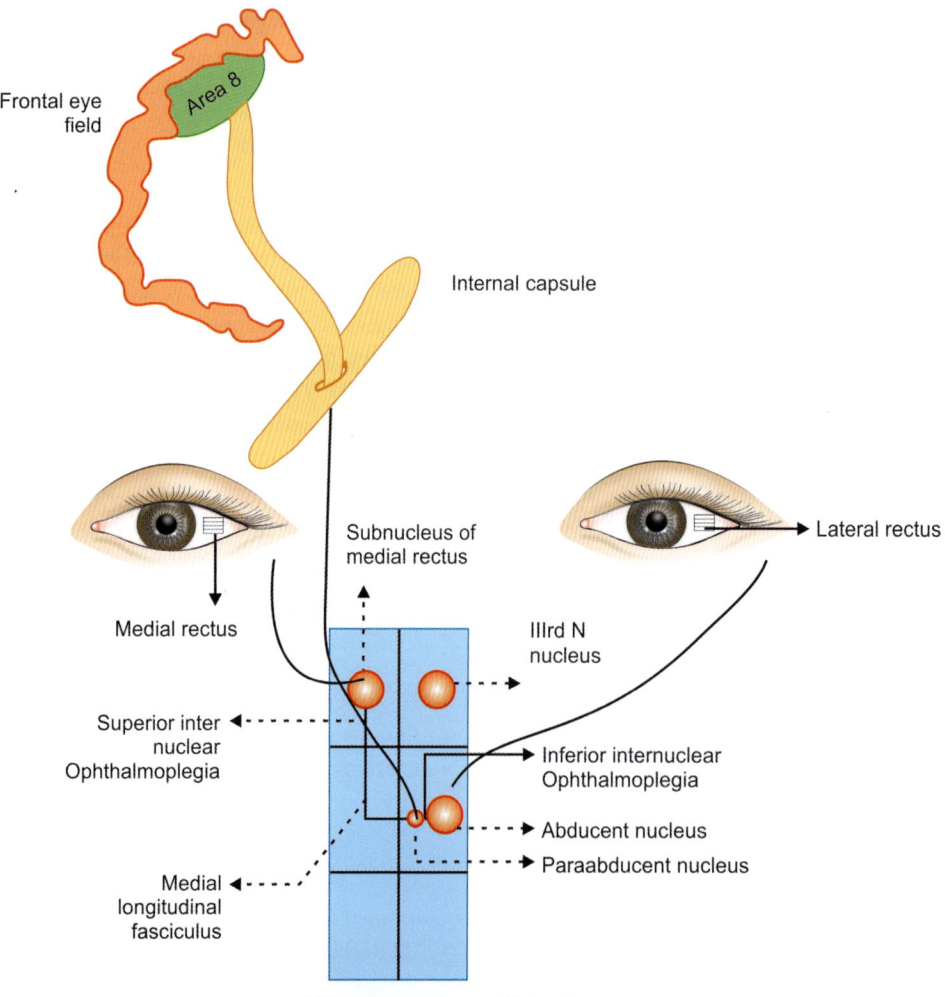

Fig. 3.20: Pathway of lateral gaze.

Pseudointernuclear ophthalmoplegia: Dysconjugate eye movement similar to internuclear ophthalmoplegia will be seen in ocular myasthenia, Miller Fisher syndrome, penicillamine-induced myopathy, abetalipoproteinemia.

Webino syndrome *(wall eyed bilateral internuclear ophthalmoplegia):* Lesion of bilateral MLF and bilateral medial rectus subnucleus—convergence also absent. Resulting in bilateral internuclear ophthalmoplegia with bilateral abduction of eye.

Wemino syndrome *(wall eyed mono-ocular internuclear ophthalmoplegia):* Lesion of unilateral MLF and ipsilateral medial rectus subnucleus resulting in unilateral abduction of eye and unilateral internuclear ophthalmoplegia.

Fisher's one and a half syndrome—*horizontal:* Lesion involving pontine paramedial reticular formation (PPRF) of one side and adjacent MLF will produce limitation of conjugate gaze to one side and absence of adduction on the same side, only horizontal movement is abduction of one eye, thus one and a half movement is absent. Vertical and convergence movements are normal. Vestibulo-ocular reflex → gaze movement is present called dissociated ipsilateral horizontal gaze palsy.

Another type of one and a half syndrome can occur in carotid disease especially at intracavernous portion—where the 6th nerve which is close to it is damaged → ipsilateral LR palsy → defective abduction and ipsilateral frontal eye field is also damaged → lateral gaze palsy, thus remaining only movement is adduction of contralateral eye.

Vertical one and a half syndrome
a. Vertical gaze palsy and mono-ocular paralytic downward movement. Lesion is selective involvement of supranuclear pathway and unilateral partial 3rd nerve palsy.
b. Downward gaze palsy and mono-ocular paralysis of elevation.

Eight and half syndrome: Seventh nerve palsy plus one and a half syndrome.

Disorders of Pursuit Movement

Occipital lobe on each side control horizontal pursuit of same side. Both lobes control vertical pursuit movement.

Occipital lobe is connected to superior colliculi and pretectal nerve for vertical pursuit.

Occipital lobe is connected to PPRF for horizontal pursuit.
a. Unilateral parieto-occipital lesion → absence of pursuit movement to opposite side.
b. Unilateral occipitomesencephalic lesion before decussation → absence of pursuit movement to opposite side.
c. Unilateral occipitomesencephalic lesion after decussation → absence of pursuit movement to same side.
d. In cerebellar lesion—pursuit movement is replaced by saccadic type called cog wheel pursuit.

Disorders of Saccadic Movement

Unilateral frontal lobe—premotor area—area 6, controls horizontal saccadic movement to opposite side

Bilateral frontal lobe—premotor area—area 6, controls vertical saccadic movement.

Saccadic movement can be elicited by keeping both the index fingers of the examiner vertically about 60 cm in front, in the same horizontal plane of patient's eyes, one on either side of mid line at about the mid lateral position of visual field. Ask the patient to fix his gaze at one finger and then shift it rapidly to the other index finger. Make him to do this alternate fixation and observe the jerky voluntary movement from one finger to the other in either direction. Simultaneously, keeping the fingers in the vertical plane in the midline, vertical saccadic movement can be tested.

Unilateral frontal lobe lesion → absence of horizontal saccadic movement to opposite side.

Lesion of frontomesencephalic pathway before decussation → absence of saccadic movement to opposite side.

Lesion of frontomesencephalic pathway after decussation→ absence of saccadic movement to same side.

Reflex Movement of Eyes

a. ***Vestibulo-ocular reflex:*** This indicates the structural integrity of brainstem—connection of 8th CN, to 3rd, 4th, 6th CN and MLF in the brainstem.
   - Irrigation of 250 mL of cold water at 30°C to one ear → eyes deviate to same side and nystagmus to opposite side.
   - Irrigation of hot water at at 45°C to one ear → deviate to opposite side and nystagmus to same side.
   - Introduction of cold water to both ears → both eyes turn downward.
   - Introduction of hot water to both ears → both eyes turn upward.

   Presence of normal response indicates the intactness of brainstem structure.

   Unilateral absence of response—unilateral brainstem lesion.

   Bilateral absence of response—severe damage of brainstem.

b. ***Oculocephalic reflex (Doll's eye movement):*** Eyes reflexly deviate opposite to the side of passive movement of head. Doll's eye movement in both direction in conscious patient with defective gaze movement, indicates intactness of nuclear and infranuclear pathways. Absence of Doll's eye movement in comatosed patient means there is structural damage of brainstem. Doll's eye movement can be elicited by holding the head of the patient with both hands and keep the eyes opened with the examiners thumb, turn the head passively from side to side through a range of 70° observe the movement of both eyes. If eyes move in a direction opposite to the side of passive movement of head, it is normal Doll's eye response.

TRIGEMINAL NERVE (FIGS. 3.21A AND B)

Neuroanatomy

Largest cranial nerve, mixed nerve, has connections with other cranial nerves—3rd, 4th, 6th, 7th and 8th.

    Large sensory part—three sensory nuclei.
    Small motor part—one motor nucleus.

Sensory nuclei:
1. Mesencephalic—midbrain—proprioceptive function
2. Chief sensory—pons—touch sensation
3. Nucleus of spinal tract—descend from pons, medulla upto C3, C4—pain and thermal sensation.

From sensory nuclei: 2nd order of neurons arise
- From chief sensory N both crossed and uncrossed trigeminothalamic tract (quintothalamic tract) terminate at the ventral posteromedial nucleus of thalamus.
- From spinal nucleus of trigeminal—crossed trigeminothalamic tract → ventral posteromedial nucleus of thalamus.
- 3rd order of neurons from thalamus → sensory cortex—inferior part of postcentral gyrus.

    Sensory somatotopic representation in spinal nucleus of trigeminal.
a. Ophthalmic area—at a lower part and mandibular at upper part.
b. Midline region of face—nose/mouth are rostrally, peripheral region of face caudally—reason for onion peel type of sensory loss in syringomyelia.

Motor nucleus:
- Situated at mid pons
- Supranuclear connection with contralateral and ipsilateral motor cortex, contralateral corticonuclear fibers > ipsilateral fibers.

Motor root: Emerges at centerolateral aspect of pons and with the sensory root which is formed by the central fibers of unipolar ganglion cells bifurcated. Gasserian ganglion lies in the Meckel's cave, cavity in the dura mater, apex of petrous bone.

Sensory Division

Ophthalmic division passes through the cavernous sinus and superior orbital fissure, supplies skin over the forehead, upper eyelid, scalp up to central suture, lacrimal gland, PNS.

Maxillary division passes through cavernous sinus, foramen rotundum—inferior orbital fissure, exits through infraorbital foramen. Supplies skin of cheek, anterior temple, upper lip, roof of mouth, soft palate and tonsil.

Mandibular division—largest—carry sensory and motor root. Exits through foramen ovale, supplies skin over jaw, lower teeth, anterior surface of pinna, anterior 2/3rd of tongue, anterior part of external auditory meatus. Secretomotor fibers of submandibular, sublingual gland is supplied through sub maxillary ganglion. Angle of mandible is supplied by—C2, C3 segment (greater auricular nerve).

Motor Supply

- Medial pterygoid, lateral pterygoid, temporalis, masseter
- Tensor tympani, tensor veli palatini, mylohyoid, anterior belly of digastric
- Medial and lateral pterygoid of one side pushes the jaw to opposite side as a common action, thus in trigeminal lesion, jaw deviate to the affected side.

Action of Muscles (Fig. 3.22)

Functions of 5th Nerve

- Sensory function of face, anterior 2/3rd of tongue and eyeball
- Motor—muscles of mastication.

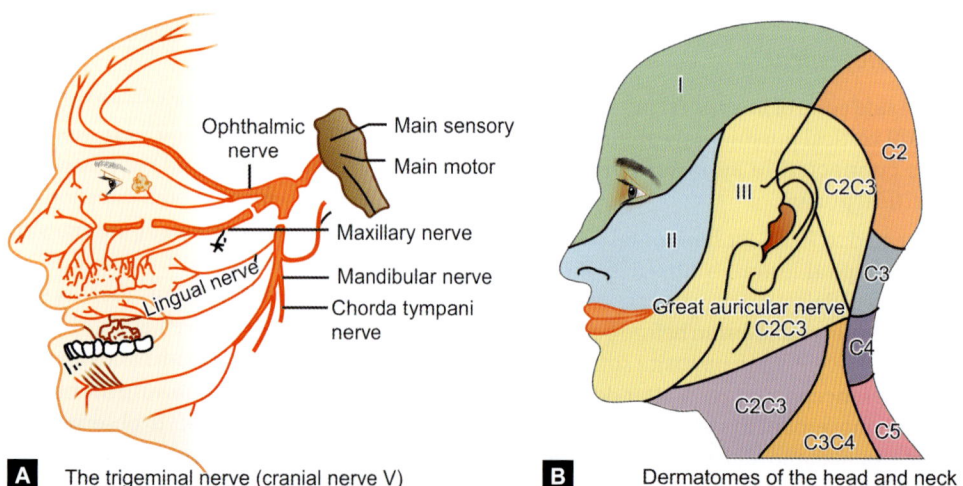

A The trigeminal nerve (cranial nerve V)
B Dermatomes of the head and neck

Figs. 3.21A and B: Distribution of trigeminal nerve.

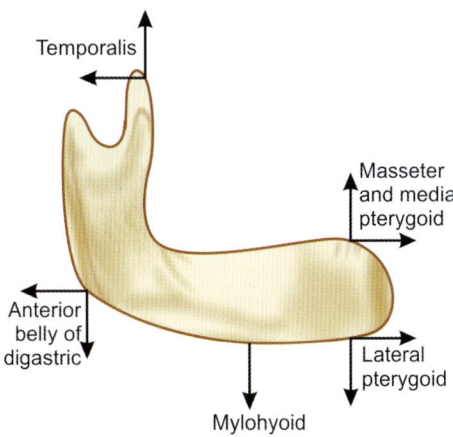

Fig. 3.22: Muscles of mastication.

Symptoms of 5th Cranial Nerve Lesion

- Dulling of sensation over face and other areas of distribution
- Neuralgic pain in face
- Difficulty in mastication and sagging of jaw
- Fatigability on mastication in myasthenia
- Trophic changes—keratitis and erosion of alae nasi
- Trismus—tonic spasm of muscles of mastication.

Clinical Examination

Motor Function

To decide motor weakness is unilateral or bilateral, LMN or UMN:
1. *Observe wasting of muscles:* Temporalis and masseter, hollowing of temple, fasciculation.
2. *Clenching the jaws:* Palpate the masseter and temporalis before clenching and while on clenching on both sides, note the contraction of muscle mass—equal and normal or reduced or absent contraction.
3. *Opening of jaws:* Note any deviation to the affected side by the push of pterygoids of normal side while opening the jaw. Opening against resistance—note any deviation.
   Deviation is appraised by noting the relation between upper and lower incisor teeth while opening and closing jaws, not by the position of lips. In case of doubt, keep a pencil or ruler from the tip of nose vertically will tell the direction of jaw. In facial palsy, there is apparent deviation of jaw due to weakness of facial muscles.
4. Side-to-side movement of jaw against resistance, in paralysis, patient moves the jaw to the paralyzed side due to the push of pterygoids from the nonparalyzed side.
5. Note the protrusion and retraction movement—minimum weakness can be detected by noting the depth of bite mark with the molar teeth on both side on a tongue blade, weak side—bite mark is decreased.
6. Other motor functions—not usually tested
   - Palpate the floor of mouth—flabbiness—weakness of mylohyoid and anterior belly of digastric.
   - Sagging of arch of palate—on the side of weakness of tensor veli palatini.
   - Tensor tympani—decreases the hearing of high tones—dysacusis of high tones.

Sensory Function

Touch, pain, thermal sensation are tested as described in chapters for examination of sensory system.
Six areas on either side are usually tested.
Forehead and upper part of nose → ophthalmic division.
Maxillary area and upper lip → maxillary division
Chin and lower jaw → mandibular division
Note the sensory loss, from peripheral part of face to central part, to look for onion peel type of sensory loss.
Skin over the angle of jaw is spared—supplied by great auricular nerve—C2, C3. Over the face midline crossing is less than elsewhere in the body.

Reflex Functions

1. *Corneal reflex*—afferent—5th cranial nerve, center—chief sensory nucleus at pons
   Efferent—7th cranial nerve
   Method—make the patient to look to opposite side at the examiners finger kept just above the opposite eye, using a wet cotton tip, touch the upper and lower part of cornea—upper part is by ophthalmic, lower part is by maxillary. Observe the prompt closure of ipsilateral and contralateral eyes—ipsilateral direct corneal reflex contralateral consensual corneal reflex.
   Unilateral trigeminal lesion—ipsilateral and contralateral responses are absent eliciting reflex on controlateral side—both eyes close.
   Unilateral facial palsy: Ipsilateral eye—absence of closure, contralateral eye closes.
2. *Conjunctival reflex:* Stimuli is given to conjunctiva, response is same as corneal reflex. Occasionally, reflex is absent if patient has high threshold for pain.
   Loss of corneal reflex is an early sign of trigeminal sensory involvement as in CP angle lesion.
   In parietal lobe lesion, there can be loss of corneal reflex—opposite side.
   Nucleus of spinal tract involvement also produce loss of corneal reflex as in Wallenberg syndrome.
3. *Jaw jerk:* Afferent and efferent are through trigeminal.
   To elicit the jaw jerk, examiner places his index finger over the middle of patient's chin, mouth is partially opened and jaw is relaxed, tap with percussion hammer over the finger, observe the sudden closure of mouth due to contraction of masseter and temporalis. Normally no elicitable response, well elicitable response is considered as exaggerated reflex, and is a sign of bilateral UMN 5th nerve lesion, above the

motor nuclei of 5th at pons, as seen in pseudobulbar palsy and motor neuron disease.

Corneomandibular reflex: Contralateral deviation of jaw due to contraction of pterygoids, when the cornea is stimulated—afferent and efferent are through trigeminal, positive reflex means ipsilateral UMN lesion of 5th cranial nerve.

Localization of Lesions of Trigeminal Nerve

a. *Supranuclear lesion:*
   - Unilateral lesion may not manifest since bilateral innervation. Mild contralateral weakness if contralateral supply is more than ipsilateral.
   - Bilateral UMN—bilateral weakness of muscles of mastication with exaggerated jaw jerk.
   - Parietal lobe and thalamic lesion—contralateral facial sensory dulling as a part of hemisensory deficit.

b. *Nuclear lesion at pons:*
   - Ipsilateral paresis, wasting and fasciculation of muscles
   - Contralateral long tract sign: Pyramidal and sensory deficit.
   - Ipsilateral facial sensory deficit.

   Nucleus of spinal tract: Dissociated sensory loss of face as in lateral medullary syndrome, due to proximity, spinothalamic tract is also involved→ dissociated sensory loss contralateral body called—crossed dissociated sensory loss. Onion peel pattern of sensory loss in syringomyelia—progressive loss of sensation from peripheral part of face to the center because of the rostral caudal somatotopic representation of face in the nucleus of spinal tract.

c. *Lesion of preganglionic trigeminal nerve root*
   - Ipsilateral facial sensory deficit → ↓ corneal reflex
   - Ipsilateral masticating paresis.
   - ± 6th, 7th, 8th, cerebellum as in CP angle lesion—accoustic neuroma, trigeminal neuroma.

d. *Lesion at Gasserian ganglion:* Tip of petrous at middle cranial fossa
   - Hemifacial or partial 5th sensory—branch involvement
   - Ipsilateral 6th CN as in
     - Gradenigo's syndrome
       Infection—otitis → meningitis
     - Secondaries
     - Osteitis
     - Aneurysm of ICA—Raeder's paratrigeminal syndrome
     - Tumor, neuroma or meningioma

e. *Lesion at Cavernous Sinus*
   - Ipsilateral ophthalmic and maxillary division
   - Ipsilateral 3rd, 4th, 6th
   - Ipsilateral Horner's syndrome ± proptosis, chemosis

f. *Lesion at superior orbital fissure*
   - Ipsilateral ophthalmic (sparing maxillary—DD from cavernous sinus)
   - ± other nerves as above

g. *Branch lesion*
   1. *Ophthalmic division*
      Sites of involvement ± other cranial nerves:
      - Middle cranial fossae
      - Petrous apex
      - Cavernous sinus
      - Superior orbital fissure
      - Face.
   2. *Maxillary division*
      Sites of involvement ± other cranial nerves:
      - Foramen rotundum
      - Pterygopalatine fossae
      - Floor of orbit
      - Infraorbital foramen
      - Numb cheek syndrome—lesion at infraorbital foramen
   3. *Mandibular division*
      Sites of involvement ± other cranial nerves + masticatory process:
      - Foramen ovale
      - Zygomatic fossae
      - Face.

Isolated mental neuropathy: Numb chin syndrome—involving chin, lower lip and mucous membrane of lower lip, seen in internal malignancy of breast lymphoma.

Tongue numbness: Ischemia of lingual nerve—in temporal arteritis.

Periodic lingual numbness: Intermittent compression of lingual nerve by sialolisthesis—submandibular swelling—profuse salivation and hemilingual numbness.

Neuromyotonia of floor of mouth: Irritation of mandibular branch—sustained muscle contraction of floor of mouth.

Etiology of Trigeminal Nerve Palsy

Motor Component

- *Bilateral upper motor neuron (UMN) lesion*: Pseudobulbar palsy, motor neuron disease (MND), upper brainstem lesion.
- *Unilateral UMN lesion*: Rarely in hemispheric lesion where contralateral innervations is more.
- *Bilateral LMN lesion*: Brainstem stroke, brainstem encephalitis, brainstem demyelination, Guillain-Barré syndrome (GBS), Myasthenia gravis, dystrophia myotonica, basal meningitis, pontine myelinolysis.
- *Unilateral LMN lesion*: Brainstem stroke, brainstem encephalitis, basal meningitis, diabetes mellitus, nonspecific mononeuritis, pontine glioma.

Sensory Component

- Herpes ophthalmicus
- Superior orbital fissure lesion

- Cavernous sinus lesion
- Raeder's paratrigeminal syndrome
- Gradenigo's syndrome
- Basal meningitis
- Trigeminal neuralgia (Fothergill's disease)
- Trigeminal neuropathy:
  - Idiopathic
  - Collagen disease
  - Tumor—neuroma
- Wallenberg's syndrome—lateral medullary syndrome
- Syringomyelia—onion peel type of sensory loss.

Other Disorders of Trigeminal Nerve

1. Hemimasticatory spasm—irritation of 5th—motor
2. Focal seizure
3. Reflex epilepsy—chewing
4. Jaw tremor in Parkinsonism
5. Trismus—spasm of muscle—tetanus and rabies
6. Complex partial seizure—chewing and tasting movement
7. Bruxism (involuntary grinding movement of teeth)—idiopathic and L dopa-induced
8. Marcus Gunn phenomenon
9. *Sturge-Weber syndrome:* Encephalotrigeminal angiomatosis
10. *Frey's syndrome:* Auriculotemporal syndrome—flushing, perspiration and warmth over the cheek and pinnae following ingestion of highly seasoned food. Secretomotor fibers of auriculotemporal to parotid is misdirected to sweat gland and blood vessels on recovery after injury.
11. Oromandibular dystonia with blepharospasm—Meige syndrome (Brueghel syndrome).

FACIAL NERVE (FIG. 3.23)

Neuroanatomy

Nuclei of facial nerve are 4
1. Motor nucleus—ventral pons—dorsal and ventral group of cells
2. Superior salivatory nucleus
3. Nucleus of tractus solitarius
4. Lacrimal nucleus.

Supranuclear connection—is unique for facial nerve—two types
1. Volitional movement
2. Reflex movement.

For volitional movement: From lower part of precentral gyrus corticonuclear fibers descend to pons and cross to opposite facial nucleus. Nucleus for the superior half of facial muscles receiving ipsilateral (I/L) and contralateral supranuclear fibers. Nucleus for the inferior half of facial muscles mainly for contralateral supranuclear fibers—UMN lesion lower half is affected.

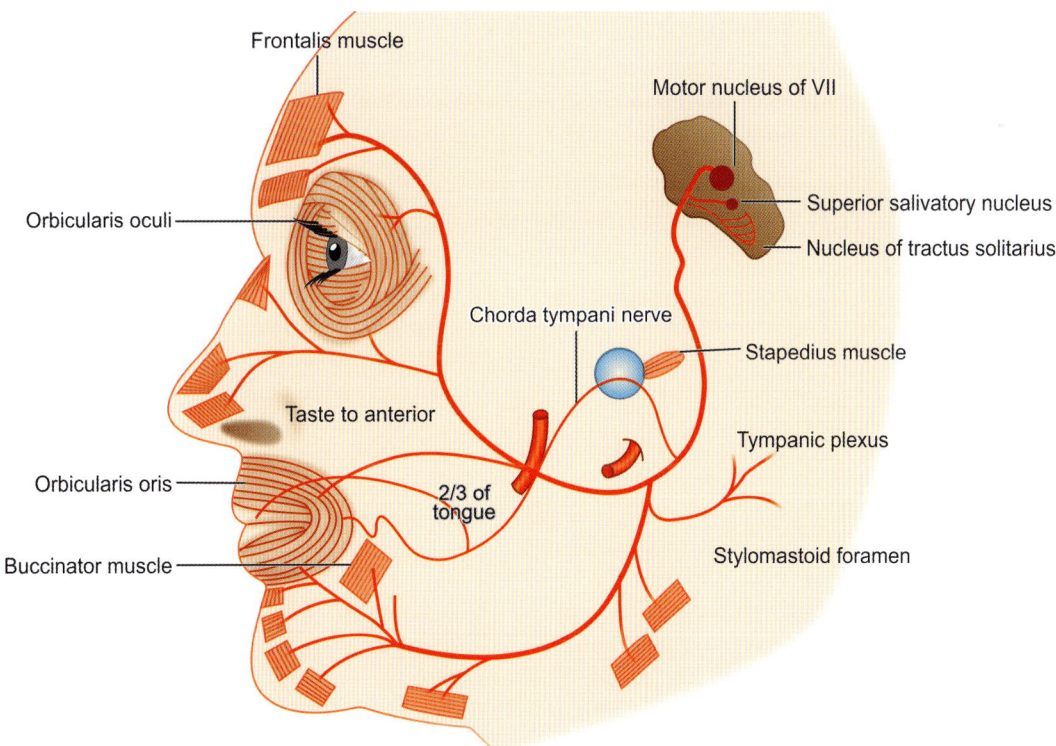

Fig. 3.23: Facial nerve.

Variation: Occasionally lower half also has ipsilateral supranuclear innervation but less than contralateral. Thus only paresis of lower half in UMN lesion, if ipsilateral supranuclear innervation also equal to contralateral, both upper half and lower half may escape in UMN lesion.

Rarely upper half will have innervation predominantly from contralateral fibers. Thus UMN lesion → extension of weakness to upper half also.

For reflex movement: Fibers from premotor area, extrapyramidal center, basal ganglia, through separate pathway, innervate the nucleus from both sides but predominantly for right cortex.

Lesion of this pathway → Mimic facial palsy

Nervus intermedius: Sensory counter part of facial nerve. Carry fibers of superior salivatory nucleus, lacrimal nucleus, and nucleus of tractus solitarius. It subserves somatic sensation of mastoid region—part of pinnae, external auditory canal, secretomotor fibers to lacrimal gland, salivary glands—sublingual and submandibular and visceral sensation—taste sensation from anterior 2/3rd of tongue.

Course

a. *Intrapontine segment*: From the first genu around the 6th cranial nerve (CN) nucleus emerge ventrolateral portion of pons with nucleus intermedius and 8th nerve.
b. *Meatal segment*: Enter the internal acoustic meatus with 8th CN.
c. *Labyrinthine segment*: Dip into the facial canal in the floor of meatal canal, reaches the medial part of tympanic cavity form the 2nd genu—geniculate ganglion—receives the nervus intermedius.
d. *Mastoid segment*: It turns back vertically downwards to emerge through stylomastoid foramen.
e. *Parotid region*: Enter deep to parotid gland, divides into temporofacial and cervicofacial. Further divide to form the final branches.
f. *Face.*

Branches (Fig. 3.23)

- Geniculate ganglion—greater superficial petrosal nerve—secretomotor fibers to lacrimal gland
- Vertical mastoid segment—nerve to stapedius—chorda tympani—5 mm above the stylomastoid foramen, carry taste sensation from anterior 2/3rd of tongue. Secretomotor fibers to submaxillary ganglion to submandibular and sublingual gland.
- Stylomastoid foramen—posterior auricular—occipitalis and auricular muscles
  - Digastric—posterior belly of digastric
  - Stylohyoid—stylohyoid muscle
- Parotid region
  - Temporofacial
    - Temporal
    - Zygomatic
    - Upper buccal
  - Cervicofacial
    - Lower buccal
    - Mandibular
    - Cervical

They supply muscles of face, scalp and platysma.

Functions of Facial Nerve

- Motor functions—muscles of facial expression
- Visceral function—taste—anterior 2/3rd of tongue
- Secretomotor function—salivation, lacrimation
- Hearing—nerve to stapedius.

Symptoms of Facial Palsy

Facial deviation, lagophthalmos (defective closure of eye), epiphora, difficulty in spitting, drooling of saliva, collection of fluid in the vestibule of mouth.

Clinical Examination

1. Motor part
2. Sensory part
3. Reflexes

Motor Part

a. **Observe for**
   - Absence of wrinkling and asymmetry of wrinkling of forehead
   - Lagophthalmos and unequal palpebral fissure
   - Blink asymmetry
   - Puffing of cheek during respiration
   - Obliteration of nasolabial fold
   - Abnormality in volitional and reflex movement like smiling and crying
   - Vesicles on the pinna, external auditory meatus
   - Fasciculation and other involuntary movement of facial muscles.

b. **Frontal belly of occipitofrontalis**
   Raise the eyebrows and wrinkle the forehead. Look for the movement of eyebrows and number of wrinkles on both sides.
   Unilateral LMN lesion—side of lesion—upward movement of eyebrow is reduced or absent, number of wrinkles is reduced or absent
   Unilateral UMN—movement of eye brow and number of wrinkles—normal
   Bilateral LMN and bilateral UMN—reduced movement of eyebrows and reduced number of wrinkles on both sides.

c. **Orbicularis oculi:** Ask the patient to close both eyes tightly and against resistance also. Compare the amount of eyelashes buried on both sides, note whether Bell's phenomenon present (rolling up of eyes while closing the eyes—synkinetic movement seen normally which will become visible when there is defective closure of eye due to weakness of orbicularis oculi). Try to open the closed eye, normally not possible, if weakness present, one can overcome the power and open.

   Bell's phenomenon is palpebral oculogyric reflex—contraction of orbicularis oculi and closing the eye, eyeball moves up, proprioceptive impulses through 7th nucleus →MLF → 3rd N → superior rectus. Ten percent of normal persons, above synkinetic movement absent.

   Decrease in palpable vibration of orbicularis oculi as the examiner attempts to open closed eyelids against resistance is an early sensitive 'lid sign' of facial palsy. Lower lid retraction is also seen in early facial palsy.

d. **Muscles attached to the angle of mouth:** Ask the patient to retract or drawback the angle of mouth and show his teeth. Note any asymmetry of retraction, deviation of angle to normal side. Note the retraction of angle of mouth both for voluntary and reflex movement like laughing and smiling. Patient may smile spontaneously after attempting to whistle, to demonstrate reflex movement.

   Affected side—retraction of angle is reduced and deviate to normal side.

   In LMN lesion, both voluntary and reflex movement is decreased.

   In UMN lesion, voluntary movement is decreased and reflex movement is normal.

   In mimic facial palsy—voluntary movement is normal, reflex movement is decreased.

e. **Orbicularis oris:** Purse the lips tightly and try to whistle or ask the patient to touch his finger with the pursed lips. If weakness present, patient is unable to do so.

f. **Buccinator:** Blow out the cheek.

   Tap the cheek with finger over the inflated cheek on either side. Escape of air will indicate weakness, normally no air will escape.

g. **Platysma:** Retraction of mouth down with clenching of teeth or pushing down the chin against resistance → longitudinal folds of skin over the neck due to contraction of platysma.

h. **Stapedius:** Observe the hyperacusis for low tone.

i. **Function of stylohyoid and posterior belly of digastric:** Usually not tested clinically. Function is to raise the hyoid bone and thyroid cartilage with retraction of tongue. Weakness of the muscles → defective deglutition and regurgitation of food.

Sensory Function

Taste sensation from anterior 2/3rd of tongue.
Primary taste sensations are—sweet—tip of tongue—sugar
Salt—tip of tongue—common salt
Sour—border of tongue—vinegar and acetic acid
Bitter—back of tongue—quinine

Explain the procedure of testing to the patient. Name of the test substances are written on a card or a piece of paper so that the patient can show the name of the test substance. Hold the tip of the tongue with cotton or gauze with examiner's left thumb and index finger. Place the solution of test substance on each half of tongue, one after another. Ask the patient to show the name of the substance in the card. Wipe the surface of tongue with cotton before using another test substance. Bitter is tested last, bitter stimuli is most sensitive.

Loss of taste sensation is called agusia.
Reduction of taste sensation is called hypogeusia.
Perverted perception of taste is parageusia.

Reflex Function

- **Corneal and conjunctival reflex** (refer 5th cranial nerve)
- **Glabellar tap**—orbicularis oculi reflex
- Percussion over the glabella is followed by reflex contraction of orbicularis oculi and bilateral closure of eyes. Afferent both 5th and 7th, efferent—7th CN. Center is pons. Normally after a few contractions, the response ceases, in bilateral UMN lesion and Parkinsonism the response persists. LMN lesion—response is absent. Persistent response is called Myerson's sign.
- **Snout reflex or orbicularis oris reflex**—Afferent 5th and efferent 7th center pons. Tapping over the upper lip or lower one produces contraction of orbicularis oris and protrusion of lips. In bilateral UMN lesion, this reflex is elicitable, in LMN lesion and normal people it is absent.
- **Palmomental reflex**—Scratching with a blunt point over the thenar area of hand—ipsilateral contraction of mentalis and orbicularis oris, wrinkling of skin of chin. This reflex is present in pyramidal lesion, UMN facial palsy, frontal lobe lesion, no localizing value.

Secretory function: Not usually tested
- Lacrimation is assessed by Schirmer's test (keratoconjunctivitis sicca), inhalation of ammonia → increase the tear flow.
- Salivation—can be stimulated by keeping flavored substance or lemon drop upon the tongue, if needed, measurement can be done with a polythene tube in the submandibular duct.

Clinical Features of Various Types of Facial Palsy

Unilateral LMN Facial Palsy

- One half of face is affected, both voluntary and reflex movements are affected
- Bell's phenomenon—present
- Taste sensation, lacrimation, salivation, hyperacusis—affected depends on the site of lesion
- Reflex—corneal, glabellar and snout absent.

Unilateral UMN Facial Palsy

- Lower half of one side is involved
- Voluntary movement is affected, reflex movement is intact
- Bell's phenomenon—absent
- Secretomotor function and taste sensation normal.

Bilateral LMN Facial Palsy

- Whole of face—both upper and lower halves are involved
- Both reflex and voluntary movements are affected
- Bells phenomenon—present
- Glabellar and snout reflex absent

Bilateral UMN Facial Palsy

- Whole of face is involved
- Voluntary movement affected, reflex movement intact
- Bell's phenomenon—absent
- Glabellar and snout reflex present.

Mimic Facial Palsy

- Only reflex movement is affected—asymmetry of facial movement present while crying and laughing
- Voluntary movement is normal
- If bilateral, expressionless face (Parkinsonism), glabellar present and snout reflex absent.

Localization and Etiology of Facial Palsy

Supranuclear Lesion

a. *Unilateral UMN*: Hemispheric and upper brainstem lesion as in stroke, meningitis encephalitis, brain abscess, demyelination, ICSOL
b. *Bilateral UMN*: Pseudobulbar palsy, motor neuron disease, upper brainstem lesion.

Unilateral LMN Facial Palsy (Table 3.7)

a. **Nuclear and fascicle:** Lesion of pons.
   - Ipsilateral LMN facial palsy + Contralateral long tract signs
   - Crossed hemiplegia
   - Millard Gubler syndrome, Foville syndrome

   Causes: Brainstem stroke, pontine glioma, brainstem encephalitis, brainstem demyelination.

b. **Infranuclear:**
   1. CP angle lesion—8th + 5th + 7th LMN + cerebellar signs—in acoustic neuroma, meningioma, arachnoiditis, cholesteatoma.
   2. Posterior cranial fossae—meningitis → unilateral LMN or bilateral LMN facial palsy.
   3. Petrous temporal bone fracture, especially transverse fracture.
      LMN facial palsy + 8th CN + bleeding from ear, CSF otorrhea.
   4. Geniculate ganglion—herpes and otogenic infection herpes of geniculate ganglion—Ramsay Hunt syndrome LMN facial palsy, otalgia, vesicles on pinna, external auditory meatus and mastoid region.
      Two types
      i. Otalgic form—pain and vesicle
      ii. Prosopalgic form—paralysis
   5. Stylomastoid foramen—Bell's palsy—idiopathic LMN facial palsy—rostral to geniculate ganglion.
      LMN facial palsy sparing taste and secretomotor function
      Cause: Edema or periosteitis of facial canal
      - Ischemia
      - Nonsuppurative inflammation—infective—non-infective
      - Segmental demyelination

Table 3.7: Comparison of LMN facial palsy at various sites.

LMN palsy site	Lacrimation	Normal hearing	Salivation	Taste	Reason
Pons	+	+	+	+	Separate nucleus in pons
CP angle	–	–	–	–	Nervous intermedius is close to motor part
Internal acoustic meatus	–	–	–	–	"
Between internal acoustic meatus and geniculate ganglion	–	–	–	–	"
Geniculate ganglion	–	–	–	–	Vesicles + in herpes
Between geniculate ganglion and stapedius	+	–	–	–	Greater superficial petrosal nerve unaffected
Between stapedius and chordae tympani	+	+	–	–	Greater superficial petrosal nerve and stapedius unaffected
Stylomastoid foramen	+	+	+	+	Above 2 branches and chordae tympani—unaffected

+, Present, –, absent

6. Parotid region—parotid disease—abscess, surgery and malignancy—complete LMN or incomplete LMN
7. At face—branch lesion—Hansen's disease—partial peripheral facial palsy—lagophthalmos
8. Other cause of LMN facial palsy—diabetes mellitus → ischemia, hypertension → hemorrhage in facial canal, migraine, disseminated sclerosis, sarcoidosis, infections—IMN, mumps, Lyme disease.

Bilateral LMN Facial Palsy

Causes:
- GBS
- Motor neuron disease
- Facioscapulohumeral muscular dystrophy
- Brainstem stroke
- Brainstem encephalitis
- Bickerstaff encephalitis
- Brainstem demyelination
- Basal meningitis
- Basilar artery aneurysm
- Congenital Moebius syndrome
- Acute lymphoblastic leukemia
- Dystrophia myotonica—(myopathic smile—horizontal smile)
- Myasthenia gravis—(vertical smile—myasthenic snarl).

Recurrent Facial Palsy

- Disseminated sclerosis
- Bell's palsy 7%
- Diabetes mellitus
- Facioplegic migraine
- Melkersson's syndrome—familial, recurrent facial palsy, facial edema, fissured tongue—lingua plicata.

Complications of LMN Facial Palsy (Bell's palsy)

- Exposure keratitis
- Hemifacial spasm
- Facial contracture (Fig. 3.24)—face deviate to the involved side
- Crocordile tears syndrome—paradoxic gustatory lacrimal reflex (Bogarad's syndrome)—tearing while strongly flavored food is taken. Fibers intended for salivation is misdirected to lacrimal gland on regeneration.
- Reverse Marcus-Gunn phenomenon (Marin-Amat syndrome)—closing of eye while opening mouth—fibers intended for the retraction of mouth redirected in regeneration and supplies orbicularis oculi also.
- Tic douloureux of chordae tympani
- Chordae tympani syndrome—increased sweating and flushing in the submental region after eating. False regeneration of secretomotor fibers to the sweat glands and blood vessels.

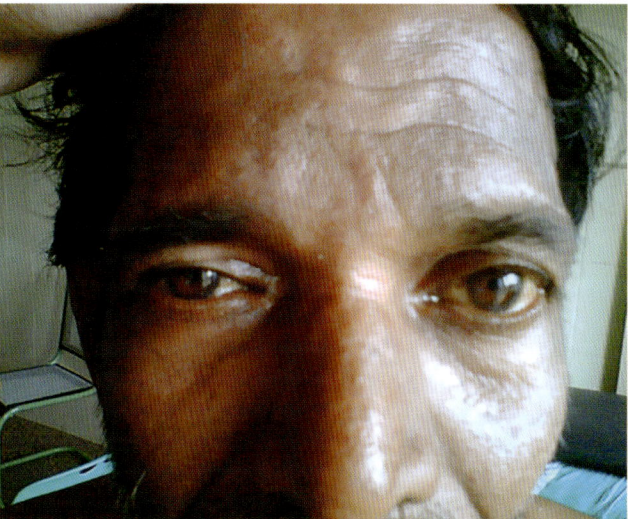

Fig. 3.24: Right side Bell's palsy (showing loss of wrinkles on right side) with facial contracture.

Abnormal Movements Related to Facial Muscles

a. Perioral tremor—alcoholics and GPI
b. Hemifacial spasm—idiopathic, posterior paralytic
c. Orofaciolingual dystonia—drug induced
d. Oromandibular dystonia—Meige syndrome
e. Tics and habit spasm—repetitive stereo-typed simple and complex movement reproduced voluntarily
f. Focal seizure—structural lesion of facial area of motor cortex.
g. Fasciculation—MND
h. Myokymia—fine undulating movements of facial muscles
i. Blepharospasm—tetanus, drug induced
j. Facial spasm—Brissaured syndrome—irritative lesion → ipsilateral facial spasm + contralateral pyramidal sign
k. Chvostek's sign—tetany, facial muscle excitability
l. Myoclonus—rhythmic involuntary facial movement ± palatal myoclonus lesion of Guillain-Mollaret triangle—formed by red nucleus, inferior olivary nucleus, dendate nucleus.

Syndromes in Connection with Facial Nerve

1. Weber's syndrome
   - Ipsilateral 3rd nerve palsy with
   - Contrlateral hemiplegia and facial palsy
2. Millard-Gubler syndrome
   - Ipsilateral LMN type of CN 6th and 7th involvement with
   - Contralateral hemiplegia
3. Foville's syndrome
   - Ipsilateral facial palsy, horizontal gaze palsy
   - Contralateral hemiparesis

4. Brissard siccard
   - Ipsilateral facial spasm
   - Contralateral pyramidal sign with or without focal seizures
5. Ramsay Hunt syndrome
   - LMN facial palsy with vesicular rash on the ear
6. Bogorad's syndrome
   - Inappropriate and sometimes excessive lacrimation provoked by eating
   - Occurs after facial paralysis
   - Due to false regeneration of secretomotor fibers.
7. Meige's syndrome
   - Oromandibular dystonia with blepharospasm
8. Melkersson syndrome
   - Recurring facial paralysis
   - Swelling of the face and lips
   - Furrows in the tongue.
9. Moebius syndrome
   - Oculofacial diplegia
   - Congenital agenesis of nucleus
10. Marin Amat syndrome
    - Inverse Marcus Gunn phenomenon
    - On opening the mouth there is closure of eyelids
    - Fibers intended for risorius supplying orbicularis oculi
11. Heerfordt syndrome
    - Uveoparotid fever
    - Fever, uveitis, swelling of parotid gland
    - Sometimes facial nerve palsy
    - Occurring in sarcoidosis

VESTIBULOCOCHLEAR NERVE

Neuroanatomy

Two parts:
1. Cochlear nerve
2. Vestibular nerve

Cochlear nerve: Carry impulses of sound from the hair cells of organ of Corti through the spinal ganglia of cochlea, enter the brainstem at CP angle, reaches the cochlear nuclei, ventral and dorsal at medulla → crossed and uncrossed fibers to trapezoid body → ascends as lateral lemniscus → nucleus of inferior colliculus → medial geniculate body → acoustic radiation—internal capsule → superior temporal gyrus—Heschl's gyrus, peripheral lesion → hearing defect, unilateral brainstem and cortical lesion will not produce because of bilateral supranuclear fibers both crossed and uncrossed fibers.

Vestibular nerve: Carry fibers from hair cells of ampulla of semicircular canal and otolith of utricle and saccule (labyrinth), vestibular nerve enter the brainstem at CP angle, reaches the vestibular nuclei at pontomedullary region—medial, lateral, superior and inferior nuclei. From medial and superior nuclei connection to cerebellum, MLF to 3rd, 4th, 6th, 9th CN and parietal and temporal lobe. Cerebellovestibular fibers to lateral vestibular nucleus (Deiter's nucleus) from there via vestibulospinal tract (uncrossed) to anterior horn cells.

Function—subserve hearing
Control of equilibrium, balance and correction of bodily displacement.

Symptoms

Cochlear

- Deafness
- Tinnitus—perception of abnormal sounds in the ear
- Auditory hallucinations—Aura—Epilepsy
- Hyperacusis—LMN facial palsy—stapedius paralysis
- Presbycusis—in elderly—progressive loss of high tone.

Vestibular

- Vertigo—sense of rotation of oneself or surroundings. It can be subjective—sense of rotation of oneself.
- Objective—sense of rotation of surroundings
- Ataxia—unsteadiness of gait
- Tendency to fall without loss of consciousness—otolithic crisis of Tumarkin
- Oscillopsia in nystagmus
- Nausea, vomiting, diaphoresis.

Terms to Remember

- Perception deafness—nerve deafness
- Conduction deafness—middle ear deafness
- Loudness recruitment—end organ damage—hair cells of organ of Corti
  Under certain type of unilateral deafness, low intensity sound appreciation is reduced in affected ear, same sound with high intensity is heard equally in both ears.
  Value—to differentiate sites of lesion of perception deafness.

Tests for Cochlear Function

Bedside Test—Whispering Test

Place a finger in the patient's external acoustic meatus on one side and move it constantly in order to produce a masking noise. Ask the patient to repeat the whispered or spoken words to him, to have a standard volume of sound, breath out and at the end of expiration, whisper few numbers like 26 or 68 for high tones, 42 or 100 for low tones. If nothing is heard the intensity of sound of whisper is increased. Normally conversational voice can be heard at 3–5 meters.

- *Rub the thumb* and index finger of examiner in front of external acoustic meatus. Note the ability to perceive.
- *Watch test:* By closing the other ear, bring the watch towards the ear, from a distance outside the range of hearing, until the patient is first able to hear a tick, the distance is compared on both sides and also with the examiners acuity of hearing.

Tuning Fork

Conduction of sound through the air to the ear drum is about twice as efficient as conduction through the bone.

Rinne test: Vibrating tuning fork with a frequency of 256 Hz is held near one external auditory meatus. Mask the other ear. Ask whether he can hear it. Then place it on the mastoid process and tell him to say the moment the sound ceases to hear. When he does so, place it again near the meatus, normally the note is still audible.

Normal: Air conduction > Bone conduction—Rinne positive

Conduction deafness: Air conduction < Bone conduction—Rinne negative.

Nerve deafness: Both air and bone conduction is reduced but, air conduction > bone conduction—reduced Rinne positive.

- **Weber test:** Tuning fork is placed on the center of forehead, ask the patient whether he can hear in both ear or better in one ear. In nerve deafness, the sound appears to be heard in the normal ear—lateralized to normal side. In conduction deafness, the sound is conducted to the abnormal ear—lateralized to abnormal side. External sound heard through the normal ear will interfere with the note of tuning fork, thus the note is better appreciated through the abnormal ear.
- **Schwabach test:** As in the Rinne test, the tuning fork is held against the mastoid process until the patient is unable to perceive any sound. The examiner then places the tuning fork over his own mastoid process and thus compares his bone conduction to that of the patient. If the examiner hears the tuning fork after the patient no longer hears it, nerve deafness is suspected.

Tests for Vestibular Function

1. *Look for spontaneous nystagmus:* Fast phase away from side of lesion.
2. *Positional nystagmus:* Hall-pike maneuver (refer nystagmus—3rd cranial nerve)
3. *Caloric Test:* Refer reflex movement of eye—3rd cranial nerve.

Directional preponderance (DP): Means, the response always for irrigation producing nystagmus is reduced in the same direction (e.g. cold water in the right ear and hot water in the left).

The DP is said to occur to the side of lesion at posterior temporal lobe.

Causes of Conduction Deafness

Diseases of external auditory meatus, middle ear, eustachian tube.

Causes of Nerve Deafness

- *Cochlear lesion:* Meniere's disease, otosclerosis, drugs like aminoglycosides, salicylates, diuretics, internal auditory artery occlusion, infection—typhus fever, typhoid fever, mumps
- *Cochlear nerve (retro-cochlear) lesion:* Old age, meningitis, CP angle lesion
- *Brainstem lesion:* Severe bilateral brainstem damage, multiple sclerosis.

Causes of Vestibular Disorders

- *Labyrinthine lesion:* Meniere's disease, labyrinthitis, streptomycin toxicity, motion sickness.
- *Vestibular nerve lesion:* Vestibular neuritis, acoustic neuroma.
- *Brainstem lesion:* Vertebrobasilar insufficiency, 4th ventricular tumor, demyelinating disorders, vertebrobasilar migraine
- *Temporal lobe lesion:* Vertiginous epilepsy.

Other Disorders of 8th CN

- *Chemodectoma* (Glomus jugulare)—tinnitus, vertigo, deafness—9th, 10th, 11th cranial nerve, vascular polyp ear, hemorrhagic tympanic membrane
- *Bonnier's syndrome*—vertigo, vomiting, tachycardia, contralateral hemiplegia, ipsilateral Deiter's nucleus lesion, and 9th and 10th cranial nerve.
- *Lermoyez's syndrome*—paroxysmal deafness of acute onset followed by vertigo, hearing returns to normal.

GLOSSOPHARYNGEAL AND VAGUS NERVE

It is customary to test 9th and 10th cranial nerve together, since they are having functions in common.

Neuroanatomy

Glossopharyngeal Nerve

- *Motor nucleus:* Nucleus ambiguus, situated upper lateral part of medulla.
  - Supranuclear fibers, both crossed and uncrossed fibers from motor cortex.
  - Motor supply to stylopharyngeus and middle constrictor of pharynx.
- *Parasympathetic nucleus:* Supply secretomotor fibers to parotid gland through otic ganglion.
- *Sensory component:*
  - Visceral sensory
  - Somatic sensory
  - Taste sensation

Visceral sensation and taste sensation of posterior 1/3rd of tongue to nucleus of tractus solitarius.

Sensory fibers—posterior tongue, pharynx, posterior soft palate tonsils and tympanic membrane → through spinal nucleus of trigeminal → sensory cortex.

Glossopharyngeal nerve emerges from medulla—posterior sulcus lateral to inferior olivary nucleus and along with spinal accessory leaves the skull through the jugular foramen.

Vagus Nerve

Contains motor, sensory and parasympathetic fibers
- *Motor nucleus:* Nucleus ambiguus in the medulla—fibers supply all the muscles of soft palate, pharynx and larynx except tensor palate by 5th cranial nerve, stylopharyngeus and middle constrictor by 9th cranial nerve. Supranuclear fibers, both crossed and uncrossed fibers, predominantly crossed fibers from motor cortex.
- *Sensory fibers:* Visceral sensation from pharynx, larynx, and esophagus → Nucleus of tractus solitarius
  Somatic sensory: Auricular branch—supply skin of concha of external ear → reaches the nucleus of spinal tract of 5th.
- *Parasympathetic supply:* Fibers from dorsal N supply GIT, heart, lung, and pancreas.

Symptoms of 9th and 10th Nerve Palsy

Three sets of symptoms:
1. Palatal weakness
   - Nasal tone of voice
   - Nasal regurgitation of fluid
2. Pharyngeal weakness—dysphagia—pooling of secretion in the throat
3. Laryngeal weakness—hoarseness of voice—stridor.

Clinical Examination of 9th and 10th Cranial Nerve

Motor part of 9th is difficult to test, thus the sensory and reflex function is assessed along with 10th cranial nerve.

Palatal Movement

a. ***Observe the soft palate at rest:*** Ask the patient to open the mouth, wait for a few moments, allow the tongue to rest on the floor of the mouth. This will usually make it possible to view the palate. Normally, position of uvula at the center and arches of soft palate are equal in position. If paralysis present on one side, there is sagging of arch on that side. Uvula remains deviated to normal side. If bilateral weakness present, both arches are seen at a lower level.
b. ***Voluntary movement:*** Ask the patient to say 'Ah', soft palate will move upward and backward, uvula remaining at the midline. Fatigability can be tested by repeat phonation.
c. ***Reflex movement—Gag reflex (glossopharyngeal reflex):*** Afferent—9th, efferent—10th, center—medulla.

   Tongue is gently depressed if needed with a tongue depressor, touch one side of the posterior pharyngeal wall with a cotton wool attached to throat swab and observe the complex reflex movement. Ask the patient the appreciation of touch sensation.

Normally—soft palate contract, move upward and backward
- Retraction of tongue
- Contraction of posterior pharyngeal wall
- Constriction of fauces of mouth.

Inference:
- 9th—isolated lesion—no reflex contraction, voluntary movement is normal. If both sides no sensation—unlikely organic
- Unilateral LMN lesion—ipsilateral weak contraction of soft palate, both for voluntary and reflex movement
  - Uvula will deviate to normal side
  - Contraction of posterior pharyngeal wall on one side will move the mucous membrane, to that side–called curtain sign (Vernet's Rideau phenomenon)
- Bilateral LMN—both voluntary and reflex movement are reduced on both side
- Unilateral UMN—may not manifest because of bilateral supranuclear innervation.
- Bilateral UMN—voluntary movement is reduced, reflex movement is better.

Taste of Posterior 1/3rd of Tongue

Testing the posterior 1/3rd of tongue is difficult by normal means, using a galvanic current of 2-4 mA touching the tongue will produce metallic taste which the patient is able to detect, then compare the two sides.

Pharyngeal Muscle

Pharyngeal muscle weakness is decided by the symptom of dysphagia both the solid and liquid and pooling of saliva in the throat. Demonstration of dysphagia and nasal regurgitation by allowing the patient to suck a mouth full of water and swallow it. The risk of aspiration into the trachea, may not pursuit to do this procedure.

Vocal Cord Abnormality

Vocal cord abnormality should be detected with the help of laryngoscope to know the laryngeal muscle weakness.

Disorders of 9th and 10th Cranial Nerve

Palatal Paralysis

I. **Unilateral LMN**
   a. *Acute:* Brainstem stroke—Wallenberg syndrome
      - Poliomyelitis, botulism, diphtheria
      - Jugular foramen syndrome
      - Diabetes mellitus, nonspecific mononeuritis
   b. *Chronic:* Early MND, syringobulbia, craniovertebral junction (CVJ) anomaly
      - Brainstem glioma, brainstem AVM
II. **Bilateral LMN**
   a. *Acute bilateral LMN:* GBS, botulism, diphtheria—nonspecific neuritis, polymyositis

b. *Chronic bilateral LMN*: MND, syringobulbia, CVJ anomaly, myasthenia, dystrophic myotonia oculopharyngeal myopathy.

III. ***Bilateral UMN***

Bilateral UMN: Pseudobulbar palsy, MND, upper brainstem lesion

Isolated 9th nerve palsy: It is rare, features are mild dysphagia, reduced gag reflex, loss of taste—posterior 1/3rd of tongue and anesthesia of glossopharyngeal distribution.

Other Disorders of 9th and 10th

a. *Palatal nystagmus/myoclonus*: It may occur with ocular or diaphragmatic myoclonus, rhythmic involuntary movement 50-240/mt. Lesion of Mollaret's triangle.
b. *Glossopharyngeal neuralgia (Tic douloureux of 9th)*: Unilateral neuralgia pain in the area of distribution of glossopharyngeal nerve and ear, associated with cough, increased salivation, syncope and reflex bradycardia.
c. *Jacobson's neuralgia (tympanic branch of 9th)*: Neuralgic pain of ear and Eustachian tube.
d. *Neuralgia of superior laryngeal nerve*: Pain in larynx and ear precipitated by talking and swallowing.
e. *Laryngeal spasm*: Noisy breathing, respiratory dyspnea and cyanosis, laryngeal inflammation and rickets—hypocalcemia.
f. *Epileptic cry*: Spasm of larynx at the onset of seizure
g. *Pharyngismus (cricopharyngeal spasm)*: Spasm of constrictors of pharynx—rabies.
h. *Globus hystericus*: Feeling of constriction of pharynx or foreign body sensation of throat
i. *Laryngeal crisis*: In tabes dorsalis.
j. **Recurrent laryngeal nerve palsy**
   - *Unilateral palsy:* Bronchogenic carcinoma, carcinoma thyroid, mitral stenosis, aortic aneurysm, Hodgkin's disease, tumors of neck.
   - *Bilateral palsy*: GBS, thyroidectomy, carcinoma thyroid, carcinoma esophagus.

ACCESSORY NERVE

Two parts: Cranial part—arising from the caudal part of nucleus ambiguous.

Spinal part—arising from upper 5 cervical segments—ventral horn of spinal cord.

Somatoptopic arrangement
- C1 and C2 → sternocleidomastoid (SCM)
- C3 and C4 → trapezius

Cranial and spinal part unite and leave the skull through the jugular foramen. Cranial part with vagus, supply pharyngeal and laryngeal muscles. Spinal part supply sternocleidomastoid and trapezius.

Supranuclear Innervation of Spinal Accessory

Both crossed and uncrossed fibers from the cortex.

Supranuclear fibers to trapezius—mainly crossed

Supranuclear fibers to SCM—mainly uncrossed.

Supranuclear fibers to SCM has double decussation, fibers from motor cortex, descend and cross to opposite side at pons, then return to the ipsilateral side below the first cervical level.

Thus hemispheric lesion → ipsilateral SCM and contralateral trapezius weakness.

Brainstem lesion → contralateral SCM, contralateral trapezius and contralateral limb weakness.

Focal seizure → ipsilateral contraction of SCM → deviation of head to opposite side.

Lower spinal accessory C3, C4—Trapezius alone, sparing SCM

Upper spinal accessory C1, C2—SCM alone, sparing trapezius.

Symptoms of Spinal Accessory Palsy

Wasting of SCM and trapezius, drooping of shoulder, involuntary movement like dystonia, head nodding.

Clinical Testing of Spinal Accessory Nerve

a. Observe for wasting, fasciculation, drooping of shoulder, displaced scapula—downward and laterally with winging of lateral border.
b. Sternocleidomastoid—place one hand against the right side of the patient's face and ask him to turn his head against it. The left sternocleidomastoid will standout prominently. Repeat this on the opposite direction. Compare the two sides for bulk and strength.
c. Trapezius—go behind the patient and compare the line and curves of trapezii and the position of scapula, make certain that the patient is sitting symmetrically upright. Then ask him to raise his shoulders towards his ear and the examiner tries to depress the shoulders forcibly. Normally one is able to resist the maneuver. Vertical fibers raise the shoulder and horizontal fibers shrug the shoulder.
d. Sternocleidomastoid—place one hand against the right side of the patient's face and ask him to turn his head against it. The left sternocleidomastoid will standout prominently. Repeat this on the opposite direction. Compare the two sides for bulk and strength (Fig. 3.25).

Clinical Disorders of Spinal Accessory Nerve

a. **Acute:** Poliomyelitis, GBS, polymyositis, jugular foramen syndrome.
b. **Chronic:** Dystrophia myotonica, MND, syringomyelia, CVJ anomaly, myasthenia.
c. **Torticollis:** Contraction of SCM → turning of face to opposite side.

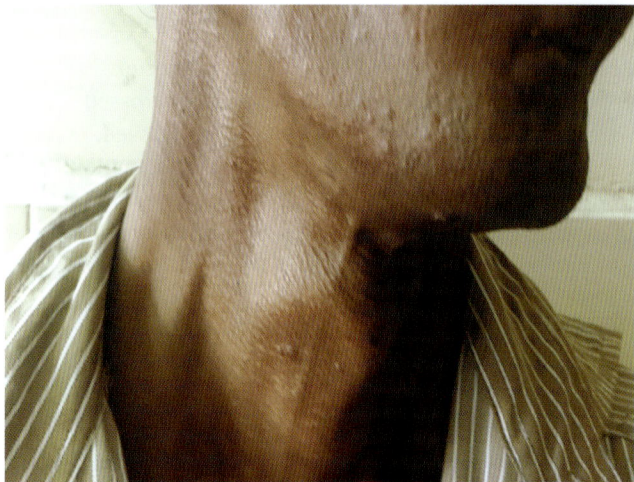

Fig. 3.25: Wasting of the sternocleidomastoid muscle.

Cause: Birth injury, congenital atrophy, paralytic, Tic and habit spasm, inflamed lymph node and focal dystonia—drug induced, encephalitis, ocular and labyrinthine lesion, conversion reaction.

d. ***Floppy head syndrome (dropped head syndrome):*** Weakness of neck extension against gravity ± neck flexion involvement as in polymyositis, GBS, myasthenia, myopathy of cervical paraspinal muscles.
Wasting of sternocleidomastoid: Goose neck appearance.

HYPOGLOSSAL NERVE

Neuroanatomy

Hypoglossal nerve arises from the hypoglossal nucleus beneath the hypoglossal trigone of 4th ventricle, travel ventrolaterally, exit form the medulla between the inferior olivary nucleus and pyramid and leaving the skull through hypoglossal foramen. It branches into lingual branches and descending hypoglossi.

Lingual branches supply—the intrinsic and extrinsic muscles of tongue except palatoglossus.

Supranuclear control of hypoglossal nerve is by both crossed and uncrossed fibers from the motor cortex, except nucleus of genioglossus which has occasionally only crossed supranuclear fibers.

Symptoms of Hypoglossal Palsy

- *Dysarthria*—both spastic and flaccid for lingual sentence, phonemes—D and T.
- *Deglutition difficulty*—1st stage of deglutition, for which the movement of tongue is required.

Clinical testing

1. Inspection—Ask the patient to open the mouth and allow the tongue to rest on the floor of the mouth, look for wasting, fasciculation, and corrugated mucosa of the surface of tongue—means atrophy of tongue. Tongue is the best site to see fasciculation since muscle fibers are directly attached to mucosa.
2. Ask the patient to protrude the tongue and do the side to side movement
   Normal—tongue in midline
   Deviation to one side—to the side of lesion—unopposed action of genioglossus.
   Difficulty in protrusion—bilateral lesion—bilateral LMN lesion → contracture and ankyloglossia—"nut in an open shell."
   Rod like tongue on protrusion—bilateral UMN lesion.
3. Ask the patient to push the inside of cheek with the tip of tongue against resistance offered by the tip of the examiner's finger, note the strength of contraction on both sides.
4. He may be asked to curl the tongue upward and downward on the lips.
5. Tapping the tongue—persistent dimple in myotonia—tapping over the protruded tongue with a small percussion hammer, wooden spatula is kept under the tongue to avoid injury.
6. Palpate the tongue—with two pieces of wet cotton
   Normal soft
   Bilateral LMN—flaccid and flabby
   Bilateral UMN—firm tongue.
7. Look for any involuntary movement like tremor, dyskinesia, and apraxia of movement.
   Fallacy: If there is facial paralysis the tongue may appear to deviate to one side due to the asymmetry of mouth. This is overcome by drawing back the corner of mouth to its normal position and compare the position of median raphe of the tongue with the central incisor.
   Few fasciculations on the surface of tongue at rest or while on protrusion is normal if no added wasting.

Clinical Disorders of 12th CN

Unilateral LMN Lesion

Tongue deviate to the affected side on protrusion. U/L wasting and fasciculation in chronic.
Lesion can be
- Acute - Poliomyelitis, brainstem stroke, median medullary syndrome, nonspecific mononeuritis, diabetes mellitus
- Chronic - Early MND, syringomyelia, foramen magnum anomaly, brainstem tumor.

Bilateral LMN

Bilateral wasting and fasciculation with weak movement can be:
- Acute—GBS, nonspecific neuritis (no wasting and fasciculation)

- Chronic
  1. Progressive bulbar palsy—MND
  2. Syringobulbia
  3. Foramen magnum anomaly
  4. Myasthenia gravis
  5. Dystrophia myotonica.

Bilateral UMN

No wasting and fasciculation, movement is weak, on protrusion it is firm rod like, firm on palpation.
- Pseudobulbar palsy
- MND
- Upper brainstem lesion.

Unilateral UMN

Deviate to one side on protrusion, no wasting and fasciculation, usually associated with same side pyramidal signs. This is due to lesion of supranuclear fibers to nucleus of genioglossus from contralateral motor cortex alone.
- Unilateral hemispheric or unilateral upper brainstem lesion as in stroke.

Difference between Pseudobulbar Palsy and Progressive Bulbar Palsy

	Pseudobulbar palsy	Progressive bulbar palsy
Lesion	UMN lesion involving corticonuclear fibers to the motor nuclei of medulla	LMN lesion involving the motor nuclei of medulla
Symptoms – Dysarthria Dysphagia, Nasal regurgitation	Spastic Less	Flaccid More
Emotional incontinence	+	–
Wasting fasciculation	–	+
Consistency of tongue	Firm and spastic	Flaccid and flabby
Jaw jerk and pyramidal signs	+	± (because in MND, combined type of lesion—both LMN and UMN)

Abnormal Movements of Tongue

1. *Tremor:*
   - Coarse, trombone like tremor of protruded tongue—neurosyphilis and alcoholism
   - Coarse tremor of Parkinsonism also affect tongue.
2. *Chorea*—alternate protrusion and retraction of tongue—jack in the box tongue
3. *Orofaciolingual dyskinesia*—phenothiazine toxicity
4. *Lingual myoclonus*—with palatal myoclonus
5. *Apraxia of tongue movement*—defective voluntary movement, automatic movement on speech, licking of lips normal
6. *Athetosis and pseudoathetosis*—deafferentation of tongue → pseudoathetosis (proprioceptive impulses of tongue is conveyed through C2 via hypoglossal nerve)
7. *Forced deviation of tongue*—part of focal seizure.
8. *Tics and habit spasm*
9. *Aphthongia*—lingual spasm occurring while speaking, similar to writer's cramp—focal dystonia.
   Lingual spasm also seen in tetanus and rabies.
   Figure 3.26 shows syndrome of multiple lower cranial nerve paralysis.

EXAMINATION OF MOTOR SYSTEM

Motor system examination is done under the following steps
- Bulk of muscle
- Tone of muscle
- Power of muscle
- Reflexes
  - Superficial
  - Deep
  - Visceral
- Coordination of movement
- Gait
- Involuntary movement.

BULK OF MUSCLE

Inspect and palpate the muscle for—normal size
- Wasting, atrophy (Fig. 3.27), fasciculation
- Contracture and deformity
- Hypertrophy—true or pseudo

Measure to assess the size of the muscle at identical points of the limbs from a bony landmark like olecranon, styloid process in the upper limb and tibial tuberosity, patella in the lower limb. A difference of 0.5 to 1.5 cm between the two sites, more on right side, is normal.

Feel of muscle—normal → semielastic
- True hypertrophy → semielastic
- Pseudohypertrophy → Tense rubbery due to increased fat content
- Wasted muscle → soft, firm if fibrosis present
- Spastic muscle → firm
- Hypotonic muscle → flabby

If wasting present—note whether:
- Neural pattern of involvement
- Radicular pattern or segmental pattern
- Proximal—distal—generalized
- Contracture
- Deformity—claw hand, wrist drop
- Claw foot, foot drop
- Pes cavus

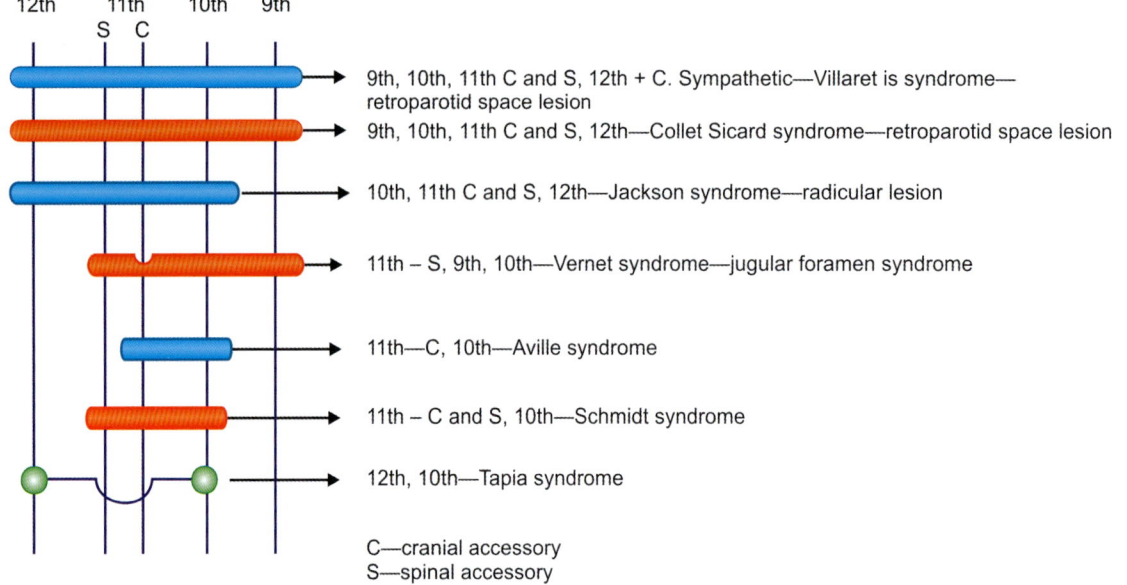

Fig. 3.26: Syndrome of multiple lower cranial nerve paralysis.

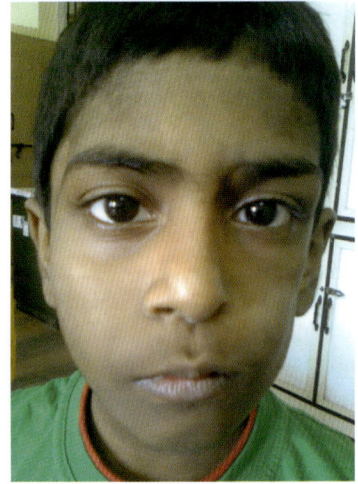

Fig. 3.27: Hemifacial atrophy (left side) in Parry Romberg syndrome.

Muscle wasting

Means loss of muscle mass followed by fibrosis.

Pathogenesis

Myogenic, arthrogenic and neurogenic
- Myogenic—muscular dystrophy, postinflammatory muscle disease like polymyositis
- Arthrogenic—Rheumatoid arthritis, osteoarthrosis
- *Neurogenic*
  - Anterior horn cell
    - Anterior root
    - Plexus
    - Peripheral nerves
  - UMN disuse
  - Parietal lobe lesion

Types of Wasting

Generalized

- Non-neurological
  - Internal malignancy
  - Thyrotoxicosis
- Neurological
  - Muscular dystrophy
  - MND

Proximal Muscle Wasting

- Muscular dystrophy
  - Facioscapulohumeral muscular dystrophy
  - Limb girdle dystrophy (Figs. 3.28 and 3.30)
- Proximal spinal muscular atrophy (SMA)—Kugelberg-Welander syndrome (juvenile proximal SMA)
- Motor neuron disease
- Proximal myopathy—thyrotoxicosis, acromegaly
- Neuralgic amyotrophy
- Posterior GBS
- Polymyositis
- Radicular lesion—proximal wasting as in cervical spondylosis, intervertebral disc prolapse (IVDP) and secondary spine.

Distal Muscle Wasting

Hand (Figs. 3.29 and 3.31)
Wasting of small muscles of hand. It is of 2 groups:
- **With pyramidal sign**

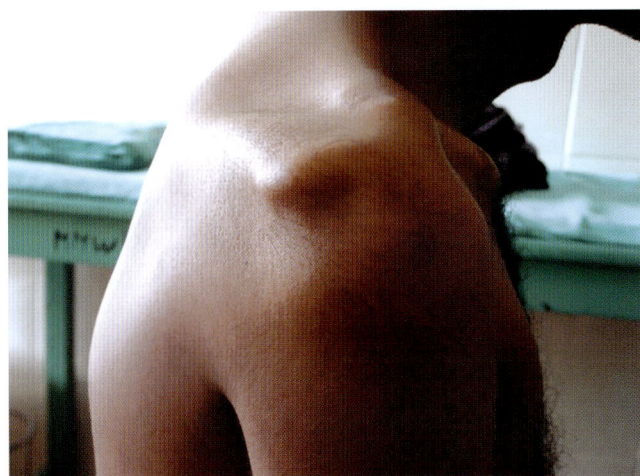

Fig. 3.28: Wasting of supraspinatus, infraspinatus and deltoid muscles in limbgirdle muscular dystrophy.

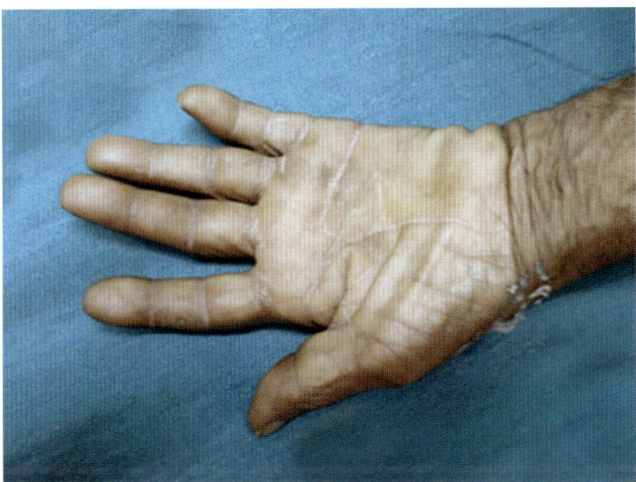

Fig. 3.29: Wasting of the small muscles of hand.

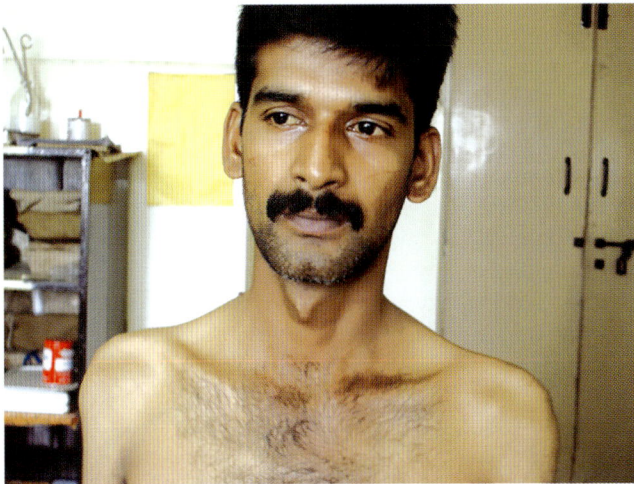

Fig. 3.30: Wasting of pectoral girdle muscles, biceps in limb girdle muscular dystrophy.

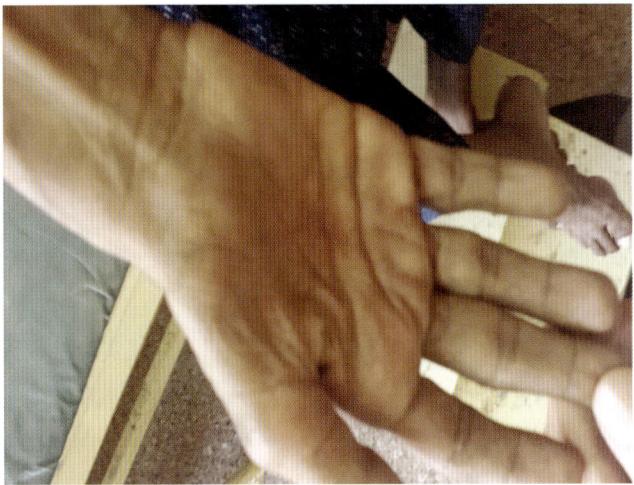

Fig. 3.31: Wasting of small muscles of hand.

- Amyotrophic lateral sclerosis
- Syringomyelia/intramedullary lesion
- Cervical spondylosis
- Extramedullary compressive myelopathy—cervical region
- Cranial pachymeningitis—syphilis—idiopathic

- **Without pyramidal sign**
   a. Myogenic—distal muscular dystrophy—bilateral dystrophia myotonica—bilateral
   b. Arthrogenic—rheumatoid arthritis—bilateral
   c. Neurogenic
      i. Peripheral nerve-
         Carpel tunnel syndrome unilateral, bilateral
         Hansen's disease—unilateral, bilateral
         Charcot-Marie-Tooth (CMT) disease—bilateral
      ii. Root—posterior GBS—bilateral
      iii. Anterior Horn cell—distal SMA—bilateral

Leg and foot—**muscle wasting (Fig. 3.32)**
- Distal muscular dystrophy—dystrophia myotonica
- Rheumatoid arthritis
- Motor—peripheral neuropathy—CMT
- Cauda equina lesion—roots of distal muscle
- Posterior GBS
- Distal SMA

Wasting of Muscles of Both Upper and Lower Limb (Fig. 3.33)

- CMT and other motor peripheral neuropathy
- Distal muscular dystrophy of Gower's
- Dystrophia myotonica
- Posterior GBS
- Distal SMA
- Rheumatoid arthritis.

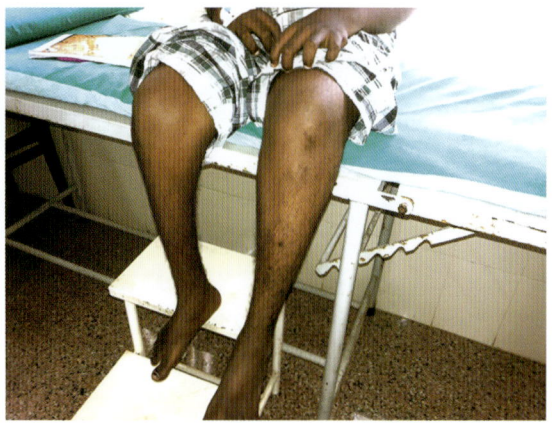

Fig. 3.32: Wasting of the leg muscle in peroneal muscular atrophy (Charcot-Marie-Tooth disease).

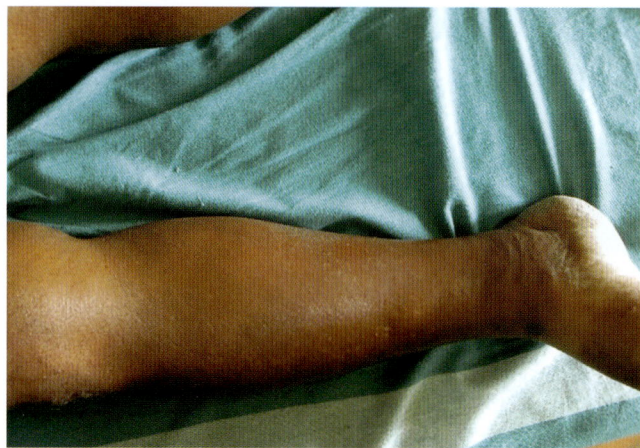

Fig. 3.34: Hypertrophy of calf muscle in hypothyroidism.

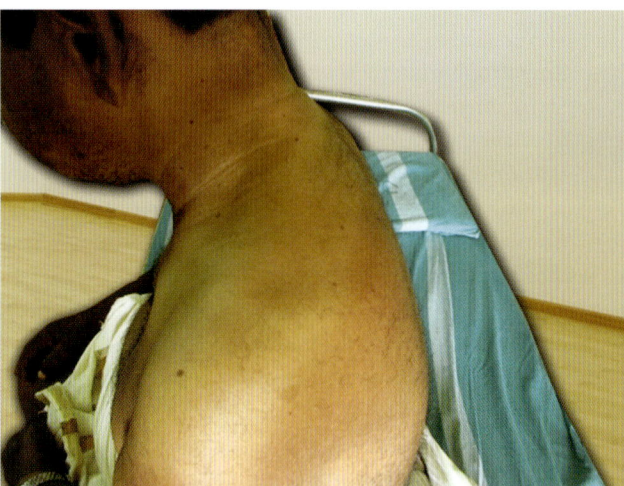

Fig. 3.33: Wasting of pectoral girdle muscles.

Hypertrophy of Muscle

- Physiological
- Hypertrophia musculorum vera of Oppenheim—benign hypertrophy of limb muscle
- Pseudohypertrophy—Duchenne muscular dystrophy—calf, glutei, thigh and shoulder muscle
- Hypothyroidism (Fig. 3.34)—Hoffmann's syndrome—calf and glutei muscle
- Acromegaly—all groups of muscles
- Congenital hemihypertrophy
- Myotonia congenita—Thomsen's disease.

Tone of Muscle

Definition: Resistance to passive movement, when voluntary control is absent. Tension of muscle is due to static reflex activity when they are relaxed, this depends on the integrity of muscle, neuromuscular junction, LMN-α, γ and internuncial neurons of spinal cord, UMN, basal ganglia and cerebellum.

Examination of Tone

Try to secure the complete co-operation of the patient, who should be comfortable and relaxed. Full range of movement at the major joints are done to assess the resistance to passive movement.

Change in tone can be observed by
- Resistance to passive movement
- Abnormal position of limbs
- Palpate the muscle for the consistency
- Lift the limb and allow to fall

Testing Tone in Upper Limb

Passive flexion and extension movement from wrist to proximal joints. Raise each arm in turn and allow to fall on to the bed noting the checking movement against the fall.

Testing Tone in Lower Limb

Roll the limb with the palm on the shin, this gives an initial assessment of the tone of hip muscles, proceed with passive flexion and extension of ankle, knee and hip joint, raise the leg and allow to fall, noting the checking movement.

Clinical abnormality of tone

- Hypotonia
- Hypertonia:
  - Spasticity
  - Rigidity
    - Lead pipe type
    - Cogwheel type
- Paratonia.

Hypotonia

Demonstrated by decrease in resistance to passive movement-hypermobility of joint—flabbiness of muscle to feel—liveless fall of limbs once the raised limb is allowed to fall.

Causes

Neurological
- LMN lesion—GBS, polio (efferent arc damage)
- Acute UMN lesion
- Cerebellar disease
- Chorea
- Myopathy—muscular dystrophy
- Myasthenia gravis
- Tabes dorsalis (afferent arc damage)
- Periodic paralysis, cataplexy, sleep paralysis.
- *Non-neurological*—mongolism—cretinism, etc.

Hypertonia

Spasticity: It is a sign of pyramidal lesion called clasp knife spasticity.

Resistance to passive movement only in the initial part of movement, then it gives way like clasp knife—quick movement is better to elicit spasticity.

In the upper limb, spasticity first appears in pronators of forearm and then in adductors of shoulder, flexors of elbow, flexors of wrist and fingers.

In the lower limb, spasticity first appears in the adductors of thigh and then in extensors of knee, plantar flexors and invertors.

Clasp knife spasticity is better demonstrated at knee joint by flexion.

Rigidity—hypertonia due to extrapyramidal lesion, i.e. resistance throughout the range of movement called lead pipe rigidity, equal resistance in both agonists and antagonists groups.

If agonist and antagonist group contract alternatively, regularly and rapidly, it is called *Cogwheel rigidity* → both rigidity and tremor present as in Parkinsonism. Cogwheel rigidity is better demonstrated by the movement of wrist joint and neck. Rigidity is better elicited with slow movement.

Paratonia

Progressive increase in resistance on movement—seen in frontal lobe lesion, called Gegenhalten phenomenon.

Myotonia

Definition: This is a state in which the contraction continues beyond the period required for a particular movement with a delay in relaxation.

Demonstration: Hand grip test—slow relaxation of hand muscles after a strong grip. Repeating the movement several times may overcome the myotonia.

Tapping with a reflex hammer over the thenar eminence will produce opposition of thumb and will persist for several seconds.

Tapping over the other muscles like deltoid or tongue → dimple that disappears slowly.

Causes:
- Myotonia congenita
- Dystrophia myotonica
- Paramyotonia

Myotatic irritability—percussion over the normal muscle → brisk feeble contraction. Myotatic irritability is increased in wasting diseases and LMN disorders.

Myoedema

A small ridge of temporary swelling is noted at the point of stimulation by percussion hammer and this persists for several seconds.

Causes—cachexia, hypothyroidism.

POWER OF MUSCLE (FIGS. 3.35 AND 3.36)

While testing muscle power the examiner should note the following:
a. Cooperation of the patient is a must, movement should be smooth, agreeable to the patient. Demonstrate the movement rather than explaining it, since the patient does not know the anatomy.
b. Examiner should remember:
   - Muscle or group of muscles tested
   - Segmental nerve supply
   - Peripheral nerve supply
   - Grade of weakness
   - Weakness constant or variable
   - Power equal or unequal on both sides
   - Test muscle should be palpated for contraction
   - Look for any painful condition—injury, infection or mechanical defect like ankylosis of joint.

Grading of Muscle Power (by Medical Research Council Scale)

Grade 0—No muscular contraction
Grade 1—Flicker or trace of contraction without movement, contraction can be palpated
Grade 2—Muscle contracts and can move the part when gravity is eliminated
Grade 3—Muscle contracts and can move the part against gravity
Grade 4—Muscle contracts and can move the part against gravity and variable amount of resistance
Grade 5—Muscle contracts and can move the part against maximum amount of resistance several times without signs of fatigue.

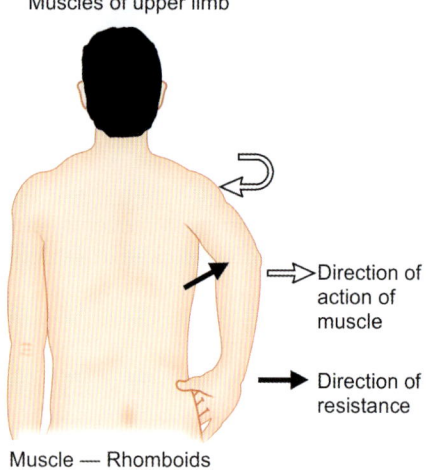

A Muscle — Rhomboids
Spinal segment — C_5
Peripheral nerve — N to rhomboids
Test — Hand on hip, the patient tries to force his elbow backwards feel the contraction of rhomboids

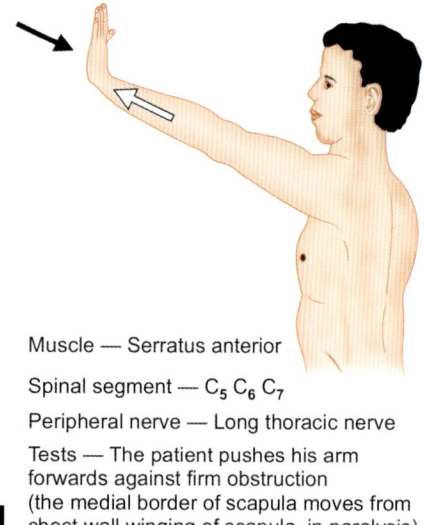

B Muscle — Serratus anterior
Spinal segment — C_5 C_6 C_7
Peripheral nerve — Long thoracic nerve
Tests — The patient pushes his arm forwards against firm obstruction (the medial border of scapula moves from chest wall winging of scapula–in paralysis)

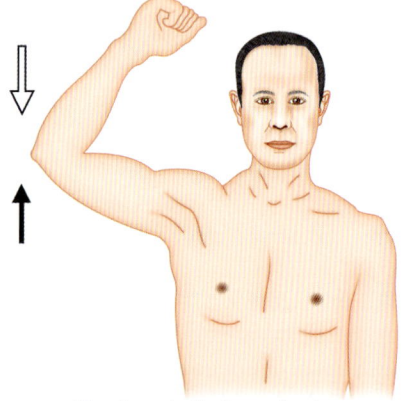

C Muscle — Latissimus dorsi
Spinal segment — C_6 C_7 C_8
Peripheral nerve — subscapular nerve
Test — Resist the patient's attempt to adduct the arm when abducted to above 90°, feel the post: fold of axilla for muscle contraction

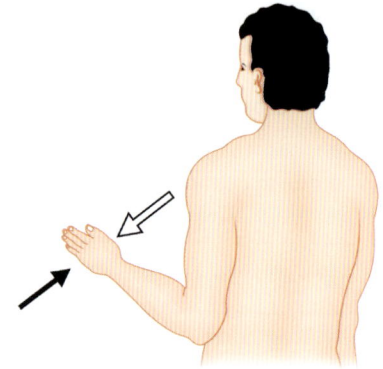

D Muscle — infraspinatus
Spinal segment — C_4 C_5 C_6
Peripheral nerve — Suprascapular nerve
Test — with the elbow flexed at the side, the arm is externally rotated against resistance on the forearm, feel the contraction of the muscle

Figs. 3.35A to D

Method of Testing

- Test of power can be carried out in two ways:
  a. The patient first completes the movement and then tries to maintain the muscle in full contraction while the examiner tries to overcome it.
  b. The examiner resists the movement throughout the whole of the patient's attempt to carry it out. This may detect even mild degrees of weakness.
- Testing muscles of upper limb
- Testing muscles of lower limb
- Testing muscles of trunk (refer Figs. 3.35 and 3.36 for testing the muscles)

Types and Pattern of Muscle Weakness

Types

a. **UMN lesion:** Pyramidal tract lesion
   - Movement is affected rather than muscles
   - Weakness is marked in extensors of upper limb and flexors of lower limb
   - Spasticity + hyper-reflexia

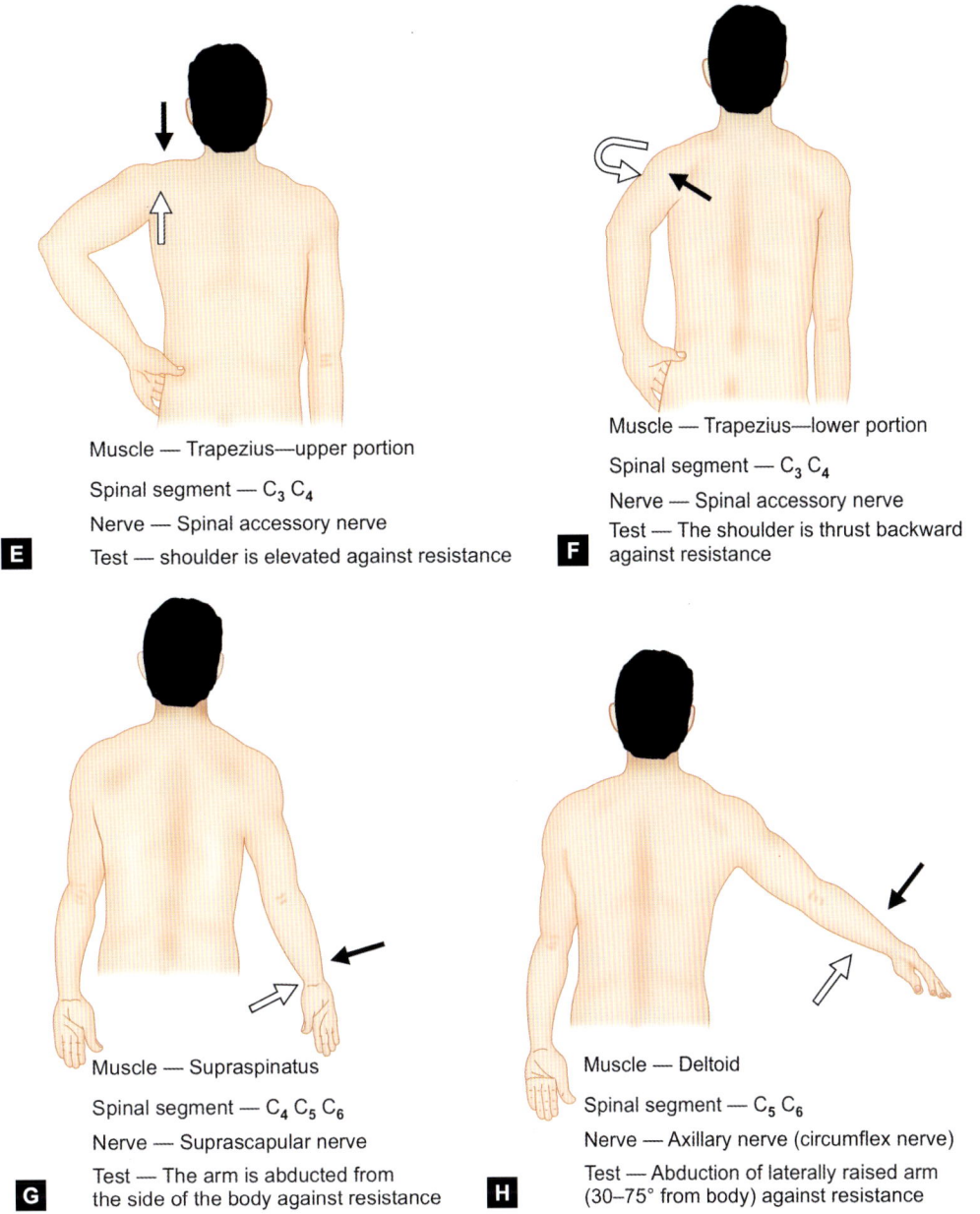

Figs. 3.35E to H

b. ***LMN lesion:*** Segmental pattern or neural pattern of muscle weakness
   - Hyporeflexia and hypotonia
   - Wasting, fasciculation and contracture
c. ***Myasthenic weakness:*** Pattern of involvement—ocular, bulbar and limb weakness.
   - Fatigability demonstrable, putting the test muscle for continuous action for 30 seconds, holding outstretched hand or looking up for 30 seconds, watch the fall of hand or drooping of eyelids.
d. ***Myopathic weakness:*** Often affects proximal muscles, pelvi femoral > pectoral girdle muscles
   - Involved muscles—atrophy or pseudohypertrophy
   - Hyporeflexia related to involved muscles
   - No fasciculation, tenderness present in polymyositis.

Pattern of Weakness

a. *Monoplegia*—paralysis of muscles of one limb—UMN or LMN/crural, brachial
b. *Hemiplegia*—paralysis of muscles of one side of the body involving upper limb, lower limb and also face → facio-brachio crural paralysis—usually UMN lesion.
c. Crossed hemiplegia—ipsilateral LMN cranial nerve palsy, contralateral limb weakness—UMN lesion—pyramidal lesion.

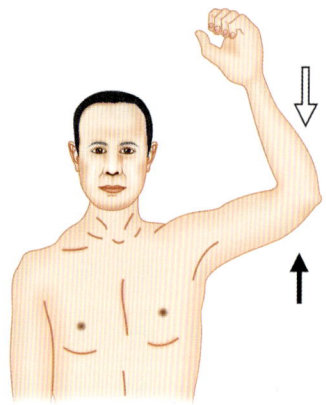

Muscle — Pectoralis major—upper portion

Spinal segment — C_5 C_6 C_7 C_8 (clavicular part)

Nerves — Lateral and medial pectoral nerves

Test — The arm is adducted from an elevated and forward position above 90° against resistance

I

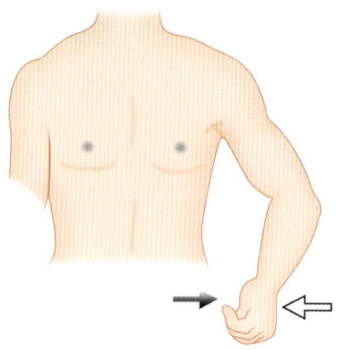

Muscle — Pectoralis major—lower portion (sternocostal part)

Spinal segment — C_5 C_6 C_7 C_8 T_1

Nerves — Lateral and medial pectoral nerves

Test — The arm is adducted from forward position below horizontal against resistance

J

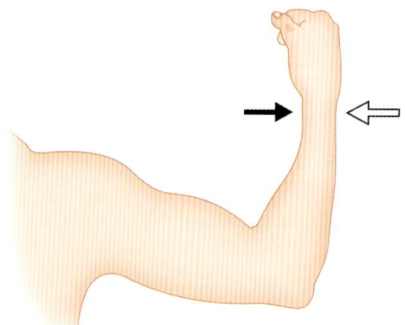

Muscle — Biceps

Spinal segment — C_5 C_6

Nerve — Musculocutaneous nerve

Test — The supinated forearm is flexed against resistance

K

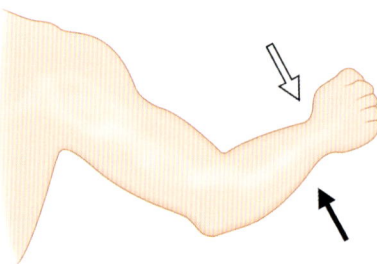

Muscle — Triceps

Spinal segment — C_5 C_6 C_8

Nerves — Radial nerves

Test — The forearm, flexed at the elbow, is extended against resistance

L

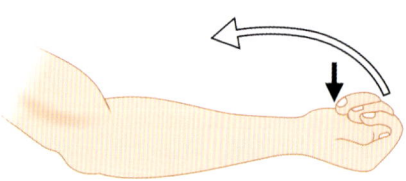

Muscle — Flexors of wrist

Spinal segment — C_6 C_7 C_8

Nerves — Median and ulnar nerves

Test — Flexion of hand at the wrist against resistance

M

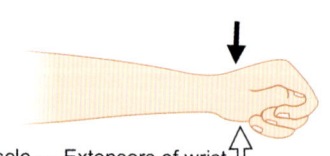

Muscle — Extensors of wrist

Spinal segment — C_6 C_7 C_8

Nerve — Radial nerve

Test — Extension of hand at the wrist against resistance

N

Figs. 3.35I to N

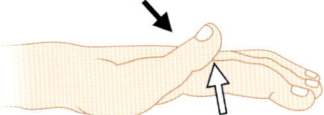

Muscle — Extensor pollicis longus
Spinal segment — C_7 C_8
Nerve — Radial nerve
Test — The thumb is extended against resistance at distal phalanx

O

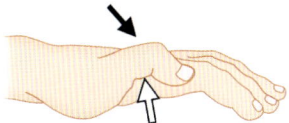

Muscle — Extensor pollicis brevis
Spinal segment — C_7 C_8
Nerve — Radial nerve
Test — The thumb is extended at the metacarpophalangeal joint against resistance, keep the distal phalanx flexed

P

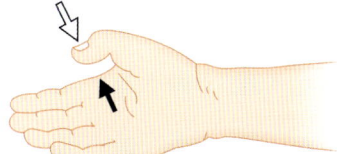

Muscle — Flexor pollicis longus
Spinal segment — C_7 C_8 T_1
Nerve — Median nerve
Test — The terminal phalanx of the thumb is flexed against resistance

Q

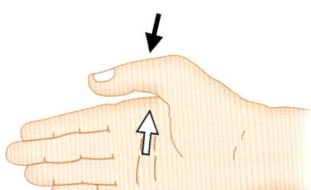

Muscle — Flexor pollicis brevis
Spinal segment — C_7 C_8 T_1
Nerve — Median nerve
Test — The proximal phalanx of the thumb is flexed against resistance, keep the distal phalanx exterted.

R

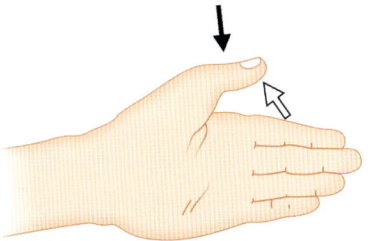

Muscle — Abductor pollicis longus
Spinal segment — C_7 C_8 T_1
Nerve — Radial nerves
Test — Radial abduction of the thumb. The patient attempts to abduct the thumb in the same plane as that of the palm

S

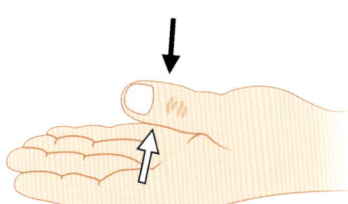

Muscle — Abductor pollicis brevis
Spinal segment — C_7 C_8 T_1
Nerve — Median nerves
Test — Palmar abduction of the thumb. The thumb is abducted against resistance in a plane at right angle to the palmar surface

T

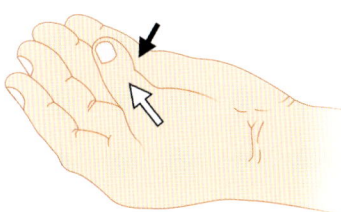

Muscle — Opponens pollicis
Spinal segment — C_8 C_1
Nerve — Median nerve
Test — The thumb is crossed over the palm against resistance to touch the top of the little finger

U

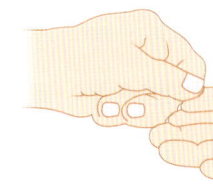

Muscle — Adductor pollicis
Spinal segment — C_8 T_1
Nerve — Ulnar nerve
Test — A piece of paper grasped between the palm and the thumb is held against resistance with the thumb nail kept at right angle to the palm

V

Figs. 3.35O to V

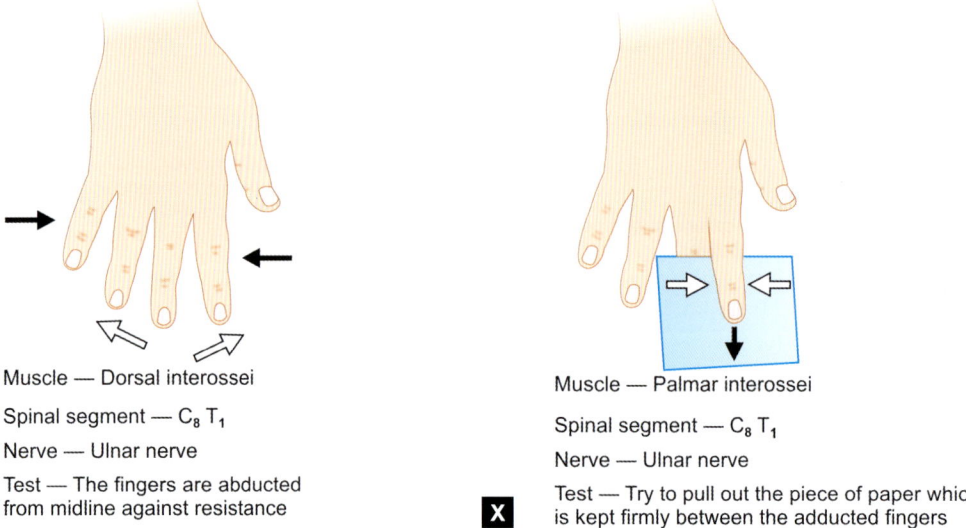

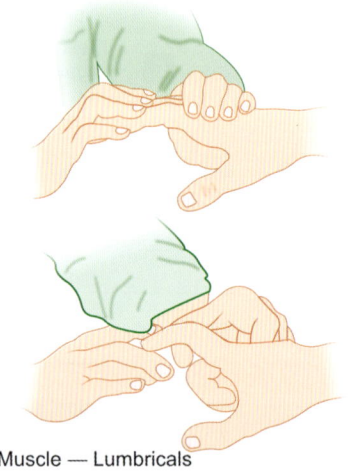

Figs. 3.35W to Y

Figs. 3.35A to Y: Method of testing—muscles of upper limb.

d. *Paraplegia*—paralysis of muscles of both lower limbs—UMN or LMN lesion.
e. *Quadriplegia*—paralysis of muscles of all the four limbs and trunk—LMN or UMN lesion.
f. *Neural pattern of paralysis*—paralysis of muscles innervated by peripheral nerve.
   I. Mononeuropathy—single nerve pattern
   II. Polyneuropathy—mononeuritis multiplex → multiple peripheral nerves in an asymmetrical pattern peripheral neuropathy—distal symmetrical pattern.

REFLEXES

Reflex is an adaptive response to the stimulation of a sense organ, which involves the center, afferent and efferent fibers to connect this center with the receptor and effector organ, response may be motor, secretory or visceral.

For the purpose of clinical examination, reflexes are classified into:
- Superficial reflexes
- Deep reflexes
- Visceral reflexes—sphincteric reflexes

Muscles of lower limb

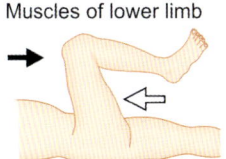
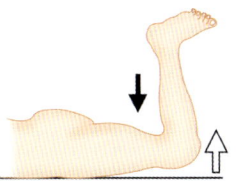
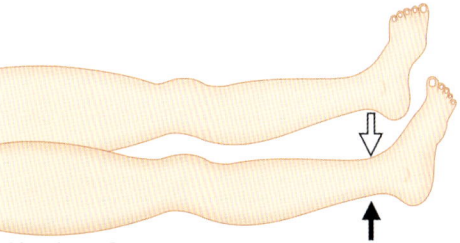

A
Muscle — Flexors of hip joint (Iliopsoas)
Spinal segment — L_1, L_2, L_3
Nerve — Femoral nerve
Test — The patient lies supine the thigh is flexed against resistance

Muscle — Extensors of hip joint (Gluteus maximus)
Spinal segment — L_4, L_5, S_1, S_2
Nerve — Inferior gluteal nerve
Test — With the subject prone, knee is lifted off the bed against resistance

B
Muscle — Gluteus maximus
Spinal segment — L_4, L_5, S_1, S_2
Nerve — Inferior gluteal nerve
Test — The patient lies supine, the heel of the straight leg is lifted with the palm of the examiner, push down the heel against resistance

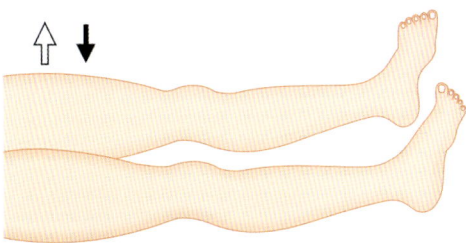
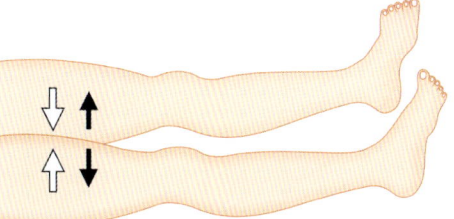

C
Muscle — Abductors of hip joint
Spinal segment — L_4, L_5, S_1
Nerve — Superior gluteal nerve
Test — The patient lies supine, both thighs are abducted against resistance

D
Muscle — Adductors of hip joints
Spinal segment — L_2, L_3, L_4
Nerve — Obturator nerve
Test — The patient lies supine, both thighs are adducted against resistance

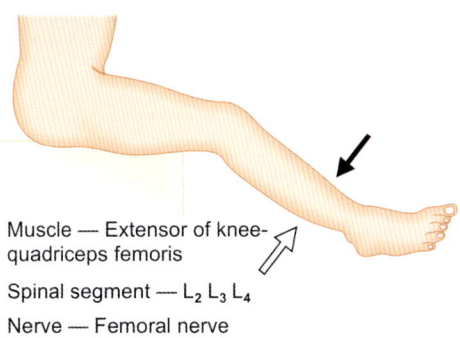
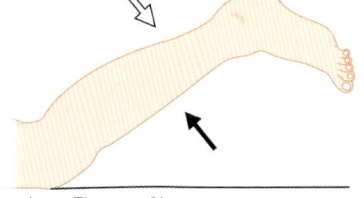

E
Muscle — Extensor of knee-quadriceps femoris
Spinal segment — L_2, L_3, L_4
Nerve — Femoral nerve
Test — The knee is extended against resistance on the leg

F
Muscle — Flexors of knee-Hamstrings group
Spinal segment — L_4, L_5, S_1, S_2
Nerve — Sciatic nerve
Test — With the patient prone, the knee is flexed against resistance

Figs. 3.36A to F

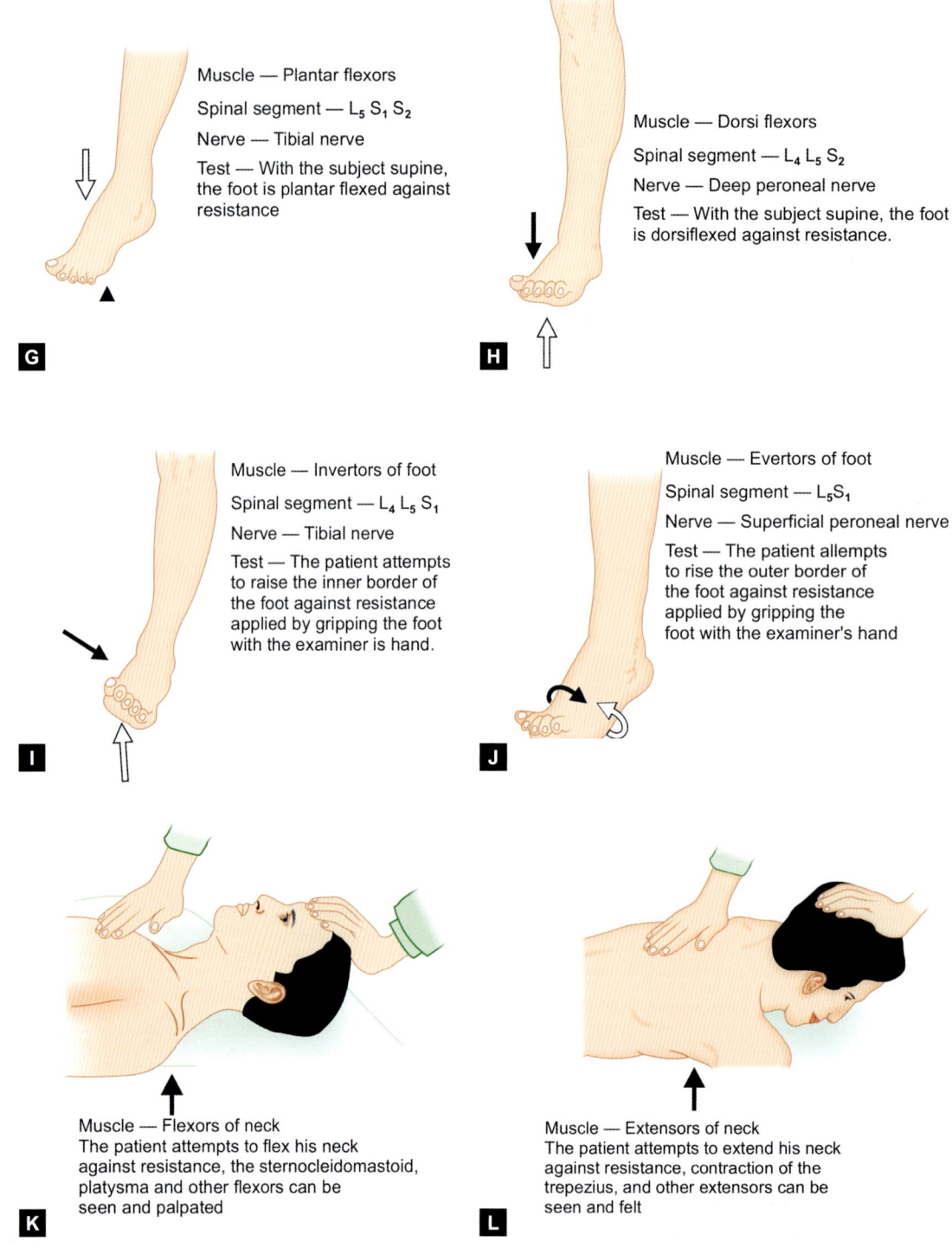

Figs. 3.36G to L

Figs. 3.36A to L: Method of testing—muscles of lower limb.

Superficial Reflexes

Reflexes elicited by stimulation of skin or mucous membrane, they are polysynaptic also, e.g. abdominal reflex, cremasteric reflex.

Corneal and Conjunctival Reflex

Refer 5th cranial nerve.

Superficial Abdominal Reflex

Center—D7 to D12 spinal segments.

Afferent—posterior root and efferent—anterior root of spinal nerves D7 to D12.

Method: The patient should lie flat, palpate the abdomen gently to assess the degree of relaxation and sensitivity of the skin. Then explain the procedure and illustrate on the chest. Any physician who has unexpectedly had his abdominal reflexes examined will appreciate the value of this warning. Lightly stroke the abdomen with a key or two point discriminator from without inwards, stimulating each of the four quadrants of the abdomen.

Normal response: Muscles in the quadrant stimulated, contract and the umbilicus moves in that direction.

Abnormal responses:
- Obese, multiparous female—Response absent.
- Pyramidal lesion—Response reduced or absent on the side of lesion
- Lesion of reflex arc—Polio, herpes—segmental loss of response.
- Paraplegia lesion anywhere between D7 and D12—Loss of reflex on involved quadrant.
- Retained abdominal reflex with pyramidal lesion—Cerebral diplegia, MND and subacute combined degeneration
- Early loss of abdominal reflex—Disseminated sclerosis
- Over response—Parkinsonism and psychoneurosis-umbilicus seems to chase the stimulus
- Easily fatigued reflex—Repeated stimulation → absent or poor response.

Cremasteric Reflex

Center—L1 and L2 spinal segment.
    Afferent—ilioinguinal nerve
    Efferent—genitofemoral nerve.

Method: Upper inner part of the thigh is stroked in a downward and inward direction, in the supine position, watch the movement of testicle and scrotum.

Normal response: The contraction of the cremasteric muscle pulls up the scrotum and the testicle upwards on the side examined.

Abnormal responses
- Absence of reflex—elderly, pyramidal lesion, any breach of reflex arc
- Local diseases like hydrocele, epididymo-orchitis
- Superficial abdominal reflex and cremasteric reflex—are absent in pyramidal lesion, these are polysynaptic reflexes, the afferent fibers extend to cortex, descending fibers to anterior horn cells are through or close to pyramidal tract. Thus in pyramidal lesion, the reflex arc is disrupted.

Plantar Reflex (Figs. 3.37 and 3.38)

Center—L5–S1 spinal segments
Afferent and efferent—L5–S1 posterior and anterior roots.

Method: One of the important clinical sign in neurology. The patient lies supine, educate the patient about the procedure, fix the ankle joint so as to avoid withdrawal of foot, the internal aspect of the sole is firmly stroked with a blunt point

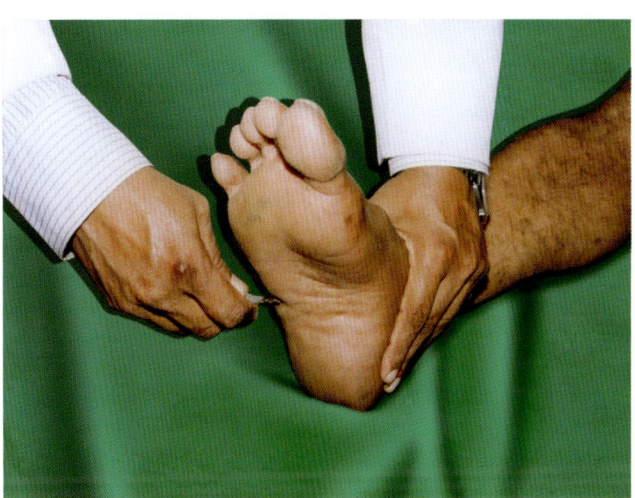

Fig. 3.37: The plantar reflex flexor response.

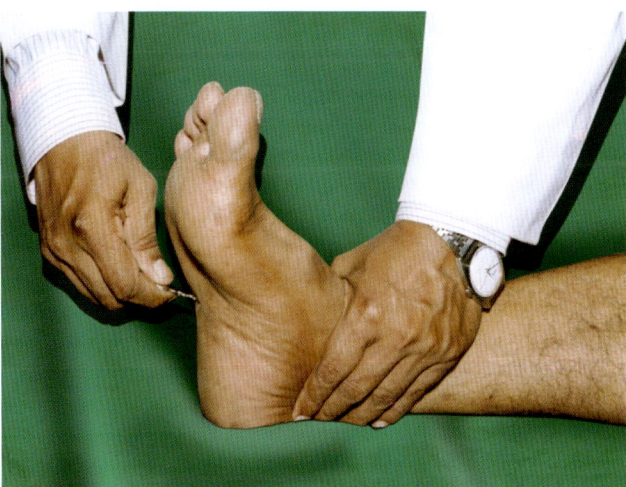

Fig. 3.38: The plantar reflex extensor response.

such as a key or end of the percussion hammer handle, from the heel to metatarsophalangeal joint, then curve medially along the metatarsal pad up to the middle metatarsophalangeal joint. The noxious stimuli is applied, which should not be too speedy or slow. Strong stimuli is given if the skin over the sole of foot is thick, otherwise no response is obtained.

Normal response: Flexor plantar response. Components of flexor plantar response are—flexion of big toe and other toes, dorsiflexion and inversion, adduction of thigh and contraction of tensor fascia lata.

Abnormal responses
a. ***Extensor plantar response***—Babinski's sign
 Components are—extension of big toe, extension of other toes and fanning, dorsiflexion and eversion, flexion of knee and hip joint. The only visible response may be dorsiflexion of big toe, contraction of other muscles can be felt by palpation.
b. ***Equivocal response***—Variation in response, it is incomplete flexor response or failure of big toe to move up or down in mild pyramidal lesion.
c. ***Zero response***—No response on stimulation, due to
 Spinal shock
 No reflex activity
 Sensory loss of receptor zone—S1 segment
 Thick skin on sole of foot
 Inflammatory disease of joints of foot-like rheumatoid arthritis.
d. ***Minimal response***—While eliciting plantar reflex, contraction of hamstring muscle (flexors of knee) can be felt.
e. ***Withdrawal response***—In individuals with over sensitive skin or sensory peripheral neuropathy, with hyperesthesia or painful stimulation—can produce rapid dorsiflexion of the ankle, flexion of knee and hip at the beginning of the delivery of stimuli.
f. ***Inversion of plantar response or peripheral extensor plantar response***—When short flexors of foot are paralyzed, the stimuli for plantar reflex will produce extensor response. This is because normally, both plantar flexors and dorsiflexors are contracting simultaneously while eliciting the reflex. Intact pyramidal system produces flexor response. Extensor response occurs when pyramidal dysfunction or damage is present. When plantar flexors are paralyzed, there is extensor response even without pyramidal lesion. Similarly when the dorsiflexors and evertors are paralyzed by an LMN lesion, reflex response will be flexor even in the presence of pyramidal lesion.
g. ***Pseudoextensor response (pseudo-Babinski's sign)***—Dyskinesia like athetosis or chorea can produce false extensor response due to dyskinetic movement of extensor group of muscles. But no hamstring muscle contraction as in true extensor plantar response.
h. ***Crossed extensor response***—Bilateral extensor response on unilateral stimulation in patient with bilateral cerebral or spinal cord lesion.

Other methods of elicitation of plantar response: Once the reflex receptor zone is widened over the lower limb, stimuli can be applied at other places of lower limb to elicit the plantar reflex.
- Chaddock's sign—Stimuli given around the lateral malleolus
- Oppenheim's sign—Apply heavy pressure with the thumb and index finger over the medial side of the shin of tibia
- Gordon's sign—squeezing or deep pain to the calf muscles
- Schaeffer's sign—Deep pressure over the tendo-Achilles.

Significance of extensor plantar response or Babinski's sign
a. Sign of pyramidal lesion above L5
b. Children below the age of 2—Before myelination is complete
c. Coma and deep sleep
d. Postictal phenomenon
e. Hepatocellular failure—Pyramidal dysfunction.

Anal Reflex

Center—S2, S3, S4
Spinal segment—inferior hemorrhoidal nerve.
Contraction of anal sphincter in response to stimulation of perianal skin by stroking or scratching. Contraction of external anal sphincter can be felt with a gloved finger at the anus.

Bulbocavernosus Reflex

Center—S3, S4; spinal segments—pudendal nerve
Pinching the dorsum of glans penis produce contraction of bulbocavernosus which can be felt by the hand placed over the perineum below the root of penis.

Loss of anal reflex and bulbocavernosus reflex is seen in lesion of reflex arc due to lower spinal cord disease.

Deep Reflexes

Muscle stretch reflex—Deep tendon reflex
Muscle stretch reflex is a monosynaptic reflex, muscle spindle is the receptor, and proprioceptive impulses carried through the afferent limb formed by peripheral nerves and posterior root, synapse with the anterior horn cell, through the anterior root and peripheral nerve which forms the efferent limb innervating the muscle. Reflex is elicited by the sudden stretch of muscle on application of stimulus to tendon or periosteum. Reflex carrying afferent fibers are large and fast conducting, vulnerable for easy damage by insult like pressure, inflammation or demyelination. This produces loss of reflex. Overstretch of muscle, stimulate Golgi tendon apparatus which inhibit the reflex activity.

Rubber percussion hammer is used to elicit the reflex. The stimulus should be quick, direct, with sufficient threshold, position of the part of the body to be tested should be optimum for the sufficient tone in the muscle for the briskness of reflex. Position of the two sides of the body should be identical to compare the reflex.

Grading of Muscle Stretch Reflex

Graded according to the response on the basis of speed of response, amplitude of movement and duration of response.
Grade 0—No response—areflexia
Grade 1+—Response present with diminished contraction—hyporeflexia
Grade 2+—Normal contraction and quick disappearance
Grade 3+—Exaggerated response—speed of response, amplitude of movement, and Duration of response is increased.
Grade 4+ —above + clonus.

Reinforcement of the Reflexes

Jendrassik maneuver: If a tendon reflex appears reduced or absent it can be physiological, the reflex response can be augmented by reinforcement—by method of Jendrassik. This will activate the γ motor neurons and increase the static reflex activity.

For testing the tendon reflexes of lower limbs the patient interlock the flexed fingers of the two hands and pulls one against the other at the moment the reflex is elicited. For upper limbs, the patient should clench his teeth tightly or while examining one arm, clench the fist of the other.

Jaw Jerk

Refer 5th cranial nerve.

Muscle Stretch Reflex of Upper Limb

Biceps Reflex (Fig. 3.39)
- Spinal segment → C5 & C6
- Peripheral nerve → Musculocutaneous nerve

Method: Keep the forearm partially flexed and partially supinated, upper limb completely relaxed and resting on the abdomen. Press the forefinger gently on the biceps tendon and strike on the finger with the hammer.

Normal response: Flexion of elbow and visible contraction of biceps muscle.

Supinator Reflex (Fig. 3.40)
- Spinal segment → C5, C6
- Peripheral nerve → Radial nerve

Method: The position of upper limb is same as that for biceps reflex. Strike the lower end of radius proximal to styloid process—2" above the wrist. Watch the movement of forearm and fingers.

Normal response: Contraction of brachioradialis and flexion of elbow, slight flexion of wrist and fingers. Other components are supination and adduction of forearm. Normally flexion of elbow and supination of forearm are well visible. All component become visible when the reflex is exaggerated.

Inversion of supinator reflex: Flexion of wrist and fingers without flexion of elbow and supination of forearm. Biceps reflex is also absent. Lesion in C5, C6 segment, UMN features below C5, C6 level.

Triceps Reflex (Fig. 3.41)
- Spinal segment → C6, C7
- Peripheral nerve → Radial nerve

Method: By holding the patient's wrist, draw the fore-arm across the abdomen, so that elbow is kept flexed at 90° and allow to lie loosely in the new position. Strike the triceps tendon at about 2" above the elbow. Care not to strike the muscle belly. Normal response—visible contraction of triceps and extension of the elbow.

Paradoxical triceps reflex: Flexion of forearm instead of extension due to damage of reflex arc of triceps and irradiation of impulses produce contraction of biceps unopposed by the triceps.

Finger Flexion Reflex
- Spinal segment → C8, T1
- Peripheral nerve → Median and Ulnar nerves

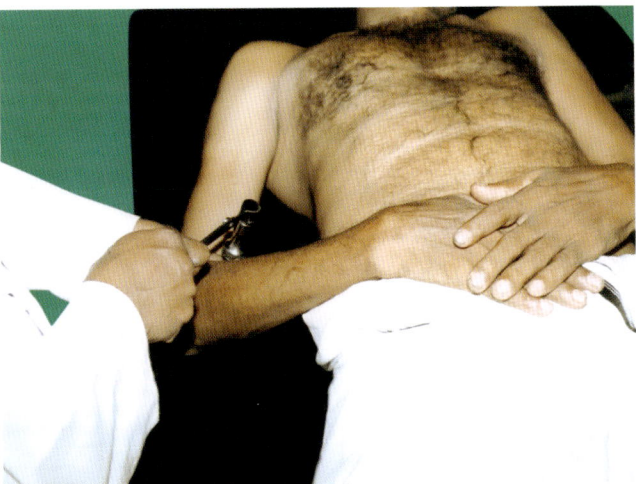

Fig. 3.39: The biceps jerk.

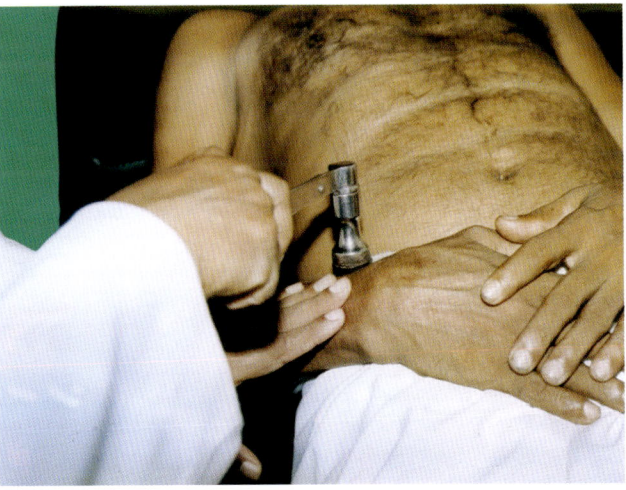

Fig. 3.40: The supinator jerk.

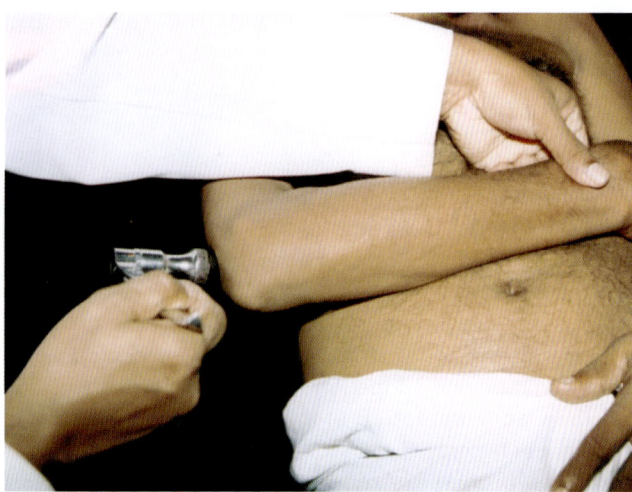

Fig. 3.41: The triceps jerk.

Method: Allow the patient's hand to rest, palm upwards on the side of the cot and the fingers are slightly flexed. The examiner places his middle and index fingers on the volar surface of the phalanges of the first four fingers, tap on his own finger with the hammer.

Normal response: Flexion of the patient's four fingers and distal phalanx of thumb. Wartenberg considered it as one of the most important reflexes of the upper limb.

Muscle Stretch Reflexes of Lower Limb

Knee Jerk (Fig. 3.42)
- Spinal segment → L2, L3, L4
- Peripheral nerve → Femoral nerve.

Method: The left arm of the right handed examiner is placed under both knees in order to flex them together to 30–45° and expose quadriceps muscle. Instruct the patient to relax the limb muscle by allowing his knee to rest completely on your hand. The patellar tendon can then be struck lightly on each side, increasing the strength of stimuli if there is no response. Light tap is best for comparing the two sides. Watch for the contraction of quadriceps and extension of knee. Another method is to seat the patient on the edge of the couch so that the legs are hanging. Pendular knee jerk can be elicited in this position in cerebellar diseases. Percussion hammer is known as knee hammer since knee jerk is the first muscle stretch reflex introduced in clinical neurology.

Normal response: Visible contraction of quadriceps muscle with extension of knee.

Abnormal responses
- *Minimal response*—contraction of vastus medialis alone.
- *Exaggerated response*—abrupt extension of the leg with increase in amplitude and duration of movement, adduction of thigh, occasionally it is bilateral, bilateral extension response also.
- *Pendular knee jerk*—three or more to and fro movements of foot and leg of the same amplitude. Normally there is progressive decline in amplitude and stop. This is seen in cerebellar disease. Hypotonicity of extensors and flexors of knee and lack of restraining influence which normally exert on each other.
- *Hung up knee jerk*—When patellar tendon is tapped while the foot is hanging free, the leg may be held in extension for a few seconds before relaxing owing to prolonged contraction of quadriceps. This is obtained in chorea.

Ankle Jerk (Fig. 3.43)
- Spinal segment → S1, S2
- Peripheral nerve → medial popliteal

Method: Correct technique will produce the normal response, otherwise it is frequently recorded as absent. The thigh is abducted and externally rotated, partial flexion of knee and partial dorsiflexion of foot. If voluntary contraction present, try to overcome by a few dorsiflexion and plantar flexion movement of foot. Also feel the gastrocnemius for the state of

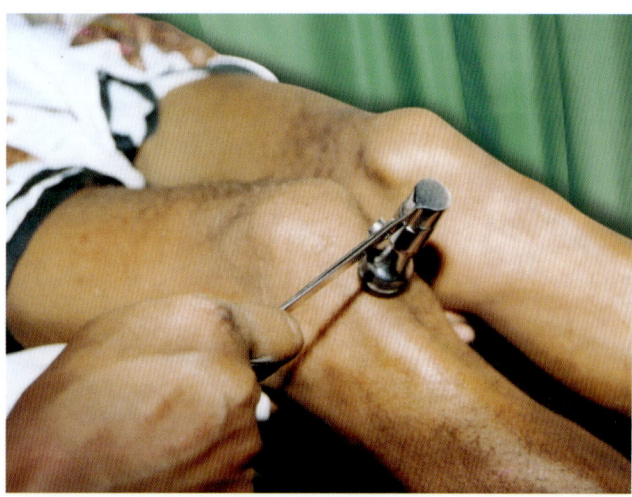

Fig. 3.42: The knee jerk.

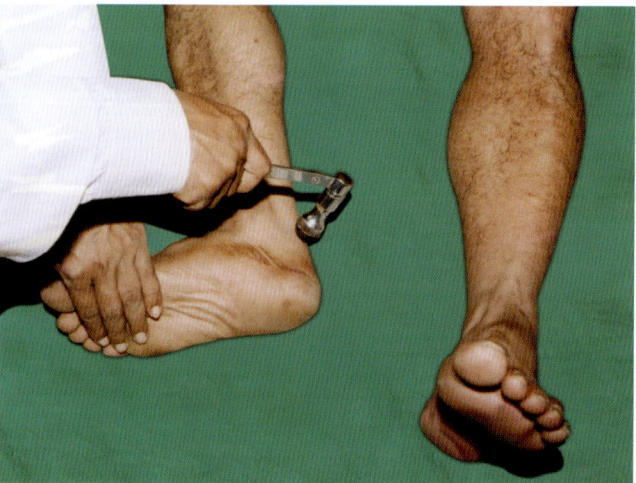

Fig. 3.43: The ankle jerk.

relaxation. The Achilles tendon is then struck, watch for the contraction of calf muscles and the movement of foot.
Normal response: Visible contraction of calf muscles and plantar flexion of foot.

Abnormal response
- *Absent response*—Lesion of reflex arc or in spinal shock, in healthy elderly person.
- *Exaggerated response*—exaggerated plantar flexion of foot
- *Minimal response*—only contraction of soleus muscle which is visible between the shin of tibia and gastrocnemius muscle
- *Myotonic reflex*—delayed relaxation in hypothyroidism called Woltman's sign.

This can be demonstrated by alternative method of elicitation of ankle jerk. Patient is asked to keep his knee up on a cushioned or blanketed chair and his feet projecting over the edge. With the foot slightly dorsiflexed, the Achilles tendon can then be struck—prolonged contraction with delayed relaxation can be seen in hypothyroidism.

Other Signs of Hyper-reflexia

Hoffmann sign: The terminal phalanx of the patient's middle finger is flicked downwards between the examiner's finger and thumb. In case of hyper reflexia, the tips of other fingers flex and the thumb flexes and adduct.

Wartenberg sign: Hook the flexed fingers of the patient with the flexed fingers of examiner. Then pull against each other's resistance. Normally the thumb extends though the terminal phalanx may flex slightly. In pyramidal tract lesions the thumb adducts and flexes strongly.

Clonus: Sudden passive stretch of a muscle tendon will produce rhythmic, involuntary muscle contractions which will persist as long as the stretch is maintained. True clonus is sustained till the stretch is over and it is a sign of UMN lesion.

I. *Ankle clonus*—The patient is in the supine position, both hip and knee are flexed at 90°, support the thigh with the examiner's left palm and with the right hand holding the foot, give a sharp and sudden dorsiflexion to stretch the tendo achilles. The foot will have clonic movement till the stretch is over.

II. *Patellar clonus*—The patient is in the supine position, keep the lower limb straight and relaxed, hold the patella between the index finger and thumb and is suddenly pushed down to stretch the quadriceps tendon. Patella will have clonic movement.

III. *Wrist clonus*—Sudden hyperextension of wrist so as to stretch the long flexors tendon will produce clonic movement of palm at wrist.

Clinical Disorders of Muscle Stretch Reflex (MSR)

About 3-10% of people without any neurological illness will have absence of one or more of the reflexes. Normal variation in reflex activity is equal in two sides means normal, until it is markedly increased or decreased.

Reduced or Absence of MSR (Hyporeflexia or Areflexia)

Due to damage of:
- Receptor
- Afferent
- Center
- Efferent
- Muscle

Receptor damage—Muscular dystrophy—reduced knee or ankle jerk due to muscle spindle damage.

Afferent lesion
- Peripheral nerve lesion
  - Peripheral neuropathy
  - Sensory
- Posterior root lesion
  - Radiculopathy
  - GBS
- Posterior root ganglion—Tabes dorsalis
- Posterior root zone—Friedreich's ataxia and SACD

Lesion of center—Spinal cord lesion
a. Syringomyelia—reflex arc damage
b. Polio }
c. MND } Anterior horn cell damage
d. SMA }

Efferent lesion
a. Anterior root lesion—radiculopathy
b. Peripheral nerve lesion
c. Peripheral neuropathy—motor.

Neuromuscular and muscle lesion
a. Muscular dystrophy
b. Myasthenia gravis
c. Periodic paralysis

Other mechanisms—paraplegia in flexion—extensor reflexes reduced.

Cerebellar lesion—reduced reflex due to hypotonia.

Common causes of hyporeflexia
a. Peripheral neuropathy
b. GBS
c. Subacute combined degeneration (SACD)
d. Tabes dorsalis
e. Friedreich's ataxia
f. Periodic paralysis
g. Cerebral or spinal shock (acute UMN lesion)

Hyperactivity of Muscle Stretch Reflex

Increased speed of response, duration and amplitude of movement.

a. *Sign of UMN lesion*—pyramidal lesion and associated damage of reticulospinal and vestibulospinal tract
b. *Psychoneurosis*—anxiety—amplitude of movement is increased

c. Tetany
d. Tetanus
e. Early phase of neuritis—increased irritability of peripheral nerve
f. Paralysis of antagonist—increased knee jerk in paralysis of antagonist hamstring muscle
g. Extrapyramidal lesion—increased tension of muscle (not always). MSR slightly increased
h. Thyrotoxicosis.

Visceral Reflexes

Reflexes concerned with swallowing, micturition and defecation.

- *Swallowing reflex*
  - Ask for dysphagia for solid, liquid food or both
  - In neurogenic dysphagia—difficulty both for solid and liquid.
  - Force of swallowing is more for solid, speed of swallowing is more for liquid, thus both are affected.
- *Defecation*
  - Any difficulty with defecation or continence
  - Anal reflex can be tested with a gloved finger
  - Stress incontinence of feces—damage to innervation of pelvic floor
- *Micturition*
  - Ask for control and initiation of micturition
  - Bladder and urethral sensation
  - Enquire about retention, urgency, precipitancy and incontinence of micturition.
  - Urge incontinence in automatic bladder
  - Stress incontinence in autonomic bladder
- *Sexual function:* Ask for any difficulty with penile erection and ejaculation.

Release Reflexes

These reflexes are present at birth or in early infancy, they disappear later when cortical control develops. Hence they are called primitive reflexes. When there is diffused cerebral damage, loss of cortical control on subcortical structures will lead to reappearance of these reflexes, called release reflexes.

Glabellar Reflex

Tap the glabella repeatedly with the examiner's finger, brought from above and behind the patient's head. This results in blinking response, normally 2-3 taps will have the response, subsequently—no response. In patients with Parkinsonism, diffused cerebral damage, bilateral UMN facial palsy, the blinking continues as long as stimuli are given.

Snout Reflex

Direct tap on the lips with the examiner's finger will produce protrusion of the lips. This is also seen in bilateral UMN facial palsy and diffuse cerebral damage.

Palmomental Reflex

Refer 7th Cranial Nerve.

Grasp Reflex

When the palm is touched on the radial border between the thumb and index finger, with the first and second fingers of examiner, the patient's fingers involuntarily flex slowly and grasp the examiner's finger.

This reflex is normally in babies under four months and it also appears in lesions of contralateral medial frontal lobe.

COORDINATION OF MOVEMENT

Coordination of motor act is mainly done by cerebellum in the presence of intact motor and sensory system, also influenced by vestibular and extrapyramidal systems. Ataxia means incoordination of voluntary movements—ataxia can be static and kinetic—static ataxia—incoordination in the resting state.

Kinetic ataxia—ataxia only on movement

Maintenance of balance and coordination of body in stance and gait is equilibratory coordination. Nonequilibratory coordination is the ability to judge distance, speed and force of movement is required for the voluntary limb movement.

Testing Nonequilibratory Coordination

Finger Nose Test

Patient is asked to abduct and extend his arm completely, ataxia is more for proximal than for distal muscle, the patient touches the tip of his index finger to his nose, then touches the tip of the examiner's finger and again touches the tip of his own nose. Examiner's finger is moved and held at different sites, in this way, distance, speed and power of movement can be tested.

Normally smooth movement, for nose and finger tip. In cerebellar disease, there is decomposition of movement, breaking the smooth movements into fragments which will be more while reaching the nose or fingertip, named as intention tremor.

Finger to Finger Test

The patient is asked to abduct to the horizontal and then bring the tips of the index fingers through a wide circle to approximate them exactly in the midline, this is done slowly and rapidly.

With unilateral cerebellar disease the finger on that side may not reach the midline and the finger of normal side crosses the midline to reach it. Also the arm on the affected side may sag under shoot, so that the finger on that side will be below on the normal side.

Heel Knee Test

In the supine position, patient is asked to place the heel of one foot on the opposite knee and then push it along the shin along a straight line to the big toe. Normally the movement of heel is smooth and uniform throughout the distance. In cerebellar disease—descend along the shin is jerky and unsteady, smooth movement is fragmented, there may be undershoot or overshoot of movement.

Testing Equilibratory Coordination

Romberg's sign is a test for the co-ordination of proprioceptive impulses, Romberg's sign is positive when there is loss of proprioceptive impulses in the legs. Conventionally, it is a test of posterior column function.

Patient is asked to stand with the feet closely approximated, first his eyes open and then closed. The patient may be able to maintain the upright posture while the eyes are open, but when the eyes are closed, he sways and tends to fall. He may attempt to prevent the swaying by placing his feet some distance apart, thus standing with a broad base.

In midline cerebellar disease, which affects equilibrium, patient may have difficulty in standing erect and maintaining a steady position with his eyes either opened or closed. He may sway from side to side or backwards to forwards.

GAIT

The act of walking or locomotion is influenced by a number of reflex mechanisms of various components of nervous system. Normal mode of walking denotes the proper integration of motor and sensory system, cerebellum, vestibular and extrapyramidal system.

Normal gait represents the heel toe phase of support and progression, pelvis rotates slightly to the side of progression, trunk moves forwards and backwards with each step, as one lower extremity is advanced, the upper extremity of the opposite side advances, this is the swinging movement of upper extremities.

Abnormalities of Gait

Spastic Gait

It is seen in unilateral and bilateral pyramidal lesion.
- **Hemiplegic gait**—Circumduction of leg due to inability to flex the hip, and dorsiflex foot against gravity, with triple flexion position of upper limb. Patient drags one foot, leaning towards opposite side, lifts the pelvis upwards in the involved side to aid in lifting the toe off the floor. Swing the entire lower limb around a semi-circle from the hip.
  Cause—hemiplegia
- **Scissor gait**—in bilateral pyramidal lesion, due to the adductor spasm of thigh, leaving legs to cross each other and each foot to trip up the other. May appear to be walking on his toes (due to calf muscle contraction) and seems to jump rapidly from the toes of one foot to other.
  Cause—Hereditary spastic paraplegia, cerebral diplegia

Ataxic Gait

- **Sensory ataxia (high stepping, stamping gait):** Caused by the interruption of proprioceptive pathways in the spinal cord. High stepping, stamping gait with broad base, heel touches the ground before the toes. Ataxia is more at night due to the lack of visual compensation for the proprioceptive loss.
  Cause—Peripheral neuropathy, tabes dorsalis
- **Cerebellar ataxia:** Broad based reeling gait, tendency to fall to one side, unable to walk on a straight line and do tandem walking.
  Titubant ataxia—ataxic gait with vertical oscillation of head and trunk. Gait ataxia is seen in lesion of upper vermis and anterior lobe of cerebellum.
- **Vertiginous ataxia:** Vertigo leading to difficulty in walking, persistent swaying to one side which is seen in vestibular lesion. At times, patient will be thrown to the floor in otolithic crisis of Tumarkin.

Spastic Ataxic Gait

Present in SACD, multiple sclerosis (MS), posterolateral sclerosis, features of both spasticity and sensory ataxia due to lesion of pyramidal system and posterior column, predominant feature depends on what structure is affected more.

High Stepping Gait—Unilateral or Bilateral

Seen in foot drop, patient lifts the foot by excessive flexion of the hip, knee to avoid injury to toes, then flops down the foot on the floor, toes touch the floor before the ball of foot and heel.
Cause—L4, L5 radiculopathy
a. Lateral popliteal nerve lesion
b. Peroneal muscular atrophy
c. Peripheral neuropathy—motor

Waddling Gait (Dystrophic Gait)

Pelvis is rotated through an abnormally large arc associated with marked lordosis and broad base of gait.
Cause
- Bilateral congenital dislocation of hip
- Proximal muscle weakness in myopathy and proximal SMA.

Festinant Gait in Parkinsonism

Gait is slow, rigid and shuffling. Body is stooped forwards with flexed attitude of upper limb and body. Upper limb is flexed at shoulder, elbow and metacarpophalangeal joint and extended at wrist and interphalangeal joints.

Kinesia paradoxa—patient with Parkinsonism is able to walk quickly with ease, than slowly.

Gait in Hyperkinesias

In chorea, athetosis, dystonia, the involuntary movement becomes more marked while walking which distort the gait.

Apraxia of Gait

Inability to use lower limbs properly in the act of walking without any sensory, motor, cerebellar and extrapyramidal defecit. Gait is slow with short steps as in normal pressure hydrocephalus

Hysterical gait—Gait is nondescript and bizarre, often marked by swaying from side to side.

INVOLUNTARY MOVEMENTS (FIG. 3.44)

Involuntary movements may involve any portion of body. They are symptoms and signs resulting from damage to various parts of motor system, cerebellum and extrapyramidal system.

The following things are to be observed while examination of involuntary movements:
a. Part of body affected
b. Constant or episodic
c. At rest, on movement or both
d. Effect of voluntary movement decrease or increase
e. Influence of sleep and emotion
f. Movement are stereotyped or not
g. Rate, rhythm and amplitude of movement.

Tremor

Definition: Involuntary rhythmic oscillatory movement produced by the alternate contraction of agonist and antagonist/group of muscles. Clinical types—static—extrapyramidal lesion/action or intention—cerebellar lesion—postural—flapping tremor, thyrotoxicosis, rubral tremor. Depends on frequency of movement—slow—up to 5/ sec.
- Moderate—5–10/sec.
- Fast—>10/sec.

Depends on Amplitude of Movement

Fine
- Toxic tremor
- Alcoholism
- Thyrotoxicosis

Medium
- Anxiety
- Benign essential tremor

Coarse
- Parkinsonism
- Senile
- Wilson's disease

Depends on No. of Joints Involved

- Single joint—simple
- More than one joint—compound
  Example: Pill rolling tremor of Parkinsonism is static, coarse and compound and it is 6 sec.

Etiology of Tremor

- Neuological
  - Cerebellar lesion—intention tremor
  - Red nucleus lesion—rubral tremor—horizontal movement of outstretched hand
  - Parkinsonism—pill rolling tremor
  - General paresis of insane (GPI) trombone tremor of tongue
  - Wilson's disease—wing beating tremor of abducted shoulder static intention tremor
- Non-neurological
  - Anxiety state, alcoholism
  - Thyrotoxicosis
  - Drugs—salbutamol
  - Benign essential tremor (heredofamilial)
  - Senile
  - Metabolic—hypoglycemia, uremia, hepatocellular failure, carbon dioxide narcosis, reduced Ca and Mg.

Chorea: Definition

Involuntary brief rapid jerky, nonrhythmic movement, semipurposeful, mainly involving distal parts of limbs, face and tongue.

Suppressed by voluntary movement, disappear with sleep and aggravated by emotion and agitation.

Site of Lesion

Caudate nucleus.

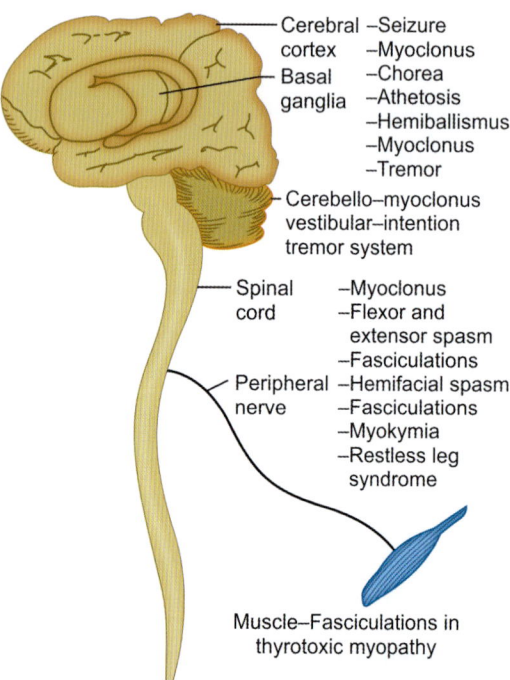

Fig. 3.44: Involuntary movements in relation to the site of lesion.

Clinical Signs

- Choreiform movements
- Hypotonia, mental instability
- *Choreac posture*—outstretched hands, hyperextended at the metacarpophalangeal joints, and wrist is flexed due to hypotonia of antagonist muscles
- *Pronator sign*—when outstretched hand is raised above the head, over pronation of forearm
- *Milking sign*—waxing and waning of the grip of individual fingers when the patient is grasping the examiner's fingers.
- *Jack in the box tongue*—protruded tongue rush back to the mouth
- Hung up knee jerk (refer reflexes).

Clinical Triad of Chorea

- Hypotonia
- Mental instability
- Choreiform movement

Variants of Chorea

Choria gravis—severe type of chorea

Paralytic chorea—marked weakness due to hypotonia

Maniacal chorea—marked emotional instability and insomnia in chorea.

Etiology

- Rheumatic fever—Sydenham's chorea
- Non-rheumatic causes
  a. Neurological—huntington's chorea—postencephalitic-CVA—apoplectiform chorea—infantile hemiplegia
  b. Infection—diphtheria, scarlet fever.
  c. Miscellaneous—chorea gravidarum—often seen with Illegitimate 1st pregnancy—senile chorea—SLE-hepatocellular failure—drugs—Phenothiazine, L-dopa, OCP, dilantin—neuroacanthosis—hypocalcemia and hypomagnesemia.

Athetosis

Mobile spasm, word meaning—unfixed or changeable
Features: This is a slow writhing movement more distal than proximal parts of limbs, may involve face and tongue.
 Fingers are extended, abducted with pronation of forearm alternate with flexion of fingers, wrist and supination of forearm.
Site of lesion: Putamen and its connection.

Etiology

- Congenital—bilateral athetosis with cerebral diplegia
- Wilson's disease → bilateral athetosis
- Infantile hemiplegia → unilateral athetosis
- Postencephalitic
- Phenothiazine dyskinesia
- Hepatic encephalopathy

Choreoathetosis

Features—are combination of features of chorea and athetosis with quick and slow component, either may predominate.

Etiology
- Wilson's disease—paroxysmal choreoathetosis—paroxysmal dystonic choreoathetosis
- Paroxysmal kinetogenic choreoathetosis—(striate epilepsy).

Pseudoathetosis

Writhing movement of limbs which are more marked when the eyes are closed due to loss of proprioceptive impulses.

Etiology
- Tabes dorsalis
- Posterolateral sclerosis
- Peripheral neuropathy
- Parietal lobe lesion

Hemiballismus

Rapid flinging movement involving the proximal part of limbs, sparing the face and trunk. It is usually acute in onset, may injure the limbs, disabling and exhausting.

Lesion—contralateral subthalamic nucleus or its connection.

Etiology—common—vascular, rarely—metastatic neoplasm.

Dystonia

Means persistence of abnormal postures.

Types
- **Torsion dystonia**—Involuntary movement leading to torsion of limbs and vertebral column. Movements are very slow due to asymmetrical distribution of hypertonia which produce torsion, eventually postures become fixed, produce contraction and deformities.
  Lesion—Caudate nucleus and putamen
  Etiology—dystonia musculorum deformans—heredofamilial
  - Kernicterus
  - Wilson's disease
  - Postencephalitic
  - Phenothiazine dyskinesia
- **Focal or segmental dystonia**
  - Flexion dystonia—Parkinsonism
  - Hemiplegia dystonia
  - Torticollis

- **Orofaciolingual dyskinesia**
  - Bizarre movement of mouth, tongue, face, jaw-like gnawing, pursing of mouth and lips, writhing movement of tongue.
  - Etiology—Phenothiazine induced
    - L-dopa
    - Adentulous person.

Myoclonus Abrupt

The brief involuntary contraction involving portion of muscle, entire muscle or group of muscles, single contraction or repetition, involving muscles of trunk and extremities, not activated by mechanical stimulation or by Neostigmine.

Lesion—Multiple like peripheral nerve, spinal cord, cerebellovestibular system, thalamus, basal ganglia and cerebral cortex.

Etiology
- Encephalitis, cerebral lipidosis, Wilson's disease, Hallervorden-Spatz disease
- C. J disease, myoclonic epilepsy, palatal myoclonus
- Intention myoclonus—anoxic encephalopathy, SSPE, dyssynergia cerebellaris myoclonica (Ramsay Hunt syndrome)
- Advanced uremia and hepatocellular failure.

Myokimia

Spontaneous transient or persistant contraction of a few muscle bundles within a single muscle especially facial muscles or orbicularis oculi, not activated by neostigmine.

Etiology—Fatigue, anemia, thyrotoxicosis, hyponatremia, uremia, tetany, facial myokimia in multiple sclerosis.

Fasciculation

Involuntary contraction of a group of muscle fibers, single muscle fiber is fibrillation. Best site to see fasciculation is tongue, can be activated by mechanical stimulation of muscle and by neostigmine.

Lesion—Irritation of anterior horn cell or motor nuclei of cranial nerves.

Etiology
- MND—Amyotrophic lateral sclerosis (ALS)/progressive bulbar palsy
- Syringomyelia
- Recovering poliomyelitis
- Cervical spondylosis—compressive myelopathy
- Thyrotoxic myopathy
- Carcinomatous myopathy
- Uremia
- Organophosphorus poisoning
- Hypo Ca, Mg, K and Na
- Benign fasciculation—fatigue

Tics

Co-ordinated, repetitive, seemingly purposive and involving a group of muscles in their synergistic relationship.

Example: Rotatory movement of head, shrugging movement of shoulder, eye closure and raising the eyebrows.

Tiquver is a person who is subjected to one or multiple tics.

Gilles de la tourette syndrome (Maladic—des—tics)—seen in preadolescent boy with multiple tics, grunts and explosive utterance of obscene nature.

Akathisia

Defined as motor restlessness, urge to move, inability to sit still.

Cause—Parkinsonism
- Phenothiazine induced
- Postencephalitic.

Restless Leg Syndrome (Ekbom Syndrome)

Urge to move due to unpleasant sensation in the legs which occur when patient sits quiet or attempts to fall asleep.

Cause—Uremia
- Peripheral neuropathy
- Pregnancy.

Involuntary Movement Depending on the Site of Origin of Lesion

a. Peripheral nerves
   - Hemifacial spasm
   - Fasciculation
   - Myokymia
   - Restless legs syndrome—Ekbom syndrome
b. Spinal cord
   - Myoclonus
   - Flexor and extensor spasm
   - Fasciculation
c. Cerebellovestibular system
   - Myoclonus
   - Intention tremor
d. Basal ganglia
   - Chorea, athetosis
   - Choreoathetosis
   - Hemiballismus
   - Dystonia
   - Tremor
e. Cerebral cortex
   - Seizure
   - Myoclonus.

EXAMINATION OF SENSORY SYSTEM

This is probably the most difficult part in neurological examination. Patient should be comfortable, co-operative and at ease during the examination. Patient must understand the procedure. It is difficult to evaluate in patient with low intelligence, language difficulty, clouded sensorium, and dysphasia and also in children.

Anatomical knowledge of sensory system especially the dermatomes and neural pattern of sensory loss is essential for the proper interpretation. Importance of sensory system evaluation will come in diseases like syringomyelia, for dissociated sensory loss, spinal cord lesion—to assess the level of lesion and peripheral nerve lesions (Figs. 3.45 and 3.46).

Modalities of Sensation for Testing

- Light touch, pain and thermal sensation—exteroceptive sensation—spinothalamic function
- Vibration, position sense, joint sense and deep pain—proprioceptive sensation—posterior column function
- Tactile localization, two point discrimination, stereognosis, graphesthesia, sensory inattention—cortical sensation—parietal lobe function.

Terms Related to Sensory System

- Anesthesia, hypoesthesia, hyperesthesia—alteration in tactile sensation—absence, ↓ or ↑ of tactile sensation
- Analgesia, hypoalgesia, hyperalgesia—alteration in pain sensation—absence, decrease or increase of pain sensation
- *Paresthesia*—feeling of abnormal sensation in the absence of a stimuli, like numbness and tingling, cold and warmth, and crawling.
- *Dysesthesia*—Perverted interpretation of sensation with a stimuli, like burning sensation to touch
- *Topesthesia*—Ability to recognize tactile localization
- *Topanesthesia*—Loss of ability to recognize tactile localization

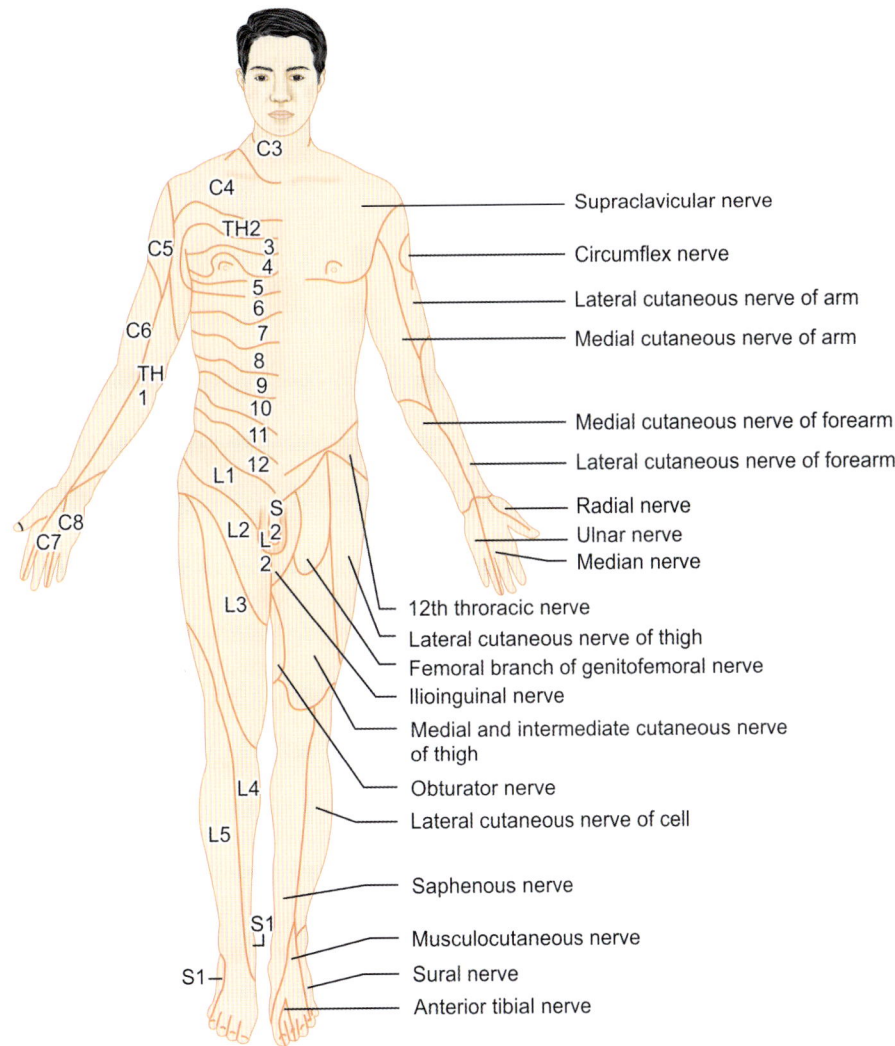

Fig. 3.45: Segmental and peripheral nerve innervation and points for testing cutaneous sensation of limbs (anterior).

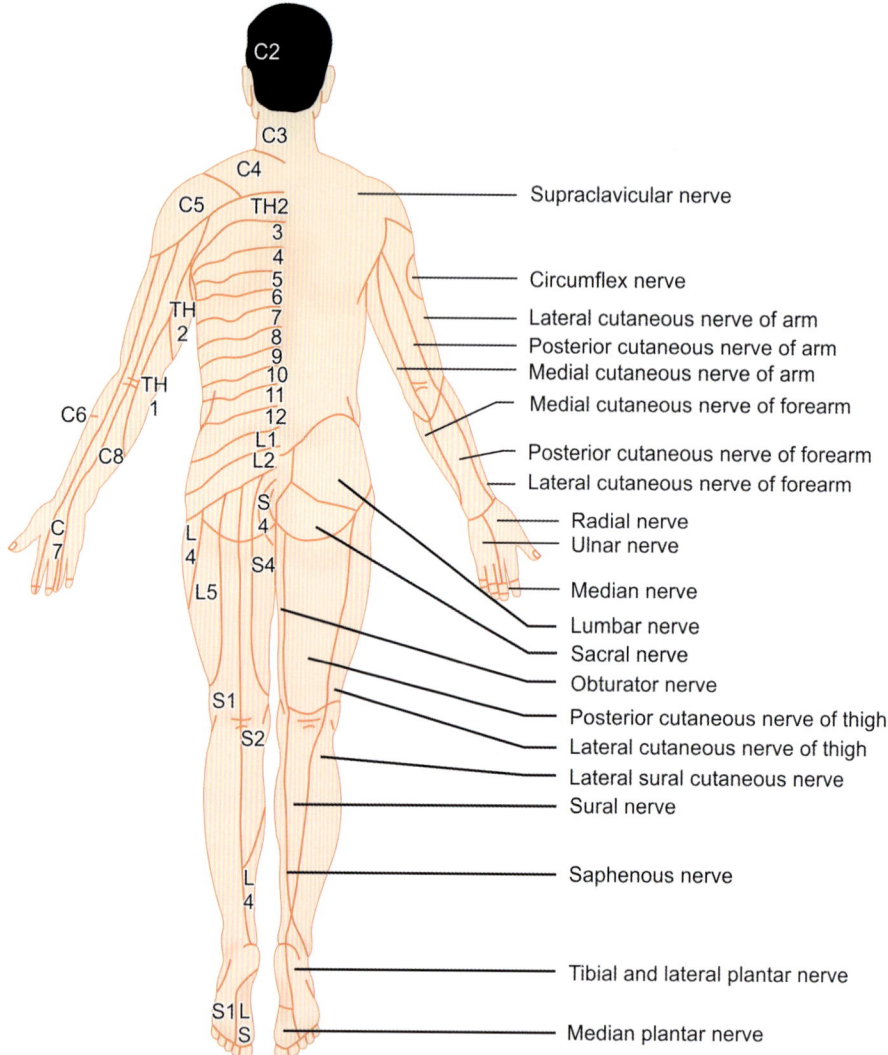

Fig. 3.46: Segmental and peripheral nerve innervation and points for testing cutaneous sensation of limbs (Posterior).

- *Graphesthesia*—Ability to recognize number or letter written on skin
- *Graphanesthesia*—Loss of ability to recognize number or letter written on skin
- *Stereognosis*—Perception of form, nature of object, identify by naming it by touch
- *Astereognosis*—Loss of stereognostic ability
- *Stereoanesthesia*—Loss of stereognostic ability due to infracerebral lesions, e.g. spinal stereoanesthesia
- *Pallesthesia*—Ability to recognize vibration sense
- *Pallanesthesia*—Loss of ability to recognize vibration sense
- *Sensory inattention or extinction*—Loss of ability to perceive sensation on one side of the body when identical areas on both sides of the body are stimulated simultaneously
- *Anosognosia*—Denial of disability
- *Hyperpathia*—Area of blunting of sensation, an effective stimuli causing disagreeable burning type of pain
- *Anesthesia dolorosa*—Intractable pain in hypoesthetic area, e.g. post herpetic neuralgia, thalamic pain.
- *Causalgia*—Neuritis with burning type of pain and trophic changes, e.g. median and sciatic nerve lesion
- *Phantom limb*—sensation of continued presence of an absent part of the body
- *Phantom sensation*—Spontaneous sensation referred to insensitive areas
- *Dissociated sensory loss*—Loss of pain, thermal sensation and touch is preserved.

Purpose of Testing Sensory System

I. To identify the modality of sensory loss
II. To identify the anatomical areas of sensory loss
III. To correlate with the known pattern of sensory loss.

Exteroceptive Sensation (Spinothalamic Tract Function)

a. **Touch**
   - Explain the procedure to the patient
   - Use a wisp of cotton wool or feather
   - Touch lightly, without pressure not to stimulate pressure sensation
   - Ask the patient to say yes each time when he feels, with closed eyes
   - Start testing face down, upper limb, trunk and lower limb in dermatome pattern
   - Hairy areas, armpit, cubital fossae are more sensitive, palm and sole are less sensitive
   - If an area of abnormal sensation is identified, it can be further delineated by repeating the test, giving continuous stimuli in a line from an area of decreased sensation to normal sensation which the patient can identify and tell.

b. **Superficial pain**
   - Use a sharp pin with a round head of 1–2 mm size
   - Procedure is explained to the patient. By using the both ends separately so that the patient can say sharp for the sharp end and blunt for the head of the pin
   - Apply sharp end and blunt ends of the pin from face downwards, when patient has closed his eyes
   - Sharp end should be applied to produce pain and not to penetrate the skin
   - On areas of loss of pain, patient says blunt even for sharp end, also ask the patient whether normal or decreased or increased pain sensation on areas of abnormal sensation when comparing to normal area.
   - Repeat the examination for anatomical delineation in areas of abnormal sensation for pain.

c. **Temperature**
   - Using test tubes containing hot water of 110° F and cold water of 45°F
   - Extremes of heat or cold will stimulate pain
   - Patient has his eyes closed, ask the patient what he feels, any difference when the other tube is used and whether he can identify the thermal stimuli
   - Compare the areas of dulling of sensation with normal area
   - Normal person can appreciate even a difference of 1°C.

Proprioceptive Sensation (Posterior Column Function)

a. **Vibration**
   - Vibrating tuning fork of 128 Hz is shown to the patient and placed on his clavicle to allow him to identify the sensation of vibration
   - He then closes his eyes, tuning fork is struck and placed on bony points, starting peripherally
   - Ask the patient to say when he ceases to feel it, if the examiner can still perceive it, means vibration perception is impaired
   - In the lower limbs, medial malleolus, lateral malleolus, tibial tuberosity and anterior superior iliac spine are used as bony points. In the upper limb, radial styloid process, olecranon, acromion process, in the trunk, over the spinous process are the bony points for testing
   - Compare the duration of appreciation on both sides and also by the examiner

Loss of vibration sense occurs earlier than the other proprioceptive sensations.

Dissociation between vibration sense and joint sense occurs in syringomyelia—loss of vibration sense earlier.

Thalamoparietal lesion does not impair the vibration.

b. **Joint sense or sense of passive movement of joint**
   - Explain the procedure to the patient with eyes open, then close his eyes.
   - Hold the sides of the digit between the forefinger and the thumb, so that the pressure above and below does not reveal the direction of movement. Better to fix the joint proximal to the joint of the moving digit.
   - Move the digit up and down, ask whether he can feel the movement, then further up and down movement done several times, instruct the patient to say the direction, avoid alternate up and down movements—otherwise the patient will say alternatively up and down without knowing the direction. One should tell the correct direction of movement at least six successive times. Movement can be done in big toe, finger, wrist and elbow also.

c. **Position sense**
   - Tell the method of testing to the patient
   - Patient's eyes should be closed, place the patient's arm in a particular position, then move it away
   - Ask him to place the limb in that position
   - Then to place the opposite limb in a similar position

The inability to do the test with eyes closed, but possible with eyes open indicates loss of proprioceptive sensation.

d. **Deep pain or pressure pain**
   - Deep pain is tested by squeezing the muscles or tendons like Achilles tendon or on calf muscles or pressure on the testicles also.
   - Abadie's sign—is loss of deep pain sense on squeezing tendo-Achilles

Proprioceptive sensation are lost in lesions of peripheral nerve, nerve root, posterior column, medial lemniscus, thalamus and thalamoparietal fibers and sensory cortex. Vibration sense is not impaired in lesions above thalamus. Loss of proprioceptive sensations will manifest as sensory ataxia and pseudoathetosis called piano playing movement, e.g. diseases with predominant posterior column involvement as in tabes dorsalis, SACD, Friedreich's ataxia.

Cortical Sensation (Parietal Lobe Function)

Test for cortical sensations are done when primary modalities of sensation are intact. Cortical component is essential for the final perception. It is a function of parietal lobe.

a. *Tactile localization*
   - Testing patient's ability to localize the tactile sensation.
   - With eyes closed apply the touch stimuli, with a wisp of cotton or tip of the finger at different sites.
   - Ask the patient to localize the site of touch.
   - Loss of tactile localization (top anesthesia) with intact exteroceptive sensation usually signifies the presence of lesion in the parietal lobe.

b. *Two point discrimination*
   - Ability to differentiate the cutaneous stimulation from one blunt point from stimulation by two blunt points.
   - Explain the test to the patient, illustrate the sensation for him by touching his finger with the two points unduly separated.
   - Use a caliper or a compass divider, keeping the eyes closed, start testing by applying one point or two points at the tip of the finger, dorsum of hand, dorsum of foot.
   - Identify the minimum distance at which the two point can be identified on both sides.
   - Normal individual identify the minimum distance of
   - 2 mm at lip
   - 2–5 mm at the pulp of finger
   - 3 cm at dorsum of hand
   - 3–5 cm at the dorsum of foot

c. *Stereognosis*
   - Ability to identify the object from the feel of its size and shape. Patient should have a normal touch and position sense, sufficient power of the muscles of hand also.
   - Patient should close his eyes and the familiar object like coin, pen or key is placed into the hand and asked to identify.
   - Compare both sides of the accuracy and speed of response.
   - Loss of stereognosis—asteregnosis
   - Lesion responsible is in the parietal lobe.
   - Spinal cord lesion with marked loss of proprioceptive sensation will have loss of stereognosis—stereoanesthesia.

d. *Graphesthesia*
   - Ability to recognize letter or numbers written on the skin with a blunt point.
   - Patient closes his eyes, letter or numerals are traced out on the palm of hand, forearm, thigh and leg.
   - Figures such as 8, 4, 5 are written first, if correct, use difficult one like 9, 6, 3, for final test, size of the digit should be > 4 cm.
   - Loss of graphesthesia (graphanesthesia) with intact exteroceptive sensation—means parietal lobe lesion.

e. *Sensory inattention*
   - It is the loss of ability to perceive sensation on one side of the body when identical areas on two sides of the body are stimulated simultaneously.
   - Explain the procedure to the patient, he should respond by saying one or two depending on the stimuli given, use the tip of index finger or cotton pin.
   - Keeping the eyes closed, deliver the stimuli to one side or both sides, identical areas simultaneously with equal pressure.
   - Normal person will perceive single stimuli and simultaneously applied stimuli as two.
   - Inability to perceive simultaneously applied stimuli as two, even though each stimuli separately is perceived, is a sign of contralateral parietal lobe lesion and may be the only sign in some cases.

Localization of Lesion of Sensory System

Peripheral Nerves (Fig. 3.52)

Neural pattern of sensory loss
- If single nerve—mononeuritis
- If multiple nerve—in asymmetrical pattern—mononeuritis multiplex
  Cause: Hansen's disease, diabetes mellitus, PAN, sarcoidosis, rheumatoid arthritis
- *In peripheral neutropathy*: Distal symmetrical sensory loss—glove and stocking type (Fig. 3.50)
  Cause: Diabetes mellitus, internal malignancy, alcoholism, nutritional neuropathy and hereditary sensory neuropathy.

Root and Plexus

- Radicular pain—if bilateral lesion, girdle pain encircling body
- Dermatome pattern of sensory loss
- Reflex loss with normal power of muscle.

Spinal Cord

- **Three types of pain**
  1. Radicular pain
  2. Local pain of spine
  3. L'hermitte's pain—sudden shooting pain spreading down to the body on flexion of neck in cervical spondylosis and disseminated sclerosis
- **Transection of spinal cord**
  - Transverse myelitis
  - All modalities of sensation lost below the level of lesion with zone of hyperaesthesia at the level of lesion
- **Hemisection of spinal cord**
  - Brown-Sequard syndrome (Fig. 3.51A)
  - Ipsilateral loss of posterior column sensation and contralateral loss of pain, thermal sensation, dissociated sensory loss

- **Intramedullary lesion** (Fig. 3.49A)
  - Tumor, syringomyelia
  - Suspended dissociated sensory loss with sacral sparing (Suspended means— above and below the area of sensory loss, have normal sensation)
- **Extramedullary lesion:** Radicular pain, contralateral dissociated sensory loss at a lower level, no sacral sparing
- **Anterior spinal artery occlusion**
  - Loss of pain and thermal sensation below the level of lesion—dissociated sensory loss, because of involvement of anterior 2/3rd of spinal cord supplied by anterior spinal artery
  - Posterior column is spared—thus touch and proprioceptive sensation are unaffected
- **Predominant loss of propioceptive sensation**
  - Posterior column lesion in tabes dorsalis, SACD, Friedreich's ataxia, compressive myelopathy with compression of posterior aspect of spinal cord
  - Loss of proprioceptive sensation → sensory ataxia, pseudoathetosis, spinal stereoanesthesia
- **Saddle anesthesia (Fig. 3.49B):** Impaired sensation of lower sacral segment as in cauda equina and conus medullaris lesion
- **Loss of vibration sense alone**
  - Early peripheral neuropathy
  - Certain cases of syringomyelia

Brainstem Lesion

- Upper brainstem lesion—hemisensory loss
- Unilateral pontine lesion—ipsilateral sensory loss face—contralateral hemisensory loss
- Lateral medullary syndrome—Wallenberg syndrome—crossed dissociated sensory loss—ipsilateral face and contralateral body (Fig. 3.48A)
- Median medullary syndrome—bilateral medial lemniscus lesion → bilateral loss of proprioceptive sensations
- Syringobulbia—onion peel type of sensory loss of face.

Thalamus

- Unilateral loss of all sensations on one-half of the body including face (Fig. 3.47)
- Spontaneous pain—thalamic pain—hyperpathia
- Partial lesion of thalamus—unilateral loss of proprioceptive sensation

Thalamoparietal Radiation

- Internal capsule—unilateral dulling of all modalities of sensation, no total loss of sensation, no hyperpathia.
- Corona radiata—localized dulling of all modalititcs of sensation, in areas corresponding—to motor deficit, since identical motor and sensory fibers are nearer—at the level of corona radiata.

Common patterns of abnormal sensation

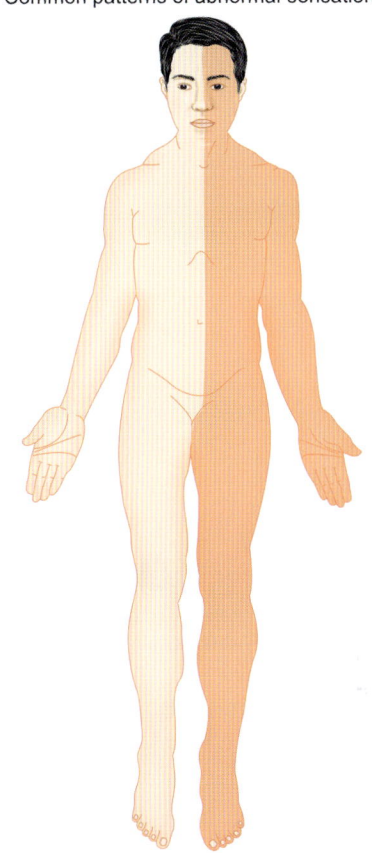

Fig. 3.47: Total hemianalgesia—thalamic or upper brainstem lesion.

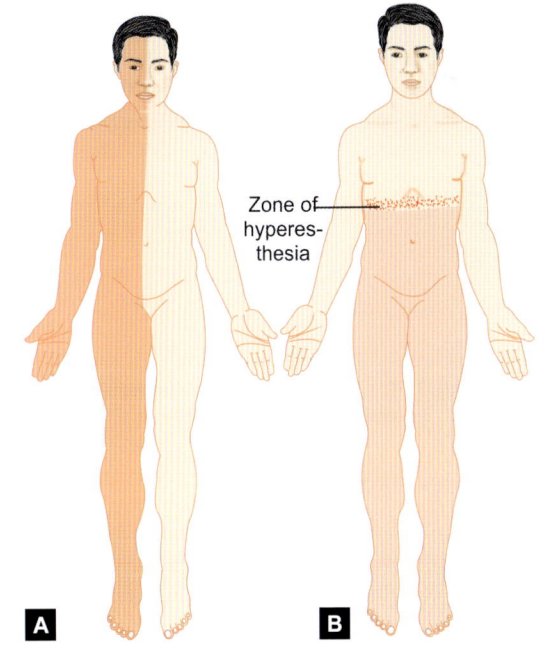

Figs. 3.48A and B: (A) Lateral medullary lesion (usually vertebral artery deficiency), (B) Transverse lesion of the cord.

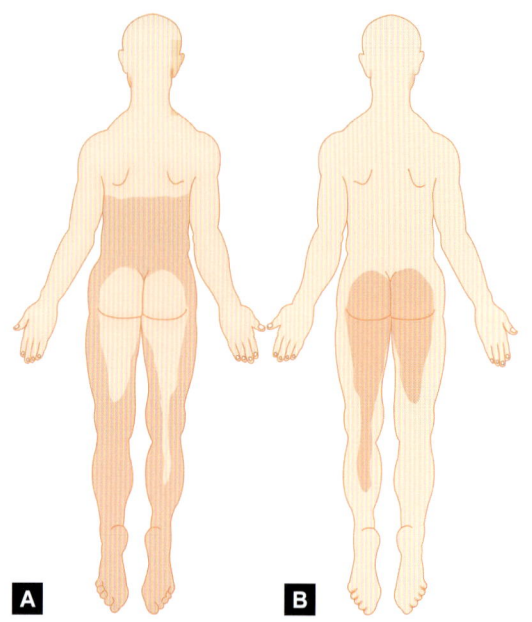

Figs. 3.49A and B: (A) Sacral sparing—cord compression. Intramedullary lesion, (B) Saddle analgesia—cauda equina or conus medullaris lesion.

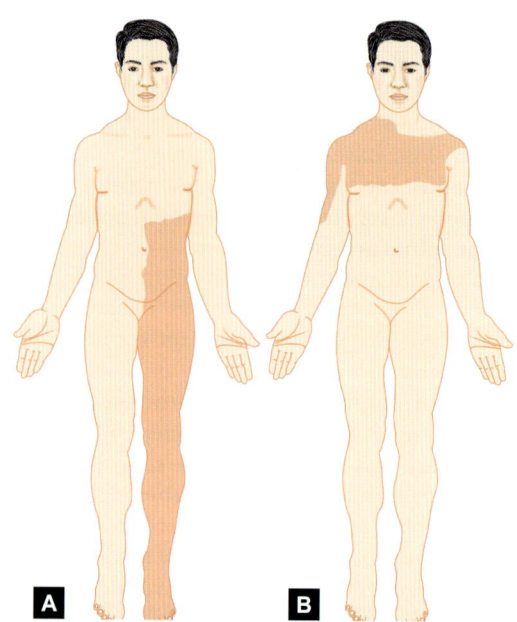

Figs. 3.51A and B: (A) Brown-Sequard lesion—hemisection of the cord, (B) Cuirasse analgesia—central cord lesion—syringomyelia.

EXAMINATION OF CEREBELLAR SIGNS

(Refer neuroanatomy of cerebellum for localization and site of lesion)

1. Skew deviation of eye
2. Nystagmus
3. Dysarthria
4. Signs in upper limb
   a. Hypotonia
   b. Finger nose test
   c. Dysdiadochokinesia of rapid alternating movement, disturbances in the reciprocal of agonist and antagonists, loss of ability to stop one act and follow it immediately to its opposite act.
   Method: Alternate pronation and supination of forearm rapidly with the elbow fixed at 90° kept to the side of chest. Clumsy movement will be seen in the side of lesion.
   d. Rebound phenomenon of Gordon Holmes
   Loss of check reflex by the antagonist leads to unchecking of antagonist.
   Method: Active flexion of forearm against resistance applied by the examiner, protect the face of the patient with the other hand, sudden release of resistance for the flexion of forearm, produce uncontrolled further flexion which is arrested by the contraction of the antagonist—triceps in normal persons.
   In cerebellar diseases unchecking of antagonist, produces further uncontrolled flexion of forearm which may hit the upper arm or face.

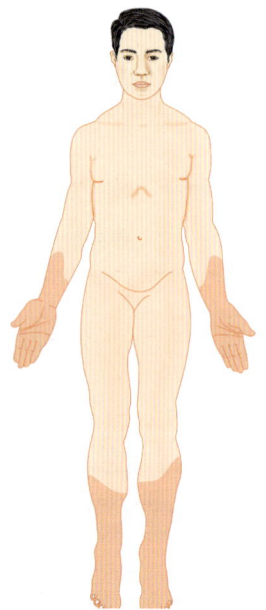

Fig. 3.50: Glove and stocking analgesia—peripheral neuropathy hysteria.

Sensory Cortex—Parietal Lobe

- Cortical type of sensory loss— loss of tactile localization, two point discrimination, sensory inattention and stereognosis.
- Primary modalities of sensation are intact in pure cortical lesions.
- Sensory seizure—paresthesia of contralateral side in irritative lesion—focal seizure—sensory aura in Jacksonian epilepsy (Figs. 3.35 to 3.40).

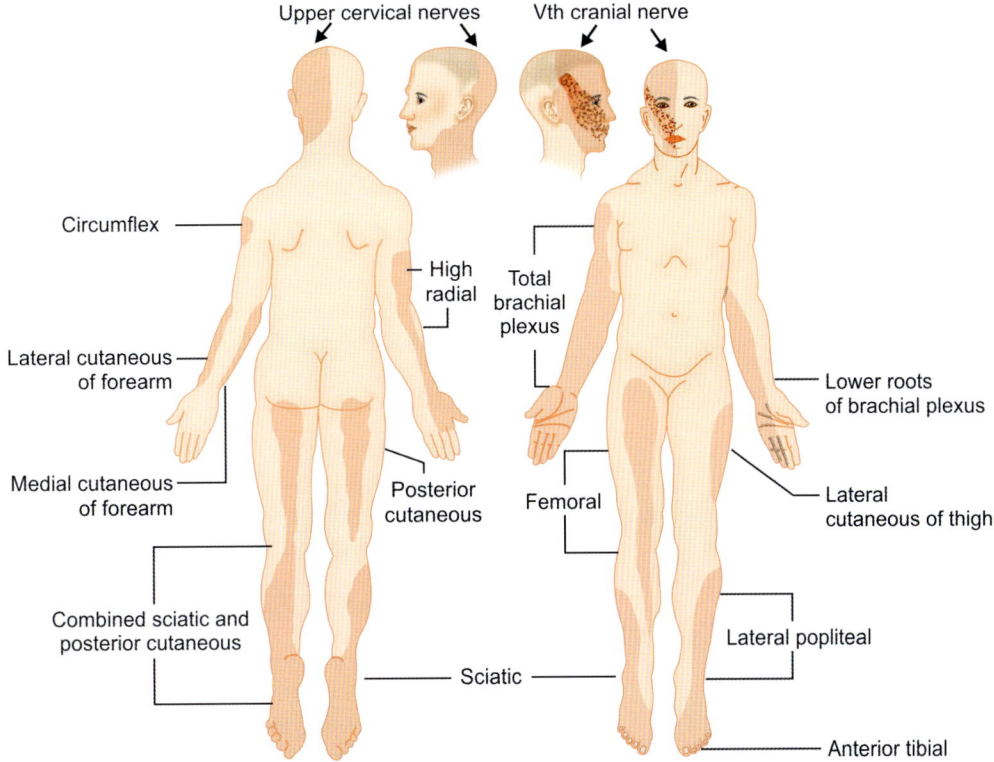

Fig. 3.52: Average areas of sensory loss resulting from the more common peripheral nerve lesions. Variation is considerable and in incomplete lesions the area involved may be greatly reduced.

e. *Dysmetria:* Inability to assess the rate, range and force of movement.
   Method: Ask the patient to take an object like pencil or pen kept away from the patient by an outstretched hand distance. Normal person will take the object by an appropriate force and distance of movement.
   In cerebellar lesion, the patient may overshoot—hypermetria, or stop short of the object—hypometria or fetch the object with great force.

f. *Barognosis:* It is the ability to recognize weight. It is tested by the use of objects of similar size, shape, but of different weights. Objects with different weights are placed in one hand one after the other and ask the patient to tell which object weighs more, with the eyes closed. This test is repeated on the other side also.
   Normal individual can distinguish minor difference of weights. In cerebellar disease there is loss of ability to distinguish weights called barognosis.

g. Finger to finger test

5. Signs in the lower limb
   a. Heel knee test
   b. Pendular knee jerk
   c. Gait ataxia (refer gait)
   d. Walking on straight line—Unable to walk on straight line and tendency to fall.
   e. Tandem walking—Loss of ability to do the tandem walking.
   Method: Tandem walking is done by placing one heel directly in front of the opposite toes with eyes open or closed. In cerebellar lesion—unable to do tandem walking even with eyes open. In sensory ataxia—unable to do tandem walking when eyes are closed.

Etiology of Cerebellar Disorders

a. **Acute cerebellar disorder**
   - CVA—cerebellar hemorrhage or infarction, brainstem stroke—Lateral medullary syndrome
   - Traumatic
   - Encephalitis—Cerebellitis by virus
     - Chickenpox
     - Measles
     - Mumps
   - Cerebellar abscess—otogenic
   - Demyelinating disease
     - Disseminated sclerosis
     - Miller Fischer syndrome
   - Drug induced—phenytoin, carbamazepine
   - Alcoholism
   - Wernicke's encephalopathy
   - Lightning/electric shock
   - Hyperpyrexia

- Hypoxic encephalopathy as in hanging
- Prolonged hypoglycemia

b. **Chronic cerebellar disorder**
   1. Hereditary ataxia—Friedreich's ataxia
   2. CV junction anomaly—Arnold-Chiari malformation
   3. Neurocutaneous syndrome
      - Von Hippel - Lindau syndrome
      - Louis Bar syndrome - Ataxia telangiectasia
   4. Metabolic disease
      - Refsum's disease
      - Hartnup disease
      - A beta lipoproteinemia (Bassen-Kornzweig syndrome)
      - Lipoprotein deficiency (Tangier's disease)
      - Wilson's disease.
   5. Chronic alcoholism
   6. Drug induced—Phenytoin
   7. Posterior cranial fossae tumors–CP angle tumors
      - Acoustic Neuromas
      - Medulloblastoma
      - Cerebellar tumors
   8. Paraneoplastic syndrome—bronchogenic carcinoma-carcinoma ovary
   9. Hypothyroidism

c. **Recurrent cerebellar disorder**
   1. Demyelinating diseases—disseminated sclerosis
   2. Hartnup disease
   3. Von Hippel Lindau syndrome—recurrent hemorrhage.

SIGNS OF MENINGEAL IRRITATION

Leptomeningeal inflammation or irritation will produce signs of meningeal irritation:
- Neck rigidity
- Kernig's sign
- Brudzinski sign

Neck Rigidity

Normally the neck can be flexed so that the chin can be placed upon the chest and can be rotated from side to side.

Resistance to the person's flexion of the neck is called neck rigidity, hold the patient's head with both hands of the examiner and try to do the flexion of the neck so as to place the patient's chin upon his chest. If neck rigidity is present there is variable resistance to passive flexion of neck, from slight flexion to no flexion, also, the rotatory movement.

Causes of Neck Rigidity

- Meningitis
- Subarachnoid hemorrhage (SAH)
- Meningism in certain fever—pneumonia, typhoid, etc.
- Cervical spondylosis
- Tetanus
- Spastic cerebral diplegia
- Cerebral coning—tonsillar herniation at foramen magnum
- Cerebellar infarct
- Retropharyngeal abscess.

Kernig's Sign

This is elicited by flexing the thigh of the recumbent patient to a right angle and then attempting to extend the flexed knee. Resistance to the extension to less than 135° is a positive Kernig's sign. Limitation of extension is due to spasm of hamstring muscles. Normally full extension of flexed knee is not possible when the hip is flexed.

Brudzinski Sign

- *Neck sign:* Passive flexion of neck is followed by flexion of both thighs and legs.
- *Leg sign:* While extending the knee in Kernig's maneuver, is accompanied by flexion of opposite hip and knee.

SKULL AND SPINE EXAMINATION

- *Note the size:* Microcephaly, macrocephaly, hydrocephalus
- *Note the shape:* Brachycephaly, dolichocephaly, oxycephaly, frontal bossing, frontoparietal bossing, craniofacial disproportion, hemangioma of face as in Sturge-Weber syndrome.
- *Palpation* for tenderness, depressed #, tender extracranial vessel—temporal arteritis and Swelling of skull—exostosis, localized bony hump in meningioma, secondaries in skull, soft mass in myeloma, eosinophilic granuloma.
- *Percussion:* Cracked pot sound in hydrocephalus.
- *Auscultation:* Over the frontal and temporal region, over the closed eye, carotids, bruit may be heard in AVM, caroticocavernous fistula, vascular meningioma and advanced Paget's disease.

SPINE

- Inspection
  - *Deformities:* Knuckle deformity, Gibbus deformity—Pott's disease
  - *Increased Lordosis:* Proximal myopathy, muscular dystrophy, generalized myasthenia
  - *Kyphoscoliosis:* Syringomyelia, multiple neurofibromatosis, Friedreich's ataxia, Morquio syndrome
  - *Epidural swelling:* Epidural abscess
  - *Short neck and low hair line:* Klippel Feil syndrome
  - *Swelling:* Meningocele, dimple on skin and tuft of hair—Satyre's tail–spina bifida occulta
- Palpation: Pain and tenderness—Pott's disease, secondary spine, localized rigidity—IVDP, paraspinal abscess-movement of spine moderately decreased in ankylosing spondylitis
- Percussion for tenderness
- Auscultation for bruit in vertebral angiomatous malformation.

Peripheral Nerves

Palpable subcutaneous peripheral nerves are examined, for thickening and tenderness.

Palpable Peripheral Nerves

- Great auricular
- Supraclavicular
- Ulnar nerve at elbow
- Dorsal branch of radial nerve at wrist
- Lateral popliteal—neck of fibula
- Sural nerve

Causes of Thickening of Peripheral Nerves

- Hansen's disease
- Primary amyloidosis
- Hypertrophic neuropathy of Dejerine Sottas
- Peroneal muscular atrophy—Charcot-Marie-Tooth disease
- Neurofibromatosis
- Acromegaly
- CIDP

EXAMINATION OF UNCONSCIOUS PATIENT

History

- *Acute*: Trauma, vascular, toxins and drugs
- *Subacute*: Metabolic, infections
- *Insidious*: Organ failure, renal, respiratory, hepatic and endocrine

History of diseases: Renal, respiratory, hepatic, endocrine—DM, CVS disease hypertension, dyslipidemia, stroke, CNS infection, intracranial space occupying lesions (ICSOL), hypertension → headache.

Examination

- General examination and vital signs—nervous system
- Other systems.

General Examination

- Injury—to head—bleeding ear, nose, black eye
- Skin—bleeding → bleeding diathesis, cerebral hemorrhage-rash → septicemia, meningococcemia—injury mark → drug addiction—dry skin → hypothyroidism, CRF—blister → phenobarb—poisoning, pseudomonas septicemia.
- Jaundice → Hepatocellular failure, septicemia, thrombotic thrombocytopenic purpurae
- Cyanosis—respiratory failure, cyanotic CHD →paradoxical embolism
- Pallor—CRF, hypothyroidism, hypopituitarism, internal bleeding and cerebral hemorrhage
- Polycythemia—polycythemia vera—cerebral thrombosis, chronic respiratory failure, cyanotic CHD
- Red color—CO poisoning
- Edema—CRF, chronic liver disease, cor pulmonale, CHF
- Clubbing—bronchogenic Ca → cerebral secondaries, nonmetastatic—SIADH, Ca ↑ cyanotic CHD interstitial lung disease
- Increased sweating—hypoglycemia, febrile illness, cerebral malaria
- Breath smell—alcoholism, kerosene—OP poisoning, fetor hepaticus, fruity odor of DKA, uremia
- Hair loss—hypopituitarism
- Thyroid—Goiter—hypothyroidism
- Pigmentation—Addison's disease.

Vital Signs

a. Temperature
   - Temperature ↑—CNS infection—meningitis, encephalitis malaria, septicemia, pontine hemorrhage, heat stroke
   - Temperature ↓ —hypothyroidism—phenobarbitone poisoning—alcoholism
b. Pulse—irregular—arrhythmia
c. Blood pressure
   - Hypertension: Hypertensive encephalopathy, stroke, CRF
   - Hypotension: Internal bleeding, septicemia, hypoadrenalism, hypopituitarism and phenobarb—poisoning.
d. Respiration
   - *Type of breathing*
     - Acidotic breathing → DKA
     - Cheyne-Stokes breathing → upper brainstem lesion
     - Neurogenic hyperventilation → midbrain lesion
     - Biot's breathing → pontine lesion
     - Chaotic breathing → medullary lesion
   - *Dyspnea:* Respiratory failure-CCF.

Nervous System Examination

- Assess level of consciousness—optic fundi—for papilledema
- Ocular movement
  - Normal gaze palsy
  - Squint
  - Sun setting appearance
  - Ocular bobbing
  - Oculocephalic reflex.
- Pupil
  - Anisocoria—brainstem lesion
  - Bilateral miosis—pontine hemorrhage
  - Unilateral mydriasis—third nerve brain herniation
  - Brain herniation
  - Bilateral mydriasis— bilateral 3rd nerve lesion brain death syndrome, atropine
- Facial muscle weakness
- Tone of the muscle
- Deep reflexes and plantar reflex
- Posture—meningitic—curled up

- decerebrate rigidity
- decorticate rigidity
- hemiplegic
- Response to pain sensation
- Meningeal signs.

Four groups depends on neurological signs		
1	No lateralizing sign No meningeal sign No brainstem damage	Metabolic, Drugs, Toxins – alcoholic Except: Morphine → miosis Phenobarb, Dilantin → ↓ oculocephalic reflex
2	No lateralizing sign With meningeal sign No brainstem damage	Subarachnoid hemorrhage Meningitis
3	With lateralizing sign No meningeal sign No brainstem damage	Hemispheric lesion Ischemic stroke ICSOL Cerebral abscess Subdural hematoma
4	With brainstem damage	Brainstem stroke, brainstem encephalitis, infratentorial ICSOL, supratentorial ICSOL with herniation

Other System Examination

- *Respiratory system:* Acute and chronic respiratory failure
- *Liver:* Hepatocellular failure—acute and chronic
- *Renal:* Renal failure
- *CVS:* Heart disease → embolism
- *Endocrine:*
  - Diabetes mellitus
  - Hypothyroidism
  - Hypoadrenalism
  - Hypopituitarism
- *Electrolytes:* Na ↑, Na ↓ and Ca ↑
- *Osmolality:* Hyperosmolality > 350

Differentiating Features of Cerebral and Metabolic Coma

	Cerebral	Metabolic
a. Motor response	Hemiplegic Decerebrate Decorticate	Normal
b. Pupil	Abnormal	Normal
c. Reflex eye movement	Abnormal	Normal

Etiology of coma: Cerebral and noncerebral causes
1. Cerebral—trauma, stroke, hypertensive encephalopathy, meningitis, cerebral malaria, encephalitis
   ICSOL
   Epilepsy
2. Noncerebral
   - Organ failure—renal, hepatic, respiratory
   - Endocrine—diabetes mellitus, hypothyroidism, hypopituitarism and hypoadrenalism
   - Electrolyte—Na ↑, Na ↓ and Ca ↑
   - Physical—hyperpyrexia, hypothermia hyperosmolality, hypoxia water intoxication

- Drugs and toxins—alcoholism, CO poisoning, narcotics
- Multisystem—septicemia—TTP.

CLINICAL EVALUATION OF HEMIPLEGIA (FIG. 3.54)

The following things to be remembered for proper localization of lesion in hemiplegia.

History

- Onset
  - Acute – Stroke
  - Subacute – Infection, meningitis, encephalitis, cerebral abscess
  - Insidious – ICSOL, c/c SDH
- Headache—acute headache—Hemorrhagic stroke—SAH—chronic headache—ICSOL, SDH hemiplegic migraine
- Altered sensorium—Brainstem lesions large hemispheric lesions, diffuse cerebral lesion—encephalitis—supratentorial lesion with herniation
- History of seizure, speech abnormality
- Cranial nerve symptoms—visual—amaurosis fugax, uniocular blindness, facial weakness, other cranial nerve symptoms
- Sensory, bowel and bladder symptoms
- History of heart disease, lung disease, hypertension, diabetes mellitus, dyslipidemia, etc.
- History of recurrence—demyelinating disease, embolic stroke, hemiplegic migraine.

General Examination

- Fever—CNS infection, pontine hemorrhage
- Pulse—arrhythmia—embolic stroke, absence of pulse—PVD
- Blood pressure—hypertension, stroke
- Polycythemia—ischemic, stroke
- Xanthomas—dyslipidemia (Fig. 3.53)

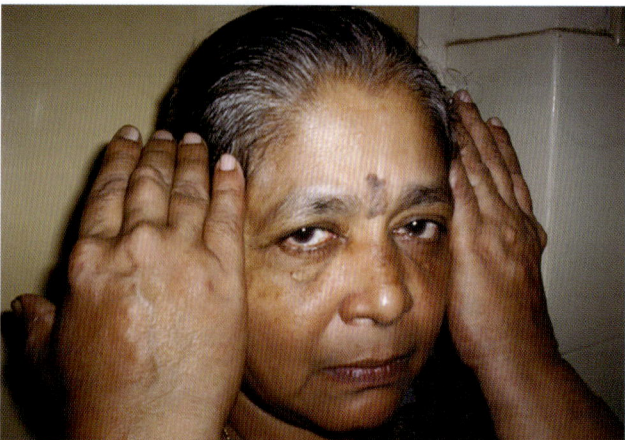

Fig. 3.53: Xanthelasma below the eyelid and xanthoma over the dorsum of the hand.

- Cyanosis—cyanotic CHD—cerebral infarction, paradoxical embolism/secondary polycythemia.

Nervous System Examination

- *Higher functions*: Level of consciousness-speech abnormality—dysphasia—cortical lesion—dysarthria—CN palsy, cerebellar
- *Cranial nerves*
  Optic nerve—uniocular blindness—internal carotid disease, homonymous hemianopia—capsular lesion
  Ocular movement—gaze palsy—premotor—frontal eye field ophthalmoplegia—brainstem lesion
  Horner's syndrome
  a. Internal carotid disease
  b. Brainstem lesion
  Other cranial nerves—LMN lesion in crossed hemiplegia in brainstem lesion—7th nerve UMN lesion-IC transient contralateral UMN lesion. Contralateral UMN 12th CN palsy.
- *Motor system*—signs of UMN lesion—contralateral pyramidal lesion areflexic flaccid weakness in acute phase.
- *Sensory system*—contralateral hemisensory deficit-dulling of primary modalities in hemispheric lesion variable to total loss in brainstem lesion.
- *Cerebellar signs*—contralateral signs in hemispheric lesion—ataxic hemiparesis due to frontopontocerebellar tract lesion—ipsilateral signs in brainstem lesions.
- *Meningeal signs*—SAH, meningitis.

Other Systems Examination

- CVS—valvular heart disease, arrhythmia, CAD, infective endocarditis. Carotid—palpation for pulsation auscultation for bruit—same side and augmentation bruit—opposite side.
- Respiratory system for pneumonia, lung abscess and bronchogenic Ca.

Localization of Hemiplegia (Fig. 3.54)

Three sites
1. Hemispheric lesion
   - Cortical
   - Subcortical—corona radiata
   - Internal capsule

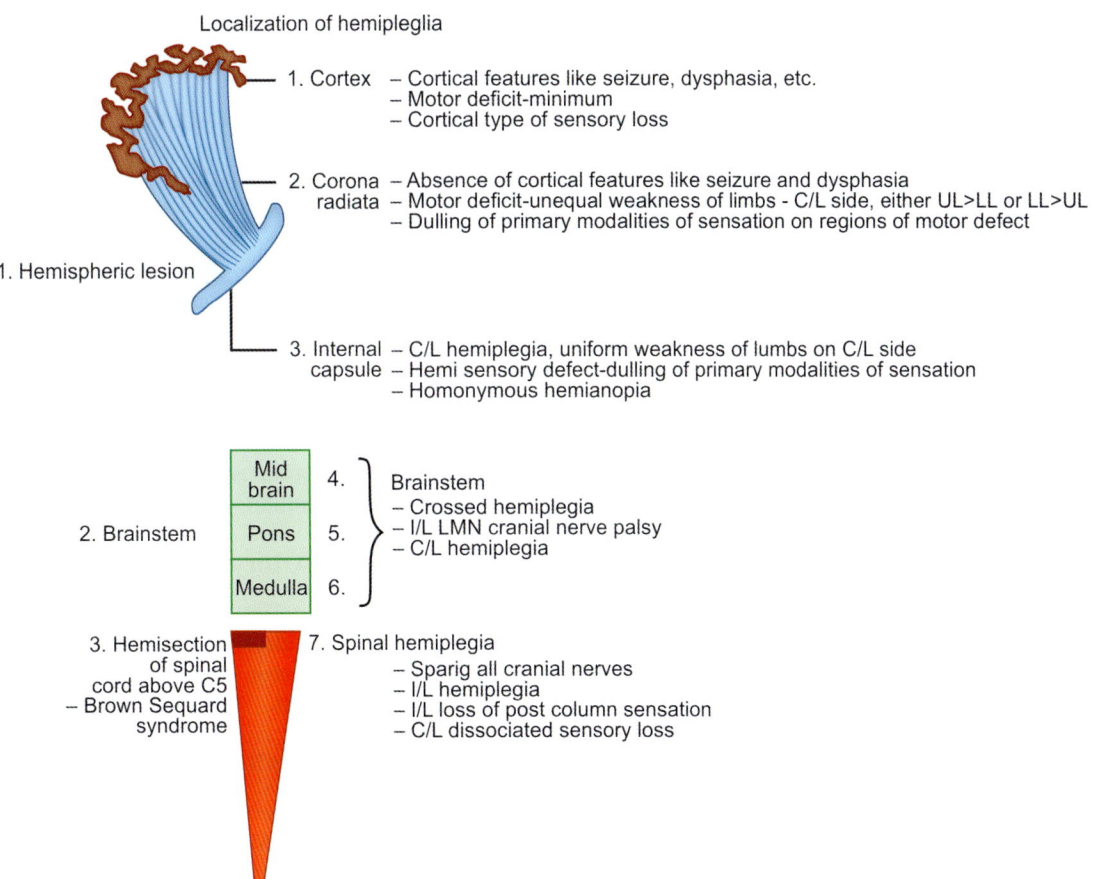

Fig. 3.54: Common sites of lesion for hemiplegia.

2. Brainstem
   - Midbrain
   - Pons
   - Medulla
3. Spinal cord—hemisection above C5 (Brown-Sequard lesion).

Hemispheric Lesion—Features

Cortical lesion
- Cortical phenomenon – seizure
- Speech abnormality
- Motor deficit → minimal motor deficit like weakness of hand.
- Sensory deficit → cortical type of sensory loss with intact primary modalities

Sub-cortical lesion (corona radiata)
- Absence of cortical signs like seizure, dysphasia
- Motor deficit → C/L unequal weakness of limbs either upper limb or lower limb is more involved with UMN signs
- Sensory deficit → dulling of primary modalities of sensation due to lesion of thalamoparietal fibers, on regions of motor deficit since identical sensory motor fibers are nearer.

Internal capsular lesion
- The commonest site of lesion for hemiplegia
- C/L hemiplegia → uniform weakness of upper and lower limb
- Hemisensory deficit – dulling of primary modality
- No total loss of sensation
- Homonymous hemianopia

Brainstem Lesion

(Midbrain, Medulla, Pons)
Crossed hemiplegia – I/L LMN CN palsy with C/L hemiplegia
For example:
- Weber's syndrome → – I/L 3rd N palsy with C/L hemiplegia
- Millard-Gubler syndrome → I/L 6th, 7th CN palsy with C/L hemiplegia.

Spinal Cord Lesion

Spinal hemiplegia: Hemisection above C5—Brown-Sequard lesion—sparing all cranial nerves—ipsilateral hemiplegia ipsilateral loss of posterior column sensation contralateral dissociated sensory loss.

Causes of Hemiplegia

1. Stroke
2. CNS infection—Meningitis, encephalitis, cerebral abscess
3. Demyelinating disease—disseminated sclerosis
4. ICSOL
5. Subdural hematoma
6. Hemiplegic migraine
7. Infantile hemiplegia

Recurrent Hemiplegia

1. Embolic stroke
2. Hemiplegic migraine
3. Demyelinating disease.

NEUROVASCULAR SYNDROMES

Anterior Cerebral Artery

- Cortical branch—crural monoplegia and organic psychosis
- Perforating branch—Heubner's artery faciobrachial weakness
- Facial and proximal muscle weakness
- Stem lesion—hemiplegia with cortical sensory loss in the leg-dissociated hemiplegia of Dimitri and Victoria
- Bilateral anterior cerebral—spasm in aneurysm rupture of anterior communicating artery → cerebral paraplegia.

Middle Cerebral Artery

- Features depend on dominant or nondominant hemisphere and upper or lower branch lesion.
- *Dominant hemisphere:* Dysphasia—varying type parietal lobe features—acalculia, fingeragnosia, left to right disorientation, dyslexia brachial monoplegia, faciobrachial weakness and hemiplegia, hemisensory deficit homonymous hemianopia, apraxia.
- *Nondominant hemisphere*—anosognosia
  - Dressing apraxia
  - Constructional apraxia
  - Motor sensory and hemianopic deficit as above
  - No dysphasia

Posterior Cerebral Artery

Weber's syndrome—cerebral peduncle and 3rd nerve lesion—hemiballismus—subthalamic nucleus—sensory stroke—thalamic lesion—organic psychosis—inferolateral temporal lobe homonymous hemianopia—occipital lobe lesion.

Internal Carotid Artery

Recurrent TIA, ipsilateral optic nerve → uniocular blindness—ipsilateral Horner's syndrome—pericarotid sympathetic fiber lesion contralateral motor sensory deficit—ipsilateral weak carotid and carotid bruit.

Vertebrobasilar System

- *Posterior inferior cerebellar artery*
  - Wallenberg syndrome (lateral medullary syndrome)
  - I/L → Horner's syndrome, palatal palsy, cerebellar signs, facial dissociated sensory loss
  - C/L → dissociated sensory loss of body

- *Anterior inferior cerebellar artery*
  (Lateral inferior pontine syndrome)
  - I/L → 6th, 7th and gaze palsy nerve deafness, auditory nerve lesion, cerebellar signs, Horner's syndrome, facial sensory loss
  - C/L → hemisensory deficit, hemiplegia, vertigo-vestibular nucleus lesion
- **Superior cerebellar artery**-(lateral superior pontine syndrome)
  - I/L → cerebellar ataxia, gaze palsy, Horner's syndrome
  - C/L → hemisensory deficit including face, vertigo-vestibular nucleus lesion.
- *Basilar artery*
  - Features
  - Combination of brainstem structures and posterior cerebral artery distribution involvement. Nuclear lesions—unilateral or bilateral multiple cranial nerve palsy long tract signs—sensory and motor—unilateral or bilateral cerebellar signs—unilateral or bilateral.

CLINICAL ASSESSMENT OF DISEASES OF SPINAL CORD

Introduction

Spinal Cord Problems Manifest as

- Quadriplegia-bilateral, above C5 lesion
- Spinal hemiplegia-unilateral above C5 hemi section
- Paraplegia-bilateral lesion between T1 and L1
- Crural monoplegia—hemisection of spinal cord between T1 and L1.

Paraplegia may occur

- With UMN features
  - When the lesion is in parasagittal region-cerebral paraplegia
  - Lesion between T1 and L1
- Manifesting with LMN features
  a. When lesion of anterior horn cells as in SMA
  b. At roots as in cauda equina and GBS
  c. Motor neuropathy as in CMT
  d. Neuromuscular-myasthenic syndrome
  e. Muscles-inflammatory myopathy, muscular dystrophy periodic paralysis.

History

- Onset—acute, subacute, insidious
- Acute—trauma, vascular
- Subacute—infection, demyelination
- Insidious—nutritional, degenerative, neoplasm.

Motor Symptoms

UMN/LMN symptoms
- UMN features-spastic weakness
- LMN features-flaccid weakness
  - Wasting
  - Fasciculation
- Gait abnormality
- Involuntary movements

Sensory Symptoms

- Pain
  - Radicular pain
  - Tract pain
  - Pain from spine.
- Loss of sensation/paresthesia
- Distribution of sensory symptoms
  - Neural pattern
  - Radicular pattern
  - Dissociated sensory pattern.

Bowel/Bladder Symptoms

- Bowel
  - Constipation
  - Incontinence
- Bladder symptoms
  - Retention
  - Incontinence
  - Urgency
  - Precipitancy
- Symptoms of spine involvement
  - Localized pain
  - Deformity
  - Difficulty in movement
  - Paraspinal swelling.

Past History

- History of febrile illness, preceding trauma/vaccination
- Family history—HSP/hereditary ataxia
- Personal history—Diet-strict vegetarian-B_{12} deficiency—Lathyrism and fluorosis (endemic areas).

Examination

General Examination

- Café-au-lait spots
- Neurofibromas
- Segmental vesicles—herpes zoster
- Cutaneous angiomatosis
- Satyre's tail

Nervous System Examination

Headache
- Parasagittal lesion—increased ICT
- GBS—increased CSF proteins—increased ICT
- Acute disseminated encephalomyelitis

Cranial Nerves
- *Optic nerve*: Optic neuritis, Devic's disease, MS
- *Ophthalmoplegia*: Miller Fischer, Guillain-Barré syndrome (GBS), hereditary ataxia.

Motor System
- Spastic weakness, hyperreflexia, extensor plantar suggests UMN lesion
- Flaccid weakness, hyporeflexia suggests LMN lesion.

Sensory System
Sensory deficit pattern and distribution reduced sensation and zone of hyperesthesia (very important for localization of spinal cord lesion).

Bowel/Bladder Features

Reflexes
Anal and bulbocavernosus reflex—lost in conus/conus-cauda lesions.

Etiology of Paraplegia

They are two groups:
1. **UMN lesion of paraplegia:** Cerebral and spinal cord
   Cerebral: Rare, usual causes are parasagittal meningioma superior sagittal sinus thrombosis bilateral anterior cerebral artery lesion trauma—parasagittal
   Spinal cord: Compressive myelopathy and noncompressive myelopathy.
   Compressive myelopathy
   - Extramedullary extradural—diseases of the spine—secondaries, Pott's disease
   - Extramedullary intradural—neurofibroma, meningioma
   - Intramedullary—ependymoma.

   Non-compressive myelopathy
   - Congenital—hereditary spastic paraplegia syringomyelia
   - Vascular anterior spinal artery occlusion, dissecting aneurysm of aorta, hematomyelia, spinal angiomatous malformation
   - Traumatic
   - Infection—syphilis-epidural abscess-herpes HIV schistosomiasis, hydatid disease, toxoplasmosis
   - Demyelinating diseases disseminated sclerosis, acute disseminated encephalomyelitis, neuromyelitis optica-Devic's disease.
   - Degenerative diseases MND—primary lateral sclerosis, hereditary ataxias
   - Nutritional subacute combined degeneration, lathyrism, fluorosis
   - Myelopathy in systemic diseases SLE, Sjogren's syndrome
   - Porto systemic myelopathy—in cirrhosis liver, myelopathy of paraneoplastic syndrome
   - Toxins and physical agents—nitrous oxide, β oxalyl amino alanine in Lathyrism, radiation
2. **LMN lesion for paraplegia**
   - Anterior horn cell—spinal muscular dystrophy
   - Anterior root—Guillian Barre syndrome
   - Cauda equina -
     - Neuropathy
     - IVDP
     - Secondary deposit
   - Lumbosacral plexus—ischemic plexopathy in diabetes and traumatic
   - Peripheral neuropathies—motor
3. **Neuromuscular junction cause** → myasthenic syndrome.
- **Muscle disease**
  - *Endocrine—proximal myopathy*
  - *Polymyositis*
  - *Muscular dystrophy—limb girdle myopathy*
- **Hysterical**
- **Recurrent paraplegia**
  - *Demyelinating disease—disseminated sclerosis*
  - *Dumpell tumor—neurofibroma*
  - *Spinal arachnoid cyst.*

Clinical Features

- Depending on the onset
  - Acute paraplegia—traumatic, vascular, hysterical
  - Subacute paraplegia—infection and demyelination, e.g. epidural abscess transverse myelitis—Guillian Barré syndrome
  - Chronic paraplegia—degenerative—primary lateral sclerosis, nutritional, neoplasm
- Pure motor paraplegia
  - Hereditary spastic paraplegia
  - Primary lateral sclerosis
  - Early cases of spondylotic myelopathy
  - CVJ anomaly
  - Extramedullary compression
- *Sensory features*: Refer localization in sensory system—spinal cord.
- LMN signs in upper limbs and UMN signs in lower limbs
  - Amyotrophic lateral sclerosis
  - Syringomyelia
  - Cervical spondylosis
  - Extramedullary compression—cervical
  - Cervical pachymeningitis—syphilitic

- Absent ankle jerk with extensor plantar
  - Subacute combined degeneration
  - Friedreich's ataxia
  - Taboparesis
- Bipyramidal signs without any definite level of lesion
  - Hereditary spastic paraplegia
  - Primary lateral sclerosis
  - Subacute combined degeneration
  - Lathyrism
  - Fluorosis
  - Early spondylotic myelopathy
  - CVJ anomaly
  - Early extramedullary compression

Paraplegia in Flexion and in Extension

Paraplegia in extension: Incomplete lesions of spinal cord involving pyramidal fibers sparing extrapyramidal fibers to anterior horn cell. The lower limbs assume extensor hypertonia → extension of knee and plantar flexion.

Paraplegia in flexion: In complete lesions of spinal cord involving both pyramidal and extrapyramidal fibers to anterior horn cell, the lower limbs have flexion of hip, knee and dorsiflexion of ankle. No UMN influence on anterior horn cell. Thus new intraspinal reflexes develop called mass reflex of Ridoch. Any type of stimuli like sound, touch, will elicit this reflex leading to flexion attitude of the lower limb with spontaneous bowel and bladder evacuation.

Progressive lesions of the spinal cord produce paraplegia in extension, later, paraplegia in flexion. In transection of the spinal cord, recovery will lead to paraplegia in flexion without undergoing paraplegia in extension.

Investigations

1. Done to localize the lesion
2. To find out the etiology

To localize the lesion:
a. X-ray spine (Fig. 3.55)
b. MRI spine

To find out the etiology:
- Compressive myelopathy-imaging
- Non compressive myelopathy
  - Infections
    - Tuberculosis → Mantoux, ESR, isolation of AFB
    - Herpes CSF → antigen/antibody
    - Syphilis → blood/CSF serology
    - HIV-serology
  - Vascular-Imaging
    - Nutritional → Serum B_{12} estimation and B_{12} kinetics
    - Demyelination—CSF Study
    - Oligoclonal band → MS, albuminocytological dissociation → GBS.

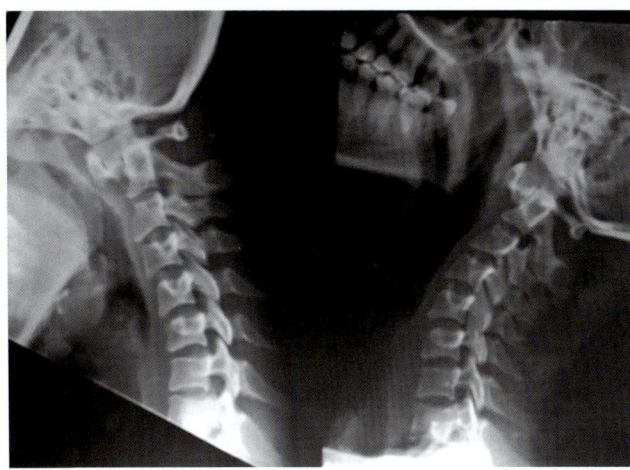

Fig. 3.55: X-ray flexion and extension of cervical spine centering at C1-showing atlanto-axial subluxation.

- Spinal block—CSF protein increased → Froin's syndrome
- Spinal SAH → AVM of spinal cord
- Fluorosis → X-ray-Hyperosteosis
- EMG → MND, Muscle disease
- NCS → Peripheral Neuropathy

Treatment

General
- Care of bowel/bladder
  - Bladder care—intermittent catheterization
  - Bowel-avoid constipation, adequate laxatives
- Skin care to prevent bed sores, frequent change of posture
- Breathing exercise to prevent hypostatic pneumonia
- Graded physiotherapy

Surgery for compressive myelopathy
- Treat infections—herpes, HIV, TB, epidural abscess
- Demyelinating-IVIg-plasmapheresis, corticosteroid
- Supplement B_{12}—in SACD
- Avoid ingestion of toxins causing lathyrism and fluorosis
- Treatment of malignancy—for paraneoplastic myelopathy
- Treatment of systemic diseases with myelopathy-like SLE, Sjogrens, cirrhosis with portal hypertension.

Neurogenic Bladder (Fig. 3.56)

a. *Parasympathetic:* Intermediolateral horn of spinal segments S2, S3, S4. They supply detrusor muscle and internal sphincter through hypogastric ganglion and pelvic nerves.
b. *Sympathetic*: From T12, L1, L2, L3.
c. *Somatic motor fibers:* From spinal segments S2, S3, S4–supply striated muscle of external sphincter through pudendal nerve.

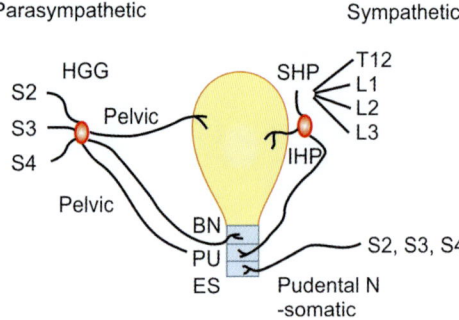

Fig. 3.56: Innervation of bladder.
Abbreviations: HGG, hypogastric ganglion; SHP and IHP, superior and inferior hypogastric plexus; BN, Bladder neck; PU, posterior urethra; ES, external sphincter

d. *Cortical fibers:* From the paracentral lobule, the inhibitory fibers descend through the corticospinal tract to the anterior horn cells of S2, S3, S4.

Micturition Reflex (Fig. 3.57)

Micturition reflex has been represented in Figure 3.57.

Symptoms of Neurogenic Bladder

a. Hesitancy—delay in the initiation of the act of micturition.
b. Urgency—inability to hold the urine once the sensation of distention of bladder is perceived.
c. Incontinence—involuntary voiding of urine, continuous—massive incontinence intermittent—dribbling incontinence
d. Retention—incomplete emptying of the bladder.
e. Distention—Abnormal increase in the capacity of bladder to hold urine.

Different Types of Neurogenic Bladder

a. *Automatic bladder (UMN bladder, Cord bladder):* Lesion above S2, S3, S4—micturition reflex arc is intact. Bladder automatically evacuates once the intravesical pressure is increased. No inhibitory influence from higher center—symptoms of urgency and precipitancy.
b. *Autonomous bladder (LMN bladder):* Lesion involving the spinal micturition center S2, S3, S4—reflex arc is disrupted. Dribbling of urine due to contraction of islets of detrusor muscle on stretch. Bladder is distended with absence of sensation.
c. Motor paralytic bladder – efferent fibers are affected → diabetes mellitus, cauda equina lesion
d. Sensory paralytic bladder – afferent fibers are affected → tabes dorsalis, cauda equina lesion.
e. *Uninhibited bladder:* Loss of voluntary inhibitory control on micturition. Urinates in inappropriate time and place. Seen in lesions of frontal lobe, dementia NPH and in children below 2 years also.
f. *Atonic bladder:* Loss of tone and contraction of bladder and its sphincters. Seen in acute spinal cord lesions like transverse myelitis, traumatic paraplegia characterized by initial retention, later becoming automatic bladder.

PERIPHERAL NEUROPATHY

Peripheral Nervous System

Definition: It is the part of nervous system outside the pia-arachnoid.

Terms Related to Peripheral Nervous System Involvement

- Mononeuropathy—features of neurological deficit confined to one peripheral nerve
- Polyneuropathy—features of neurological deficit confined to more than one peripheral nerves.

Types

- Peripheral neuropathy—distal symmetrical involvement
- Mononeuritis multiplex—asymmetrical involvement of 2 or more peripheral nerves.

Peripheral Neuropathy: Etiology

- Congenital—hereditary motor sensory neuropathy
- Infection
  - Hansen's disease
  - Diphtheria
  - HIV
  - Infectious mononucleosis
  - Lyme disease
- Demyelination
  - AIDP
  - CIDP
- Drugs
  - INH
  - Nitrofurantoin
  - Antineoplastic drugs

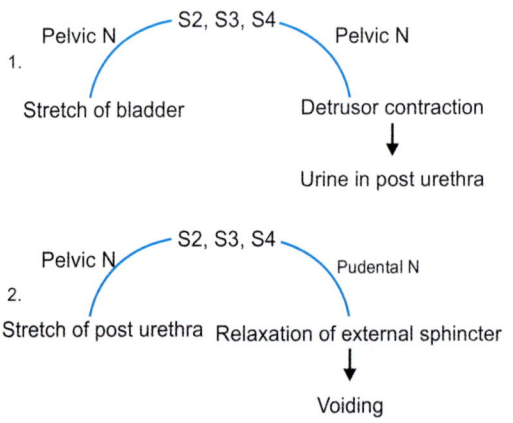

Fig. 3.57: Micturition reflex.

Table 3.8: Difference between intramedullary and extramedullary lesion.		
Clinical features	Intramedullary	Extramedullary
Spontaneous pain	Burning type: poorly localized	Radicular type and distribution; early and important symptom
Sensory deficit	Suspended dissociated sensory loss	Contralateral loss of pain and temperature; ipsilateral loss of proprioceptive; Brown-Sequard type
Changes in pain and temperature sensations in Saddle areas	Sacral sparing	No sacral sparing
LMN involvement	Marked and widespread; with atrophy and fasciculations	Segmental
UMN involvement	Late and minimal	Early and prominent
Muscle stretch reflexes	Changes- late and minimal	Early hyperreflexia
Pyramidal signs	Late	Early
Trophic changes	Marked	Usually not marked
Spinal subarachnoid block and changes in spinal fluid	Late and less marked	Early and marked (Froin's syndrome)
Bowel and bladder dysfunction, sexual dysfunction	Early	Late

Table 3.9: Differences between lesions of conus medullaris and cauda equina.		
Clinical features	Conus medullaris (S3, S4, S5, Co1)	Cauda Equina (L2 root down)
Spontaneous pain	Not common or severe; bilateral and symmetric; in perineum or thighs	May be most prominent symptom; severe; radicular type; unilateral/asymmetric; in perineum, thighs and legs; distribution in the lumbosacral nerves
Sensory deficit	Saddle distribution; bilateral; Usually symmetric; Dissociation of sensation	Saddle distribution; unilateral and asymmetric; all forms affected; no dissociation of sensation
Motor deficit	Symmetric; not marked; fasciculations may be present	Asymmetric; more marked; atrophy may occur; usually no fasciculations
Reflex loss (DTR)	No reflex loss	Patellar and Achille's reflex may be absent
Bladder and rectal symptoms	Early and marked	Late and less marked
Trophic changes	Early	Less
Sexual functions	Erection and ejaculation Impaired	Impairment less
Onset	Sudden and bilateral	Gradual and unilateral

- Toxins
  - Mercury
  - Arsenic
- Alcoholism
- Metabolic
  - Diabetes mellitus
  - Porphyria
  - Amyloidosis
  - Bassen-Kornzweig syndrome
  - Tangier's disease
- Nutritional
  - B_{12} deficiency
  - B_6 deficiency
  - Pantothenic acid deficiency
- Collagen vascular diseases
  - SLE
  - Progressive systemic sclerosis
  - Sjögren syndrome
- Endocrine
  - Hypothyroidism
  - Graves' disease
  - Acromegaly
- Malignancy-Paraproteinemia
- Critical illness neuropathy
- Paraneoplastic
- **Mononeuritis multiplex**
  - Hansen's disease
  - Polyarteritis nodosa

- Rheumatoid arthritis
- Sarcoidosis
- Paraneoplastic

Investigations
- Nerve conduction study
- Nerve biopsy
- Electromyography
    - Hansen's disease—nerve biopsy—AFB
    - CSF—albuminocytological dissociation—AIDP, CIDP
    - Serum protein electrophoresis
    - Vitamin B_{12} assay
    - Urine porphobilinogen—porphyria
    - Serology—collagen vascular disease

Thickened Peripheral Nerves
- Hansen's disease
- Dejerine Sottas disease
- Neurofibroma
- CIDP
- CMT
- Acromegaly

Management of peripheral neuropathy
- Infection—appropriate antimicrobials
- Demyelination—IVIg, plasmapheresis
- Methylprednisolone
- Avoid toxins, alcohol and drugs
- Metabolic—DM-glycemic control
- Nutritional B_1, B_6, B_{12} supplementation
- Collagen vascular diseases—corticosteriods, immunosuppressants
- Endocrine—hormone supplementation
- Malignancy—treat accordingly
- Physiotherapy.

Classification of Nerve fibers

Fiber type	Conduction velocity	Diameter	Functions	Myelin
A fibers				
Alpha	70–120 m/s	12–20 μm	Motor–skeletal muscle	Yes
Beta	40–70 m/s	5–12 μm	Sensory—touch, pressure, vibration	Yes
Gamma	10–50 m/s	3–6 μm	Muscle spindle	Yes
Delta	6–30 m/s	2–5 μm	Sharp and localized pain, temperature, touch	Yes
B fibers	3–15 m/s	<3 μm	Preganglionic autonomic	Yes
C fibers	0.5–2 m/s	0.4–1.2 μm	Pain-diffuse deep, temperature, postganglionic autonomic	No

Small Fiber Neuropathies
1. Painful neuropathies
    - Diabetic small fiber neuropathy
    - Alpha lipoprotenemia-Tangier's disease
    - Fabry's disease
    - HIV and ART
2. Neuropathy with dissociated sensory loss
    - Hansen's disease
    - Amyloidosis

Large Fiber Sensory Neuropathy/Ataxic Neuropathy
- Sjögren's syndrome
- Vitamin B_{12} neuropathy (dorsal column involvement)
- Cisplatin neuropathy
- Pyridoxine toxicity
- Friedrich's ataxia.

Small and Large Fiber Neuropathy—Global Sensory Loss
- Carcinomatous sensory neuropathy
- Hereditary sensory neuropathy
- Diabetic sensory neuropathy
- Xanthomatous neuropathy of primary biliary cirrhosis.

Peripheral Neuropathy with Cerebellar Involvement
- Abetalipoproteinemia
- Tangier's disease
- Refsum disease

Disease and Treatment-associated Peripheral Neuropathy
- Diabetes mellitus and insulin
- Rheumatoid arthritis and gold
- Alcohol and antabuse
- HIV and stavudine
- Malignancy and antineoplastic drug—cisplatin
- Hansen's disease—dapsone.

Myelopathy with Peripheral Nerve Involvement
- B_{12} neuropathy
- Paraneoplastic
- Demyelination
- SLE
- Sjögren's syndrome
- Adrenomyeloneuropathy.

Peripheral Neuropathy with Cranial Nerve Involvement
- Guillain-Barré syndrome
- Diabetes mellitus
- Sarcoidosis
- Hansen's disease
- Diphtheria
- Vitamin B_{12} deficiency.

CHAPTER 4

Examination of Cardiovascular System

SYMPTOMATOLOGY

1. Dyspnea
2. Palpitation
3. Chest pain
4. Cyanosis
5. Edema
6. Syncopal attack
7. Cough and hemoptysis
8. Fatigue

Dyspnea

See section on General Examination in Chapter 2.

Palpitation

Awareness of one's own heartbeat.

Mechanism

- Increase in the rate of contraction
- Increase in the force of contraction
- Change in the rhythm of contraction.

Clinically Two Types

- Exertional palpitation—with organic heart disease, anemia, etc.
- Paroxysmal palpitation—episodes of palpitation at rest and nonexertional fast, chaotic irregular—atrial fibrillation fast, regular—paroxysmal tachyarrhythmia.
  - Paroxysmal supraventricular tachycardia (PSVT) and ventricular tachycardia (VT)
  - Thyrotoxicosis
  - Pheochromocytoma
- PSVT is characterized by abrupt onset and abrupt offset lasting for several minutes with fatigability and followed by polyuria.
- Patient should try to replicate the rhythm of the palpitation by tapping on a table to know whether regular or irregular.
- Skipped beat → flopping sensation is due to atrial extra systole or ventricular extra systole. Strong beat of overfilled heart following extra systole produces the awareness of heartbeat.

Drugs causing palpitation:
- Caffeine
- β agonists—salbutamol
- Atropine, etc.
  The most common cause of palpitation is anxiety neurosis.

Chest Pain

It is the most important symptom in cardiovascular diseases.
  It can be due to—cardiovascular origin or non-cardiovascular origin
- Cardiovascular origin
  - Myocardium pain
  - Pericardial pain
  - Aortic pain
- Non-cardiovascular origin
  - Chest wall pain
  - Respiratory system-pleura
  - Upper airway mediastinum-esophagus and other tissues
  - Psychogenic
- Myocardial pain—resulting from imbalance between blood supply and demand of myocardium.
  - Factors are—vascular, myocardial or combination of both.

Features
- Site—retrosternal
- Character—constricting, heaviness to unbearable pain.
- Body language of pain
  - Fist over the central chest—Levine's sign
  - Pressing with palm over the central chest
  - Rotatory movement of the hand over the central chest
  - Radiation—to neck and jaw, left arm, right arm and epigastrium

- Associated with—sweating, palpitation
- Precipitated by exercise, emotion, exposure to cold
- Relieved by rest or by nitrates usually within 5 minutes.

Depends on duration
- Angina—more than 2 minutes to less than 20 minutes
- Myocardial infarction—more than 30 minutes
- The angina pain is usually not less than 1 minute and not more than 20 minutes
- Functional classification of angina (by Canadian Cardiovascular Society):

Class 1: Angina resulting from strenuous or prolonged exertion at work.
Class 2: Angina resulting from walking or climbing stairs rapidly, walking uphill.
Class 3: Angina resulting from ordinary physical activity like dressing oneself and taking bath.
Class 4: Angina present at rest or inability to carry out day to day activity without pain.

Causes of Angina

- Coronary disease
  - Atherosclerotic and nonatherosclerotic
  - Vasculitis, vasospasm, embolism
  - Congenital anomaly
- Noncoronary disease
  - Aortic stenosis
  - Hypertrophic obstructive cardiomyopathy (HOCM) and mitral value prolapse (MVP)
  - Hyperviscosity—polycythemia
  - Right ventricular (RV) angina—pulmonary arterial hypertension (PAH)
  - Systemic hypertension and left ventricular hypertrophy (LVH)
  - Severe anemia
- Pericardial pain:
  - Central chest pain for hours to days relieved by sitting and leaning forward. Aggravated by lying down
- Aortic pain:
  - Due to dissecting aneurysm of aorta
  - Acute, excruciating, tearing type of chest pain
  - Site of pain depends on the site of dissection
  - May radiate to back
  - Added with features of ischemia elsewhere like ischemic stroke, acute paraplegia, ischemia of limb.

Three vascular accidents in the chest causing severe pain:
  - Acute myocardial infarction (MI)
  - Dissecting aneurysm
  - Pulmonary embolism

Cyanosis

See section on General Examination in Chapter 2.

Edema

See section on General Examination in Chapter 2.

Syncopal Attack

It is a transient loss of consciousness due to decreased cerebral blood supply.
- Cardiac syncope is due to decrease in the cardiac output.
- Presyncope/Near syncope—feels dizzy, weak and tends to lose postural tone, no loss of consciousness.

Decrease in cerebral blood supply for
- 5 sec → presyncope
- 10 sec → loss of consciousness
- 15 sec → seizure.

Causes of cardiac syncope:
- Aortic stenosis, HOCM, severe PAH, tetralogy of Fallot (TOF)
- Bradyarrhythmias—complete heart block
- Sick sinus syndrome → Stokes Adams syncope
- Tachyarrhythmias—ventricular tachycardia, PSVT

Heart rate <40 and >160 will produce hemodynamic symptoms in normal person.

Cough and Hemoptysis

- **Cough**
  - Due to recurrent respiratory tract infection (RTI) as in mitral valvular disease
  - Left to right shunt
  - Nocturnal cough in paroxysmal nocturnal dyspnea (PND)
  - Cough with pink frothy sputum in pulmonary edema.
- **Hemoptysis** in cardiovascular diseases are due to:
  - *Pulmonary* edema—pink frothy sputum
  - Mitral stenosis—bronchopulmonary apoplexy due to rupture of bronchopulmonary venule.
  - PAH as in Eisenmenger syndrome → pulmonary infarct.
  - Infective endocarditis—right ventricular—ventricular septal defect (VSD) and tricuspid valvular endocarditis—vegetation → pulmonary infarct
  - Patent ductus arteriosus (PDA) with end arteritis - vegetation → pulmonary infarct
  - Congestive heart failure (CHF) → deep vein thrombosis (DVT) → pulmonary infarct
  - Post-MI → DVT → pulmonary infarct

Fatigue

Fatigue in heart disease are due to:
- Low output state—obstructive valvular lesion:
  - AS
  - PAH
- Diffuse myocardial damage:
  - Ischemic heart disease (IHD), cardiomyopathy
- Decreased blood volume and electrolyte imbalance
  - Diuretics
  - β blocker
  - Added anxiety and depression.

HISTORY IN CARDIOVASCULAR DISORDERS

- Presenting symptoms in chronological order are as follows:
  - Dyspnea
  - Palpitation
  - Chest pain
  - Cyanosis
  - Edema
  - Syncopal attack
  - Cough and hemoptysis
  - Fatigue
  - Fever
  - Symptoms of rheumatic fever: Arthritis, rash, abnormal movements.
- History of presenting complaint
  - Detailing of each symptom—(see section on Symptomatology)
- Past history
  - Enquire about the presence of diabetes mellitus, dyslipidemia hypertension, etc.
  - Rheumatic fever
  - Sexually transmitted diseases
  - Other illness
- Family history
  - Hypertension
  - Coronary artery disease (CAD)
  - Diabetes mellitus
  - Obesity
  - Rheumatic and congenital heart disease, dyslipidemia
- Personal history
  - Appetite, diet
  - Alcoholism
  - Smoking
  - Occupation
  - Exercise
- Treatment history
  - Drugs for—CAD, hypertension, diabetes mellitus, and dyslipidemia.

GENERAL EXAMINATION IN CARDIOVASCULAR SYSTEM

- **Dyspnea**
  - Dyspnea—Orthopnea and resting dyspnea suggest cardiac failure
  (See section on General Examination in Chapter 2).
- **Cyanosis**
  - Central cyanosis—cyanotic CHD
  - Differential cyanosis—PDA with Eisenmenger syndrome
  - Mixed cyanosis—Pulmonary edema and shock in acute MI
  - Peripheral cyanosis—shock, severe PAH, right heart failure.
  (See section on General Examination in Chapter 2).
- **Edema**
  - Dependent edema—sign of right heart failure
  - Pitting bilateral pedal edema/sacral edema
  (See section on General Examination in Chapter 2).
- **Clubbing**
  - In cyanotic CHD, infective endocarditis, aortic aneurysm, subclavian aneurysm
  - Unilateral clubbing atrial myxoma—rare.
- **Anemia**
  - Can aggravate all heart diseases
  - Anemia and heart disease together seen—in infective endocarditis and hypothyroidism
  - Anemia → Congestive heart failure.
- **Polycythemia**
  - Primary polycythemia—hyperviscosity angina coronary thrombosis
  - Secondary polycythemia—in cyanotic CHD
- **Markers of infective endocarditis**
  - Osler's node—reddish purple tender nodule in distal pad of finger and toe
  - Janeway lesion—coalesced nontender hemorrhagic lesion of palm and sole.
  - Splinter hemorrhage—linear subungual hemorrhage-distal third of nail.
- **Markers of rheumatic fever**
  - Polyarthritis—major joints
  - Erythema marginatum—in 10%, evanescent ringed lesion with raised red margin, seen over the chest, abdomen and proximal part of limbs.
  - Subcutaneous nodule—in 10-15%, firm painless felt over bone and tendons—extensor aspect of elbow, knee, margin of scapula—occipital region.
  - Erythema nodosum—nonspecific lesion, erythematous tender lesion over the shin.
- **Somatic abnormalities with heart disease**
  - Polydactyly (Fig. 4.1) and syndactyly—VSD
  - Hypertelorism—increase in the interpupillary distance—pulmonary stenosis (Fig. 4.2)
  - Arachnodactyly (Fig. 4.3)—Long thin fingers—atrial septal defect (ASD)
  - Atriodigital anomaly—fingerisation of thumb—ASD
  - Holt Oram syndrome
  - Turner's syndrome—Dwarfism, primary amenorrhea-coarctation of aorta
  - Noonan's syndrome—triangular facies, somatic features of Turner-Pulmonary stenosis
  - Mongolism—endocardial cushion defect/VSD

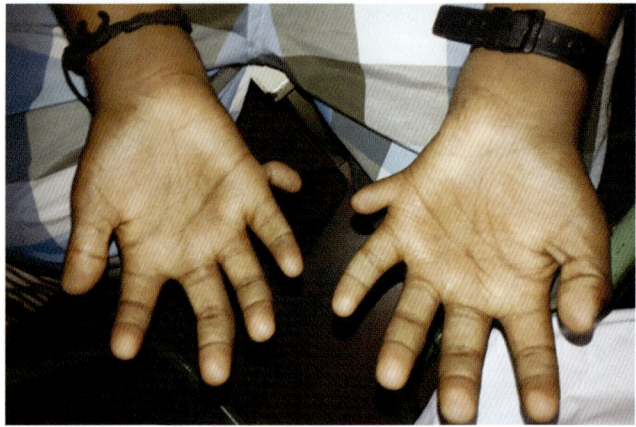

Fig. 4.1: Polydactyly in Lawrence-Moon-Bardet-Biedel syndrome.

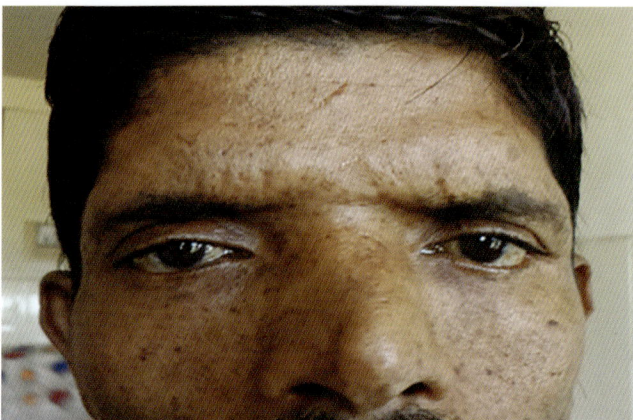

Fig. 4.2: Hypertelorism—increase in the interpupillary distance.

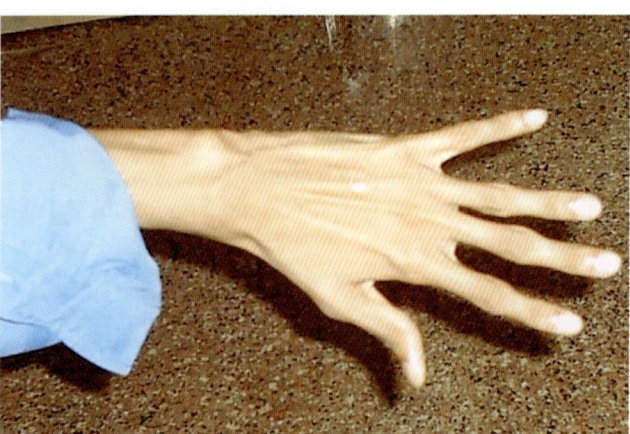

Fig. 4.3: Arachnodactyly—Long thin fingers in a patient with Marfan's syndrome.

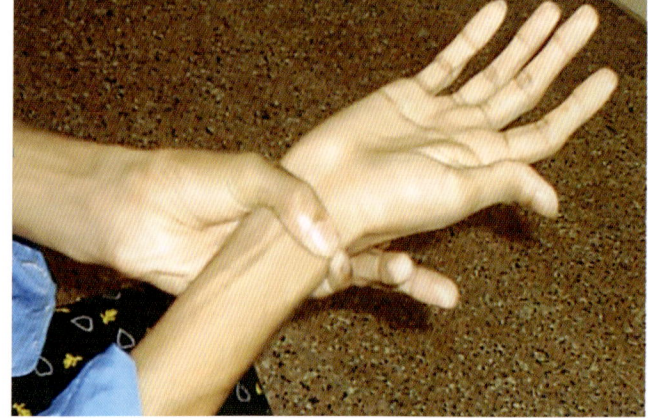

Fig. 4.4: Wrist sign in a patient with Marfan's syndrome.

- Ellis Van Crevald syndrome—dwarfism, chondroectodermal dysplasia—VSD
- William's syndrome—Elfin facies—mental retardation, hypercalcemia and supravalvular AS
- Pierre Robin syndrome—micrognathia, glossoptosis—coarctation of aorta
- Marfan's syndrome (Fig. 4.4)—dissecting aneurysm, ASD, MVP, AR, etc.
- TAR syndrome—thrombocytopenia, absent radius with ASD.
- **Skin**
    - Pigmentation—hemochromatosis → cardiomyopathy
    - Flushing—carcinoid syndrome → right sided valvular lesion
    - Markers of systemic lupus erythematosus (SLE) and progressive systemic sclerosis (PSS)—myocardial and pericardial involvement
    - Markers of rheumatic fever and infective endocarditis
        - Xanthomas—s/c nodule
        - Xanthoma tuberosum
        - Tendon-xanthoma tendinosum
        - Palm and sole—eruptive xanthoma
        - Dyslipidemia→ CAD
    - Markers of heritable connective tissue disease—Ehler Danlos → aortic valvular disease.
- **Thyroid**—for evidence of hypo- and hyperthyroidism → heart disease.
- **Fever in heart disease**
    - Infective endocarditis, RTI
    - Rheumatic activity
    - Pericarditis—TB, pyogenic, viral
    - Collagen vascular disease
    - Infarction—myocardial and pulmonary
    - Atrial myxoma—rare.
- **Locomotor system**—for evidence of
    - Rheumatic fever → valvular heart disease
    - Rheumatoid arthritis → Aortitis–AR
    - Ankylosing spondylitis → Aortitis–AR
    - Psoriatic arthritis → Aortitis–AR
    - Reiter's syndrome → Aortitis–AR.

CVS Examination

- Pulse
- Blood pressure
- Jugular venous pressure and pulsation
- Examination of precordium
- Inspection
- Palpation
- Percussion
- Auscultation

PULSE

It is defined as a pressure wave propagated along the arterial wall from the root of aorta as a result of ejection of blood with every cardiac contraction.

- **Normal arterial waves:**
  - Percussion wave—produced by the ejected amount of blood into the arterial system
  - Tidal wave—generated along the arterial wall
  - Dicrotic wave—formed by the recoil of the vessel

Clinically the pulse is usually examined at the radial artery.

While examining, note the following:

- Rate
- Rhythm
- Volume
- Character
- Condition of the vessel wall
- Peripheral pulsations
- Radial femoral delay

Normal pulse can be expressed as "Rate 72/min, regular in rhythm, volume and character—normal, vessel wall is soft, all pulsations felt equally, no radial femoral delay".

Method—Patient is in the supine position, support the right hand of the patient with the right hand of the examiner. Slight flexion of the wrist will allow feeling the radial artery better. Use the middle 3 fingers of the examiner's left hand to feel the radial pulse (Fig. 4.5).

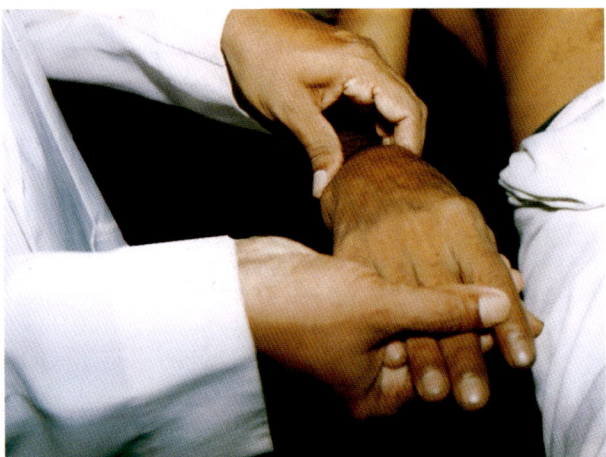

Fig. 4.5: Palpation of radial pulse.

Rate

- Normal rate is 60–100/min
  - Bradycardia - < 60/min
  - Tachycardia - > 100/min

Pulse rate should be counted for one full minute by palpating the radial artery.

Abnormalities

- **Sinus bradycardia**
  - Physiological
    - Athletes—increased vagal tone
    - Sleep—decrease in sympathetic activity
  - Pathological
    - Hypothyroidism
    - Obstructive jaundice
    - Increased intracranial pressure—Cushing phenomenon
    - Sick sinus syndrome
    - Drugs–β blocker, digoxin
- **Sinus tachycardia**
  - Physiological
    - Exercise, infants, emotion
  - Pathological
  - Fever, thyrotoxicosis
    - Pheochromocytoma
    - CHF, pericardial disease
    - Hypovolemic shock
  - Drugs
    - β agonists
    - Salbutamol
    - Nifedipine-Ca channel blocker
    - Atropine, caffeine

Rhythm

It is the regularity with which one beat follows the other.

Clinical Abnormalities

- **Occasionally irregular—extrasystole**
- **Regularly irregular**
  - Regular extrasystole
  - Sinus arrhythmia
  - Inspiration increase in heart rate. Expiration decrease in heart rate due to change in vagal tone.
- **Irregularly irregular**
  - No two beats are alike
  - Atrial fibrillation, multiple extrasystole
  - Paroxysmal atrial tachycardia (PAT) with varying block.

Difference between AF and Multiple Extrasystole

	AF	Multiple extrasystole
a wave	Absent	
Pulse deficit	> 10	<10
On exertion	Persist or increase	Diminish or disappear

Volume of pulse

Amplitude of expansile movement of the vessel wall during the passage of pulse wave that depends on the pulse pressure.

Pulse Pressure

- 30–60 – normal volume
- < 30 – decrease volume
- > 60 – increase volume

Clinical Abnormalities

- Low volume
- High volume
- Varying volume
- Pulsus alternans
- Pulsus paradoxus

Low Volume—Causes

- Hypovolemia
- Obstructive valvular lesion–AS
- Severe PAH
- Pericardial effusion
- Low output in myocardial damage—CAD, cardiomyopathy

High Volume

- The basic mechanism is rapid run off of blood from arterial system either to heart, corresponding vein or to capillaries.
  - At cardiac level → AR
  - At aortic level → PDA
  - At arterial level → Arteriovenous fistula
  - At capillary level → opening up of all capillaries on demand
  - Anemia, high fever, thyrotoxicosis, beri-beri, cirrhosis liver

Varying Volume

- *Varying volume* is a combination of low, normal, or high volume pulse in varying manner because of varying duration of diastolic filling.
  - Atrial fibrillation—varying volume with irregular pulse—Total irregularity of pulse
  - Ventricular tachycardia—varying volume with regular pulse. Atrial support to ventricular filling is variable.

Pulsus Alternans

- High and low volume of alternate pulse due to alternate high and low stroke volume, which is seen in left ventricular failure (LVF).
- Mechanism–is reflex mediated, → Initiated by an extrasystole in LVF → Sensed by the sensitive baroreceptors of the carotid sinus → Left ventricular contraction following an extrasystole is strong due to more diastolic filling during compensatory pause → stroke volume increases→ pulse volume is increases. This is sensed by the baroreceptors of the carotid sinus which in turn send inhibitory impulse to atria via carotid vagoatrial reflex weak contraction of atria, ventricular filling decreases → stroke volume decreases → pulse volume decreases, which is again sensed by the baroreceptor → facilitator impulses via carotid sympathetic atrial reflex → atrial contraction is increases → ventricular filling is increases → stroke volume is increases → pulse volume is increases. This reflex activity occurring alternatively → produce high and low pulse volume.
  - Pulses alternans can be felt by palpation but definite demonstration is by sphygmomano-meter. Occlude the pulse by raising the pressure, then slowly reduce the pressure. Initially the Korotkoff sounds due to the passage of the high volume pulse is heard, further reduction will allow the passage of the weak beat also. This will produce sudden doubling of the Korotkoff sounds–Gallavardin sign.

Pulsus Paradoxus–Kussmaul's Pulse

- It is an exaggerated narrowing of the pulse volume during inspiration as evidenced by inspiratory fall of systolic BP > 10 mm Hg during quiet breathing.
- In normal person also, inspiratory filling of LV is less, stroke volume is less, pulse volume is less, but may not be clinically detectable.
- **Mechanisms**
  - In pericardial diseases like constrictive pericarditis, cardiac chambers are held in rigid pericardium, inspiratory increased filling of RV is taking place at the expense of the LV volume. Thus, LV volume is decreased→ filling is decreased→ stroke volume decreases→ pulse volume decreases. Ventricles cannot increase its size during diastole due to thickened pericardium or due to increased intrapericardial pressure as in pericardial effusion.
  - During inspiration, there is a fall in negativity of pressure in all the structures inside the chest. Considering the fall in pressure in LA and pulmonary vein, the fall in pressure is more in pulmonary vein than in LA which is kept inside the rigid pericardium, thus the pressure gradient between pulmonary vein and LA is decreased

→ LA filling is decreased → LV filling is decreased → stroke volume is decreased→ pulse volume is decreased.
- During inspiration there is stretch of pericardium by the downward movement of diaphragm, this will further decrease the volume of the cardiac chambers including LV → impeding the filling further → stroke volume is decreased→ pulse volume decreases.
- **Demonstration:** Pulses paradoxus is demonstrated accurately by using sphygmomanometer-demonstrating systolic pressure fall >10 mm Hg during inspiration. Patient should be in quiet breathing, by raising the pressure occlude the arterial pulse, slowly release the pressure, initially one will hear the Korotkoff sounds only during expiration. On further reduction, Korotkoff sounds during inspiration also start hearing. The difference in pressure between expiration and inspiration is <10 mm Hg normally. In pulses paradoxus, it is >10 mm Hg.
  - Expiration-Korotkoff sounds—11111 11111 11111 11111
  - Inspiration-Korotkoff sounds—11111 11111 11111 11111 11111 11111 11111
  - Difference in systolic pressure in expiration and inspiration >10 mm Hg.

Causes
- Constrictive pericarditis
- Cardiac tamponade in pericardial effusion
- Airway obstruction.

Reverse Pulses Paradoxus

Inspiratory rise in pulse volume and arterial pressure.

Causes
- HOCM
- Isorhythmic AV dissociation
- Intermittent positive pressure ventilation.

Anisosphygmia

Difference in pulse volume on identical vessels of both sides, may indicate occlusive arterial disease like coarctation of aorta, Takayasu's disease.

Character of Pulse

The wavy pattern of pulse is not felt normally since it is obliterated by the normal vascular tone. Normal character of the pulse (Fig. 4.6) is smooth upstroke, peak and a smooth downstroke.

Clinical Abnormalities

- Collapsing pulse
- Bisferiens pulse
- Anacrotic pulse
- Dicrotic pulse
- High volume jerky pulse in HOCM.

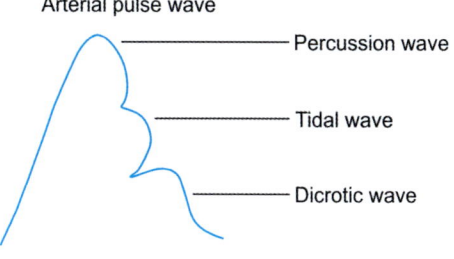

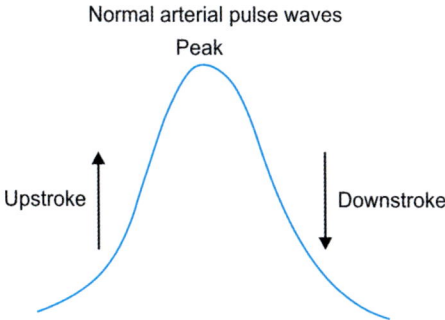

Fig. 4.6: Normal characters of pulse.

Collapsing Pulse: Corrigan's Pulse, Water Hammer Pulse (Fig. 4.7)

Features
- Abrupt upstroke, ill-sustained peak, abrupt downstroke and collapsing feel of pulse under the palpating hand.
- The thrust produced by the abrupt upstroke of the pulse will resemble the thrust produced by the tilting of the water hammer toy.
- Abrupt downstroke of the pulse produces the collapsing feel.

Method
- Collapsing pulse should be palpated with the palm of the hand.
- Feel both radial and ulnar arteries proximal to the wrist.
- Then raise the hand above the head by supporting the elbow of the patient with the other hand.

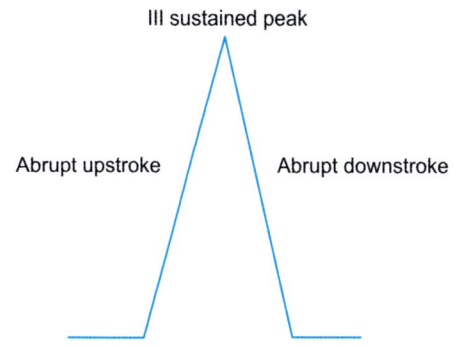

Fig. 4.7: Collapsing pulse.

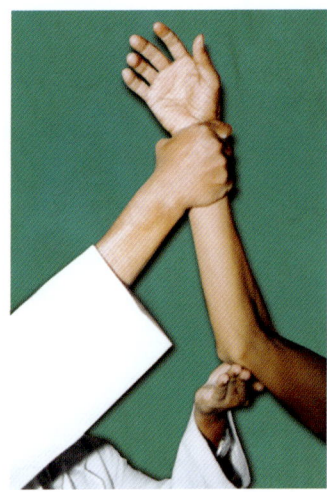

Fig. 4.8: Demonstration of collapsing pulse.

- Normally, only the radial artery is distinctly felt, no appreciable difference when the hand is elevated.
- In collapsing pulse, both radial and ulnar arteries are distinctly felt with an abrupt thrust and collapse of the vessel under the palm when the hand is elevated (Fig. 4.8).

Mechanism
- Same as the production of the high volume pulse, as rapid run off of blood from arterial system, as discussed earlier.

Causes
- High volume collapsing
  - Aortic regurgitation
  - PDA
  - Arteriovenous fistula
  - Anemia
  - Thyrotoxicosis
- Normal volume collapsing
  - Mitral regurgitation
  - VSD
  - Beri-beri.

Bisferiens Pulse (Fig. 4.9)

It is high volume double peaked pulse.
Causes: AS-AR, severe AR

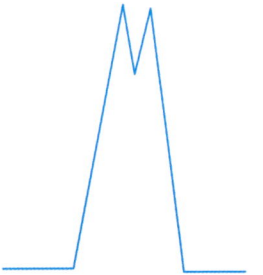

Fig. 4.9: Bisferiens pulse.

- It is better felt over the proximal vessels like carotid and brachial artery.
- *Method:* With the fingers, try to press and occlude the brachial artery. On slowly releasing the pressure, one may feel the double peaking of the pulse.

Anacrotic Pulse (Fig. 4.10)

It is a low volume pulse with slow upstroke, sustained peak and a slow downstroke, also a palpable notch in the ascending limb of pulse.
Cause: Aortic stenosis—here the percussion wave is delayed the tidal wave.

Dicrotic Pulse (Fig. 4.11)

It is double-peaked pulse due to the palpability of dicrotic wave. Hypotonia of the vessel wall in toxic fever will lead to the appearance of dicrotic wave.
Cause: Enteric fever, malaria, septicemia

High Volume Jerky Pulse (Spike and Dome Pulse) in HOCM (Fig. 4.12)

This is the only obstructive lesion producing high volume pulse due to the dynamic obstruction of LV outflow tract. This resembles bisferiens pulse.

Mechanism
- Initial phase—no obstruction—stroke volume is increased.
- Maximum ejection phase—obstruction—stroke volume decreased.
- Late phase-relaxation—obstruction decreases, stroke volume increases.

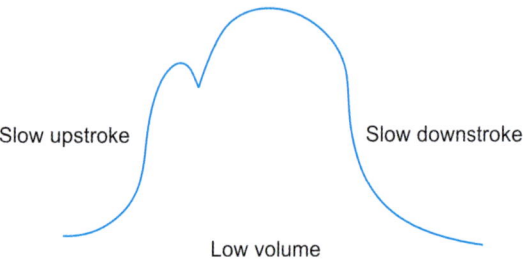

Fig. 4.10: Anacrotic pulse.

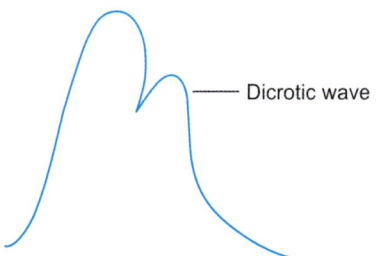

Fig. 4.11: Dicrotic pulse.

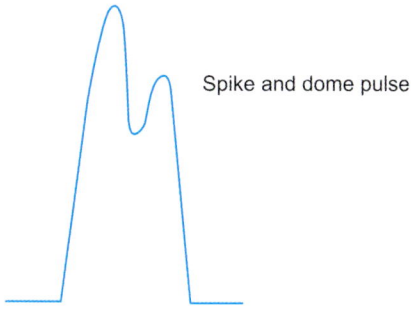

Fig. 4.12: High volume jerky pulse in HOCM.

Condition of the vessel wall: It is assessed by the palpation of the radial artery:
- Normal–soft
- Thickened vessel–firm to hard and cord like
- Thickening of the vessel
- Atherosclerosis
- Monckeberg's medial calcific sclerosis.

Method: Radial artery is palpated with the middle three fingers, occlude the artery proximally using the ring finger, empty a column of blood using index finger and roll the vessel free of blood, by the middle finger over the distal radius.

Peripheral Pulsations

- *Normal:* All pulsations felt equally. Feel the following peripheral arteries:
  - Brachial artery—cubital fossa
  - Carotid artery—carotid triangle in the neck
  - Femoral artery—groin
  - Popliteal artery—popliteal fossa
  - Dorsalis pedis—proximal part of 1st interosseous space—dorsum of the foot
  - Posterior tibial—behind the medial malleolus.
- Absence of peripheral pulsations
  - Peripheral vascular disease
  - Aortoiliac arteritis—decrease lower limb pulsation
  - Abdominal aorta arteritis—decrease lower limb pulsation
  - Coarctation of aorta—decrease and delayed femoral pulsation
  - Takayasu's disease—decrease upper limb pulsation.

Radiofemoral Delay

Normal: Radial and femoral pulsations felt equally and synchronously.

Timing of pulsation after cardiac cycle:
- Carotid–30 milli sec
- Brachial–60 milli sec
- Femoral–75 milli sec
- Radial–80 milli sec.

Delay of femoral beyond radial pulse is abnormal, seen in coarctation of aorta.

Mechanism: In postsubclavian COA, blood flow occurs though anterior intercostal branch of internal mammary from subclavian—to the posterior intercostals—branch of descending aorta. Thus, blood has to travel a long distance to reach the femoral vessel, thus producing delay to feel.

JUGULAR VENOUS PRESSURE AND PULSATION

Jugular Venous Pressure

It is defined as vertical height in centimeters from sternal angle to the upper level of the venous column. Examination of Jugular venous pressure is an important clinical sign in assessing the functional status of the heart. Raised jugular venous pressure is the first sign to appear and last sign to disappear in right heart failure.

Sternal angle is selected as an anatomical landmark since there is a constant distance of 5 cm from the center of right atrium to sternal angle. Height of jugular venous column + 5 cm will give the central venous pressure.

Normal jugular venous pressure:
- In the lying position—venous column is well visible at neck
- At 45° - lying position—venous column is visible at the root of the neck
- In the sitting position–venous column is not visible at neck
- Normal height is 2–4 cm
- >4 cm is considered abnormal
- Venous column of the internal jugular vein is observed in between the two heads of the sternocleidomastoid.

Measurement of Jugular Venous Pressure (Fig. 4.13)

- If the venous column is not well visible in the sitting position, keep the patient in the lying position inclined at 45°-the head and thorax should be in a line without flexing the neck. The idea of keeping the patient at 45° is to bring out the minimal elevation of jugular venous pressure. Keep one scale horizontally at the upper limit of venous column, and then measure the vertical height from sternal angle with another scale; this will give the jugular venous pressure in centimeters.
- If the jugular venous pressure is raised and well visible in the sitting position, there is no need to keep the patient at 45°. In the sitting position, measure the vertical height of the venous column by using two scales as mentioned earlier.

Raised Jugular Venous Pressure (Fig. 4.14)
- Early sign of right heart failure
- Nonpulsatile—engorged jugular in SVC obstruction (Fig. 4.15)

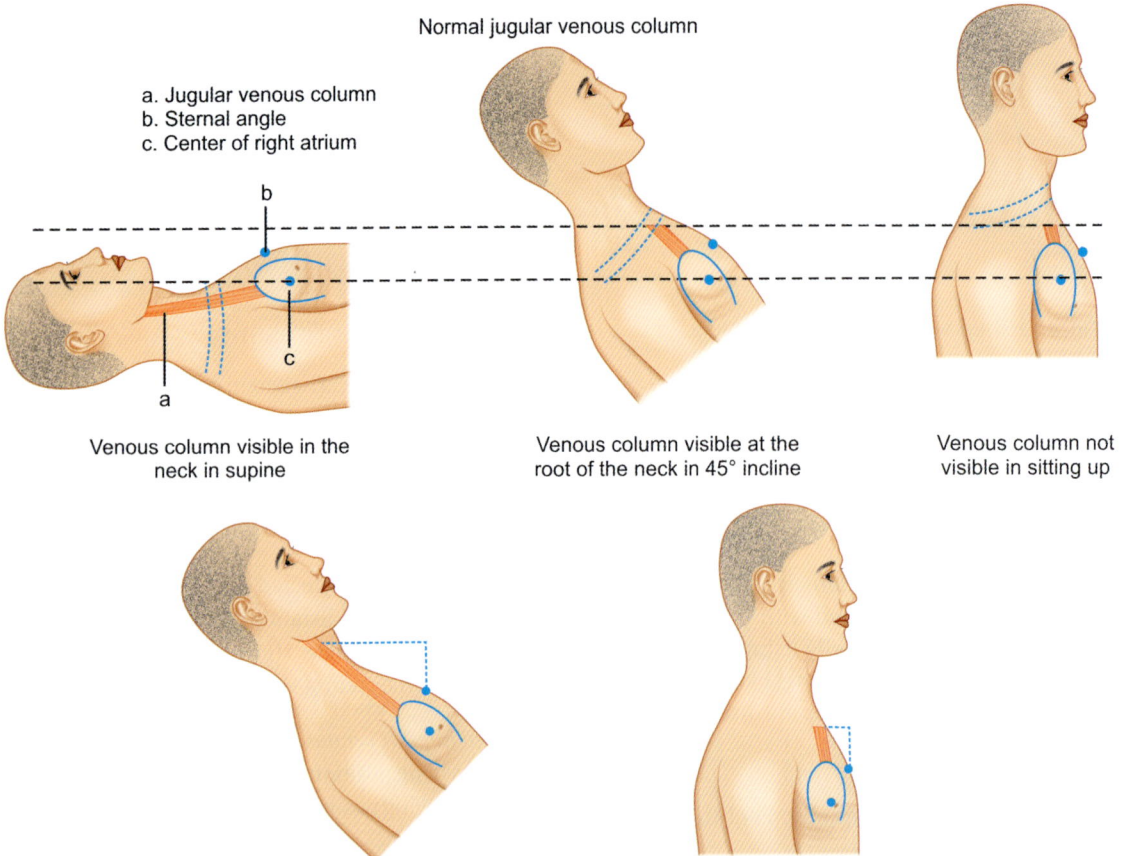

Fig. 4.13: Measurement of jugular venous pressure.

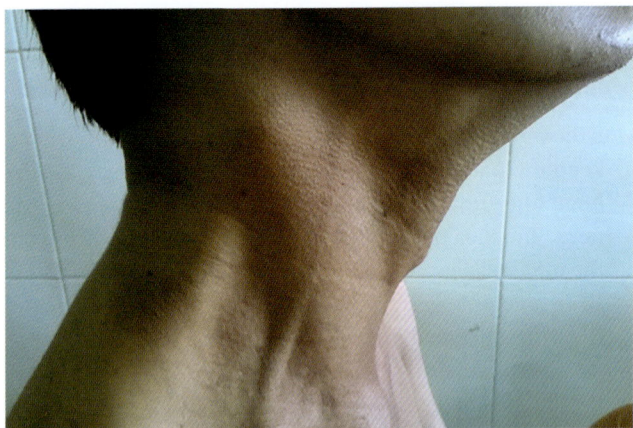

Fig. 4.14: Raised jugular venous pressure.

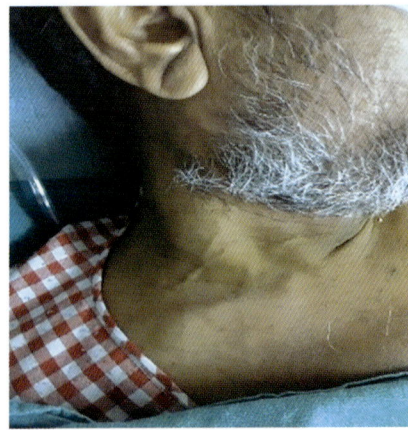

Fig. 4.15: Raised nonpulsatile engorged jugular vein.

- Raised JVP without heart failure
  - Anemia, Pregnancy
  - A/c glomerulonephritis
  - Excessive intravenous fluid
- Rarely—right atrial myxoma, tricuspid stenosis.

Decreased Jugular Venous Pressure
Hypovolemia/shock.

Hepatojugular Reflex

By applying firm pressure over the abdomen for 15–30 seconds, an extra amount of visceral venous blood is shifted to the right side of the heart.
This will produce:
- In normal person: Momentary rise of JVP <3 cm, healthy right ventricle pump out the extra load of blood.

- In patients with impending CHF—persistent elevation of JVP until the pressure is relieved.
- In patients already in CHF—further elevation of JVP.
- In patients with IVC obstruction—no hepatojugular reflex.

Jugular venous pulsations: In the neck, both arterial and venous pulsations are present. The difference is:

	Venous pulsation	Arterial pulsation
Site	Root of neck between the two heads of sternocleidomastoid	Upper part of neck in the carotid triangle
Pulsation	Wavy pulsation, two visible positive wave	Single systolic wave
Respiration	Inspiratory fall and expiratory rise	No change
On inspection and palpation	Better seen than palpable	Better palpable than seen

Physiology of Jugular Venous Pulsation

Jugular venous pulsations are direct reflections of the pressure changes of the right atrium through the superior vena cava (Fig. 4.16).

Three positive and two negative waves are present.

Positive waves:
1. a wave—produced by the active contraction of right atrium, visible as sharp short lived flickering wave and asynchronous with carotid pulsation.
2. c wave—closure of tricuspid valve → mild rise of pressure in right atrium.
3. v wave—rise in pressure due to slow venous return to right atrium. Clinically, it is a slow sinuous wave, synchronous with carotid pulsation.

Negative waves:
1. x descend—atrial relaxation following atrial contraction → fall in atrial pressure.
2. y descend—fall in atrial pressure when the tricuspid valve is opened.

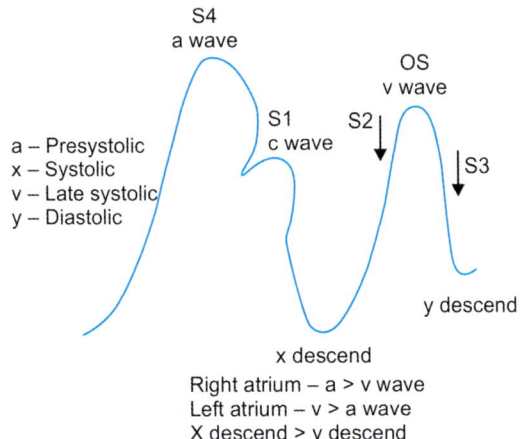

Fig. 4.16: Heart sounds in relation to jugular venous pulsation.

Method

Clinically, only 2 waves, positive waves 'a' and 'v', are detectable. Keep the neck in neutral position in patients with elevated jugular venous column in sitting position, look for the pulsation, identify 'a' and 'v' depending on the character, further confirmed by palpating the opposite carotid, by putting the examiner's hand behind the patient's neck.

Asynchronous pulsation is 'a' wave; synchronous pulsation is 'v' wave.

Clinical Abnormalities of Jugular Venous Pulsation

A Wave

Prominent 'a' wave—is due to forcible atrial contraction, against noncompliant right ventricle, in RVH or against pulmonary valve in pulmonary stenosis or against tricuspid valve in tricuspid stenosis.

Causes:
- PAH
- Pulmonary stenosis
- Tricuspid stenosis
- ASD with mitral stenosis
- Tricuspid atresia
- Right ventricular endomyocardial fibrosis (RV EMF)
- *Giant 'a' wave—Cannon wave* is due to contraction of right atrium against closed tricuspid valve.
- Irregular cannon wave—complete AV block, VT
- Regular cannon wave—junctional rhythm
- Occasional cannon wave—extrasystole
- *Absence of a wave*—atrial fibrillation.

V Wave—Prominent V Wave

Causes:
- Tricuspid regurgitation—venous return and regurgitant stream of blood produce rise in pressure in atrial diastole.
- ASD with MR—left atrial prominent v wave is reflected to right through ASD
- TAPVC (total anomalous pulmonary venous connection) blood from the pulmonary veins also draining to right atrium.
- Ruptured sinus of Valsalva (RSOV) to right atrium—right atrial diastolic filling increases.

X Descend

- Prominence of x descend in cardiac tamponade
- Absence of x descend in atrial fibrillation.

Y Descend

- Sharp y descend in constrictive pericarditis and TR
- Slow y descend in tricuspid stenosis
- Reduced y descend in cardiac tamponade.

Sharp and deep y descend manifest as diastolic collapse of jugular-called *Friedreich's sign*.

Kussmaul's sign: Inspiratory rise of jugular venous column seen in pericardial disease and chronic right heart failure.

EXAMINATION OF PRECORDIUM

Conventional method of examination, by inspection, palpation, percussion, auscultation, was invented by the father of Clinical Medicine-Sir William Osler, as "look the patient, touch the patient, tap the patient and listen the patient", is still remaining the best method of examination.

Inspection of Precordium

Part of the chest wall overlying the heart is called the precordium
- **Shape of the precordium**
  - Precordial bulge—RV enlargement, early in childhood.
- **Visibility of apex beat**
  - Apical impulse is the outermost and the lowermost point over the precordium where a distinct impulse is seen or felt during each cardiac cycle.
  - Apical impulse is formed by the forward movement of the anatomical apex of LV which produces an impulse on the chest wall during each cardiac cycle.
  - Normally visible in the 5th left intercostals space inside the midclavicular line.
  - Apical impulse not visible—thick chest wall, behind the rib, pericardial effusion, left pleural effusion, etc.
- **Displaced apex**—cardiomegaly,
  - RV enlargement displaces the apex horizontally and outward
  - LV enlargement shifts the apex downward and outward
  - Displaced heart by pleuropulmonary disease and gross kyphoscoliosis.
- **Diffuse apex**—in ventricular aneurysm
  - Epigastric pulsation—seen in
    - RV enlargement
    - Aortic pulsation in thin individual
    - Aortic aneurysm
    - Vascular tumors of the liver.
- **Intercostal pulsation**
  - Normally at rest—no visible intercostal pulsation
  - Visible pulsation at rest suggest ventricular enlargement
  - RV enlargement → left parasternal pulsation, gross RV enlargement as in ASD → pulsation over the entire precordium
  - LV enlargement → pulsation of part of precordium.
- **Second left intercostal space pulsation**
  - Pulmonary artery pulsation—seen in pulmonary hypertension, pulmonary artery aneurysm, hyperkinetic pulmonary blood flow as in ASD and idiopathic dilatation of pulmonary artery.
- **Suprasternal pulsation—causes**
  - Unfolding of aorta
  - Aortic aneurysm
  - Aortic regurgitation
  - Coarctation of aorta.
- **Position of the trachea**
  - Trail's sign (Prominence of sternal head of sternomastoid due to the shift of trachea to the same side)
  - Pleuropulmonary disease with mediastinal shift produces displacement of the heart.
- **Carotid pulsation**—prominent pulsation seen in:
  - Aortic regurgitation—Corrigan's sign
  - Coarctation of aorta
  - Kinked carotid—pseudoaneurysm/Students aneurysm
  - Systemic hypertension
  - Other hyperdynamic state.
- **Sternoclavicular pulsation**—present in:
  - Aortic regurgitation
  - Aortic aneurysm
  - Subclavian aneurysm
  - Right sided aortic arch.
- **Right hemithorax pulsation**
  - Right 2nd intercostals space pulsation—aortic aneurysm-Potain's sign
  - Marked cardiomegaly
  - Displaced heart by respiratory disease
  - Dextrocardia.
- **Pulsation over the interscapular space**
  - Visible pulsation of the posterior intercostal vessel in coarctation of aorta—Suzman's sign.

Palpation of Precordium

- To confirm inspection findings
- Palpation of apex beat
- Left parasternal heave.

Pulsation

- Pulmonary area and other intercostal spaces
- Thrill and shocks of heart sounds
- Position of trachea.

Apex Beat

Normal apex beat:
- Site—5th left intercostal space 1 cm inside the midclavicular line
- Confined to one intercostal space
- Size of apical impulse—2 cm
- Palpating finger is lifted, but not above the plane of the adjoining ribs

- Apex beat is occurring at the end of the isometric contraction phase of cardiac cycle
- *Factors affecting the apical impulse formation*: LV size, LV filling, force and duration of contraction.

Method: Patient should be in supine position for localization of apex beat.

Change in position of the patient can displace the apex beat to 1–2 cm from normal position. First, palpate the apex with the palm, then digital localization with the fingertip. Watch the amplitude and duration of the lift of the palpating finger. If the apical impulse is not palpable in supine position, keep the patient in left lateral position and palpate the apex beat, to know whether the heart is in the left hemithorax.

Clinical abnormalities of apex beat
- **Forcible apex beat**
  - Palpating finger is lifted above the plane of the adjoining rib, but it is ill-sustained.
  - Apical impulse is shifted outward and downward.
  - Apical impulse is palpable in more than one intercostals space.
  - Mechanism is diastolic overload of LV → increase in force of contraction.
  - Causes—AR, MR, PDA, VSD and hyperdynamic state.
- **Heaving apical impulse**
  - Palpating finger is lifted above the plane of the adjoining rib and it is sustained
  - Apical impulse is felt in normal position
  - Confined to one intercostal space
  - *Mechanism:* Pressure overload of LV →increase in force and duration of contraction
  - *Causes:* Aortic stenosis, systemic hypertension, and HOCM.
- **Tapping apex beat**
  - Palpating finger is not lifted.
  - The distinct palpable shock of accentuated 1st heart sound is felt as tap by which the apex beat is located.
  - *Mechanism:* Tapping apex beat is present only in mitral stenosis, where the LV size and LV filling is less. Therefore, the impulse produced by the LV is less which cannot be felt by the palpating finger, instead the accentuated 1st heart sound produced at the mitral valve is transmitted to the apex giving the feel of tap. Later, PAH and RV enlargement produces clockwise rotation of the heart pushing the LV further posteriorly, thus, further impeding the forward movement of the anatomical apex.
  - *Cause:* Mitral stenosis.
- **Impalpable apex beat**—Causes:
  - Thick chest wall
  - Behind the rib
  - Pericardial effusion
  - Left pleural effusion
  - Left pneumothorax
  - Emphysema
- **Bifid apex beat**
  - Two impulses felt during each cardiac cycle
  - Apical impulse + palpable shock produced by the presence of 3rd or 4th heart sound.
- **Triple or wavy apex beat** is a feature of HOCM
  - Systolic bifid apical impulse + palpable shock of 4th heart sound.
- **See saw apex beat**
  - Diffuse apex beat confined to more than one intercostal space
  - When 2 fingers are placed over each intercostal space, there is upward movement of one finger and downward movement of the other finger
  - *Cause:* Ventricular aneurysm.
- **Displaced apical impulse**
  - Dextrocardia (Fig. 4.17)
  - Push and pull of pleuropulmonary disease.

Apical Impulse formed by RV

Precordial surface of heart is mainly occupied by grossly enlarged RV as in ASD, which will produce the apical impulse also.

Left Parasternal Heave

It is the systolic elevation of left lower costal cartilages produced by the contraction of hypertrophied and dilated right ventricle.

Method: Keep the ulnar border of hand over the 3rd, 4th, 5th left intercostal spaces by the side of the sternum. Systolic elevation of the left lower costal cartilages is felt as an impulse.

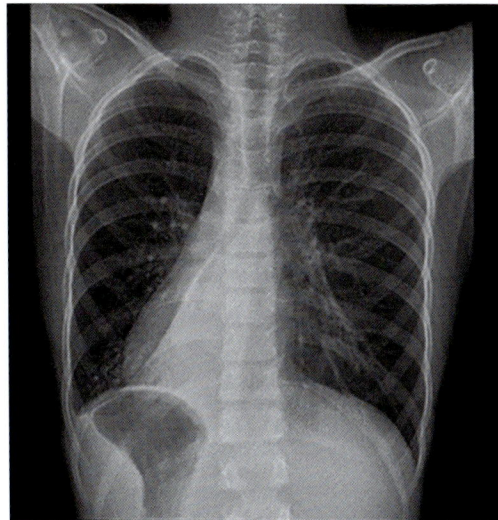

Fig. 4.17: X-ray showing dextrocardia and situs inversus.

Causes
- Right ventricular hypertrophy
  - Pressure overload of RV → left parasternal heave-sustained impulse as in PAH, pulmonary stenosis.
  - Volume overload of RV → left parasternal lift → forcible impulse as in ASD and tricuspid regurgitation.
  - Left atrial enlargement as in MR rarely produces left parasternal lift.
  - Occasionally marked LV enlargement as in AR → counter clockwise rotation of heart → left parasternal region occupied by the enlarged LV → left parasternal lift. Left parasternal impulse is also produced by aneurysm of descending aorta.

Pulsation of Major Vessels

Pulmonary artery pulsation can be felt over the pulmonary area with the pulp of fingers.

Causes:
- Pulmonary artery dilatation in PAH
- Idiopathic dilatation of pulmonary artery
- Aneurysm of pulmonary artery.
- *Aortic pulsation:* In dilated aorta or aneurysm of ascending aorta, the pulsation of aorta can be felt over the right 2nd and 3rd intercostal space.
  - Potain sign—pulsation of the right 2nd intercostals space in aneurysm of ascending aorta.

Palpable Shock of Accentuated Heart Sounds

Palpable impulse produced by the accentuated heart sound is called shock. Accentuation means pathological loudness of heart sounds.
- First heart sound → palpable shock over mitral area in mitral stenosis
- *Pulm*onary component of second heart sound → palpable shock over pulmonary area → in PAH
- Aortic component of second heart sound → palpable shock over aortic area in aneurysm of aortic root, systemic hypertension
- Third heart sound → palpable shock over mitral area in MR, LVF
- Fourth heart sound → palpable shock over mitral area in AS, HOCM.

Mitral events can be better felt keeping the patient in left lateral position.

Aortic events are better felt, keeping the patient in sitting, leaning forward and breath held in expiration.

Thrill

- Thrill means palpable murmur
- 3 types—systolic, diastolic and continuous
- Low pitched murmurs of stenotic lesions will produce thrill than the high pitched murmurs of incompetent lesions
- Over the apex
  - Diastolic thrill → (thrill ending in apical impulse)-MS
  - Systolic thrill → (thrill along with apical impulse)-MR
- Left sternal border-systolic thrill → VSD, AS
- Pulmonary area
- Systolic thrill → pulmonary stenosis, large ASD, Supracristal VSD,
- Continuous thrill → PDA, RSOV
- Aortic area
- Systolic thrill—AS
- Rarely diastolic thrill—acute severe AR.

Pericardial rub—can be palpated as leathery rub.
Bruit over the carotid—can be felt in aortic stenosis.
Venous hum at the root of the neck-can be felt in anemia
Bruit over the interscapular region—dilated posterior intercostal artery in coarctation of aorta.

Percussion of Heart Borders

"The art of percussion was invented by Leopold Auenbrugger when he was a medical student."

Usually right border, left border of the heart and 2nd left intercostal space are percussed.

Upper border of the heart is occupied by the major vessels, hence it cannot be percussed out.

Lower border is close to diaphragm and left lobe of the liver, thus difficult to percuss.

Right border of heart—is percussed out in the right 4th intercostals space towards the sternal margin. The direction of enlargement is maximum in the right 4th intercostal space, thus minimal enlargement can be made out in this space.

Method

Percuss the upper margin of the liver, 5th right intercostals space by tidal percussion:
- Make sure the 4th space is resonant, then percuss toward the right sternal margin.
- The right border corresponds to right sternal margin/retrosternal.

Left border of the heart—is percussed in the space where the apex beat is felt and a space above it, to get two points to make a border. Percussion is done from axilla towards the apex. If the apex beat is not palpable, percuss the 5th left intercostals space and a space above it. Left border usually corresponds with apex beat. Dullness beyond the apex beat is present in pericardial effusion.

Percussion of 2nd left intercostals space—normally it is resonant, dilated pulmonary artery will produce dullness. Percussion is done from left midclavicular line to the sternal border in 2nd left intercostals space.

Nowadays, percussion, as a clinical method is seldom used and it is being replaced by X-ray chest and echocardiography.

Auscultation

Auscultation is the most important part in cardiovascular examination. One should gain the skill by experience obtained by constant repetition. Diagnosis of heart disease especially congenital and valvular heart disease, were mainly depending on the auscultatory finding before the advent of echocardiography.

Stethoscope was invented by Theophille Hycynth Lennec.

Ideal stethoscope should have tube length of 25 cm, double tube is better, the size of the tube-0.3 cm, two chest pieces diaphragm with a diameter of 4 cm, bell with a diameter of 2.5 cm, and well-fitting ear pieces. Bell is used to hear low-pitched sounds and murmurs (30–150 Hz), one should not press the bell too much since the skin will act as a diaphragm. Diaphragm is used for high-pitched sounds and murmurs; it will filter out low pitched sounds of less than 300 Hz.

The beginner will have difficulty in identifying the auscultatory findings. One should understand the physiological events in cardiac cycle; identify the 1st and 2nd heart sounds for differentiating the systolic and diastolic phase and events occurring therein. Remembering the quality of sounds and murmurs are easy for the recognition of the findings, than the other features in description.

Auscultatory Areas

- Mitral area—corresponds to apex beat—5th left intercostals space (LICS) 1 cm inside the midclavicular line
- Tricuspid area—lower left sternal border of 5th LICS
- Pulmonary area—2nd LICS close to sternum
- Aortic area—2nd right intercostals space (RICS) close to sternum
- 2nd aortic area—3rd LICS close to sternum

These areas are named because the events occurring in each valve is heard in isolation.

Observe the following things on auscultation:
- Heart sounds—first and second heart sounds
  - Added sounds—third and fourth heart sounds
  - Opening snap, ejection click
  - Non-ejection click
- Murmurs
- Pericardial rub.

Heart sounds: Mechanism of production
- Closing of valves—S_1 and S_2
- Filling of ventricles—S_3
- Atrial sound—S_4
- Opening of the valves—opening snap, ejection click.

First Heart Sound

- Physiology—2 components—mitral and tricuspid
- Produced by the closure of the mitral and tricuspid valves, mainly contributed by anteromedial cusp of mitral valve
- Features are—low pitched, loud and long duration
- Site of hearing—better in mitral area than the other areas
- Intensity of the 1st heart sound depends on the position of the valve cusp at the onset of the ventricular systole, if the valve cusps are wide apart; they close with a loud sound. If the valve cusps are near to closure, at the onset of ventricular systole, they close with a soft sound.

Clinical Abnormalities First Heart Sound

- **Accentuation of first heart sound:**
  - Pathological loudness is called accentuation.
  - Sinus tachycardia—diastole is less, cusps are wide apart.
  - Mitral stenosis—Cusps are wide apart because of high left atrial pressure, which is not allowing the physiological closure to occur.
  - Short PR interval (<0.1 sec–pre-excitation syndrome)-ventricular activation immediately after atrial activation-thus the mitral cusps are wide apart.
  - Tricuspid component accentuation → S_1 accentuation e.g. ASD - only L → R shunt with S1 accentuation TAPVC (Total anomalous pulmonary venous connection) and Ebstein's anomaly.
- **Soft first heart sound:**
  - Sinus bradycardia—increase diastole, cusps are nearly closed position.
  - Mitral regurgitation—improper close of mitral valve → increase LV filling allowing early closure
  - Aortic regurgitation—increased LV filling from aorta and left atrium → premature closure of mitral valve
  - Prolonged PR interval - 1° AV block–lengthy diastole, cusps are nearly closed position.
- **Varying intensity first heart sound:**
  - Atrial fibrillation and multiple extrasystole → varying diastolic period → varying time for physiological closure of mitral valve.

Cannon sound: Explosive type of accentuated 1st heart sound in complete AV block.

Second Heart Sound

The most difficult thing in auscultation is to identify the abnormalities of S_2.

Physiology—2 components—aortic and pulmonary.
1. Aortic—1st component and loud—heard in all areas
2. Pulmonary—2nd component and soft, heard only over pulmonary area.

Normal second heart sound—high pitched, normal split—2 components separately heard during inspiration and as single component during expiration over the pulmonary area. Distance between the 2 components during inspiration is 0.04 sec, during expiration is 0.02 sec. Human ear can appreciate, when the distance between the 2 components is 0.03 or more.

Normal second heart sound is expressed as–normal in intensity and normal split with respiration.

Clinical Abnormalities of S_2

- **Accentuation of aortic component**
  - Systemic hypertension
  - Aortic aneurysm and syphilitic aortitis
  - Dilated aorta
- **Accentuation of pulmonary component**
  - Pulmonary hypertension
  - Dilated pulmonary artery

  Criteria for accentuation—when the 2nd component of S2 is equal or more than the 1st component, the 2nd component is heard in all areas.
- **Wide split of 2nd heart sound**
  - Two components heard separately both during inspiration and expiration but better during inspiration
  - Due to delayed pulmonary component or early aortic component.
  - Delayed pulmonary component:
    - Volume overload – ASD - prolonged RV contraction
    - Obstruction – pulmonary stenosis – prolonged RV contraction
    - Electrical delay – RBBB – delay in RV contraction.
  - Early aortic component
    - Duration of LV contraction is decreased
    - MR and VSD.
- **Reverse or paradoxical split of 2nd heart sound**
  - Aortic component is delayed beyond the pulmonary component.
  - Clinically 2 components heard separately both during inspiration and expiration, but better during expiration
    - Prolonged LV contraction and delay in aortic component
    - Volume overload in PDA
    - Pressure overload in AS
    - Electrical delay in LBBB
- **Wide and fixed split of 2nd heart sound**

  Two components of S_2 are heard both during inspiration and expiration with a fixed distance. It is a hallmark of ASD.

  Mechanism: Wide split

  Volume overload → prolonged RV contraction → delayed pulmonary component.

  Mechanism: Fixed split

  During inspiration - more filling of RV - increased venous return → decreased L → R shunt → more filling of LV - both pulmonary and aortic components are equally delayed.

  During expiration - less venous return → less filling of RV →increased L → R shunt → less filling of LV - both pulmonary and aortic components are equally early.

  Thus inspiratory delay of pulmonary component with paradoxical movement of aortic component will lead on to delay of both components in inspiration and both components early in expiration keeping a fixed distance.

- **Single second heart sound**

  It can be due to:

  A_2 abnormality
  - Absence of aortic valve—aortic atresia
  - Masking of aortic component—By systolic murmur of PS, VSD, MR.

  P_2 abnormality
  - Absence of pulmonary valve—in pulmonary atresia
  - Masking of pulmonary component by—Systolic murmur of AS
  - Inaudible pulmonary component—TOF (tetralogy of Fallot)
  - Single valve—in PTA (persistent truncus arteriosus)
  - Synchronous closure of both valves—Eisenmenger VSD and TOF.

Third Heart Sound

Ventricular filling sound.

Mechanism

More than normal amount of blood reaching the ventricle during rapid filling phase, produce stretch on myocardium → tense chordae and papillary muscle which produce S_3.

Features

- Low pitched, 0.12 sec after S_2 in diastole, produced both in LV and RV.
- Physiological: 3rd heart sound–in children and adults up to 30–35 years.
- Pathological: 3rd heart sound
  - LV S_3–MR, LVF
  - RV S_3–TR, RVF.
- Three sounds heard during each cardiac cycle → triple rhythm.
- Triple rhythm with sinus tachycardia → gallop rhythm imitating the sounds of galloping horse.
- LV S_3 gallop → is an important auscultatory sign of LVF.
- S_3 is a sign of systolic dysfunction of ventricle.
- Early S_3 is heard in RV EMF-sudden limitation of ventricular filling.
- Pericardial knock—an early S_3 in constrictive pericarditis.

Fourth Heart Sound

Atrial sound.
- *Mechanism:* Forcible atrial contraction to fill the non compliant ventricle in ventricular hypertrophy or infarct, will produce stretch on the myocardium → tense chordae and papillary muscle → S_4
- *Physiology:* It is a low pitched sound in presystole—just before 1st heart sound.
- *Causes:*
  - LA S_4—systemic hypertension, AS (left ventricular hypertrophy)
    - LV myocardial infarction

- RA S_4—pulmonary hypertension, pulmonary stenosis (right ventricular hypertrophy)
  - RV myocardial infarction.

Opening Snap

- *Mechanism:* It is a high-pitched diastolic sound produced by the sudden halt of the opening process of the diseased mitral or tricuspid valve.
- *Features:* High pitched sound, widely conducted, distance between S_2 and OS is less than 0.12 sec.
  - OS-Mitral–mitral stenosis
  - Tricuspid–tricuspid stenosis-rare.

Mitral opening snap: Importance
- Heard medial to mitral area with diaphragm
- High pitched widely conducted
- S_2-OS distance-lesser → severe MS
- Presence of OS indicates mobility of valve cusp
- OS persist with AF in MS
- Presence of OS with mid-diastolic murmur (MDM) → mitral stenosis
- Absence of OS—mild MS, calcific/fibrosed mitral valve, MS with AR.

Difference between Mitral Opening Snap and S_3 (LV)

	Mitral opening snap	S_3 (LV)
Site	Medial to mitral area, Conducted to other areas	Mitral area
Pitch	High pitched	Low pitched
Distance from S_2	<0.12 sec	>0.12 sec
Mid-diastolic murmur	Mitral stenosis	Flow murmur (absence of mitral stenosis)

Ejection click

It is a high pitched opening sound from aortic and pulmonary valves.
Two types: Vascular or valvular mechanism
- **Vascular:** Dilated vessel conduct the normal opening sound to the surface:
  - Pulmonary ejection click in:
    - Dilated pulmonary artery in PAH
    - Idiopathic dilatation of pulmonary artery
  - Aortic ejection click
    - Aneurysm of aortic root
    - Systemic hypertension.
- **Valvular:** Sudden halt of the opening process of diseased valve → ejection click.
  - It indicates the site of the lesion, not the severity of the lesion.
  - Pulmonary ejection click in pulmonary stenosis-it is inconstant EC better during expiration, inspiratory diastolic opening of pulmonary valve in pulmonary stenosis, thus in inspiration, no ejection click is produced.

- Aortic ejection click-valvular aortic stenosis—it is constant both during inspiration and expiration, better heard over the apex.

Nonejection Click (Fig. 4.18)

It is a mid-systolic click in mitral/tricuspid valve prolapse followed by late systolic murmur. It is produced by the stretch on the chordae and papillary muscles by the prolapsed cusp of the mitral/tricuspid valve.

Multiple sounds are heard in Ebstein's anomaly-split S_1, split S_2, OS and S_4.

Murmurs

Definition: It is an auditory vibration of variable duration, intensity and pitch produced by the turbulent blood flow.

Mechanism:
- Laminar flow is distorted to turbulent flow
- Increased velocity of blood flow
- Change in caliber of vessel or chamber—narrowing or dilatation
- Backward flow—incompetence of valve, VSD, PDA
- Loose structure in the line of blood flow—band, ruptured papillary muscle
- Decrease in the viscosity of blood.

Note the Following for the Description of Murmur

- Site of maximum intensity → indicates site of lesion
- Timing-systolic/diastolic/continuous
- Duration-systolic-pansystolic, ejection systolic, early and late systolic, diastolic-early diastolic, mid diastolic, presystolic
- **Intensity-grading of murmur by Levine and Harvey**
  - *Grade 1:* Very faint murmur detected on auscultating 2 or more cardiac cycle
  - *Grade 2:* Faint murmur detected in the 1st cardiac cycle on auscultation
  - *Grade 3:* Loudest murmur without thrill
  - *Grade 4:* Murmur with thrill
  - *Grade 5:* Murmur with thrill-heard even with the edge of diaphragm

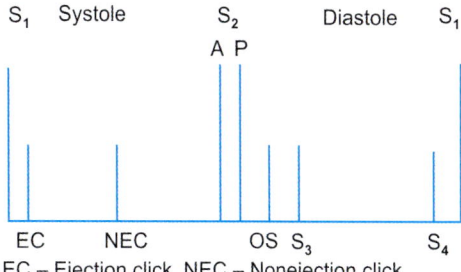

EC – Ejection click, NEC – Nonejection click
OS – Opening snap, S_3 – Third heart sound
S_4 – Fourth heart sound

Fig. 4.18: Heart sounds in cardiac cycle.

- *Grade 6:* Loudest murmur with thrill–audible with the chest piece held off the chest wall. Usually widely conducted, can be heard over the acromion, olecranon, occiput, etc.
- Pitch
  - Stenotic murmurs - low pitched–AS, MS
  - Regurgitation murmurs—high pitched–MR, AR
- Quality–musical murmurs
- Mitral
  - Rheumatic valvulitis–MR
  - Infective endocarditis → "Seagull murmur"–ruptured papillary muscle
- Aortic
  - Systolic—calcific aortic stenosis
  - Diastolic—syphilitic–retroversion of anterior cusp
- Conduction—selective propagation of murmur from the site of maximum intensity to another site with same intensity
- Transmitted murmur—with less intensity
  - MR—pansystolic murmur conducted to axilla
  - AS—ejection systolic murmur → carotid
- Variation with respiration
  - All right-sided murmurs increase with inspiration–Carvallo's sign
  - Aortic murmurs increase with expiration
- Posture
  - Mitral murmur—left lateral position
  - Aortic murmur—sitting, leaning forward
  - MVP—Murmur increase on standing
  - HOCM—Systolic murmur decrease in squatting.

Dynamic auscultation–Done in following situation:

Maneuver	Lesion		
	HOCM	MVP	AS
Valsalva	Louder	Longer	Softer
Squatting	Softer	Shorter	Louder
Hand grip (isometric)	Softer	Shorter	Softer

Systolic Murmurs

- Pansystolic murmur (Fig. 4.19)
- Ejection systolic murmur (Fig. 4.20)
- Early systolic murmur
- Late systolic murmur.

Pansystolic Murmur

Features
- No gap between S1 and murmur
- Uniform intensity throughout systole
- High pitched

Causes
MR, TR, VSD.

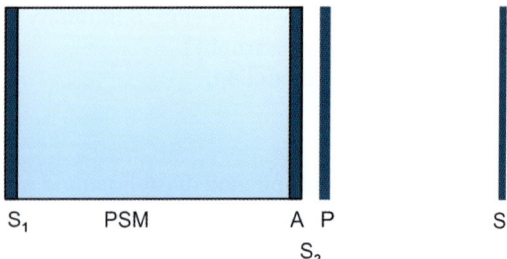

Fig. 4.19: Pansystolic murmur.

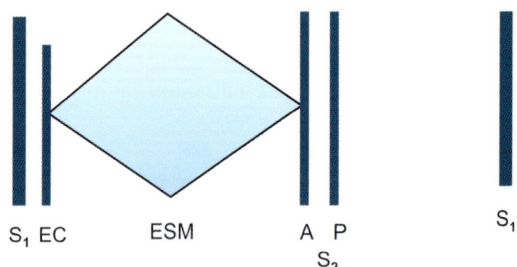

Fig. 4.20: Ejection systolic murmur.

Ejection Systolic Murmur

Features
- Distinct gap between the murmur and S_1
- Crescendo-decrescendo–Diamond shaped
- Low pitched.

Causes
- Aortic ejection systolic murmur
  - AS
  - Aortic sclerosis
  - Aortic aneurysm, flow murmur
- Pulmonary ejection systolic murmur
  - Pulmonary stenosis,
  - TOF
  - ASD, hemic murmur.

Late Systolic Murmur

Systolic murmur occurring in the 2nd half of systole.

Causes
- MVP
- Papillary muscle dysfunction
- Coarctation of aorta
- HOCM.

Early Systolic Murmur

Systolic murmur occurring in the early phase of systole

Causes
- Acute MR,
- Organic TR,
- Papillary muscle dysfunction-LV EMF.

Diastolic Murmurs

- Early diastolic (Fig. 4.21)
- Mid-diastolic (Fig. 4.22)
- Late diastolic-presystolic
- Pandiastolic.

Early Diastolic

It is a high pitched blowing decrescendo murmur starting from 2nd heart sound.

Causes-AR and PR

Clinical difference	AR	PR
High pitched decrescendo murmur	+	+
Position of patient best heard	Sitting and leaning forward	Supine
Respiratory variation Better	Expiration	Inspiration
Conduction	Conducted down to 2nd aortic area, mitral area along left sternal border (LSB)	Localized
Murmur follows	Aortic component of S_2	Pulmonary component of S_2
Pulmonary hypertension	Usually absent	Usually present
Peripheral signs of AR	Present	Absent

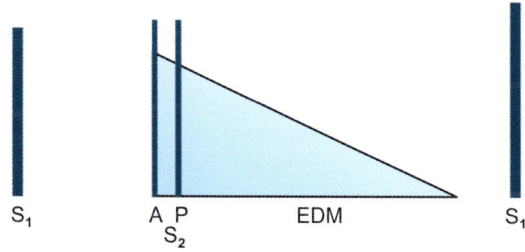

Fig. 4.21: Early diastolic murmur.

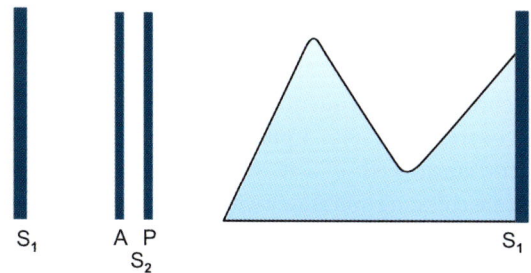

Fig. 4.22: Mid-diastolic and presystolic murmur.

Mid-diastolic Murmur

It is a low pitched rough and rumbling murmur occurring at mid-diastole.

Causes–Mitral mid-diastolic and tricuspid mid-diastolic
- Mitral mid-diastolic murmur
  - With obstruction
    - Mitral stenosis.

Other causes of obstruction
- Functional-Austin Flint murmur in AR
- Valvulitis-Rheumatic-Carey Coombs murmur
- Vegetations
- Thrombus
- Myxoma
  - Without obstruction
    - Increased flow-MR, PDA, etc.
    - Normal flow-dilated ventricle
- Tricuspid mid-diastolic murmur-
  - Tricuspid stenosis
  - Flow murmur
    - Tricuspid regurgitation
    - ASD
    - TAPVC.

Late Diastolic/Presystolic Murmur

It is a murmur occurring late in diastole due to active atrial contraction in: Mitral stenosis and tricuspid stenosis.

Pandiastolic Murmur

It is a decrescendo diastolic murmur heard throughout diastole.

Causes
- Pulmonary regurgitation-in PPH
- ASD and PDA Eisenmenger
- AR.

Continuous Murmur

It is a systolic murmur extending beyond 2nd heart sound.

Mechanism of Production

- **High pressure system communicating with low pressure system**
  - Intracardiac
    - RSOV to RV, RA, pulmonary artery
    - Coronary artery fistula to cardiac chamber
  - Extracardiac
    - PDA, aortopulmonary septal defect
    - Pulmonary AVF, systemic AVF
    - Anomalous left coronary artery from pulmonary artery.
- **Narrowing of vessel**
  - Coarctation of aorta
  - Peripheral pulmonary artery stenosis
  - Carotid stenosis.

- **Increased blood flow through vessels**
  - Venous hum-Devil's murmur-root of neck
  - Venous hum (Cruveilhier-Baumgarten murmur)–umbilicus - in portal hypertension
  - Intercostal arteries–coarctation of aorta
  - Bronchopulmonary anastomoses–pulmonary atresia–TOF
  - Internal mammary artery–mammary souffle in pregnancy.
- **Continuous murmur with cyanosis**
  - TOF with PDA
  - Pulmonary atresia with bronchopulmonary anastomoses
  - Pulmonary AVF.
- **Continuous murmur with systolic > diastolic**
  - PDA
  - Peripheral pulmonary artery stenosis
  - Bronchopulmonary anastamoses.
- **Continuous murmur with systolic < diastolic**
  - Coronary AVF
  - Pulmonary AVF
  - RSOV.
- **Systolodiastolic murmur**
  - Murmurs heard both in systole and diastole because of 2 different lesions
  - *Causes*
    - AS and AR
    - VSD and AR
    - MR and AR.

Differential diagnosis of murmur depending on the site

Apical: Mid-diastolic murmur
- Mitral stenosis, Austin flint murmur
- Carey Coombs mumur
- Flow murmur—MR, PDA
- Obstruction of mitral valve
  - Vegetation
  - Thrombus
  - Myxoma
  - Ritan's murmur of complete AV block
  - Cor triatriatum

Apical systolic murmur
- MR - Pan systolic
- VSD - Pan systolic (transmitted murmur)
- TR - Pan systolic (clockwise rotation of heart)
- AS - Ejection systolic murmur

Systolic murmurs of Left sternal border
- Upper sternal border (Pulmonary area)
  - Pulmonary stenosis
  - TOF
  - ASD
  - Supracristal VSD
  - Hemic murmur
  - PDA with hypertension
- Mid sternal border
  - VSD
  - AS
  - MR - Post cusp
- Lower sternal border
  - TR
  - VSD
  - MR—post cusp/transmitted murmur
- Systolic murmur: Aortic area
  - Aortic stenosis
  - Aortic sclerosis
  - Aortitis
  - Aortic aneurysm
  - Flow murmur.

Named Murmurs

- Gibson's murmur—continuous murmur of PDA
- Carey Coombs murmur—MDM of rheumatic valvulitis
- Graham-Steel murmur—EDM of pulmonary regurgitation → PAH
- Austin Flint murmur—MDM in aortic regurgitation.

Pericardial Rub

Pericardial rub is produced due to the sliding of the two inflamed layers of the pericardium.
- It is triphasic—systolic, presystolic and diastolic
- Site—left sternal border-3rd and 4th intercostals space
- Cause—pericarditis
  - Pericardial effusion-pericardial rub persist in spite of the effusion unlike in pleural effusion, since both layers of the pericardium dip deep into the AV groove which cannot be separated by the fluid in effusion, thus the rub is persisting.
  - In acute MI, pericardial rub indicates transmural infarction.

Method of Auscultation

- Patient in supine position or in propped up position, if orthopnea present.
- The conventional sequence of auscultation of areas -Mitral area → tricuspid area → pulmonary area → aortic area → second aortic area.
- Start auscultating mitral area with bell, then with diaphragm, for better appreciation, patient can be put in left lateral position also.

- Look for abnormality of S_1 and presence of S_3, S_4, OS and mitral systolic and diastolic murmur, conduction of systolic murmur to axilla.
- *Tricuspid area:* Look for diastolic and systolic murmurs of tricuspid valve disease, augmentation with inspiration in the sitting position.
- *Pulmonary area:* Identify the abnormality of S_2, in intensity and split, ejection click, systolic, diastolic and continuous murmur.
- *Aortic area:* Position of the patient—sitting, leaning forward and breath held in expiration—look for intensity of aortic component, aortic, systolic and early diastolic murmur.
- *Second aortic area:* Sometimes aortic events are better heard in the 2nd aortic area and the position of the patient is as above.

CLINICAL FEATURES OF COMMON CARDIOVASCULAR DISORDERS

Valvular Heart Disease

Mitral Stenosis

- Normal mitral valve area—4-6 cm^2.
- Mitral apparatus consists of cusp, ring, chordae tendinae, papillary muscle, LA-myocardium, LV-myocardium.
- Two cusps–large anteromedial and a small posterolateral cusp.

Etiology

- Rheumatic valvulitis
- Very rarely—congenital
- Other causes of LA inflow obstruction
- Large vegetation
- LA thrombus
- LA myxoma
- 60% recall rheumatic history
- Rest—subclinical.

Pathophysiology

- Hemodynamic obstruction when valve area is less than 2.5 cm^2
- Mild stenosis <2.5 cm^2 → LA pressure >
- Moderate stenosis-1.5 cm^2 → LA pressure > 10 mm
- Severe stenosis-1 cm^2 → LA pressure > 25 mm
- Critical stenosis-0.5 cm^2.

Hemodynamic

- Mitral stenosis → decrease LV filling → low output state → increase LA pressure → increase pulmonary venous pressure → *Pulmonary* arterial hypertension → RVH → RV failure

- Pulmonary hypertension in MS:
  - Passive pressure from LA to pulmonary vascular system → increase in pulmonary arterial pressure → reactive changes in pulmonary arterioles → secondary thrombotic occlusions of pulmonary vessels.

Clinical Features

- Symptoms of pulmonary venous congestion
  - Progressive exertional dyspnea
  - PND
  - Hemoptysis
  - Orthopnea
- Symptoms of low output
  - Fatigue
- Symptoms of complications like
  - Recurrent RTI
  - Embolic phenomenon.

Signs

- *Mitral facies:* Rare-due to dilated veins of cheeks
- Pulse: Normal or decrease in volume in severe stenosis/pulmonary arterial hypertension
  - Irregular if AF present
- JVP: Increased if RVF present
  - a wave increase—pulmonary hypertension
  - a wave absent if AF present
  - v wave increase—if TR present
- Precordium
  - Tapping apex beat
  - Apical diastolic thrill
  - Palpable shock of increase S_1
  - Left parasternal heave
  - Palpable pulmonary artery and
  - Palpable shock of S_2
- Auscultation—Accentuation of S_1 (Fig. 4.23)
  - MDM
  - Presystolic murmur with accentuation
  - Opening snap
- Auscultatory features of MS sounds like-
  - Fout -ta-ta-rou
  - Fout-S_1↑, ta-S_2, ta-OS, rou-MDM

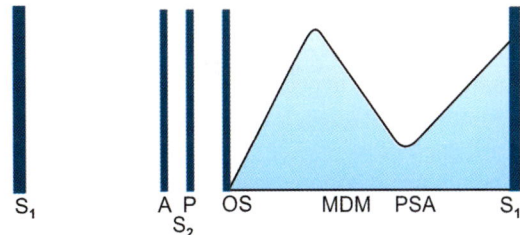

Fig. 4.23: Auscultatory signs of mitral stenosis.

- If PAH + - P2 ↑, pulmonary EC, TR murmur Graham Steell murmur and RA S_4
- Dulling of S_1-calcified valve, AR and MR.

Mechanism of Presystolic Accentuation

- Presystolic contraction of LA
- Physiological narrowing of mitral valve in presystole.

Absence of Presystolic Accentuation

- Atrial fibrillation
- Presence of MR
- Flabby LA
- ASD
- After surgery
- Junctional rhythm
- Under estimation of mitral stenosis
  - Presence of ASD
  - Systemic hypertension
  - Aortic valvular disease.

Differential Diagnosis of MDM—Apex (Refer MDM)

Precipitating factors of congestive heart failure in MS:
- Anemia, pregnancy, atrial fibrillation, RTI, rheumatic activity
- Pulmonary embolism, thyrotoxicosis, undue exertion
- Other added anomalies—MR, aortic valvular disease
- ASD-Lutem-Bacher's syndrome
- PDA-CoA.

Investigations

ECG

Left atrial enlargement, RVH, RA enlargement (if PAH +), atrial fibrillation.

X-ray Chest

- Evidence of LA enlargement
  - Straightening of left border
  - Shadow within shadow
  - Visibility of LA appendage
  - Lifting up of left main bronchus
  - Indentation in barium swallow-lower part
  - Sheep nose appearance of heart.
- Pulmonary venous hypertension
  - Prominence of upper lobe veins
  - Perihilar flare
  - Kerley's A and B lines—engorged septal lymphatics
  - Interlobar effusion
  - Ground glass appearance of lung field
  - Hydrothorax.

- Pulmonary arterial hypertension
  - Main pulmonary artery dilatation
  - Right pulmonary artery dilatation
  - Proximal branches dilatation
  - Peripheral pruning-Oligemia.
- Calcification of mitral valve
  - Echocardiography—for
    - Valve morphology and valve area
    - LA size and thrombus
    - Subvalvular structures
    - Added MR
    - Pulmonary artery pressure.

Complications of Mitral Stenosis

Can be—pulmonary, cardiac and general
- **Pulmonary**
  - Pulmonary edema
  - Recurrent RTI
  - Hemoptysis
  - Pulmonary hypertension
  - Pulmonary infarction—RA thrombus/DVT in CHF
  - Pulmonary hemosiderosis.
- **Cardiac**
  - Atrial fibrillation
  - Thromboembolism
  - CHF/LA thrombus (due to stasis, atrial fibrillation, MacCallum patch)
    - Ball valve thrombus—LA
    - Infective endocarditis—rare.
- **General**
  - Ortner's syndrome—cardiovocal paralysis
  - Cardiac cirrhosis of liver
  - Cardiac cachexia
  - Stunting of growth—juvenile RHD.

Common complications are:
- Recurrent RTI
- Hemoptysis
- Pulmonary edema
- Atrial fibrillation
- Thromboembolism
- PAH and CHF.

Complications unrelated to severity:
- Atrial fibrillation
- Thromboembolism
- Infective endocarditis—rare.

Indicators of Severity of Mitral Stenosis

Symptoms, cardiac enlargement, S_2-OS interval, length of the murmur.

Management

Medical

Prophylaxis—rheumatic prophylaxis
- IE prophylaxis
  - Prompt treatment of all infections
  - Antibiotic cover for surgical procedure.
- Drugs- for
  - Atrial fibrillation
  - CHF
  - Thromboembolism
  - RTI.

Surgical

Indications
- Symptomatic
- Moderate to severe mitral stenosis
- Mitral valve area < 1.5 cm^2
- First successful surgical relief of MS-achieved by Cutler and Levine at the Peter Bent Brigha hospital on 20-5-1923.

Procedures
- BMV
  - Balloon mitral valvuloplasty
  - Symptomatic, pure mitral stenosis, No LA thrombus
  - Noncalcified and nonfibrosed valve, No MR.
- CMV
  - Closed mitral valvotomy
  - Symptomatic, pure mitral stenosis, No LA thrombus
  - Noncalcified and nonfibrosed pliable valve, No MR.
- OMV
  - Open mitral valvotomy
  - Presence of LA thrombus, fibrosed valve.
- MVR
  - Mitral valve replacement
  - Grossly damaged valve and subvalvular structures, presence of MR.

MITRAL REGURGITATION

- It results from in co-ordination of any structure of the mitral apparatus.

Etiology

Depends on Pathogenesis

- Deformity of valve cusp
  - RHD
  - Congenital
  - Infective endocarditis
- Dilatation of the valve ring—functional MR
  - LV enlargement
    - Aortic valvular disease
    - Hypertensive heart disease
    - Cardiomyopathy
    - Myocarditis
    - CAD
  - MAC—mitral annular calcification
- Dysfunction of chordae and papillary muscle (subvalvular MR)
  - IHD
  - Infective endocarditis
  - Congenital—anomalous insertion of chordae
  - Mitral valve prolapse
  - Marfan's syndrome

Depends on Anatomy

- Anterior cusp lesion—usual
- Posterior cusp lesion—rare.

Depends on Duration

- Acute:
  - IHD
  - Rheumatic valvulitis
  - Infective endocarditis.
- Chronic:
  - Mitral valve prolapse
  - RHD
  - Cardiomyopathy
  - Congenital.

Common Causes

- MVP, RHD, IHD (most common)
- Cardiomyopathy
- Infective endocarditis
- Congenital.

Pathophysiology

Hemodynamic abnormality depends on the severity of leak from LV to LA. Diastolic overload of LV → LVH → LV enlargement → LV dysfunction → symptoms—Dyspnea, PND, palpitation, hemoptysis, recurrent RTI. LA enlargement → pulmonary venous hypertension → PAH → RV enlargement and dysfunction → CHF → congestive hepatomegaly, pedal edema.
- Low output state-fatigability
- LA enlargement pulls posterior leaflet away—increase MR
  The aphorism MR begets MR
  MR → LV enlargement
  ↓   ↑
  LV enlargement ← MR

Clinical Features

Symptoms

- Mild exertional dyspnea and palpitation
- Once LV dysfunction → progressive exertional dyspnea, PND, orthopnea, hemoptysis.

Signs

- Pulse—normal/normal volume collapsing
- JVP
  - Normal/raised if CHF +
  - Pulsation-a wave increase →PAH
  - a wave absent → atrial fibrillation
  - v wave increase → TR +
- Precordium
  - Forcible apex, systolic thrill, cardiomegaly ±
  - Left parasternal heave—RV enlargement/LA enlargement
- Auscultation (Fig. 4.24)
  - S_1 soft, pansystolic murmur
  - S_2 Normal/wide split-early A_2
  - $P_2 \uparrow$ — If PAH present
  - S_3+, Mid-diastolic murmur (severe MR)
- Severity
  - Symptoms ± Class 3/4 cardiomegaly
  - S_3 and MDM.

Other Types of MR

- Acute MR
  - Early systolic murmur
  - S_4
  - Pulmonary edema
- Posterior cusp lesion MR
  - Systolic murmur, conducted medially and to aortic area
  - S_1-Normal
- Papillary muscle dysfunction MR
  - Early, mid or late systolic murmur
- MVP MR-NEC + Late systolic murmur
- Ruptured papillary muscle MR
  - Systolic murmur—cooing quality
  - "Seagull murmur"
- Complete heart block with MR
  - Corrected transposition of great arteries.

Complications

- Pulmonary edema, hemoptysis, recurrent RTI
- Atrial fibrillation, → thromboembolism
- Infective endocarditis-with mild MR
- PAH, CHF and Ortner's syndrome.

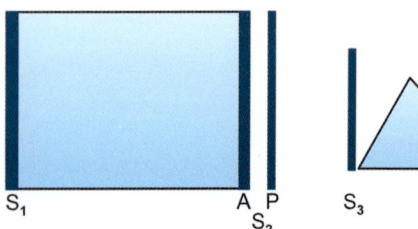

Fig. 4.24: Auscultatory signs of mitral regurgitation.

Investigations

- Routine blood and urine examination
- Blood culture and RFT—infective endocarditis
- X-ray chest:
  - Evidence of left atrial enlargement (LAE), pulmonary venous and arterial hypertension
  - Calcified valve
- ECG:
  - LVH
  - LAE
  - Atrial fibrillation ±
  - IHD ±
- Echocardiography
  - Morphology of mitral valve and subvalvular structures
  - LV enlargement and end systolic diameter
  - Ejection fraction and LV dysfunction, LAE, MVP, regional wall motion abnormality (RWMA) in CAD
  - Vegetation in IE
  - Calcification in MAC.

Management

- Rheumatic prophylaxis, infective endocarditis prophylaxis
- Class 1 and 2
  - Follow-up with medical treatment
  - Drugs for—CHF, RTI, AF and thromboembolism
  - Vasodilator-ACEI—in chronic MR
- Surgery
  - Class 3/4
  - Echo evidence of ejection fraction (EF) < 60%, left ventricular end systolic (LV ESD) > 4.5 cm
  - LAE > 5.5 cm
- Surgical procedures
  - MVR
  - Mitral valvuloplasty—repair of mitral valve in Flail leaflet and ruptured chordate
  - Mitral annuloplasty—annular dilatation.

MITRAL VALVE PROLAPSE

Pathogenesis

- Normal LV size with large mitral apparatus or
- Small LV size with normal mitral apparatus → prolapse of anterior cusp or posterior cusp to LA of 2 mm or more.

Clinical Features

- Usually asymptomatic
- Palpitation and chest pain
- Mid systolic NEC with late systolic murmur
- On dynamic auscultation, murmur increase on standing, murmur decrease on squatting.

Complications

- Infective endocarditis
- Fatal arrhythmias
- Acute MR → pulmonary edema
- Embolic phenomenon.

Management

- IE prophylaxis
- β blockers → bradycardia → LVE → decrease prolapse
- Antiplatelet if TIA present
- Mitral valve repair.

Clinical Comparison of Mitral Valvular Disease

MS (Pure MS)	MS mr (Dominant MS and mild MR)	MR ms (dominant MR and mild MS)	MR (Pure MR)
Tapping apex S_1 increase, MDM Presystolic murmur with accentuation OS +	All findings of MS + Systolic murmur apex, conduction ±	All findings of dominant MR + with MDM S_1 - N/ increase No S_3, OS ±	Forcible apex Apical systolic thrill, S_1 decrease, PSM S_3 + short MDM

AORTIC STENOSIS

- Normal aortic valve area–2.5–3.5 cm²
- Hemodynamic effect when the valve area is 1 cm² or less.
- Symptoms - < 0.7 cm²
- Critical stenosis - < 0.5 cm².

Etiology

- Rheumatic heart disease
- Congenital
- Valvular
- Supravalvular
- Subvalvular
- Calcific aortic stenosis
- Atherosclerotic—AS after 65 years of age
- HOCM—dynamic obstruction

Pathophysiology

- LV outflow tract obstruction → low and fixed output
- Progressive LV hypertrophy and dilatation → diastolic dysfunction
- Mismatch of supply and demand of blood → ischemia of myocardium
- Low output → fatigability, syncope, etc.

Clinical Features

Symptoms

- Exertional angina
- Syncope
- Exertional—diversion of blood to skeletal muscles → decrease cerebral blood supply
- Nonexertional—transient ventricular arrhythmias
- Exertional dyspnea diastolic dysfunction of LV
- Sudden cardiac death.

Signs

- Pulse—anacrotic pulse
- BP—pulse pressure is decreased
- Precordium
  - Heaving apex, systolic thrill—aortic area
  - Cardiomegaly ±
  - Ejection systolic murmur—better heard (Fig. 4.25) in aortic area/2nd aortic and occasionally in mitral area conducted to carotid
  - Ejection click—in valvular aortic stenosis
  - S_2—dull A_2 in valvular AS
  - Paradoxical split
  - S_4 +
- *Severity of AS* depends on
  - Symptoms +, cardiomegaly
  - Lengthy ESM with late peaking
  - Paradoxical split of S_2
  - Presence of S_4
  - Transvalvular pressure gradient > 50 mm Hg
  - Valve area < 0.75 cm².

Complications

- Angina
- Syncope
- Ventricular arrhythmia
- Sudden cardiac death
- Infective endocarditis
- CHF.

Differential diagnosis of aortic systolic murmur-(Refer Murmur)

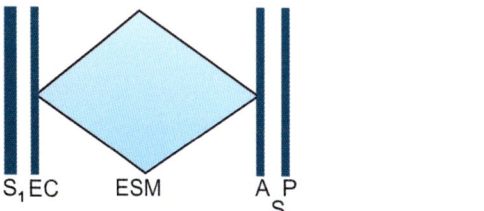

Fig. 4.25: Auscultatory signs of aortic stenosis.

Investigations

- ECG—LVH with strain pattern
- X-ray chest
  - Post-stenotic dilatation (in valvular AS)
  - Calcification of aortic valve
- Echocardiography
  - Valve morphology
  - LVH
  - LV function—diastolic and systolic
  - Cardiac catheterization—to assess the pressure gradient
  - Coronary angiography—to rule out CAD.

Prognosis

- Lifespan
  - Presence of angina—4 years
  - Presence of syncope—3 years
  - Presence of CHF—2 years.

Management

Medical

- Rheumatic and infective endocarditis (IE) prophylaxis
- Drugs for arrhythmia, angina, and CHF if present.

Surgical

Indications

- All symptomatic severe AS
- Asymptomatic AS with LV dysfunction
- Ventricular tachycardia
- Marked LVH
- Valve area < 0.6 cm^2.

Procedures

- Aortic valve replacement (AVR)
- Balloon aortic valvotomy is done as a bridge procedure to AVR, high risk for AVR and harboring other systemic diseases like malignancy.

AORTIC REGURGITATION

Etiology

- Rheumatic heart disease
- Aortic diseases
- Congenital with VSD
- Bicuspid AV
- Infective endocarditis
- Syphilitic
- Arthropathies
  - Ankylosing spondylitis
  - Rheumatoid arthritis
  - Reiter's syndrome
  - Psoriatic arthritis
- Aortic diseases
  - Root aneurysm
  - Dissecting aneurysm
- RSOV
- Atherosclerotic
- Severe systemic hypertension
- Marfan's syndrome
- Ehlers Danlos syndrome
- Mucopolysaccharidosis
- Traumatic.

Causes of Acute AR

- Dissecting aneurysm
- RSOV
- Prolapse of AV valve in VSD
- Infective endocarditis in bicuspid AV valve
- Rheumatic valvulitis
- Traumatic.

Pathophysiology

Hemodynamic effect depends on the severity of AR. Diastolic filling of LV increase → LV dilatation and hypertrophy → stroke volume increase → systolic pressure is increased. Peripheral vascular resistance is decreased due to reflex vasodilatation to decrease the regurgitation → low diastolic pressure → wide pulse pressure.

Two streams of blood from aorta and LA to LV,↑ the diastolic filling → premature closure of mitral valve → functional narrowing of mitral valve → MDM of Austin Flint. Increased stroke volume → ejection systolic murmur. The hallmark of the lesion is early diastolic murmur.

Clinical Features

Symptoms

- Mild exertional dyspnea and palpitation
- Angina
- Hemodynamic effect—mean aortic pressure is decreased
- Added CAD
- Syphilitic coronary ostial stenosis
- Dissecting aneurysm blocking coronaries
- Syncope—if ventricular arrhythmia present
- Progressive exertional dyspnea and PND—If LV dysfunction present.

Signs

Two groups—peripheral and precordial.

Peripheral signs

- Wide pulse pressure, collapsing pulse
- Prominent carotid pulsation-Corrigan's sign
- Locomotor brachii

- Alfred de Musset's sign—systolic nodding of head (systolic extension of neck)
- Pistol shot sound—systolic sound on auscultating over major vessels
- Duroziez's murmur—systolic murmur on proximal pressure, systolic and diastolic murmur on distal pressure while auscultating with diaphragm on femoral artery
- Traube's double tone-systolic and diastolic murmur on auscultating over major vessel without pressing
- Hill's sign—exaggerated systolic pressure in lower limb
  - Mild AR: 20-40 mm Hg
  - Moderate AR: 40-60 mm Hg
  - Severe AR: >60 mm Hg
- Visible retinal artery pulsation-Becker's sign.

Precordial signs
- Forcible apex beat, cardiomegaly ±
- S_1 soft, early diastolic murmur on aortic area conducted down along left sternal border (Fig. 4.26)
- Ejection systolic murmur on aortic area
- MDM: Austin Flint murmur on mitral area
- S_2: A_2 ringing in syphilitic AR
- A_2 dull in rheumatic AR.

AR with EDM Conduction along Rt. Sternal Border

- Syphilitic AR
- Dissecting aneurysm
- Marfan's syndrome
- RSOV.

Severity

- Mild AR
  - Early diastolic murmur
  - No wide pulse pressure and peripheral signs
- Moderate AR
  - Early diastolic murmur + wide pulse pressure, no peripheral signs
- Severe AR
  - Early diastolic murmur + wide pulse pressure + all peripheral signs,
    - Hill's sign > 60 mm Hg
    - Duration of murmur > 2/3rd of diastole

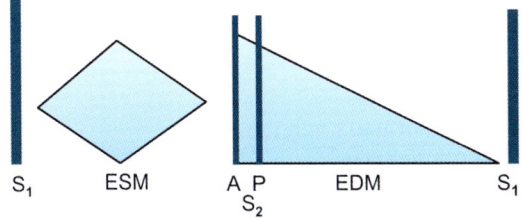

Fig. 4.26: Auscultatory signs of AR.

- Austin flint murmur +
- AR with ejection systolic murmur

Clinical difference between flow murmur and AS

	Flow murmur	Aortic stenosis
Pulse	Collapsing	Bisferiens
Pulse pressure	Wide	Not wide
SBP	Markedly increased	Not ↑
DBP	< 40 mm Hg (Muffling of Korotkoff sound continuous with pistol shot sound)	> 60 mm Hg
Apex	Forcible	Heaving
Systolic thrill	Absent	Present
ESM	Short	Lengthy
Conduction to carotid	+	+

- AR with elevated diastolic pressure (> 60 mm Hg)
  - AR with CHF
  - AR with CoA
  - AR with AS
  - AR with systemic hypertension.

AR with MDM-Clinical difference between Austin Flint and mitral stenosis

	Austin Flint murmur	Mitral stenosis
S_1	Soft	Normal/↑
Opening snap	Absent	±
Thrill	Absent	Present
MDM	Lengthy	Short
Pulmonary hypertension	Usually absent	±
Atrial fibrillation	Absent	±

Complications of AR

Ventricular arrhythmia, infective endocarditis, LV failure.

Investigations

ECG-Volume overload, LVH.

X-ray chest:
- Cardiomegaly with LV contour—"Sitting Duck" appearance
- Calcification of ascending aorta—syphilitic
- Calcification of valve—calcific aortic stenosis and bicuspid aortic valve
- Echocardiography for—morphology of aortic valve and aorta
  - LV size and LVH
  - LV function-ejection fraction.

Management

Medical
- Rheumatic and infective endocarditis prophylaxis
- Treatment of primary disease like infective endocarditis, etc.
- Drugs for—ventricular arrhythmia and CHF vasodilator like ACEI to ↓ regurgitation.

Surgical
- Indications
  - Symptomatic severe AR
  - Asymptomatic severe AR with
  - Echo features—End systolic diameter of LV > 55 mm, ejection fraction < 50%.
- Procedure: Aortic valve replacement.

TRICUSPID VALVULAR DISEASE

Tricuspid Regurgitation
- Size of the valve area is 7 cm^2.

Etiology
- Secondary to pulmonary hypertension—mitral valvular, Eisenmenger syndrome, primary pulmonary hypertension
- Congenital—Ebstein's anomaly
- Infective endocarditis—drug abuse, gonococcal
- RHD
- Carcinoid syndrome
- RV EMF
- RV infarction.

Clinical Features
- Symptoms—fatigue and weakness
- Symptoms of primary heart disease.

Signs:
- Prominent v wave-venous Corrigan
- Left parasternal heave-if PAH +
- Pan systolic murmur ↑ with inspiration
- RV S$_3$ ±
- Signs of PAH in secondary TR
- Systolic pulsation of liver.

Investigations
- ECG—RVH, RAE
- X-ray chest:
  - Cardiomegaly—RA and RV prominence
  - Features of PAH ±.

Management
- Drugs—RV failure present
- Treatment of primary disease—IE, mitral valvular disease, etc
- Surgical—annuloplasty/TVR.

Tricuspid Stenosis
Rare valvular lesion usually seen with mitral valvular disease.

Causes
- RHD (with MS)
- Congenital
- Carcinoid syndrome.

Clinical Features
- *Symptoms:*
  - Low output state → fatigability
  - Dyspnea ← ascites and hepatomegaly.
- *Signs:*
  - Prominent a wave
  - JVP ↑
  - MDM ↑ with inspiration
  - Opening snap ± Ascites
  - Congestive hepatomegaly with presystolic pulsation.

Investigations
- ECG—RAE, no RVH
- X-ray chest—RAE, SVC prominent.

Management
- Drugs for-CHF.
- Surgery
  - Diastolic pressure gradient > 5 mm Hg
  - Tricuspid valve area < 1.5–2 cm^2
  - Tricuspid valve replacement—if TR present.

PULMONARY VALVULAR DISEASE

Pulmonary Stenosis

Etiology
- Congenital
  - Valvular
  - Subvalvular—infundibular and subinfundibular
  - Supravalvular—pulmonary trunk and peripheral
- Carcinoid syndrome
- RHD—very rare.

Clinical Features
- *Symptoms*
  - Fatigue
  - Mild exertional dyspnea
  - Syncope ±.
- *Signs*
  - Pulse—Normal/↓ volume
  - Prominent a wave
  - Left parasternal heave +
  - Systolic thrill—pulmonary area
  - Ejection systolic murmur—pulmonary area

- Inconstant pulmonary ejection click
- S_2—wide split, dull and delayed P_2
- RA S_4
- Continuous murmur—peripheral pulmonary artery stenosis
- Added anomalies
- TOF, ASD, transposition of great vessels (TGV), congenital Rubella Noonan's syndrome, William's syndrome Leopard syndrome and Turner's syndrome.

Investigations

- ECG—RAD, RVH with strain, RAE
- *X-ray chest*:
  - Cardiomegaly—RV type and Pulmonary oligemia
  - Prominent main pulmonary artery
  - Poststenotic dilatation—may extend to right pulmonary artery and left pulmonary artery imitating primary pulmonary hypertension
  - Segmental hypovascularity in peripheral stenosis
  - Stencilled heart border → pulmonary oligemia.
- *Echocardiography*:
  - Valve morphology, site of lesion
  - RVH and RV function.
- *Severity of lesion*:
  - Lengthy murmur, dull and delayed P2
  - S1-EC ratio—less
  - RA S4
  - Prominent a wave
  - Cardiomegaly
  - Pressure gradient:
    - Mild 30–50 mm Hg
    - Moderate- 50–100 mm Hg
    - Severe - > 100 mm Hg

Complications

- Infective endocarditis → medical valvotomy
- Right to left shunt—at atrial level (PFO) → cyanosis
- Right ventricular failure
- Rarely hemoptysis—thrombosis of peripheral stenosis.

Management

- *Medical:*
  - Infective endocarditis prophylaxis
  - Drugs for RV failure
  - Follow-up of-mild to moderate lesion with medical treatment.
- *Surgery:*
  - Severe lesions
  - Balloon valvuloplasty
  - Transventricular pulmonary valvotomy-Brock's operation
  - Pulmonary valve replacement.

Pulmonary Regurgitation

Etiology

- Most common—secondary to PAH
- Congenital—absence of Pulmonary valve in TOF
- Marfan's syndrome
- IDPA (idiopathic dilatation of pulmonary artery)
- Infective endocarditis—in PS (2nd common cause)
- Carcinoid syndrome
- After surgery.

Clinical Features

Symptoms are due to the primary disease.

Signs:
- Early diastolic murmur ↑ on inspiration on pulmonary area
- Pan diastolic murmur occasionally in PAH of Primary pulmonary hypertension, Eisenmenger ASD & PDA
- In organic PR—diastolic murmur is delayed, low pitched and crescendo decrescendo
- Features of primary heart disease → PAH.

Investigations

- ECG—RVH-if PAH present
- *X-ray chest:*
  - RVE, prominent main pulmonary artery
  - RVE and RVH
- Doppler echo to detect PR.

Management

Medical
- Infective endocarditis prophylaxis
- Drugs for RV failure, treatment of primary disease like IE
- Treatment of lesion for PAH.

Surgery
- Seldom required for pulmonary regurgitation
- If intractable RV failure present, pulmonary valve replacement. TVR-if TR present.

COMMON CONGENITAL HEART DISEASES

Two Groups

- **Acyanotic**
  - With shunt—L → R shunt-ASD, VSD, PDA
  - Without shunt-with obstruction—congenital AS, PS, CoA
  - Without obstruction and shunt—dextrocardia-IDPA (idiopathic dilatation of pulmonary artery).
- **Cyanotic**
  - With pulmonary oligemia—TOF, PS with R → L shunt,
  - Pulmonary hypertension—Eisenmenger syndrome
  - With pulmonary plethora—TAPVC, TGV, PTA.

General Features of CHD

- L → R shunt—recurrent RTI, absence of cyanosis
  - Hyperkinetic precordium, flow murmurs
  - Pulmonary plethora in CXR
- R → L shunt—central cyanosis, clubbing and polycythemia
  - Anoxic spell, squatting and growth retardation
  - With PS—ejection systolic murmur
    - Dull and delayed P_2/single S_2
    - Oligemic lungs.
- With PAH—clinical and chest X-ray evidence of PAH
- With pulmonary plethora-CHF and CXR-evidence of pulmonary plethora
- With obstruction—absence of cyanosis
  - Absence of hyperkinetic precordium
  - Heaving cardiac impulse
  - Stenotic systolic murmurs
  - Absence of flow murmur
  - Delay in corresponding component of S_2
  - L → R shunt.

ATRIAL SEPTAL DEFECT

- Commonest congenital heart disease in adults
- Developmentally 3 types (Fig. 4.27):
  - Below fossa ovalis
  - At fossa ovalis
  - Above fossa ovalis

Below fossa ovalis: Ostium primum—defective fusion of the septum primum with endocardial cushion resulting in ASD with mitral valve or tricuspid valve abnormality-Usually ASD with MR.

At fossa ovalis: Ostium secundum-commonest, defective closure of the foramen ovale by septum secundum.

Above fossa ovalis—Sinus venosus type: Defect in the primitive interatrial septum at the roof of the atrium-ASD with partial anomalous pulmonary venous connection.

Pathophysiology

L → R shunt at atrial level → RV volume overload → RVH and RV enlargement →↑ blood flow through the pulmonary valve → hyperkinetic pulmonary blood flow. LV is spared

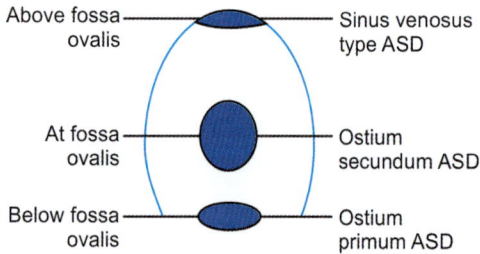

Fig. 4.27: Types of atrial septal defect.

hemodynamically–small and underfilled. Increased blood flow through tricuspid valve and pulmonary valve → mid diastolic and ejection systolic murmurs. In ASD, at the site of the defect-no murmur because of low pressure gradient.

Clinical Features

Male: Female ratio-1: 4.
Symptoms of recurrent RTI, dyspnea and palpitation.
Signs: To produce clinical signs the shunt ratio is 2: 1
- Pulse—normal/low volume, absence of cyanosis
- Precordial bulge
- Cardiomegaly, left parasternal heave
- Systolic thrill over pulmonary area (large shunt)
- Pulmonary ejection systolic murmur
- S_2-wide and fixed split, S_1 accentuated
- Tricuspid mid-diastolic murmur (flow murmur) ±.

Severity: Cardiomegaly, pulmonary systolic thrill and tricuspid flow murmur.

Associations of ASD: Arachnodactyly, fingerization of thumb (Holt Oram syndrome)
- Marfan's syndrome, mitral stenosis (Lutem Bacher syndrome)
- TAPVC, TGV, PS (Fallot's Triology)
- MVP, 1° AVB-familial ASD, left sided superior vena cava.

Complications

Recurrent RTI, supraventricular arrhythmia-AF and SVT.
- Pulmonary hypertension and Eisenmenger-delayed development of pulmonary hypertension—because, L → R shunt start only after regression of the pulmonary vasculature and right ventricular (RV) to a low pressure system as in adult. The mechanism of pulmonary hypertension is—hyperkinetic blood flow → reactive pulmonary hypertension→ thrombotic occlusion.
- Occasionally, pulmonary hypertension and Eisenmenger syndrome develop early in ASD because RV involution occur earlier than the pulmonary vascular regression. Thus the shunt may start early preventing full regression of the pulmonary vascular system to adult pattern allowing persistence of the fetal pulmonary vasculature.
- Pulmonary artery dilatation → cardiovocal paralysis (Ortner's syndrome), IE is very rare.

Clinical Evaluation of ASD

- *Cyanosis in ASD*:
  - Pulmonary hypertension → R → L shunt
  - Large ASD-IVC type-rare
  - Pulmonary stenosis (PS) with R → L shunt at ASD
  - To rule out total anomalous pulmonary venous connection (TAPVC)

Type of lesion with ASD	Cyanosis	JVP	A wave	Thrill	EC	PSM	RV S₃	MDM	S₂–Wide and fixed
Mild to moderate ASD	–	N	N	–	–	+	–	–	+
ASD–large L → R shunt	–	N	N	+	+	+	+	+	+
ASD with mild PS	–	N	↑	+	+	+	–	–	+
ASD with PAH	+	N/↑	+	–	+	–	– RA S₄	– PR and TR murmur	+
ASD and MS	–	↑	+	+	+	+	+	+	+
ASD and TS	–	↑	+	–	–	+	–	+	+

- *Raised JVP in ASD*:
  - Pulmonary hypertension with RV failure
  - PS and RV failure
  - MS and TS (without cyanosis)
  - Left ventricular failure (LVF) in old age ASD
- *Prominent a wave in ASD*:
  - Pulmonary hypertension, MS
  - PS and TS
- Systolic thrill in ASD–PS, MS and large shunt in ASD
- Mid-diastolic murmur (MDM) in atrial septal defect (ASD): Large L → R shunt → Tricuspid flow murmur
  - Tricuspid stenosis
  - Mitral stenosis (Both mitral and tricuspid diastolic murmur)
- *MR in ASD*:
  - Rheumatic MR, ostium primum ASD
  - MVP and cleft mitral valve.

Investigations

- *ECG*: RAD, right bundle branch block (RBBB), right ventricular hypertrophy (RVH)–Ostium primum → LAD + RBBB
- *CXR*: Main pulmonary artery dilatation, pulmonary plethora, cardiomegaly–RV type
  - Aortic knuckle less prominent.

Management

Medical
- Drugs for RTI, CHF and supraventricular arrhythmia

Surgery
- If shunt is > 1.5:1 (Pulmonary: Systemic flow),
  - Umbrella closure or
  - Amplatzer device.
  - Timing of procedure → preschool age (3–5 yrs)
- If shunt is less, follow up with medical management.

VENTRICULAR SEPTAL DEFECT

- Interventricular septum developed from:
  - Primitive interventricular septum.
  - Bulbospiral septum–Conus septum
  - Endocardial cushion

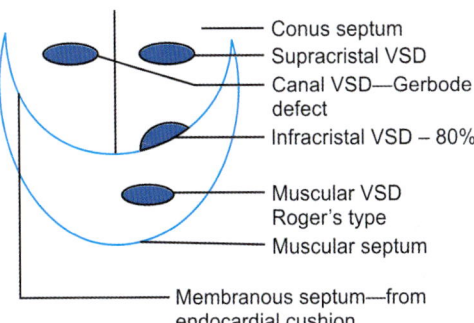

Fig. 4.28: Development of interventricular septum and types of VSD.

- **Types of ventricular septal defect (VSD)** (Fig. 4.28)
  - Defective fusion of muscular septum with conus septum–infracristal VSD–80%
  - Defect in muscular septum–muscular VSD–Maladie De Roger–5%
  - Defect in conus septum–supracristal VSD–5%
  - Defect in membranous septum from endocardial cushion–Canal VSD–5%
  - Multiple defect–5%.

Pathophysiology

L → R shunt at inter ventricular level → hyperkinetic pulmonary blood flow → diastolic overload of LV → hypertrophy and RV hypertrophy also. Murmur is produced at the site of defect, flow murmur at mitral valve.

Anatomical Severity of VSD (Rogers)

- 2–4 mm—mild
- 5–9 mm—moderate
- 10–15 mm—severe
- 15–30 mm—severe with pulmonary arterial hypertension (PAH)

Clinical Features

- Male: Female ratio = 1:1
- Features depend on the age, size of defect and pulmonary vascular resistance.

- *Symptoms:*
  - Muscular type—asymptomatic
  - Significant shunt—recurrent RTI, palpitation, exertional dyspnea
- *Signs*
  - Pulse—normal/normal volume collapsing,
  - Jugular venous pressure (JVP) normal
  - Forcible apex beat—left parasternal heave
  - Systolic thrill—3rd and 4th left intercostal space
  - Pansystolic harsh murmur—Grade 4 or >.—3rd and 4th left intercostal space
  - Mitral diastolic flow murmur if shunt is large.
  - In muscular VSD, shunt is small—loud murmur and thrill without hemodynamic change.
  - In supracristal VSD—the murmur heard over 2nd and 3rd left intercostal space
  - In canal VSD—Gerbode defect-LV → RA shunt, prominent v wave, RA enlargement, systolic murmur
  - Gasul's type of VSD—hypertrophy of RV outflow tract in VSD mimicking the hemodynamics of VSD with PS.

Associated Anomalies

Tetralogy of Fallot (TOF), TGV, double outlet right ventricle (DORV), right sided aortic arch, polydactyly, syndactyly and mongolism, etc.

Complications

- Recurrent respiratory tract infections, infective endocarditis, congestive heart failure (CHF), acute AR-prolapse of aortic cusp, pulmonary hypertension → Eisenmenger syndrome
- Pulmonary hypertension in VSD
- Persistence of fetal pulmonary vasculature—more with VSD than other L. → R shunt
- Hyperkinetic pulmonary blood flow—reactive pulmonary hypertension-plexogenic pulmonary arteriopathy thrombotic occlusion

Thus Eisenmenger syndrome is early with VSD among the L → R shunt.

Investigations

- *ECG*: Biventricular hypertrophy, LAD in canal VSD
- *CXR*: Cardiomegaly ±, pulmonary plethora,
- Echocardiography-Color Doppler study-detect the location, size of defect and associated anomalies
- Catheterization and angiography—to assess the state of pulmonary vascular resistance.

Management

- Medical
  - IE prophylaxis
  - Drugs for CHF, arrhythmia and RTI
- Spontaneous closure of VSD: If the defect is < 5 mm - muscular VSD
  - Mechanism—Septal muscle will grow & close. Prolapsed Aortic valve/septal cusp of tricuspid valve gets adherence to defect and close
- Surgery
  - Significant shunt (shunt 2:1or >)
    - Surgical closure is required.
    - Timing of surgery: 1 year of age or 10 kg weight.
    - Procedure → closure with pericardial patch.
  - VSD with CHF
    - Drug treatment → Surgery at 1 year of age
    - Poor response to drug treatment → Surgery at early with risk.
- *Small VSD* → Observe for spontaneous closure.

PATENT DUCTUS ARTERIOSUS

Develops from left 6th dorsal arch maintaining communication with dorsal aorta as ductus. Normal length of the ductus- 10 mm, diameter-6 mm, > 4 mm diameter size is required to produce continuous murmur.

Closure of the ductus-functional closure starts immediately after birth, completes within 15 hours after birth. Anatomical closure-within 2-4 weeks.

Function of ductus after birth—for a few hours R → L shunt then after 3 hours L → R shunt, till complete functional closure.

Window ductus means small ductus connecting aorta to pulmonary artery.

Etiology

- Premature infants, congenital rubella, respiratory distress syndrome, high altitude.

Clinical Features

Male: Female ratio = 1:3
Asymptomatic, recurrent RTI, exertional dyspnea and palpitation.

Signs:
- High volume collapsing pulse, forcible apex beat
- Continuous thrill over pulmonary area, cardiomegaly ±
- Continuous murmur peaking at S_2 over pulmonary area
- Systolic > diastolic component
- Murmur is also known as Gibson's murmur, machinery murmur or "Train in the tunnel" murmur.
- Multiple clicks present—produced by vibration of ductus due to continuous flow of blood from aorta to pulmonary artery. This will differentiate the ductus murmur from other continuous murmurs.

- S_2—Normal/paradoxical split.
- Mitral diastolic flow murmur and aortic systolic flow murmur ±.

Severity of PDA

Symptoms, wide pulse pressure, cardiomegaly, mitral diastolic murmur and paradoxical split of S_2.

Associated Anomalies

- Coarctation of aorta, compensatory ductus in TOF, TGV, and pulmonary atresia
- Congenital rubella syndrome
- Aortic stenosis.

Complications

- Recurrent RTI, Congestive heart failure, infective endocarditis-vegetation at the pulmonary end of ductus → Pulmonary embolism.
- Pulmonary hypertension-Eisenmenger syndrome with differential cyanosis.
- Aneurysm of the ductus, cardiovocal paralysis

Differential diagnosis of continuous murmur (refer murmur).

Investigations

- *ECG*: Volume overload, left ventricular hypertrophy (LVH), left atrial enlargement (LAE)
- *CXR*: Cardiomegaly-LV type, pulmonary plethora-R > L, Aortic knuckle prominent, calcification of the ductus
- *Echocardiography*: LA enlargement, LV enlargement and 2D echo detects large ductus, Color Doppler echo for small ductus.

Management

Medical

- IE prophylaxis, drugs for CHF
- Administration of indomethacin in 1st 2-7 days to reduce PGE synthesis → closure of the ductus—for babies weighing < 1000 g premature babies and term infants with ductus.

Surgical

- Significant shunt → 1 year of age
- If CHF → drug treatment and surgery at 1 yr of age
- Surgery at the time of detection even if ductus is small
- Procedure: Coil embolization

Clinical Comparison of L → R Shunt

Features	ASD	VSD	PDA
Pulse	N/↓ volume	N/NV collapsing	High volume collapsing
Cardiomegaly	+	±	±
RV impulse	+	+	–
LV impulse	–	+	+
Murmur	Pulmonary ESM	PSM	Continuous murmur
Flow murmur	Tricuspid MDM	Mitral MDM	Mitral MDM
S_2	Wide and fixed	N/Wide split	N/Paradoxical split
X ray–chest Aortic knuckle Pulmonary plethora Calcified ductus	↓ + –	N + –	↑ + ±
Electrocardiography	RBBB and RVH	Biventricular hypertrophy	LVH

EISENMENGER SYNDROME

R → L shunt developing due to pulmonary hypertension on a L→ R shunt

- Relation to size of shunt:
  - PDA >5 mm
  - ASD >3.5 cm
  - VSD >1 cm
- Mechanism of pulmonary hypertension in L → R shunt
  - *Persistence of fetal pulmonary vasculature:* Normally adult pattern is attained within 2 years after birth, Due to L → R shunt, the pressure reflected to the pulmonary vascular system will not allow the normal regression. This is more with VSD, not with ASD because in ASD, shunt will start only after full regression.
  - *Hyperkinetic pulmonary:* Blood flow
  - *Reactive pulmonary:* Vascular changes-plexogenic pulmonary arteriopathy, 6 grades of changes by Heath and Edward-
    - Muscularization of pulmonary arterioles
    - Cellular intimal proliferation
    - Intimal fibrosis and fibroelastosis
    - Pulmonary arteriolar dilatation—plexiform lesion
    - Rupture of dilated vessels and pulmonary hemosiderosis
    - Necrotizing arteritis
    - Thrombotic occlusion of pulmonary vessels

Clinical Evaluation of Eisenmenger Syndrome

- *Somatic abnormality*
  - Polydactyly or syndactyly—VSD
  - Arachnodactyly, thumb abnormality—ASD
  - Congenital rubella syndrome—PDA
- *Age of onset*:
  - Early—in VSD
  - Late—in ASD
- *Pulse volume*:
  - Low in Eisenmenger syndrome due to PAH
  - High in PDA Eisenmenger due to persistence of previous structural damage
- Central cyanosis—differential in PDA, occasionally in left upper limb also
- Jugular venous pulsation—prominent a wave, marked in ASD
  - Less prominent in VSD/PDA
- Cardiomegaly—marked in ASD, normal size heart in VSD
- S_2—single in VSD, fixed split in ASD, normal split in PDA
  - Appreciable split of S_2 exclude VSD Eisenmenger
- Pan diastolic murmur—PDA and ASD

Differential Diagnosis of Eisenmenger Syndrome

- Primary pulmonary hypertension with R → L shunt due to opening of foramen ovale.
- *TOF*: D/D of VSD Eisenmenger because of Single S_2 and normal sized heart
- Interstitial lung disease with pulmonary: Hypertension-Cor pulmonale, differential diagnosis of Eisenmenger because of cyanosis, clubbing and pulmonary hypertension.

TETRALOGY OF FALLOT

Constitute 10% of the congenital heart disease and is one of the most common cyanotic heart disease.

Components of TOF

- Infundibular PS
- VSD (large infracristal)
- Dextroposition of aorta
- RVH

Embryology

Asymmetric septations of truncus arteriosus by the bulb spiral septum leading onto the four abnormalities.

Hemodynamics

The deciding lesion for the severity is PS. LV pressure is reflected to RV both chambers acting as a single one and ejecting blood to aorta. RV has 2 outflow tracts, either to pulmonary artery or to aorta. If PS is severe more blood from RV will go aorta. If PS is less more blood from RV will go to pulmonary circulation. The murmur at the PS is less in severe lesion and more in mild lesion. VSD is silent and does not produce any sign. Pulmonary component of S_2 is inaudible and also synchronous closure of the pulmonary and aortic valve producing single S_2.

Clinical Features

Symptoms

- Central cyanosis
- Cyanotic spell or anoxic spell—due to the spasm of the infundibulum of the RV which is sensitive to circulating catecholamine rise in catecholamine may occur when the child is crying, etc.
- Syncope and seizure
- Squatting while on exercise—peripheral vascular resistance is ↓ on exertion and R → L shunt is ↑ → anoxia to tissues. By adopting squatting position→ kinking of femoral arteries → ↑ peripheral vascular resistance → reducing R → L shunt. Kinking of the femoral veins prevent venous return from the periphery which is more desaturated. There is shift of visceral venous blood which is less desaturated to the heart in the squatting position.
  All these mechanisms help the patient for the relief of anoxia due to the exercise.
- Headache—polycythemia and cerebral complications.

Signs

- Central cyanosis: Usually appear one year after birth because of—patency of ductus, presence of HbF which has less affinity to O_2 and easily released to tissues, progressive anatomical abnormality like infundibular hypertrophy
- Clubbing and polycythemia
- JVP—normal
- Mild prominence of a wave ±
- No cardiomegaly
- Silent precordium—absence of pulsation
- Systolic thrill ± (mild TOF)
- Loud single S_2
- Pulmonary ejection systolic murmur—length of the murmur is inversely proportional to the severity of the lesion
- Aortic EC, aortic systolic flow murmur
- Pulmonary phasic EC ±
- Continuous murmur if present due to compensatory PDA, bronchopulmonary anastomosis in severe Fallot, and after BT shunt.

Associated Anomalies

- *Congenital* absence of pulmonary valve and PR, AR, ASD (Fallot's pentalogy)
- Right sided aortic arch, compensatory PDA, absence of left pulmonary artery.

Severity

- Presence of symptoms, cyanosis, short ejection systolic murmur
- RAD > 150° in ECG, prominent aortic knuckle in chest X-ray.

Complications

- Anoxic spell, syncope and seizure, infective endocarditis, paradoxical embolism, polycythemia → cerebral thrombosis and abscess, growth retardation.
- CHF—rare, precipitated by anemia, IE AR, systemic hypertension, etc.
- Platelet dysfunction and bleeding tendency
- Increased incidence of pulmonary tuberculosis.

Investigations

- ECG—RAD, RVH with early transition
- CXR: Normal size heart with RV contour and uplifted cardiac apex producing the appearance of boot shaped heart—"Coeur en Sabot" appearance
  - Concavity at the site of main pulmonary artery
  - Pulmonary oligemia—differential oligemia, L > R due to change in the direction of the RV outflow tract → more blood to right lung
  - Diffuse reticular pattern of vascular marking or bush like vessel shadow near hilum if bronchopulmonary anastomosis present.
- *Echocardiography*:
  - Aortic enlargement, aortic septal discontinuity
  - Aortic over riding of the interventricular septum
  - VSD lie below aortic valve cusp.
  - Main pulmonary artery (MPA) hypoplastic
- Catheterization and angiography—to confirm diagnosis, amount of right to left shunt and the details of anatomical abnormality

Differential diagnosis of TOF
- Trilogy of Fallot—PS with R → L shunt at atrial level
- Pentalogy of Fallot—Tetralogy + ASD
- PS with single ventricle, TGV, DORV
- Pink Fallot (mild Fallot)—differential diagnosis are: PS and supracristal VSD.

Management of TOF

- *Medical*: Infectious endocarditis prophylaxis, correction of polycythemia if PCV > 65%
- *Anoxic spell*: Knee chest position, IV morphine-0.1 mg/kg body weight IV bicarbonate-2 mL/kg and prophylaxis-Propranolol-0.025-0.05 mg/kg body weight.

Surgery
- Palliative—in infancy if marked pulmonary hypoplasia present.
- BT shunt (Blalock-Taussig shunt)—left subclavian to pulmonary artery shunt
- Ascending aorta to right pulmonary artery shunt (Waterston Cooley operation)

- Total correction: If RV outflow tract anatomy and size of pulmonary artery satisfactory, total correction is done in infancy itself.

COARCTATION OF AORTA

- 7% of the congenital heart disease
- Male: Female = 2:1

Definition

Narrowing of lumen of aorta along its course. Common site is after left subclavian at the site of Ligamentum arteriosus.

Pathogenesis

Obliterative process extending to aorta
- *Congenital* defective development of isthmal portion of aorta (the part between the left subclavian and the ductus).

Etiology

- Congenital
- Acquired—aortitis.

Clinical Features

Asymptomatic, headache and epistaxis due to hypertension
- Symptoms of CHF in infancy
- Leg fatigue and muscle cramps—ischemia of legs
- Symptoms of complications like cerebral hemorrhage, infective endarteritis.

Signs:
- Underdeveloped lower limbs
- Hypertension in the upper limbs—mechanical, ↑ Renin angiotensin,
- ↑ Peripheral vascular resistance
- Radio-femoral delay—delayed and weak femoral pulse
- Prominent suprasternal and carotid pulsation
- Visible pulsation of dilated intercostals—interscapular region-Suzman's sign
- S_2-A_2↑, paradoxical split of S_2
- Aortic ejection click, LA S_4.
- Murmurs due to—coarctation, added anomaly like bicuspid aortic valve, collaterals
- Late systolic murmur—coarct site-left interscapular region
- Continuous murmur—interscapular region-from dilated intercostal arteries.
- Auscultatory Triad in Coarctation—A_2↑, EC, late systolic murmur.

Sites of Coarctation–Isthmal

- Pre subclavian
- Lower dorsal
- Subphrenic.

Anastomosis in Coarctation

- Anterior intercostals from internal mammary of subclavian artery anastomose with posterior intercostals of descending aorta
- Internal mammary branch, musculophrenic gives 7th, 8th, and 9th anterior intercostal artery
- Superior intercostal branch of costo cervical from subclavian artery gives 1st two posterior intercostal arteries
- 1st two posterior intercostal arteries.

Added Anomalies

- Bicuspid aortic valve, AS, AR, PDA, VSD, MS
- Turner syndrome, Marfan's syndrome, Pierre Robin syndrome, William's syndrome
- Berry aneurysm of cerebral vessels, polycystic kidney.

Complications

- CVA—cerebral hemorrhage
- LVF—in infancy and after 40 years
- Infective end arteritis, dissecting aneurysm of aorta, aneurysm of intercostal artery.

Investigations

- *ECG*: LVH, LBBB ±
- *CXR*: Double aortic knuckle—due to aortic knuckle and dilated left subclavian artery
  - Dock's sign-Rib notching—from 3rd to 8th rib—after the age of 6-12 years
  - Odman's sign: Erosion of the post surface of sternum by the dilated internal mammary artery
  - Barium swallow: Double indentation due to pre and postcoarct dilatation 3 sign or reverse E sign.
- *Echocardiography*:
  - 2D echo—detect the coarctation and the added anomaly
  - Doppler study—flow velocity at the site of coarctation
  - Catheterization and angiography—anatomy of the arch vessels, length of the coarctation and other anomalies.

Management

Medical-For hypertension and CHF
- *Surgical correction*: Usually between the age of 4-6 years
- Postoperative complications like arteritis of abdominal vessels, paraplegia, paralytic Ileus, and postoperative hypertension.
- Re stenosis—balloon dilatation

PULMONARY HYPERTENSION

- Normal pulmonary: Artery pressure is 25/10 mm Hg
- Mean pulmonary artery pressure is 15 mm Hg
- Pulmonary hypertension means > 30/15 mm Hg or Mean pulmonary artery pressure > 20 mm Hg.

Causes of Pulmonary Hypertension

- **Passive pulmonary hypertension**
  - Mitral valvular disease
  - Late phase of aortic valvular disease and IHD. Here left atrial pressure ↑→ pulmonary venous pressure ↑ →concomitant rise in pulmonary arterial pressure
- **Hyperkinetic pulmonary hypertension—**
  - L → R shunt TAPVC, PTA (persistent truncus arteriosus. Increased pulmonary blood flow → rise in pulmonary vascular pressure.
- **Obstructive/obliterative pulmonary: Hypertension—**
  - *Primary pulmonary* disease—COPD, diffuse parenchymal disease of lung

Features	Pink Fallot	Pulmonary stenosis	Supracristal VSD
Posterior exercise cyanosis	+	–	–
Clubbing	Mild	–	–
JVP-a wave	–	+	–
LV impulse	–	–	+
RV impulse	–	+	±
Cardiomegaly	–	+	±
Systolic thrill	±	+	+ – 2nd and 3rd LICS
Systolic murmur	ESM ↑ with inspiration	ESM ↑ with inspiration	PSM–better in expiration
S_2	Single	Wide split, dull and delayed P_2	Normal split/wide split–early A_2
Ejection click	Aortic ±	Phasic pulmonary click	Absent
Electrocardiogram	RAD, RVH with early transition	RAD, RVH with strain	Biventricular hypertrophy
X-ray–chest	No cardiomegaly Pulmonary: Oligemia, and absence of main pulmonary artery shadow	Cardiomegaly, posterior stenotic dilatation of MPA, pulmonary oligemia	Cardiomegaly ±, pulmonary plethora

- Thromboembolic pulmonary hypertension—Castleman Bland syndrome
- Parasitic disease of lung
- More than 2/3rd of pulmonary vasculature obliteration → pulmonary hypertension
- **Reactive pulmonary: Hypertension**
  - Persistent passive pulmonary hypertension and hyperkinetic pulmonary blood flow → reactive changes in the pulmonary vasculature (arterioles), muscularization and intimal thickening → narrowing of the vessel, called Plexogenic pulmonary arteriopathy in L →R shunt.
- **Vasoconstrictive pulmonary: Hypertension**
  - Alveolar hypoxia as in chronic obstructive pulmonary disease (COPD), high altitude
  - Hypoxia has vasoconstrictive effect on pulmonary vascular system
- **Primary pulmonary: Hypertension**
  - Pulmonary: Hypertension without any identifiable cause, seen more in females in the 3rd and 4th decades.

Clinical Features of Pulmonary Hypertension

- Fatigue and syncope due to low output state
- Hemoptysis—thrombotic occlusion of the pulmonary vessels in late phase of pulmonary hypertension
- Symptoms of primary heart disease
- *Signs*:
  - Pulse—low volume, peripheral cyanosis, central cyanosis in Eisenmenger syndrome
  - JVP-prominent a wave
  - Precordium—pulsation of pulmonary artery, palpable P_2, left parasternal heave
  - Dullness of 2nd LICS
  - Auscultation—accentuation of P_2, constant EC, TR murmur, Graham steell murmur, RA S_4

Investigations

- *ECG*—RAD, RVH, RAE and features due to primary heart disease
- *CXR* (Fig. 4.29)
  - Main pulmonary artery dilatation, right pulmonary artery dilatation, dilatation of proximal branches and peripheral oligemia.
  - Cardiomegaly and chamber enlargement depends on the primary heart disease.
  - Lung field—for evidence of diffuse parenchymal disease/COPD.
- *Echocardiography*
  - For L → R shunt, mitral valvular disease, RVH, RAE and dilatation of MPA
- *Cardiac catheterization*
  - To identify underlying heart disease
- *Pulmonary* function test
  - Lung scan and pulmonary angiography in appropriate cases to find out primary pulmonary diseases

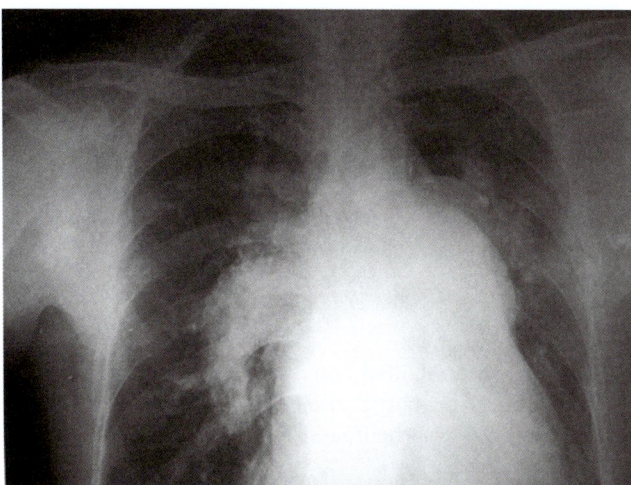

Fig. 4.29: Chest X-ray showing pulmonary artery hypertension–Eisenmenger syndrome.

Management: Depends on the cause of pulmonary hypertension.

PERICARDIAL DISEASES

Depends on the Duration

- Acute < 6 weeks
- Subacute–6 weeks to 6 months
- Chronic > 6 months.

Clinical Types

- Acute pericarditis
- Pericardial effusion—acute and chronic (Fig. 4.30)
- Cardiac tamponade
- Constrictive pericarditis
- Causes of pericardial disease.

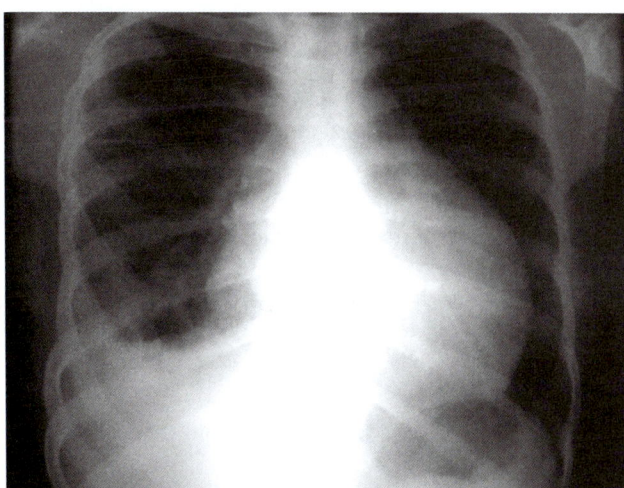

Fig. 4.30: X-ray showing pericardial effusion.

Causes of Pericardial Disease

Infection

- Viral—coxsackie
- Bacterial—pyogenic, tuberculosis
- Parasitic amoebic
- Mycotic.

Noninfectious

- Uremia
- Hypothyroidism
- IHD—transmural infarction
- Malignancy—primary and secondary
- Hypersensitivity—rheumatic fever
- Collagen disease
- Post cardiac injury syndrome
- Postinfarction-Dressler's syndrome
- Postcardiotomy
- Serum sickness.

Causes of Cardiac Tamponade

- Postoperative, traumatic
- Tuberculosis, malignancy.

Causes of Constrictive Pericarditis

- Tuberculosis, uremia
- Rheumatoid arthritis, postradiation
- Hemorrhagic and pyopericardium
- Fungal infection: Histoplasmosis/nocardiosis

Causes of Hemorrhagic Pericardial Effusion

- Malignancy-Primary and secondary
- Postoperative, tuberculosis
- Uremia, Post cardiac injury syndrome
- IHD—acute MI on anticoagulant.

Clinical Features

Symptoms and signs due to infection and inflammation of pericardium, hemodynamic features and primary disease.

Symptoms

- Due to infection/primary systemic disease
- Pericardial pain
- Hemodynamic-dyspnea (↓ in tidal volume)
- Palpitation-sinus tachycardia/arrhythmia

Signs

- Due to pericardial inflammation and effusion
- Pericardial rub-usually triphasic
- ↑ in cardiac dullness
- Distant heart sounds, pericardial knock in constrictive pericarditis
- Ewart's sign – dullness – Left infrascapular region which decreases on leaning forward
- Due to hemodynamic effect - ↑ Intrapericardial pressure → ↓ venous filling of heart →↑systemic venous pressure → ↓ in the arterial pressure.
- Pulse-sinus tachycardia, pulsus paradoxus
- Signs of ↑ systemic venous pressure
- JVP-↑—Kussmaul's sign and Friedreich's sign
- Jugular venous pulsation—M pattern in constrictive pericarditis/cardiac tamponade. M pattern is due to prominent x descent and y descent
- Square root sign-RV pressure tracing shows characteristic dip-and-plateau waveform
- Congestive hepatomegaly, ascites, pedal edema
- Beck's triad-↑ in systemic venous pressure, silent heart, ↓ in arterial pressure in cardiac tamponade.

Investigations

ECG

- ST elevation-concave up in acute cases—ST-T down in chronic cases
- ↓ voltage of QRST in pericardial effusion.

CXR

- Stenciling of heart border-water bottle shape-in pericardial effusion
- Shaggy heart borders with normal sized heart and occasional pericardial calcification in constrictive pericarditis.

Echocardiography

- For pericardial fluid and thickening of pericardium
- Catheterization and angiography-if required
- Study of pericardial fluid-to find out the etiology.

Management

- Aspiration of pericardial fluid
- Treatment of etiological factor
- Pericardiectomy in constrictive pericarditis and drugs for atrial fibrillation.

INFECTIVE ENDOCARDITIS

It is a microbial infection of endocardium in proximity of damage due to congenital/acquired heart disease. It is of two types:
1. Acute IE-septicemic process
2. Subacute IE-immunological process.

Pathology

- Basic lesion is vegetation, consisting of platelet, fibrin and bacteria which may produce thromboembolism, damage to valve, precipitate CHF, and lead to immune complex deposit.

- Site of vegetation-atrial surface of mitral valve, ventricular surface of aortic valve, right ventricle in VSD, pulmonary end of ductus, etc.

Etiological Factors

- Predisposing factors: Heart disease—mild MR and AR, PS, VSD, PDA, bicuspid aortic valve, CoA, MVP, prosthetic heart valve and rare in MS and ASD
- Precipitating factors—infections and surgical procedures
- Presence of bacteremia
    - Acute IE: Virulent organism-*Staphylococcus aureus*, Strepto-β hemolytic streptococci, Pneumococci, etc.
    - Subacute IE: Low virulent organism—Streptoviridans, *Streptococcus faecalis*, *Streptococcus bovis*
    - Other organisms: Coagulase negative Staphylococci prosthetic valve/postoperative
    - HACEK group of organisms
    - Fungi - *Candida* species and *Rickettsia*.

Clinical Features

- *Infection and septicemia*: Fever, pallor, loss of weight, clubbing, splenomegaly, patechiae, Roth's spot in retina
- *Embolic phenomenon*
    - Cerebral → focal neurological deficit
    - Peripheral → vascular occlusion
    - Visceral → mesenteric occlusion, splenic and renal infarct
    - Pulmonary embolism and hemoptysis in RV endocarditis, VSD and tricuspid valve endocarditis
- Immune complex phenomenon → Vasculitis, Osler's node, Jane way lesions, splinter hemorrhage, Glomerulonephritis-focal and diffuse, mycotic aneurysm
- Cardiac signs → Changing murmurs, musical murmurs, acute valvular lesions
- Precipitation of CHF
- Signs of predisposing heart disease.

Clinical Presentations of Infective Endocarditis

1. Pyrexia of unknown origin (PUO): Prolonged fever and murmur of susceptible heart disease
2. Acute LVF-VSD-AR, large vegetation, fungal endocarditis
3. Embolic phenomenon—central, peripheral, visceral
4. Fever and hemoptysis—VSD, PDA, TV endocarditis
5. Mycotic aneurysm—SAH
6. Acute IE—septicemia and multiorgan failure
7. Acute infective endocarditis, pneumonia and meningitis- Austrian syndrome
8. Febrile encephalopathy +/- seizures—small vessel disease of the brain
9. Prosthetic valve damage and ring abscess
10. Immune complex nephropathy and progressive renal failure
11. Splenic abscess.

The Duke Criteria

The Duke criteria has been developed on the basis of clinical, laboratory and echocardiographic findings for the diagnosis of infective endocarditis.

Requirement for diagnosis of endocarditis:
- Two major criteria or
- One major and three minor criteria or
- Five minor criteria

Major Criteria

1. Positive blood culture
    - Typical microorganisms for infective endocarditis from two separate blood cultures: Viridians streptococci, *Streptococcus bovis*, HACEK group, *Staphylococcus aureus* or
    - Community acquired enterococci in the absence of primary focus or
    - Persistently positive blood culture, defined as recovery of a microorganism consistent with infective endocarditis:
        - Blood cultures drawn >12 hr apart or
        - All the 3 or a majority of 4 or more separate blood cultures with first and last drawn at least 1 hr apart
        - Single positive blood culture for *Coxiella burnetii* or phase I IgG antibody titer or > 1:800
2. Evidence of endocardial involvement: Positive echocardiogram
    - Oscillating intracardiac mass on valve or supporting structures or in the path of regurgitant jets or in implanted material in the absence of an alternative anatomic explanation or
    - Abscess or
    - New partial dehiscence of prosthetic valve or
    - New valvular regurgitation (increase or change in preexisting murmur not sufficient)

Minor Criteria

1. Predisposition: Predisposing heart condition or injection drug use
2. Fever >/= 38.00C (>/= 100.40F)
3. Vascular phenomena: Major arterial emboli, septic pulmonary infarcts, mycotic aneurysm, intracranial hemorrhage, conjuctival hemorrhage, Janeway lesions
4. Immunologic phenomena: Glomerulonephrits, Osler's nodes, Roth's spots, rheumatoid factor
5. Microbiologic evidence: Positive blood culture but not meeting major criterion as noted previously or serologic evidence of active infection with organism consistent with infective endocarditis.

Investigations

- Blood culture—3 samples -3 different sites–one hour interval
- CBC, ESR Hb, Urine-RE, RFT

- ECG and CXR—for primary heart disease
- Echocardiography—for primary heart disease and vegetation.

Management

- General measures—for fever, CHF
- Specific treatment—appropriate antibiotic for 4-6 weeks.
- Surgery—acute valvular lesions, ductus with uncontrolled infection
- IE prophylaxis—prompt treatment of all infections, antibiotic cover for surgical procedures.

CLINICAL EVALUATION OF HEART FAILURE

Definition

Insufficient cardiac output to meet the demands of the body despite normal venous pressure.

Pathophysiology

- Structural changes
- Neurohumoral changes
- Hemodynamic changes.

Structural Changes

Myocardial remodeling: This is brought about by myocyte hypertrophy, myocyte slippage and myocardial interstitial fibrosis. The stimuli for myocyte hypertrophy is mechanical stretch and for fibrosis, it is humoral.

- Myocyte loss—by necrosis or apoptosis
  - Apoptosis—by ↑ in tumor necrosis factor (TNF) α
  - Necrosis—by β-adrenergic stimulation, Angiotensin II, and aldosterone.

Neurohumoral Changes

Activation of sympathoadrenal system-Heart rate ↑→ stroke volume, ↑vascular resistance ↑(↑ in afterload) → induce arrhythmia, down regulation of β-receptor, damage of myocyte and remodeling of myocardium.

Activation of renin angiotensin aldosterone system- decreased CO →↑ renin→↑ angiotensin II →↑ vasoconstriction (↑ afterload) →↑ aldosterone→Na-H_2O retention →↑preload. Angiotensin II and aldosterone → myocyte damage.

Cytokines and other humoral factors

- TNF α → stimulate nitric oxide synthetase → nitric oxide↑→ negative inotropic action → Endothelin I - From endothelial cells → vasoconstriction →↑ in afterload.
- ANP →↓ systemic vascular resistance, ↑ natriuresis → ↓ activation of neurohumoral system. Neutral endopeptidases degrade ANP.

Hemodynamic Changes

- Left heart failure →↑ left atrial pressure→ pulmonary venous congestion →↑ pulmonary capillary pressure → pulmonary edema. These changes leads to progressive exertional dyspnea, PND, orthopnea, acute dyspnea, cough and hemoptysis.
- Right heart failure →↑ right atrial pressure → systemic venous congestion→↑ JVP →↑ visceral congestion → congestive hepatomegaly and pedal edema.
- Edema in heart failure—right heart failure →↑ capillary hydrostatic pressure RAAS activation → Na-H_2O retention
- Sympathetic activation → RAAS activation → Na-H_2O retention.

Etiology and Types of Heart Failure

Acute and Chronic Heart Failure

- Acute heart failure
  - Acute MI
  - Aortic valvular disease
  - Acute AR
  - Mitral valvular disease
  - Myocarditis
- Chronic heart failure
  - Slowly pregressive cardiac failure in valvular heart disease,
  - Cardiomyopathy
  - CAD

Systolic and Diastolic Heart Failure

- Systolic heart failure
  - Dilated ventricle with failure of systolic function
  - Low output and symptoms of hypo perfusion as in dilated cardiomyopathy
  - Presence of S_3 - systolic failure
- Diastolic heart failure
  - Compliance failure of the ventricle which is concentrically hypertrophied and features related to the elevation of filling pressure as seen in HOCM,
  - Hypertensive heart disease
  - AS
  - Acute MI
  - Presence of S_4 → diastolic failure

High Output and Low Output Failure

- High output failure
- Causes: Anemia, hyperthyroidism, c/c AR
- There is hemodynamic burden placed on the heart to pump abnormally large quantities of blood to meet the demand of the tissues.
- Low output failure
  - Causes: Cardiomyopathy, IHD, AS, myocarditis
  - Heart fails to generate adequate output despite high filling pressure.

Forward and Backward Failure

- Forward failure
  - Inadequate pumping of blood into the arterial system resulting in Na and H_2O retention due to activation of RAAS
- Backward failure
  - Failure of the ventricle to fill adequately causing elevation of pressure in the atria and venous system → → capillary hydrostatic pressure→ edema.

Left sided and Right Sided Heart Failure

- Left sided heart failure
  - Present with pulmonary edema
  - Manifesting as orthopnea, basal crepitation and S_3 gallop rhythm
  - Causes → Aortic valvular disease, Mitral valvular disease, hypertensive heart disease, and IHD
- Right sided heart failure
  - Present with → JVP, Congestive hepatomegaly and peripheral edema
  - Causes → Left heart failure → Right heart failure, PPH, PS, Tricuspid valvular disease, RVMI and RV EMF

Biventricular Failure

- Feature of both right and left heart failure
- Causes
  - Persistent left heart failure will lead to right heart failure
  - Dilated cardiomyopathy
  - Myocarditis
  - Biventricular EMF

Etiology of Heart Failure

- CAD, hypertensive heart disease
- Rheumatic heart disease, congenital heart disease
- Cardiomyopathy, myocarditis
- Primary pulmonary disease → cor pulmonale
- Extra cardiac high output state—anemia, thryrotoxicosis, etc.
- Fluid over-load states—AGN, acute on chronic renal failure.

Clinical Features

Symptoms

- Exertional dyspnea. PND, orthopnea
- Cough, hemoptysis, fatigue
- Anorexia and abdominal discomfort

Signs

- Orthopnea, pedal edema
- sinus tachycardia, pulsus alternans
- ↑JVP, Cardiomegaly ±
- S_3 gallop, basal crepitation
- Tender hepatomegaly
- Signs of LVF—orthopnea, basal crepitation, and S_3 gallop
- Signs of RVF—↑ JVP, tender hepatomegaly, pedal edema.

Precipitating Causes for Cardiac Failure

- Anemia, RTI, pregnancy, tachyarrhythmias, IE
- Pulmonary embolism, thyrotoxicosis
- Rheumatic activity, etc.

Clinical difference of acute heart failure and acute exacerbation of bronchial asthma/COPD		
	Acute heart failure	Acute exacerbation of bronchial asthma/COPD
History	Harboring heart disease	Episodes of cough and wheeze
Dyspnea and distress	+++	+
Central cyanosis	Usually absent	Present – late phase
Polycythemia	Absent	Present
Cardiomegaly	Usually present	Absent (except in corpulmonale)
Significant murmurs	Present	Absent (except in cor pulmonale)
Lung signs	Basal crepitation > bronchospasm symptoms > signs	Bronchospasm > crepitation signs > symptoms
CXR	Cardiomegaly, chamber enlargement + signs of pulmonary venous hypertension	Cardiomegaly usually absent. Tubular heart, emphysema and prominent bronchovascular marking
ECG	Chamber hypertrophy, ischemic changes and arrhythmia	RVH, P – Pulmonale in cor pulmonale

Investigations

ECG:
- Finding depends on the primary heart disease, chamber hypertrophy, chamber enlargement and ischemic changes.

CXR:
- Cardiomegaly ±, chamber enlargement, evidence of pulmonary venous hypertension.
- Normal size heart with cardiac failure—acute MI and MS.

Echocardiography
- To assess systolic and diastolic function of the ventricle, ventricular size, regional wall motion abnormality of IHD, valve morphology, intracardiac shunt, global hypokinesia in dilated cardiomyopathy, etc.

- Catheterization and angiography: For hemodynamic assessment and confirming primary heart disease.
- *Imaging of ventricular function*: By radionuclide angiography and cardiac MRI.

Management

Treatment of heart failure may be divided into 3 components:
- Treatment of state of congestive heart failure
- Treatment of precipitating factors for heart failure
- Treatment of primary heart disease.

Treatment of State of CHF

- Pharmacological measures
    - Principles
        - Control of Na and fluid balance
        - Inotropic support
        - Vasodilatation
- Standard drugs
    - Triple drug therapy
    - Diuretics
    - Digoxin
    - ACE inhibitors/ARB
- *Other inotropic agents:*
    - Dopamine–dobutamine
    - Phosphodiesterase inhibitors–Milrinone
    - Ca channel sensitizers–Pimobendan
    - Newer drugs for heart failure
    - Endopeptidase inhibitors–Ecadotril
    - Anti TNF α–Entanercept
    - Endothelin I antagonist–Bosentan
- β-blockers-
    - Reverse cardiac remodeling, thus included along with triple drug therapy
    - Gradually escalating doses of β-blocker such as carvedilol or bisoprolol
- Anti-arrhythmic: Amiodarone
- Anti aldosterone
    - Spironolactone—to prevent aldosterone induced myocardial fibrosis and vasculopathy
- Non pharmacological measures: Ultra filtration,
    - Revascularization
    - Implantable cardioverter defibrillator–ICD
    - Circulatory assist devices
    - Cardiomyoplasty.

Refractory Heart Failure

When severe symptoms of heart failure persist despite therapy with diuretics, vasodilators and digoxin, improvement can, however, be frequently achieved after further evaluation and intensification of therapy.

Reevaluate the Patients for:

- **Cardiovascular factors**
    - Silent ischemia, arrhythmias
    - IE, silent valvular lesions
    - Pulmonary embolism and myocarditis
- **Extracardiac factors**
    - Anemia, infections
    - Thyrotoxicosis, alcoholism
    - Salt intake and drugs with salt retention
    - Electrolyte disturbance
    - Diseases of other systems
- **Therapeutic factors**
    - Poor drug compliance
    - Sub optimal dose of drugs

Measures of Therapy

- Correction of the above factors, if present
- Intensification of drug therapy
- Cardiac transplantation—final line of treatment.

CHAPTER 5

Examination of Respiratory System

FUNCTIONAL ANATOMY

Respiratory Airways

- Upper respiratory tract extends from external nares to the junction of the larynx with the trachea at the vocal cords. It includes the nasal cavity, the nasopharynx, posterior nasal spine (PNS), oropharynx and the larynx.
- Lower respiratory tract includes trachea, lobar bronchus, segmental bronchi to 23 generations of tracheobronchial tree ending in alveolar sacs.
- Right bronchus is in line with the trachea, thus aspirated material will go to the right lower lobe.
- Less than 1 mm size bronchiole is devoid of cartilage.
- Small airway size is less than 2 mm.
- 16th generation of tracheobronchial tree is terminal bronchiole. Above this is called the conducting zone known as the dead space, capacity of 150 mL.
- 17th generation onwards is called the respiratory zone having the capacity of 3L.
- The narrowest lobar bronchus is the left lower lobe bronchus and more susceptible for bronchiectatic changes because of easy obstruction.
- The lining epithelium
  - Pseudostratified ciliated columnar—trachea and major bronchi
  - Columnar epithelium—bronchioles
  - Cuboidal epithelium—respiratory bronchiole onwards
  - Alveolar sac lined by thin squamous cells called pneumocyte type I—for diffusion of air. Type II pneumocyte lining the alveoli is granular, secretes the surfactant. These cells are cuboidal and divide to form the pneumocyte type 1.
- Alveoli communicate with each other with Pores of Kohn's for equalization of pressure.
- Non-communicating alveoli are responsible for the spontaneous pneumothorax in healthy people, due to rupture, because of the rapid rise of intrapulmonary pressure in maneuvers like isometric exercise.
- The membrane for diffusion of air consists of alveolar wall and capillary wall with a thickness of 0.5 microns.

Bronchopulmonary Segments (Table 5.1)

Table 5.1: Bronchopulmonary segments.			
Right main bronchus and segments		Left main bronchus and segments	
Upper lobe	Apical Posterior Anterior	Upper lobe	Apical Posterior Anterior
Middle lobe	Medial Lateral	Lingula	Superior Inferior
Lower lobe	Apical Medial basal Anterior basal Lateral basal Posterior basal	Lower lobe	Apical Medial basal Anterior basal Lateral basal Posterior basal

Lobe of Azygos Vein

Sometimes the medial part of the upper lobe is partially separated by a fissure of variable depth containing the terminal part of the azygos vein enclosed in the free margin of a mesentery derived from the mediastinal pleura forming the lobe of azygos vein—It can be a site for bronchiectasis.

Sequestration of Lung

Isolation of a part of lung from the rest during development having separate blood supply and bronchus. There are two types—Intrapulmonary and Extrapulmonary—site for bronchiectasis.

Surface Marking of the Lobes

Oblique fissure: Starts from 2nd thoracic spine, courses obliquely downwards and anteriorly to the 6th rib in mammary line crossing the mid-axillary line in the 5th intercostal space, below this fissure is lower lobe.

Horizontal fissure: Starts from 4th right sternocostal junction, tracing back to oblique fissure in mid-axillary line.

PLEURA

It has two layers:

Parietal pleura: Supplied by somatic sensory from intercostal nerves and phrenic nerve—pain sensitive.

Visceral pleura: Supplied by autonomic nervous system—pain insensitive.

Mediastinal and central parietal pleura are supplied by phrenic nerve, thus pain from these areas radiate to neck and shoulder.

Mediastinal pleura is thinner on the left side, thus mediastinal and esophageal diseases will produce left pleural involvement. The normal amount of pleural fluid is 5–10 mL in each pleural cavity.

Pleural Fluid Dynamics (Table 5.2)

Table 5.2: Pleural fluid dynamics.

Parietal pleura capillary	Pleural space	Visceral pleura capillary
← OP 34 cm	Negative pressure 8 cm	OP 34 cm →
	+	
→ HP 30 cm	OP 5 cm	HP 11 cm ←
← 4 cm	→ 13 cm ←	23 cm →
	→ 9 cm →	10 cm →

Fluid from parietal pleura capillary → pleural space → visceral pleura capillary [OP—osmotic pressure, HP—hydrostatic pressure]

Protective Mechanisms of Respiratory System

- Reflexes—sneezing and cough
- Mucociliary system
- Surfactant and other proteins
- Alveolar macrophage—phagocytosis
- Lymphatic system

Clearance of Deposited Particles

- Impaction—nasopharynx—size >5 microns—particles swallowed
- Sedimentation—small airways—size 1–5 microns—mucociliary system transport particles
- Diffusion—alveoli—size <0.1 micron—alveolar macrophage and lymphatics.

Relation of ribs to the lobes of the lung
First 4 ribs—upper lobe—pump handle movement
   5th and 6th rib—middle lobe right. Lingual lobe left—more lateral movement
   7th–10th ribs—lower lobe—mainly lateral movement (bucket handle movement).

SYMPTOMATOLOGY

- Cough
- Sputum
- Hemoptysis
- Dyspnea
- Wheeze
- Chest pain
- Hoarseness of voice
- Stridor
- Fever and sweating

Cough

Definition: Cough is a sudden expiratory thrust with phonation and momentary loss of rhythm of respiration. It is also the most important protective reflex of the respiratory system.

Reflex arc

Afferent: Receptors in the pharynx, larynx, trachea, bronchi, in the distribution of 5th, 9th, sup. laryngeal and 10th nerve.

Center: Cough center, Medulla.

Efferent: Recurrent laryngeal nerve, intercostal nerves and phrenic nerve.

Phases of Cough

Inspiratory phase: Deep inspiration preceding cough.

Compressive phase: Contraction of the muscles of respiration with closed glottis.

Expulsive phase: Glottis opened and rapid flow of air through upper airways.

Acute cough: More the 8 weeks, sub acute cough-3-8 weeks—acute upper respiratory tract infection (URTI), acute lower respiratory tract infection (LRTI), congestive cardiac failure (CCF).

Chronic cough: >3 weeks—chronic obstructive pulmonary diseases (COPD), lung malignancy, bronchial asthma, gastroesophageal reflux disease (GERD), suppurative lung disease and drug induced cough.

Types of Cough

Dry cough—nonproductive; early URTI and LRTI, interstitial lung disease and drug-induced—ACE inhibitor.

- Productive cough—URTI, LRTI, suppurative lung disease, COPD, PT.

- Brassy cough—cough with metallic sound produced by compression of trachea.
- Paroxysmal cough—prolonged bout of cough followed by long inspiratory whoop—whooping cough.
- Bovine cough—cough with absence of phonation—recurrent laryngeal. N. palsy.
- Postural cough—lung abscess, bronchiectasis and bronchopleural fistula.
- Nocturnal cough—paroxysmal nocturnal dyspnea (PND), tropical pulmonary eosinophilia and postnasal drip.
- Barking type of dry cough—acute laryngitis.

Sputum

Normal amount of tracheobronchial secretion is ≤100 mL/24 hours.

Normal sputum contains tracheobronchial secretion, cells and microorganisms. It is colorless, mucoid, loose and non-sticky. It is removed by the mucociliary action to the upper airway, then coughed out or swallowed.

Note the Following things with the Sputum

- Color
- Quantity
- Odor
- Consistency

Large quantity sputum—in bronchiectasis, lung abscess, bronchopleural fistula and alveolar cell carcinoma. In bronchiectasis, the sputum will form 3 layers on keeping in a container—serous, mucoid and purulent.

Foul-smelling sputum—lung abscess, bronchiectasis, and infection with anaerobic organisms.

Serous sputum—clear watery and frothy—bronchoalveolar cell Ca-Pink frothy sputum—Pulmonary edema.

Mucoid sputum—grayish white sputum—bronchial asthma, chronic bronchitis.

Purulent/mucopurulent sputum—yellowish or greenish sputum—bacterial infections of respiratory tract.

Rusty sputum—purulent sputum tinched with blood → rust color—lobar pneumonia.

Sticky and tenacious sputum—jelly-like sputum—acute asthma, COPD.

Hemoptysis

Expectoration of blood is called hemoptysis and is a sinister symptom of lung disease.

Types

- Depending on severity—
  - Rusty sputum—tinge of blood in sputum
  - Blood streaked with sputum—from upper respiratory tract
  - Blood mixed with sputum—from lower respiratory tract
  - Frank hemoptysis—expectoration of blood alone
  - Severe hemoptysis >200 mL/24 hours
  - Massive hemoptysis >500 mL/24 hours or 250 mL in single bout
  - Spurious hemoptysis—blood from nasopharynx
- Common causes of hemoptysis:
  - Acute respiratory tract infection—URTI and LRTI
  - Pulmonary tuberculosis
  - Bronchogenic carcinoma
  - Suppurative lung disease
  - Mitral valvular disease

Causes Depending on the Anatomical Site for Hemoptysis

- **Upper airway source**—Infection, bleeding diathesis
- **Tracheobronchial source**—Bronchitis, bronchiectasis, bronchogenic Ca, adenoma, endobronchial TB and foreign body
- **Parenchymal source**—Pneumonia, lung abscess, tuberculosis, aspergilloma, Good Pasteur's syndrome, Wegener's granulomatosis, idiopathic pulmonary hemosiderosis, lung flukes—endemic hemoptysis [Paragonimus westermani], hydatid disease.
- **Pulmonary vascular source**
  - Increased pulmonary venous pressure—Mitral stenosis and acute left ventricular failure (LVF)
  - Pulmonary arterial hypertension and thrombosis
  - Pulmonary infarction
  - Pulmonary arteriovenous malformation (AVM)
- **Miscellaneous**
  - Trauma, bleeding diathesis, anticoagulant therapy, pulmonary endometriosis
  - Iatrogenic—bronchoscopy, biopsy, etc.

Dyspnea

Dyspnea in respiratory disease can be due to—

- Ventilatory defect—COPD
- Diffusion defect—parenchymal disease—interstitial lung disease (ILD)
- Perfusion defect—pulmonary vascular disease—pulmonary embolism

Anatomical defect → dyspnea

- Tracheobronchial diseases
- Lung parenchymal diseases
- Pleural diseases
- Thoracic wall deformity

Clinical types of dyspnea in respiratory disease—

- Acute dyspnea—acute asthma and acute exacerbation of COPD, tension pneumothorax
  - Massive pulmonary embolism
  - Upper respiratory obstruction—edema and foreign body (FB)

- Exertional dyspnea—COPD, interstitial lung disease
  - Chest wall deformity, etc.
- Orthopnea—acute asthma and acute exacerbation of COPD
  - Bilateral diaphragmatic paralysis
- Nocturnal dyspnea—nocturnal asthma.

Two pulmonary diseases with exertional dyspnea without clinical signs are early interstitial lung disease and multiple pulmonary infarction.

Common respiratory causes for dyspnea:
- COPD, bronchial asthma
- Interstitial lung disease
- Diffuse pulmonary TB
- Pneumoconiosis
- Chest wall deformity—Gross kyphoscoliosis

Wheeze

It is a musical sound produced by the passage of air through narrow bronchi as in COPD, bronchial asthma and acute RTI in children.

Chest Pain

Three types of chest pain in respiratory disease:
- Upper retrosternal pain—in tracheitis
- Retrosternal pain—in mediastinal disease—mediastinitis, mediastinal emphysema—oppressive character resembling cardiac pain, radiate to neck and arms, unrelated to exertion
- Pleuritic pain—most important cause, localized catchy type of pain more at the end of inspiration, increased by respiratory movement and cough, less with shallow breathing. Patient prefers to lie on the affected side to reduce the chest wall movement.

Causes of pleuritic pain
- Pleurisy
- Pneumothorax—stretch on pleura
- Pulmonary infarction
- Infiltration of pleura by malignancy
- Traumatic

Hoarseness of Voice

Indicates laryngeal disease—varies from slight hoarseness to aphonia.

Causes
- Infection—acute laryngitis, diphtheria, TB
- Abuse of voice
- Edema—angioedema
- Neurological—recurrent laryngeal nerve palsy due to intrathoracic malignancy, mitral valvular disease, aortic aneurysm, L → R shunt.

Stridor

Laryngeal stridor: High pitched crowing sound with each inspiration

Causes

Foreign body, laryngeal spasm
- Edema, infection, tumor
- Bilateral vocal cord paralysis

Tracheal stridor: Croaking inspiratory sound or continuous sound increased by coughing, associated with inspiratory dyspnea and indrawing of the suprasternal notch.

Causes: Obstruction of the tracheal lumen by tumor or foreign body.

Fever and Sweating

- RTI is one of the commonest causes for fever. Lobar pneumonia produces continuous type of fever with rapid rise of temperature.
- Prolonged fever is seen with TB, lung malignancy.
- Pulmonary infarct.
- Increased night sweating—feature of pulmonary TB.

HISTORY TAKING IN RESPIRATORY DISEASES

Presenting Symptoms in Chronological Order

- Cough—wheezing
- Sputum—hoarseness
- Hemoptysis—stridor
- Dyspnea—fever

History of Presenting Complaints

- Detailing the symptoms (refer symptomatology)
- Enquire about presence of AIDS, epilepsy, cardiovascular and upper GI disease like GERD.

Past History

- Respiratory disease in the past
  - Nasobronchial allergy
  - Childhood TB, measles, whooping cough → bronchiectasis
- H/o loss of consciousness → aspiration, lung abscess in epilepsy, alcoholism and anesthesia, etc.
- H/o chest injury

Family History

- Bronchial asthma
- Pulmonary tuberculosis
- Emphysema—α 1 antitrypsin deficiency

Personal History

- Smoking—COPD, lung malignancy
- Alcoholism—aspiration and LRTI

Treatment History

Details of drugs for respiratory disease
- Antituberculous drugs, bronchodilators, corticosteroids
- Immunosuppressants—increased infection with bacterial, fungal and tuberculosis
- Drug pneumopathy—lung fibrosis—busulfan, bleomycin.

Occupational History

- Exposure to industrial dust—coal miner's, asbestos, silica dust—pneumoconiosis
- Persons in contact with pets—pigeon, parrots, etc.—extrinsic allergic alveolitis (Bird fancier's lung), psittacosis
- Exposure to allergen—pollen, cotton dust, feather, fungal spore—asthma.

GENERAL EXAMINATION IN RESPIRATORY SYSTEM

1. **Dyspnea at rest**—acute exacerbation of COPD, acute asthma, tension pneumothorax, inspiratory dyspnea in upper respiratory obstruction.
2. **Central cyanosis**—COPD, diffuse parenchymal disease of lung.
3. **Clubbing (Fig. 5.1)**
   - Bronchogenic carcinoma
   - Suppurative lung disease
   - Empyema
   - Interstitial lung disease
   - Pulmonary tuberculosis—post-TB bronchiectasis TB empyema and diffuse fibrosis of the lung
   - Hypertrophic osteoarthropathy—mostly seen in bronchogenic Ca.
4. **Lymph node enlargement:**
   - Scalene lymph node—in bronchogenic Ca, tuberculosis, sarcoidosis.
   - Other groups of cervical lymph nodes—in Tuberculosis, Hodgkin's lymphoma.
   - Generalized lymph node—in non-Hodgkin lymphoma (NHL), TB, AIDS.
   - Palpation of scalene lymph node—scalene lymph node lies in a pad of fat on the surface of scalenus anterior muscle. Careful palpation is required to feel the enlarged lymph node. Stand behind the patient who is seated, partially flex the neck to relax the cervical muscle, palpatory finger must dip behind the medial part of clavicle to feel the lymph node. Nodes more than 0.5 cm, firm to hard in consistency, are always pathological.
5. *Nicotine staining of the finger*—gives clue to the habit of smoking.
6. Pedal edema—in cor pulmonale.
7. Puffiness of face—in COPD, SVC obstruction in superior mediastinal lesions.
8. Anemia—in chronic infections like TB.
9. Polycythemia—secondary polycythemia in COPD, diffuse parenchymal disease of the lung—ILD.
10. Skin—erythema nodosum—primary TB, sarcoidosis, fungal disease-histoplasmosis
    - Lupus vulgaris
    - Tinea versicolor-increased sweating in PT
    - Metastatic nodule
    - Acanthosis nigricans—bronchogenic Ca.

EXAMINATION OF RESPIRATORY SYSTEM

Consists of:
a. Rate of respiration
b. Rhythm of respiration
c. Type of respiration
d. Examination of upper respiratory tract
e. Examination of chest
   - Inspection
   - Palpation
   - Percussion
   - Auscultation

Rate of Respiration

Normal—18/min (16–20/min)

Tachypnea >22/min

Causes
- Exercise, fever, pneumonia, anoxia
- Upper brainstem damage, salicylism
- Acidosis, psychogenic

Bradypnea

Reduction in rate of respiration of <10/min

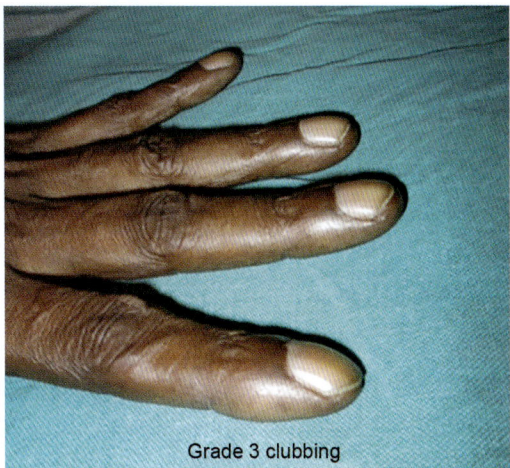

Grade 3 clubbing

Fig. 5.1: Clubbing.

Causes

Narcotic poisoning—phenobarbitone, morphine
- Hypothyroid coma
- Lower brainstem damage
- Hypothermia, alkalosis
- Increased intracranial pressure.

Rhythm of Respiration

Abnormal pattern of breathing:
- Cheyne-Stokes breathing—periods of apnea alternate with periods of hyperapnea—seen in LVF, upper brainstem damage, increased intracranial pressure
- Biot's/ataxic breathing—breathing which is irregular in time and depth—seen in brainstem damage and meningitis
- Apneustic breathing—postinspiratory pause in breathing—seen in pontine lesions
- Kussmaul's breathing—deep rapid breathing—seen in metabolic acidosis.

Type of Respiration

- Abdominothoracic—male
- Thoracoabdominal—female

Examination of Upper Respiratory Tract

- Nose (Fig. 5.2) and Sinuses—deviation of the nasal septum, sinus tenderness and nasal polyp
- Oral cavity—for evidence of gum and tooth infection
- Pharynx—nasopharynx and orophaynx - postnasal drip, infection and ulcers (in SLE and Wegener's granulomatosis)
- External ear—external acoustic meatus, drum and pinna—for infection
- Larynx—examination is done by indirect and direct laryngoscopy.

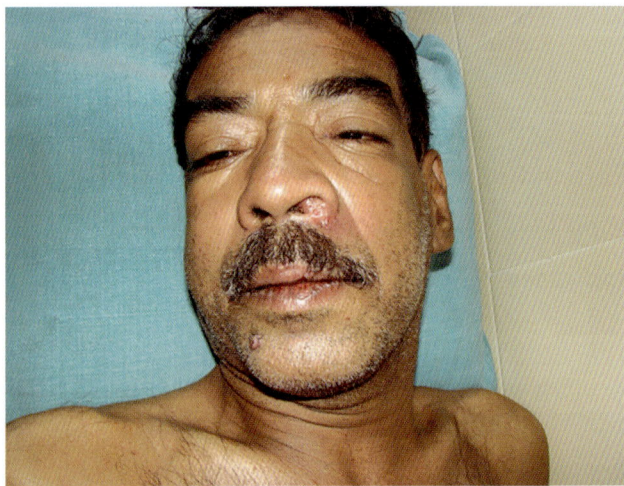

Fig. 5.2: Rhinosporidiosis of left nostril.

Importance of upper respiratory tract examination:
- Both upper respiratory and lower respiratory tract are affected in nasobronchial allergy
- URT I → LRTI/lung abscess
- Kartagener's syndrome—sinus aplasia and bronchiectasis
- Wegener's granulomatosis—ulcers of URT and lung parenchymal involvement.
- Laryngeal examination—to evaluate hoarseness of voice, stridor, inspiratory dyspnea as in laryngeal TB, laryngeal tumor, foreign body in larynx, laryngeal edema, vocal cord paralysis.

EXAMINATION OF CHEST

Inspection

Shape of Chest

- Normal—bilaterally symmetrical, truncated cone shaped, transverse diameter > anteroposterior diameter and vertical is the highest
- Normal ratio of transverse—anteroposterior is 7:5
- Abnormal shape -
  - Flat chest—ratio of transverse: anteroposterior is 2:1.
  - Barrel shape—in emphysema—ratio is 1:1
  - Pectus Carinatum—pegion chest—forward protrusion of the sternum and adjacent costal cartilage in childhood respiratory disease and rickets.
  - Pectus excavatum—funnel chest depression at lower end of sternum—developmental defect—displaces heart and reduces ventilation, it is seen in Marfan's syndrome.
  - Thoracic kyphoscoliosis—reduce ventilatory capacity of lung.
  - Harrison's sulcus—symmetrical horizontal groove along the costal margin seen in respiratory disease in childhood and rickets.
  - Rachitic and scorbutic rosary—beed like enlargement of costochondral junction in rickets and scurvy—scorbutic rosary is painful.
  - Tietze disease—congenital costochondral prominence.

Position of Trachea

Shift of trachea produces prominence of sternal head of sternocleidomastoid on the side to which the trachea is shifted. It is called Trail's sign.

Causes of tracheal shift—
  - Pleural disease—shift to opposite side
    - Pleural effusion
    - Pneumothorax
  - Pulmonary disease—shift to same side—
    - Fibrosis and Collapse of lung
  - Goiter—Shift of trachea to opposite side

Position of the Shoulder

Drooping of the shoulder
- Look for the following
    - Lower end of scapula is at a lower level
    - Spine—scapular distance is reduced
    - Medial border of scapula is more prominent on the affected side
- Causes of Drooping
    - Fibrosis
    - Collapse of the lung
    - Trapezius paralysis

Supraclavicular and Infraclavicular Fossa

Hollowing—in fibrosis and collapse of the lung and malnutrition.

Unilateral Flattening of the Chest

Fibrosis and collapse of lung.

Apical Impulse

Displacement—seen in push and pull of the pleuropulmonary disease.

Movement of the Chest

Movement of the chest wall should be noted. Look carefully for asymmetry of chest wall movement anteriorly and posteriorly. Assessment of the expansion of the upper lobes is better achieved by inspection form behind the patient, looking down at the clavicles during moderate respiration.
- Equal on both sides—normal
- Reduced movement on one side—pleural disease pulmonary disease
- Bilaterally reduced movement—in emphysema.

Skin Over the Chest

- Scar—intercostals drainage of empyema and pneumothorax
- Engorged veins—in SVC (superior vena cava) (Fig. 5.3) and IVC (inferior vena cava) obstruction
- Sinuses—TB and systemic fungal infection
- Metastatic nodule
- Swelling due to empyema necessitans.

Palpation

To Confirm Inspection Finding

- *Position of the trachea:* Position of the trachea is most important in deciding the upper mediastinal shift. From in front of the patient, the forefinger of the right hand of the examiner is pushed up and backwards until the trachea is felt. If the trachea is displaced to one side, its edge, rather than its middle will be felt and a larger space will be present, on the side opposite to the side of shift. Slight flexion of the neck will allow a better feel of the trachea (Fig. 5.4 and 5.5).

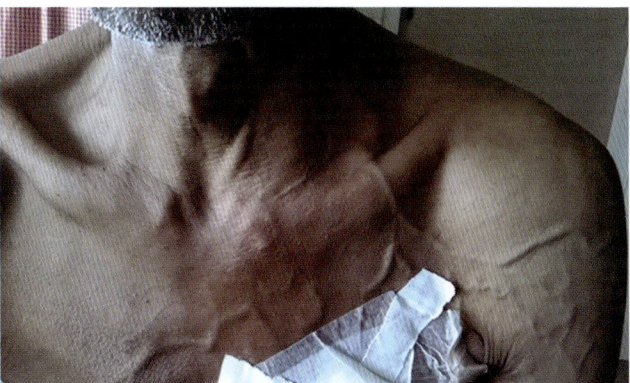

Fig. 5.3: Engorged veins over the chest in a patient with SVC obstruction.

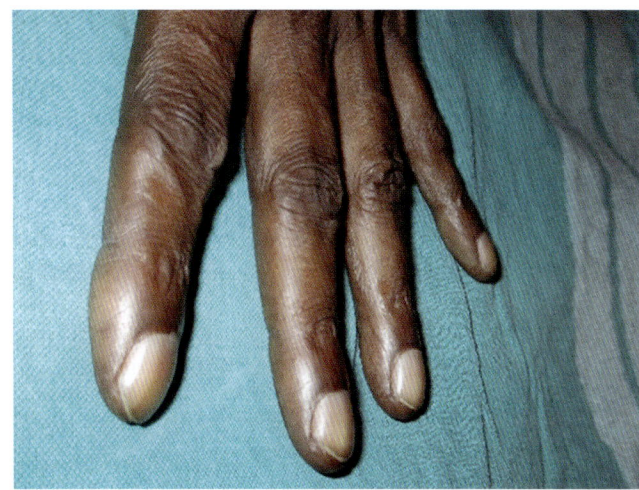

Fig. 5.4: Nicotine staining of the finger.

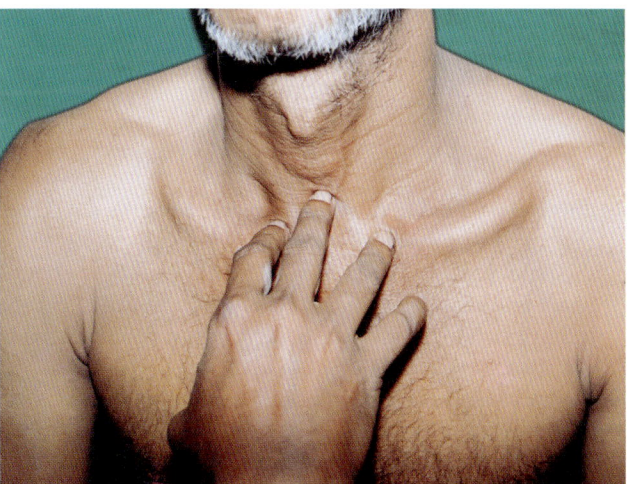

Fig. 5.5: Palpating the position of the trachea.

A slight deviation of the trachea to the right may be found in healthy people. Shift of the trachea means upper mediastinal shift, due to the push and pull of pleuropulmonary disease.
- *Position of the apex*: Lateral and medial shift of the apex will indicate lower mediastinal shift. Palpate for the cardiac impulse over the right hemithorax in the sitting and leaning forward position will also give clue to the lower mediastinal shift to the right side.

  Respiratory diseases for the shift of the apex
  - Pleural disease—pleural effusion and pneumothorax → shift of the lower mediastinum to the opposite side
  - Pulmonary disease—fibrosis and collapse of the lung → shift of the lower mediastinum to the same side
  - Impalpable apex—emphysema, left sided pneumothorax and pleural effusion.
- *Movement of the chest*: Place the hands firmly on the chest wall with the fingers extending around the sides of the chest. The thumbs should almost meet in the midline and should be lifted slightly off the chest so that they are free to move with respiration. As the patient takes a big breath in, the thumbs should move symmetrically apart at least 5 cm. Movement is assessed by noting the excursion of the thumbs from the midline and the feel over the palms. Movement should be assessed anteriorly and posteriorly, both upper and lower parts. Reduced expansion on one side indicates a lesion on that side (Figs 5.6 to 5.9).

  Lower lobe expansion is assessed from the back, upper and middle lobe expansion from the front of the chest.

  Causes of diminished movement
  Bilateral diminished movement
  - Emphysema
  - Ankylosing spondylitis
  - Interstitial lung disease

  Unilateral diminished movement
  - Pneumothorax
  - Pleural effusion
  - Consolidation
  - Fibrosis
  - Collapse of the lung.

Vocal Fremitus

- This is the palpable vibration transmitted to the chest wall through the air passages from the larynx, on speaking. Place the palm or the ulnar border of the hand on the patient's chest and make the patient to say 1, 2, 3 or 99. Feel the intensity of the vocal fremitus on corresponding areas of the chest.

  Vocal fremitus is decreased in pleural effusion, pneumothorax and emphysema.

  Vocal fremitus is increased in consolidation and collapse of the lung, which is in direct contact with bronchus or trachea.

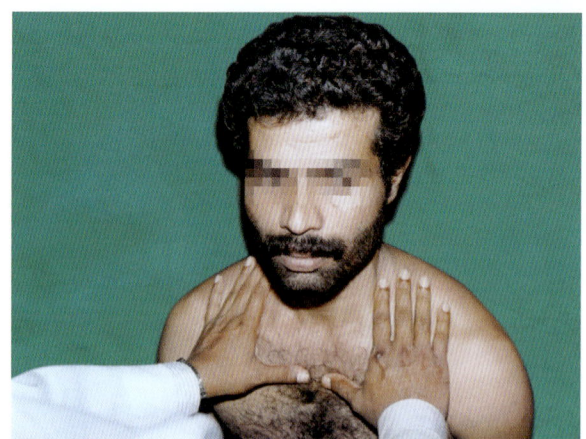

Fig. 5.6: Palpating the respiratory movement of upper anterior chest.

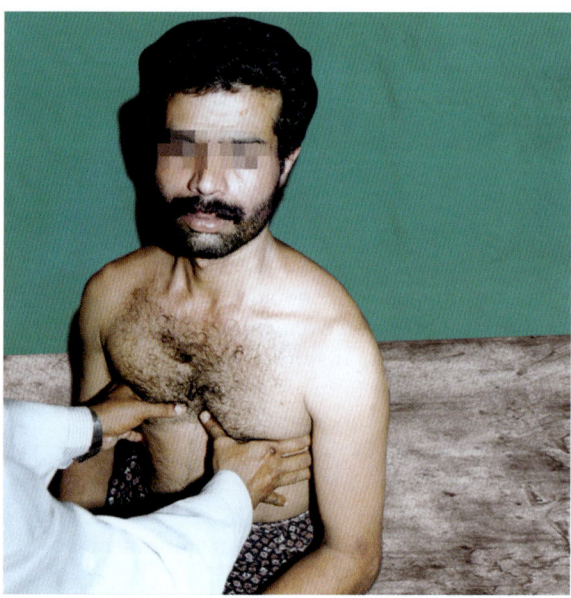

Fig. 5.7: Palpating the respiratory movement of lower anterior chest.

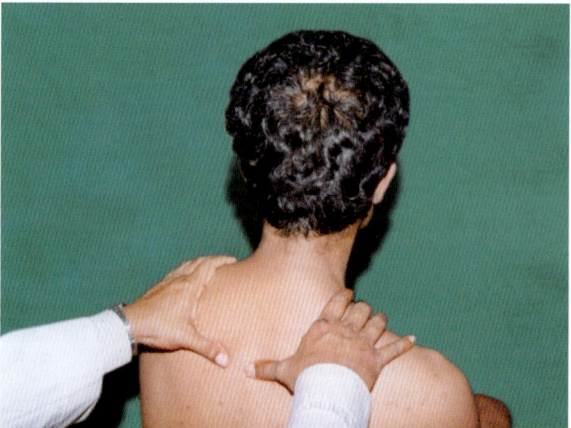

Fig. 5.8: Palpating the respiratory movement of upper posterior chest.

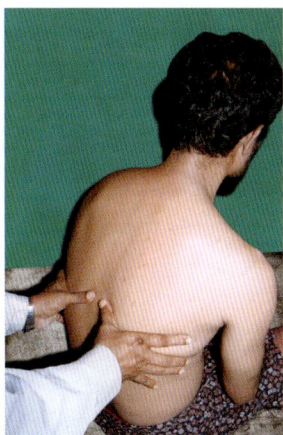

Fig. 5.9: Palpating the respiratory movement of lower posterior chest.

Measurement of Chest Expansion

This is done by using a measuring tape. In males the measurement is done at the level of nipple and in females, below the breast.

Measurement is noted both during inspiration and expiration.

Normal expansion is 5–8 cm, < 2 cm is always pathological, < 1 cm—seen in emphysema, and ankylosing spondylitis.

Hemithorax size is also measured from the vertebral spine to the midsternal line. Reduced hemithorax size is a feature of fibrosis or collapse of the lung.

Palpation of the Chest Wall

- Following things can be noted by palpating the chest wall
  - Rhonchial fremitus—palpable rhonchi
  - Palpable pleural rub
  - Tenderness of the chest wall in
    - Empyema
    - Tumor infiltration
    - Osteomyelitis and fracture of rib
    - Costochondritis—Tietze syndrome
  - S/c nodules—metastatic nodule, sarcoid
  - Nodule and neurofibroma
  - Subcutaneous emphysema
    - Spongy crepitant feel on palpation.
    - It is present in injury to chest wall, pneumothorax, rupture of esophagus
  - Local rise of temperature in s/c abscess and osteomyelitis of rib.

Percussion

Position of the Patient (Figs 5.10A to D)

- The best position of the patient for percussion is sitting posture. Supine position is desirable for tidal percussion.

- Anterior percussion: Patient sits erect with the hands by his side.
- Posterior percussion: The patient bends his head forward and keeps his hands over the opposite shoulders. This position keeps the scapula further away so that more space is available for percussion.
- Lateral percussion: The patient sits with his hands held over the head.

Purpose of Percussion

- To note the degree and dulling of resonance.
- To map out the area of abnormal percussion note.

Rules of Percussion

- The pleximeter—the middle finger of examiner's left hand should be kept tightly over the intercostal space of the chest wall without any air space in between.
- The plexor—middle finger of the examiner's right hand is used to hit the middle phalanx of the pleximeter.
- The movement of the right hand should be sudden, originating from the wrist.
- The line of percussion should be perpendicular to the border to be percussed.
- The pleximeter should be kept parallel to the border to be percussed.
- Percuss from the area of normal resonance to the area of abnormal resonance.

Areas of Percussion (Table 5.3)

- Direct percussion—over bone [clavicle]
- Indirect percussion—over other areas
- *Anterior chest wall: Supraclavicular area—Kronig's isthmus*
  - Over the clavicle
  - Infraclavicular area
  - Mammary area
  - Inframammary area
- *Kronig's isthmus:* It is a band of resonance of 5–7 cm size connecting the anterior and posterior resonance separated by nuchal and shoulder muscles.
  - In apical tuberculosis and malignancy, this area will become dull.
- *Lateral chest wall: Axillary area*
  - Infra-axillary area
- *Posterior chest wall:*
  - Suprascapular area
  - Interscapular area
  - Infrascapular area
- *Observe the following while percussing:*
  - Compare the percussion note on corresponding areas on both sides.
  - Percuss out the cardiac dullness (refer CVS examination).
  - Hepatic dullness is percussed on the right side by tidal percussion.

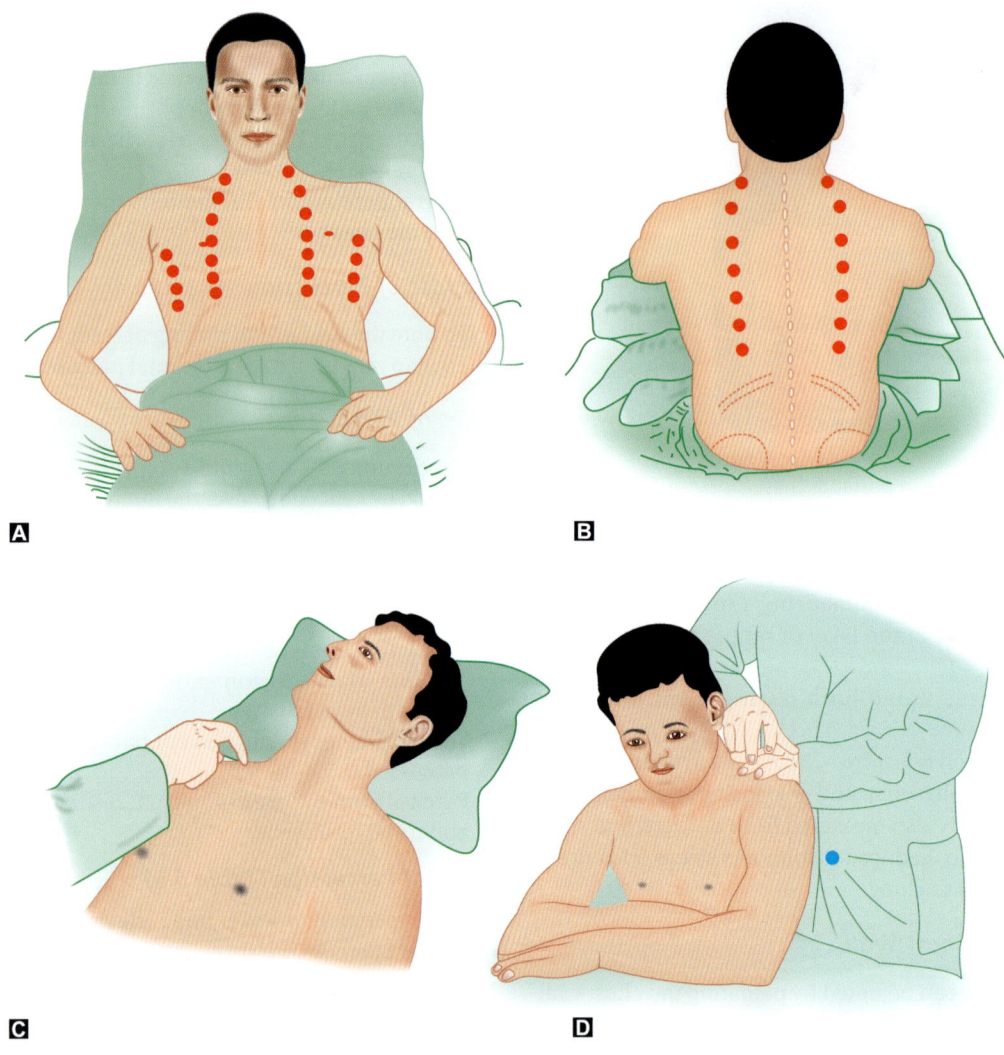

Figs. 5.10A to D: Sites for percussion. (A) Anterior and lateral chest wall; (B) Posterior chest wall; (C) Direct percussion on clavicle; (D) Percussion of apex of lung.

\multicolumn{3}{c}{Table 5.3: Anatomical areas for examination.}
Areas	Surface marking	Lobe

Anterior aspect
  Supraclavicular areas
  Infraclavicular area
  Mammary area
  Inframammary area
	• Above the clavicle
	• Clavicle to 3rd rib
	• 3rd–6th rib
	• 6th rib to costal margin
		• Apical segment—upper lobe
		• Anterior part of upper lobe
		• Anterior part of middle lobe right and lingular lobe left
		• Part of middle lobe—right
		  Lingular lobe—left and lower lobe on both sides

Lateral aspect
  Axillary area
  Infra-axillary area
	• Up to 6th rib
	• 6th rib to costal margin
		Lateral aspect of upper lobe
		Lateral aspect of middle lobe right
		Lingular left—above
		Lateral aspect of lower lobes on both sides—below

Posterior aspect
  Suprascapular area
  Interscapular area
  Infrascapular area
	• Above the upper border of the scapula
	• Between the medial border of the scapula and vertebral spine—D_2–D_7
	• Below the angle of the scapula—D7 to 11th rib
		• Apical segment of upper lobe
		• Apical segment of the lower lobe—posterior aspect
		• Basal segment of the lower lobe—posterior aspect

Tidal Percussion

On deep inspiration, the previous dull note in the 5th right Intercostal space in the midclavicular line becomes resonant. It indicates that the dullness is due to liver which is pushed down by the right hemidiaphragm on deep inspiration. If the dullness persists on deep inspiration, suspect underlying pleuropulmonary disease, diaphragmatic paralysis and subphrenic abscess.

Types of Percussion Notes

- Resonance—normal lung field
- Hyper resonance—pneumothorax and emphysema
- Impaired percussion note—fibrosis, congestive phase of consolidation, infiltrative lesions of the lung
- Dullness—consolidation, collapse, mass lesion, thickened pleura
- Stony dullness—pleural effusion
- Tympanitic resonance—over hollow viscus—Traube's space.

Traube's Space

It is a semi lunar area in the left inframammary region bounded by base of the lung above, costal margin below, spleen on left side and left lobe of the liver on the right side. The content is the fundus of the stomach. Percussion note over this area is tympanitic.

Obliteration of Traube's space: Left sided pleural effusion
- Massive pericardial effusion
- Massive splenomegaly
- Enlarged left lobe of the liver
- Growth—fundus of the stomach.

Upward shift of the Traube's space:
- Left diaphragmatic paralysis
- Left lower lobe fibrosis
- Left lower lobe collapse.

Other Features of Percussion of Clinical Importance

1. **'S' shaped curve of Ellis:** In pleural effusion, the highest level of dullness is in the axilla. In the anterior and posterior, the dullness is at a lower level and tends to assume the shape of the letter 'S'.
   Mechanism: In pleural effusion, there is passive collapse of the lung towards the hilum. The retraction of the lung, due to fluid collection, is more laterally than anteriorly and posteriorly. Thus, thick column of the fluid is present on the lateral aspect with a high level of dullness.
2. **Horizontal level of dullness:** In hydropneumothorax—horizontal level of dullness is percussed out in the sitting position anteriorly, laterally and posteriorly.
3. **Shifting dullness:** The patient in sitting position. Percuss anteriorly and note the upper level of the dullness. Then keep the patient in supine position, proceed the percussion downwards. The dull area will become resonant. On percussing laterally from the resonant area, the shifted dullness can be demonstrated. This is a definite feature of hydropneumothorax.
4. **Crack pot resonance:** A type of tympanitic note, can be elicited over a large communicating cavity.

Auscultation

General Principles

- Using the diaphragm of stethoscope listen to the breath sounds, in identical areas anteriorly, posteriorly and axilla.
- Demonstrate the type of breathing required to the patient by the examiner.
- Patient should take deep and slightly faster breathing through the open mouth.
- Better to use bell for auscultation above the clavicle to the lung apices.
- Avoid auscultation within 2-3 cm from the midline in the upper part of posterior chest, since the breath sounds in these areas normally have a bronchial character.
- Auscultation over hairy areas may produce friction sounds.

Purpose of Auscultation

- To note the
  - Breath sounds—intensity and character
  - Vocal resonance—normal, reduced or increased
  - Adventitious sounds—crepitation, rhonchi, pleural rub, pleuropericardial rub
  - Other auscultatoy features of clinical importance
    - Whispering pectoriloquy
    - Post tussive crepitation
    - Post tussive suction
    - Succussion splash
    - Coin sound

Breath Sounds

Normal breath sound—vesicular breath sound.

Breath sounds heard throughout inspiration and early part of expiration with rustling quality and no pause between inspiration and expiration.

Breath sounds are produced throughout the respiratory passages and the range of frequency is between 200 and 2000 Hz. Breath sound at trachea is low pitched—400 Hz, as it reaches the distal part, it will become high pitched, 1700 Hz in the terminal bronchiole. This high pitched breath sound at alveolar duct is modified by the functioning alveoli into the vesicular breath sound and conducted to the chest wall (Fig. 5.11).

Abnormal breath sounds—Bronchial breathing

Characterized by breath sounds throughout inspiration and expiration, pause in between inspiration and expiration, aspirate in quality.

Quality is the most important identifying feature.

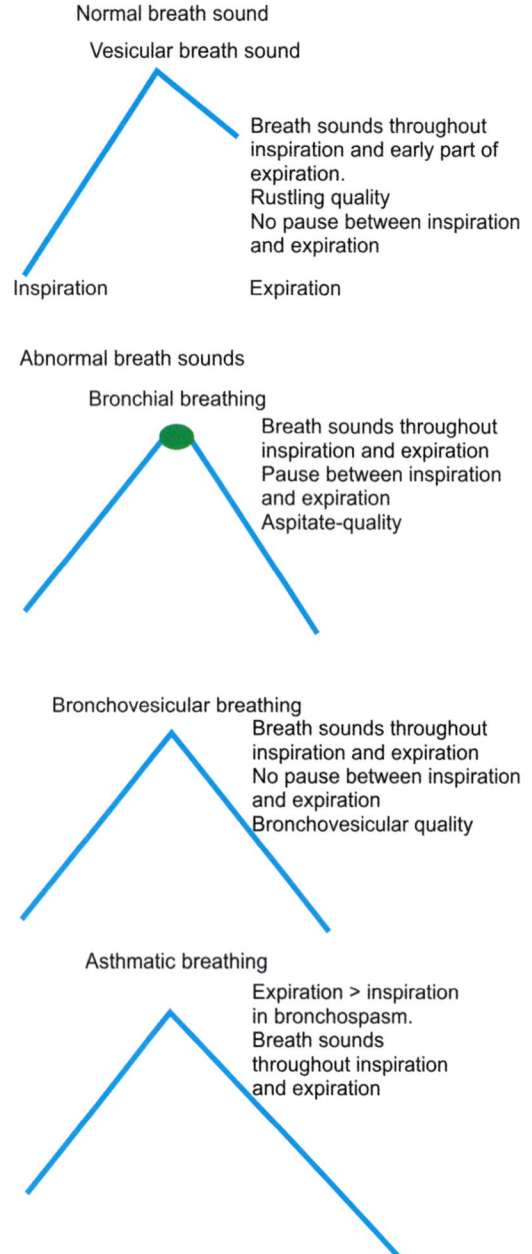

Fig. 5.11: Types of breath sounds.

Depends on the Pitch: Four Types of Bronchial Breathing (Fig. 5.12)

Tubular breathing: It is a high pitched bronchial breathing in consolidation.

Mechanism: High pitched sounds at alveolar duct is conducted to the chest wall without modification by the alveoli due to consolidation.

Cavernous breathing: It is a low pitched bronchial breathing in lung cavity.

Mechanism: High pitched sounds at alveolar duct will become low pitched in the cavity and conducted to the surface without modifications.

Amphoric breathing: It is basically a low pitched bronchial breathing with super added high pitched overtones producing metallic quality on auscultation.

Mechanism: The high pitched sounds at alveolar duct will become low pitched in the large communicating cavity. The reflected sounds from the wall of the cavity is high pitched producing the combination of low pitched sounds with high pitched over tones in amphoric breathing. This is present in large communicating cavity and bronchopleural fistula.

Medium pitched bronchial breathing: Usually heard over the area of fibrosis due to the proximity of the bronchus.

Bronchovesicular breath sound: It is characterized by breath sounds heard throughout inspiration and expiration without a pause in between. This type of breath sound is normally heard over the right infraclavicular and right interscapular region because of the proximity of the bronchus.

Breath sound characterized by prolonged expiration: As in COPD and bronchial asthma—due to bronchospasm.

Variation in Intensity of Breath sounds

- Bilateral reduction in intensity
  - Emphysema
- Unilateral reduction in intensity
  - Pleural effusion
  - Pneumothorax
  - Thickened pleura
  - Collapsed lung with complete bronchial obstruction.

Vocal Resonance

This gives information about the lung's ability to transmit vibrations of sounds. Normal lung filters high pitched components and transmit low pitched components of speech up to 200 Hz. Auscultate over the chest while the patient speaks the syllables like 1, 2, 3 or 99 and watch the intensity, character of the sounds over corresponding areas of the chest on both sides.

Vocal resonance—normal—means as if the syllables are produced at the chest wall.

Vocal resonance—increased—means as if the syllables are produced between the chest wall and ear piece-as in consolidation.

- Bronchophony—means the syllables are produced right into the ear—in consolidation and cavity.
- Aegophony—bronchophony with a nasal or bleating quality—in consolidation with mild pleural effusion and cavity.

Vocal resonance—reduced—means, the intensity of the VR is less when comparing to the identical area of the opposite side as in pleural effusion, pneumothorax, emphysema.

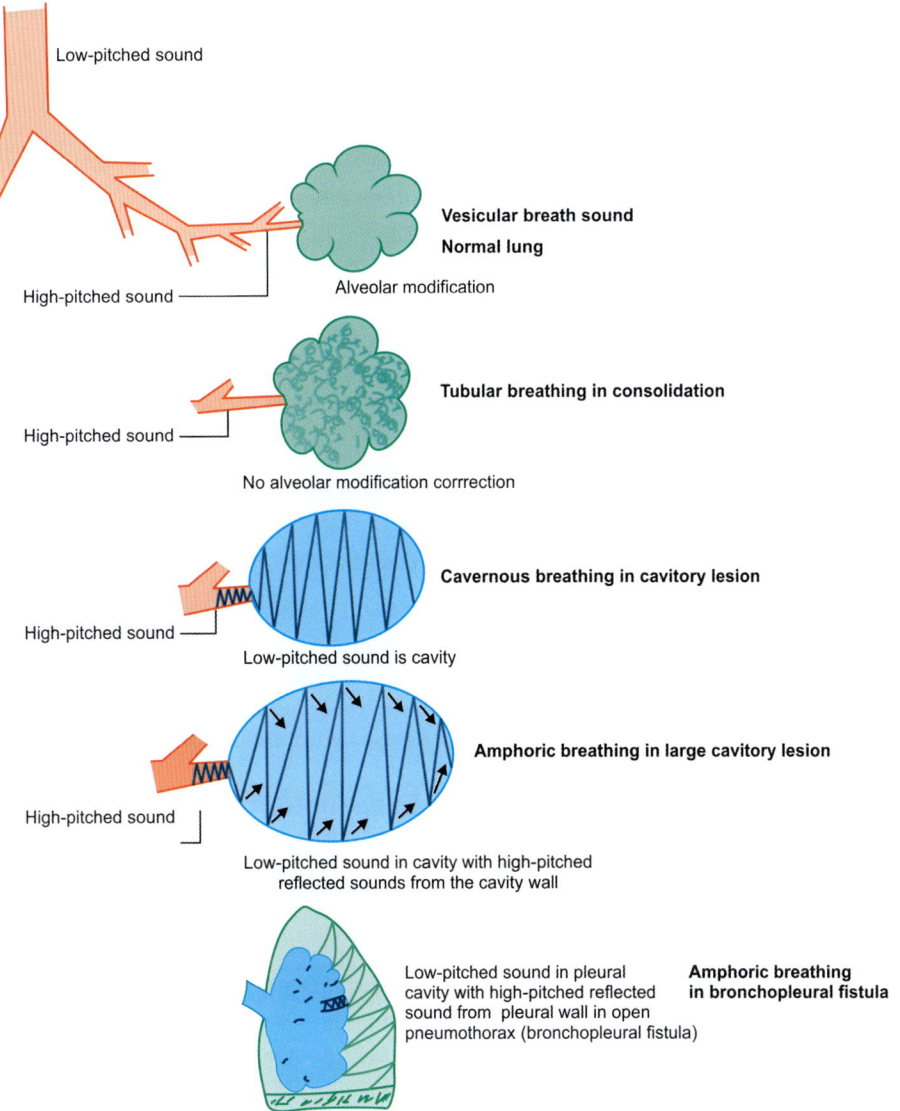

Fig. 5.12: Mechanism of bronchial breathing.

Adventitious Sounds

Crepitation (Crackles)

These are noncontinuous sounds with a crackling quality better heard during inspiration.

Mechanism: By the mixing of air and fluid in the respiratory passage.

By the separation of sticky alveolar or bronchiolar walls during inspiration.

Three types of crepitations:
1. Fine crepitations—in early stage of consolidation and fibrosing alveolitis
2. Medium crepitations—in pulmonary edema
3. Coarse crepitations—resolving pneumonia, bronchiectasis and lung abscess.

Crepitation depends on the timing of respiratory phase:
- Inspiratory
  - Early inspiratory—bronchitis—airway disease.
  - Late inspiratory—fibrosing alveolitis, early consolidation—parenchymal disease
  - Pan inspiratory—bronchiectasis and pulmonary edema.
- Expiratory and inspiratory
  - Bronchiectasis and pulmonary edema.

Coarse crackles/crepitation (death rattle) can occur as a terminal event in gross pulmonary edema.

Rhonchi

It is a dry continuous sound produced by the passage of air through narrow bronchus and heard better in expiration.

Depending on pitch: Two types
1. Low pitched (Sonorous)—arising from large airways.
2. High pitched (Sibilant)—arising from small airways.

Causes of Rhonchi
- Bronchial asthma
- COPD
- LVF (cardiac asthma)
- Tumor—fixed monomorphic rhonchi—localized
- Foreign body—fixed monomorphic rhonchi—localized
- Tropical pulmonary eosinophilia.

Pleural Rub

It is a superficial grating sound produced by the rubbing of inflamed parietal and visceral pleura. It is best heard with firm pressure of the chest piece at the end of inspiration and beginning of expiration. It is associated with pain, not altered by coughing.

Pleuropericardial Rub

It is due to the inflamed mediastinal pleura rubbing with pericardium or the inflamed pericardium rubbing with the mediastinal pleura. The grating sound is related to the cardiac cycle but increased by inspiration and disappears on holding the breath.

Table 5.4: Clinical difference between pleural rub and crepitation.	
Rub	Crepitation
Superficial and loud	Not superficial or loud
Continuous	Discontinuous
Localized	Widespread
Unaffected by cough	Affected by cough
Presence of pain	Absence of pain

Other Auscultatory Features of Clinical Importance

Whispering Pectoriloquy

Normally whispered syllables are indistinctly heard over the chest. Whispered sounds lack the low frequency component since the vocal cords do not oscillate. In pneumonic consolidation, the whispered syllables are distinctly heard over the chest while on auscultation since the high frequency component is well transmitted by the consolidated lung to the surface. This is called whispering pectoriloquy.

Post-tussive Suction

It is a pathognomonic sign of cavitary lesion. It is a sucking sound heard over the chest wall during inspiration following a bout of cough, over the area of thin walled superficial communicating cavity.

Post-tussive Crepitation

Crepitations appearing after a bout of cough, this is usually present in early infiltrative lesions of TB.

Succussion Splash

It is a tinkling sound produced by the mixing of air and fluid in hydropneumothorax while shaking the patient. First percuss out the air fluid level in hydropneumothorax, keep the chest piece over that area. Then shake the patient suddenly by holding the opposite shoulder of the patient. This is a pathognomonic sign of hydropneumotho- rax, also heard occasionally over a large cavity with fluid.

Coin Sound

It is the metallic quality of a coin sound produced on one side of the chest that can be appreciated on the diametrically opposite side of the chest wall by use of a stethoscope on that side. It is present in pneumothorax and the air filled portion of the hydropneumothorax.

Examination of Other Systems in Respiratory Disorders

Nervous System
- Horner's syndrome—bronchogenic Ca
- Hoarseness of voice—recurrent laryngeal nerve—Lt. > Rt., bronchogenic Ca
- Phrenic nerve palsy—diaphragmatic paralysis—intrathoracic neoplasm.
- Lower brachial plexus lesion—small muscle wasting—Pancoast's tumor
- Intercostal neuralgia—secondary deposit—spine
- Flapping tremor—altered sensorium and Papilledema—respiratory failure with hypercapnia
- Seizure—brain secondary
- Cerebellar degeneration—nonmetastatic manifestation-bronchogenic carcinoma
- Myasthenic syndrome—Eaten Lambert syndrome—nonmetastatic manifestation
- Peripheral neuropathy—nonmetastatic manifestation-bronchogenic carcinoma.

Eye
- Optic neuritis—ethambutol
- Phlycten—primary complex—tuberculosis
- Choroid tubercle—miliary tuberculosis
- Chemosis and edema—SVC obstruction
- Uveitis, iritis—ankylosing spondylitis, acute sarcoidosis
- Scleritis and scleromalacia—rheumatoid arthritis

CVS

- Pulmonary hypertension, RVH, right heart failure—cor pulmonale
- JVP ↑—cor pulmonale and SVC obstruction
- SVC obstruction—nonpulsatile engorged jugulars
- Dilated veins over the chest
- Pericardial disease—tuberculosis, bronchogenic Ca

GIT

- Halitosis—lung abscess
- Hepatomegaly—cor pulmonale, secondaries in liver, miliary TB, amyloidosis, lymphoma
- Splenomegaly—miliary TB, amyloidosis, lymphoma
- Ascites—right heart failure, TB
- Epididymo-orchitis—TB
- Inguinal hernia—chronic cough-COPD, etc.

Endocrine

- Gynecomastia—bronchogenic Ca, anti-TB drug—Pyrazinamide
- Cushing syndrome—ectopic ACTH—bronchogenic Ca—small cell
- Acromegaly—ectopic GH—bronchogenic Ca—small cell
- Pseudo hyperparathyroidism—ectopic parathormone—bronchogenic Ca
- Carcinoid syndrome—bronchial
- SIADH—small cell—bronchogenic Ca

Renal System

- Nephrotic syndrome—bilateral hydrothorax
- CRF—uremic lung

CLINICAL FEATURES OF COMMON RESPIRATORY DISEASES (TABLE 5.5)

Pneumonia

It is defined as the inflammation of the lung which is characterized by exudates into the alveoli. Associated with recent radiological shadow which is either segmental, lobar or multilobar.

Classification

- Primary—community acquired pneumonia (CAP)
- Secondary—defect in defense mechanism
  - Bronchopneumonia
  - Aspiration pneumonia
  - Hospital acquired pneumonia (HAP)
  - Pneumonia in immunocompromised patient (ICP)

Pathophysiology

- Microbes

Table 5.5: Signs in common respiratory diseases.

Pathology	Mediastinal shift	Movement of chest	Percussion note	Breath sounds	Vocal resonance	Added sounds
Consolidation	Midline	↓	Dull	Tubular	↑	Crepitation
Fibrosis	Same side	↓	Impaired	↓ or bronchial	Variable	Fine crepitation
Collapse—major bronchus obstruction	Same side	↓	Dull	↓	↓	Nil
Collapse – peripheral bronchus obstruction	Same side	↓	Dull	Tubular	↑	Crepitation ±
Cavity	Midline or Same side if fibrosis+	↓	Impaired	Cavernous	↑	Crepitation fine/coarse
Bronchiectasis	Midline	↓	Impaired	Vesicular/bronchial	Normal/↑	Coarse leathery crepitation
Emphysema	Midline	B/L ↓	Hyper resonant	B/L ↓	Normal/↓	Rhonchi
Bronchial asthma	Midline	Normal or B/L ↓	Resonant	Vesicular with prolonged expiration	Normal	Rhonchi—inspiratory and expiratory
Pleural effusion	Opposite side	↓	Stony dull	↓/absent	↓/absent	Nil
Pneumothorax	Opposite side	↓	Hyper-resonant	↓/absent or amphoric breathing	↓/absent	Nil

- CAP
  - Pneumococci – 30%
  - Legionella – 5%
  - Chlamydia – 10%
  - Mycoplasma – 9%
- HAP
  - Enteric anaerobic
  - Oral anaerobes
  - Pseudomonas
  - *Staphylococcus aureus*
- ICP
  - Pneumocystis carinii
  - Atypical mycobacteria
  - *H. influenza*
  - *S. pneumonia*

Uncommon Organism (Table 5.6)

- Klebsiella
- *Staphylococcus aureus*
- *H. influenzae*
- Virus
- Fungi

Source of infection:
- Aspiration, inhalation (< 5 microns)
- Hematogenous, direct spread—intubation
- Contiguous spread—from adjacent focus of infection.

Stages of Pneumonia

- Stage of congestion—24-48 hours
- Stage of red hepatization—2-4 days
- Stage of gray hepatization—4-8 days
- Stage of resolution—2-3 weeks

Clinical Features

Fever—rapid rise of temperature, cough with purulent or rusty sputum, tachypnea, pleuritic chest pain.

Signs:
- Febrile, tachypnea, tachycardia, herpes labialis
- Respiratory system—no mediastinal shift, dull note on percussion, tubular bronchial breathing, ↑ VF and VR, bronchophony, egophony, whispering pectoriloquy
- Auscultatory triad of consolidation—Tubular bronchial breathing bronchophony and whispering pectoriloquy.

Features depending on the organism
- Mycoplasma pneumonia—insidious onset, erythema nodosum, myocarditis, rash, meningoencephalitis and hemolytic anemia
- Legionella pneumonia—Myalgia, GI symptoms, hepatitis, hyponatremia, hypoalbuminemia
- Chlamydia—Sinusitis, laryngitis, pharyngitis, normal TLC, liver transaminases elevated
- Klebsiella pneumonia—marked systemic symptoms, upper lobe with multilobar involvement, purulent dark sputum
- *Staph. aureus*—multilobar, septicemia, abscess in other organs.

Time table for recovery
- Acute symptoms like tachypnea, high fever disappear within 4 days
- All symptoms usually disappear within 7 days
- Lung signs disappear within 2 weeks
- Radiological signs disappear within 3-4 weeks.

Bad prognostic signs
- Age > 60, respiratory rate > 30
- Hypotension, multilobar pneumonia
- Underlying lung disease
- Uremia, Diabetes mellitus
- Laboratory features—hypoxia, leukopenia < 4000, leukocytosis > 20,000, hypoalbuminemia
- Positive blood culture

Complications

- Local—lung abscess, empyema, pneumothorax
- General—hyperpyrexia, circulatory failure (fluid loss, septicemia, myocarditis)
- Septicemia and multiorgan failure
- Distant—myocarditis, pericarditis, acute infective endocarditis, meningitis, meningism, toxic hepatitis, arthritis.

Causes of Unresolved Pneumonia

- Systemic causes—extremes of age, immunocompromised patients, diabetes mellitus, internal malignancy
- Local causes—pneumonia on bronchiectasis, lung malignancy and obstruction of bronchus.

Investigations

- To establish diagnosis
- To find out the organism
- To find out defect of defense mechanism
- To look for complications
- CXR—homogenous opacity, lobar pattern with air bronchogram
- Sputum—gram stain and culture (good specimen of sputum > 25 polymorph and <10 epithelial cells/low power field)
- Blood culture—in septicemia
- Serology—antibody to mycoplasma, chlamydia, legionella
- Legionella antigen in urine
- Pneumococcal antigen in serum and sputum
- Cold agglutinin in mycoplasma
- PFT and ABG
- Pleural fluid study
- Invasive procedures—BAL, transtracheal aspiration
- Fiber optic bronchoscopy

Management

- General—control of fever, fluid balance, analgesics for pleuritic pain, etc.
- Specific treatment—appropriate antibiotics.

Table 5.6: Antibiotic therapy in pneumonia.	
Organism	Antibiotic
Pneumococci	Benzyl penicillin—10–20 million units/day or for 7–10 days 3rd/4th generation cephalosporin-Ceftriaxone—1gm IV BID or β lactam + β lactam inhibitor Amoxyclav
Staph. aureus	Vancomycin—1 g IV infusion BID or (15 mgm/kg) Linazolidine - 600 mg BID or Cefdinir—300 mg BID
Klebsiella Legionella	Gentamicin + ceftazidime/ciprofloxacin > 14 days Erythromycin/clarithromycin—2–3 weeks or Newer fluoroquinolones
Mycoplasma Chlamydia	Fluoroquinolones, levofloxacin, gatifloxacin Erythromycin/tetracycline

Treatment of complications: Like ventilatory support—respiratory failure other organ support in multiorgan failure.

Lung Abscess (Suppurative Pneumonia)

It is a cavity containing pus and necrotic debris.
- Primary—in normal lung due to aspiration.
- Secondary—complication of other diseases of lung like pneumonia, infarction, cyst.

Causes

- Pneumonias—*Klebsiella, Staphylococcus, H. influenzae*, anaerobic organisms
- Aspiration
- Obstruction
- Infection of pulmonary infarct
- Infected emboli
- Open negative syndrome
- Pulmonary cyst with infection
- Sub diaphragmatic abscess and liver abscess rupturing to lung

Predisposing Factors

Defect in defense mechanism
- Vocal cord paralysis
- Anesthesia
- Coma
- Cricopharyngeal achalasia
- Ineffective expectoration—postoperative
- Defective mucociliary action
- Upper respiratory infection—sinusitis

Clinical Features

- Fever, cough with foul smelling sputum
- Hemoptysis, halitosis, clubbing, pleuritic pain
- Chest examination—signs of consolidation/cavity
- Crepitation, pleural rub

Investigations

- CXR—thick walled cavity with fluid level
- Sputum—culture and sensitivity
- To find out the defect in defense mechanism

Management

- Appropriate antibiotic for 4–6 weeks
- Chest physiotherapy and postural drainage
- Surgery—failure of medical therapy, presence of obstructive lesion

Fibrosis of Lung

Anatomical Types

- Parenchymal
- Peribronchial
- Vascular
- Pleural

Etiology of Parenchymal Fibrosis

Tuberculosis, ankylosing spondylitis, collagen vascular disease (rheumatoid arthritis, progressive systemic sclerosis), drugs, radiation, pneumoconiosis.

Drugs → fibrosis—Busulfan, Bleomycin, Methotrexate, Amiodarone.

Upper lobe fibrosis: Tuberculosis, ankylosing spondylitis, silicosis, coal worker's pneumoconiosis, drugs, radiation.

Lower lobe fibrosis: Rheumatoid arthritis, systemic sclerosis, asbestosis, idiopathic fibrosing alveolitis (Hamman Rich syndrome).

Clinical Features

Symptoms of chronic respiratory illness, cough, sputum dyspnea and features of primary disease.

Signs

- Mediastinal shift to the affected side, chest wall abnormality, movement decreased, impaired percussion note, VF and VR variable, breath sound reduced or medium pitched bronchial breathing.
- Right lower lobe fibrosis—elevation of hepatic dullness, medial shift of apex, palpable cardiac impulse over right hemithorax.

- Left lower lobe fibrosis—elevation of tympanitic resonance above 5th LICS, lateral shift of the apex.

Differential Diagnosis

Collapse of the lung: Features of reduction in lung volume with absence of chest wall abnormality ± evidence of obstruction of bronchus like as mass lesion, lymph node enlargement, and superior mediastinal obstruction.

Investigation

- CXR—nonhomogeneous opacity—with reduction in lung volume, crowding of ribs (Fig. 5.13)
- PFT, ABG-for primary disease.

Management

- Principles—treatment of primary disease—functional support of lung—like ambulant oxygen therapy.
- Control of infection/relapse of TB, drugs for bronchospasm.

Cavitary Lesion

It is an air containing space within the lung parenchyma surrounded by a wall whose thickness is > 1 mm.

Causes

- Infectious—*TB, Staph.*, Pneumococci, *Klebsiella*, anaerobic organism, *Legionella, Pneumocystis carinii, Melioidosis,* Fungal—Histoplasmosis, Blastomycosis
- Noninfectious—Malignancy, Wegener's granulomatosis, infected cyst and bullae.

Clinical Features

- Depends on—size, depth of cavity and communicating or not

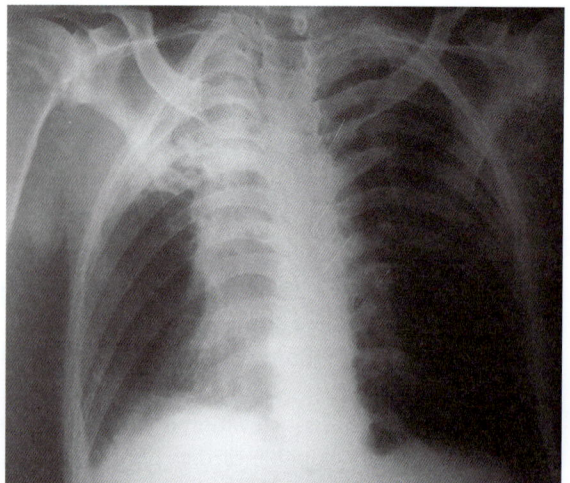

Fig. 5.13: X-ray showing right upper lobe fibrosis with mediastinal shift.

- Mediastinal shift if fibrosis present
- Cavernous breathing/amphoric breathing—large cavity
- Whispering pectoriloquy
- Post tussive suction—pathognomonic sign
- Crepitations
- Auscultatory triad of cavity—
  - Cavernous breathing
  - Post tussive suction
  - Whispering pectoriloquy

Healing of Tuberculous Cavity

- Closed cavity healing—fibrosis and occlusion at the bronchocavitary junction → absorption of air in the cavity → collapse and healing
- Concentric fibrosis of cavity—fibrosis occurring in the wall of cavity in layers in concentric manner → disappearance of cavity
- Open cavity healing—bronchial epithelium grows and lines the cavity, cavity is sterile for AFB due to anti TB drugs. This is called open negative syndrome which can lead on to
  - Aspergilloma
  - Secondary infection and abscess
  - Hemoptysis—rupture of loose vessel in cavity.

Cavity may also persist in spite of the recoil of the lung due to increased intracavitory pressure. Fibrous lesion at the bronchocavitary junction will act as a valve like mechanism → increase the intracavitory pressure.

Thick walled cavity—lung abscess, bronchogenic Ca, fungal cavity and WG.

Thin walled cavity—infected bullae and tuberculosis.

Collapse of Lung (Atelectasis)

It is the reduction in the size of lung parenchyma usually secondary to complete obstruction of airway.

Types of Collapse

- Active collapse—complete obstruction of airway
- Passive collapse—pleural effusion, pneumothorax
- Compressive collapse—mass lesion pressing the surrounding lung
- Cicatrical collapse—fibrosis and shrunken lung
- Adhesive collapse—surfactant deficiency and parenchymal collapse.

Clinical Features of Active Collapse of Lung

- Depends on—lung, lobe or the segment affected
- Features for evidence of obstruction like mass lesion, lymph node
- Features of SVC obstruction ±
- Neurological signs—Horner's syndrome, hoarseness of voice, diaphragmatic paralysis.

Investigations

- CXR—homogenous opacity with reduction in lung volume (Fig. 5.14) ± evidence of mass lesion/mediastinal lymph node-presence of pleural disease like pleural effusion, pneumothorax
- CT—chest—to identify the cause of the collapse lung like mass lesion, lymph nodes.

Management

- Measures to remove the obstruction—by bronchoscopy/surgery.

Causes of SVC Obstruction

- Bronchogenic Ca
- Lymphoma
- Thymoma
- Other mediastinal tumors
- Nonmalignant—mediastinal fibrosis in histoplasmosis
- Aortic aneurysm, postradiation
- SVC thrombosis due to prolonged CV line

Bronchiectasis

It is persistent irreversible dilatation of medium sized bronchi of more than 2 mm usually 5th-9th generation of bronchial tree.

Etiology

- Infectious—measles, whooping cough, childhood TB, HIV, adult PT
- Noninfectious—Immunodeficiency, neutrophil abnormality, obstructive lesions, allergic bronchopulmonary aspergillosis

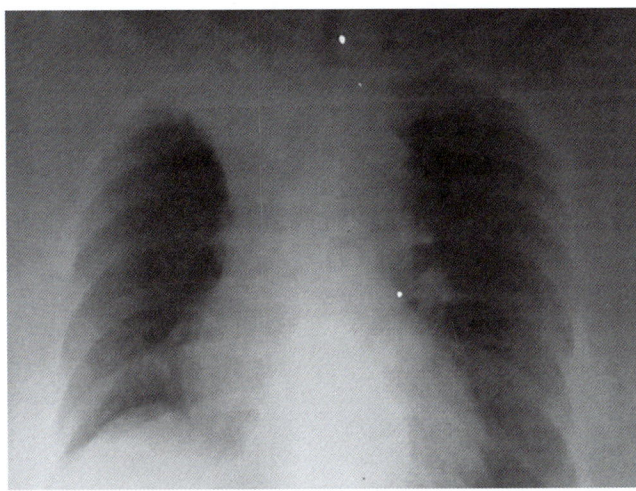

Fig. 5.14: Chest X-ray showing collapse right upper lobe.

- Congenital—tracheobronchomegaly—defect in all structures of the bronchial wall—Mounier-Kuhn syndrome
- Bronchomalacia—absence of cartilage of bronchus –William Campbell syndrome
- Kartagener's syndrome—sinus aplasia, bronchiectasis and situs inversus
- Young syndrome—obstructive azoospermia with bronchiectasis
- Yellow nail syndrome—yellow nail, bronchiectasis, pleural effusion and lymphedema
- Cystic fibrosis
- Pulmonary sequestration

Pathological Process

Obstruction → stagnation → infection → destruction → dilatation.

Morphological Types

- Cystic—involving terminal bronchus
- Fusiform—medium sized bronchus
- Cylindrical—lobar bronchus

Clinical Features

- Chronic cough with large quantity of foul smelling sputum
- Postural cough, hemoptysis, recurrent RTI—pneumonia
- Clubbing, halitosis
- Chest examination—coarse leathery crepitation—pan inspiratory and expiratory
- Evidence of fibrosis or consolidation
- Site—in the order of frequency-left lower lobe, right middle lobe and lingular lobe

Bronchiectasis sicca—manifesting as recurrent hemoptysis without expectoration of large quantity of sputum, seen in upper lobe bronchiectasis, no pending of sputum because of easy drainage, usually post-tuberculous.

Complications

- Hemoptysis, recurrent LRTI—pneumonia, fibrosis, lung abscess
- Pneumothorax, pleural effusion, hydropneumothorax
- Pulmonary hypertension, Cor pulmonale, respiratory failure
- Amyloidosis, metastatic abscess—cerebral

Bad Prognostic Signs

- Multilobar, cystic bronchiectasis
- COPD, respiratory insufficiency
- Cor pulmonale

Investigations

- CXR—increased bronchial markings, ring shadows, evidence of fibrosis, evidence of PAH

- Sputum—macroscopically—three layered sputum, serous, mucous and purulent, culture and antibiotic sensitivity
- Bronchography—bronchiectatic changes, site and extend can be studied
- PFT and ABG analysis
- HRCT—diagnostic lesions can be detected
- Ciliary function assessment—a pellet of saccharide is placed on the anterior chamber of nose. The time taken for it to reach the pharynx, so that the patient can taste it, is noted. Normally it is not more than 20 minutes. In ciliary dysfunction, it will be more.

Management

- Postural drainage, chest physiotherapy
- Mucolytics and hydration
- Bronchodilators—if bronchospasm present
- Control of infection by appropriate antibiotic
- Surgery for localized disease

Bronchial Asthma

Definition: Inflammatory disease of airways characterized by episodic reversible bronchial obstruction, clinically manifesting as paroxysm of dyspnea, cough and polyphonic wheeze.

Pathophysiology

- Changes in the airway—
  - Airway inflammation
  - Airway obstruction
  - Airway hyper-responsiveness
  - Airway remodeling
- Biphasic response to allergen
  - Early asthmatic reaction—mediators from mast cells → airway narrowing by smooth muscle contraction, mucosal edema and mucous—IgE mediated
  - Late asthmatic reaction—sensitized T cells → interleukins and leukotrienes → recruitment of inflammatory cells and eosinophils → inflammation → airway obstruction.

Etiological Types

- Extrinsic asthma—
  - Atopic—early onset
  - Features are—onset in childhood, atopic individuals, IgE mediated, other allergic disorders like allergic rhinitis and eczema
- Intrinsic-asthma—
  - Non-atopic, late onset
  - Features are—onset at any age, usually in adults, no external allergen.

Factors Precipitating Asthma

- Allergens—inhaled allergens—pollen, house dust mite
  - Ingested allergens—fish, nuts, etc.
  - Occupational allergen—grain dust, cotton fiber
- Respiratory infections—viral, bacterial
- Cold air, tobacco smoke
- Exercise
- Drugs -
  - Analgesic
  - Aspirin, NSAID
  - β blockers
  - Emotional stress

Clinical Features

- Episodic dyspnea, cough and wheeze
- Wide spread polyphonic rhonchi, inspiratory and Expiratory
- Silent chest in fatal asthma.

Clinical Types

- Chronic persistent asthma.
  - *Stage 1*: Patient with intermittent asthma intermittent symptoms less than once per week, night symptoms less than 2 times per month, in between normal. FEV1 and PEF > 80%, variability < 20%.
  - *Stage 2*: Patient with mild persistent asthma. Symptoms more than once per week, but less than once per day, night symptoms more than 2 times a month. FEV1 and PEF > 80 % with variability 20–30%.
  - *Stage 3*: Patient with moderate persistent asthma. Symptoms daily, affect activity, night symptoms more than once per week, FEV1 and PEF 60–80% and variability > 30%.
  - *Stage 4*: Patient with severe persistent asthma. Continuous symptoms, frequent exacerbations, frequent night time asthma, physical activity limited, FEV1, PEF < 60%, variability > 30%.
  - Acute severe asthma
    Features: Severe breathlessness—cannot speak in sentences
    - Heart rate > 110/minute
    - Respiratory rate > 25/minute
    - Pulsus paradoxus
    - PEFR < 50%
- Life threatening signs
  - Silent chest/cyanosis
  - Bradycardia/hypotension
  - PEFR < 33 %
  - ABG - $PO_2 < 60$, $PCO_2 > 50$, pH < 7.35

Differential diagnosis of acute severe asthma
- Acute LVF—cardiac asthma
- COPD with acute exacerbation

- ARDS
- Tension pneumothorax
- Bronchiolitis
- Upper respiratory obstruction

Nocturnal Asthma

It is defined as overnight fall of more than 20 % in FEV1. It may be due to:
- Circadian reduction in plasma cortisol at night
- Decrease in circulating catecholamines
- Increase in vagal tone
- Airway cooling
- Increased allergens in bedroom
- GERD

Exercise Induced Asthma

It is asthma induced by exercise and due to unstable mast cells. The excursion of respiratory tract on exercise degranulates the mast cells.

Diagnosis of Bronchial Asthma

- Compatible clinical history + either/or
  - More than 15% improvement in FEV1/PEFR following administration of bronchodilator
  - More than 15% spontaneous change in FEV1/PEFR during 1 week of home monitoring

Investigations

- CXR—
  - To rule out other causes of wheeze
  - To rule out presence of pneumothorax and pneumonia in acute severe asthma
- PFT—
  - Obstructive type of lung disease, FEV1 following 2 puffs of β agonists shows an increase by 15% or greater than the previous level
  - PEFR—serial recording of PEFR may show overnight fall (morning dip and subsequent rise during the day).
- Blood—eosinophilia
- Sputum—eosinophils
- Serum IgE—increased in atopic asthma.

Management

- Principles of treatment
- Avoidance of allergen
- Avoidance of precipitating factor
- Hyposensitization
- Drugs

Drugs in Bronchial Asthma

- Prophylactic—sodium chromoglycate—5-10 mg-MD inhaler-QID
- Nedocromil sodium—2-4 mg-MD inhaler-QID
- Ketotifen—1-2 mg/day
- Bronchodilators
- Methyl xanthines—theophylline, aminophylline
- Sympathomimetics—β_2 agonists
- Short acting—salbutamol, terbutaline
- Long acting—salmeterol
- Anticholinergic—ipratropium bromide by MDI, tiotropium by MDI
- Antiinflammatory—corticosteroid
- Inhalational—beclomethasone, budesonide, fluticasone
- Systemic—oral prednisolone
- Leukotriene antagonist—montelukast, zafirlukast
- Lipoxygenase inhibitor—zileuton.

Treatment of Chronic Persistent Asthma

Concept of step up and step down drug treatment in asthma.

Step Up Treatment

- Step 1: Occasional use of β_2 agonists like salbutamol or terbutaline as inhalation
- Step 2: Inhaled short acting β_2 agonist + regular inhaled anti-inflammatory agent, inhaled steroid—beclomethasone/budesonide up to 800 µg/day or fluticasone 400 microgram/day.
- Step 3: High dose inhaled corticosteroid—800- 2000 µg/day + long acting β_2 agonist—salmeterol-50 µg twice daily or sustained release theophylline
- Step 4: High dose inhaled corticosteroid and regular bronchodilators. Inhaled short acting β_2 agonist SOS + inhaled corticosteroid 800-2000 µg/day + inhaled long acting β_2 agonist—salmeterol
- Sustained release oral theophylline ± montelukast ± inhaled ipratropium—in sequential therapeutic trial
- Step 5: Step 4 + Oral corticosteroid therapy—the lowest therapeutic dose to control symptom.

Rescue oral corticosteroid—is required to regain control of symptoms in a dose of 30-60 mg/day until 2 days after control is established.

Step Down Therapy

In general, it is better to start with a treatment regimen which is likely to achieve disease control rapidly and then step down rather than to start with inadequate treatment and then step up. Patient compliance is also better when symptom control is achieved rapidly. Consider step down if good symptom control for 3 months or more. Withdrawal of anti-inflammatory treatment if patient is well for at least 6 months.

Treatment of Acute Severe Asthma

- Oxygen inhalation—40-60%
- Nebulizer—β_2 agonist—
  - Salbutamol—2.5-5 mg
  - Terbutaline—5-10 mg—repeat every 30 minutes if necessary
- Systemic corticosteroid—IV hydrocortisone 200 mg or oral prednisolone 40 mg

- If severity persist—ipratropium bromide—0.5 mg added to the nebulized β_2 agonist
- IV aminophylline—250 mg in 20 mL in 20 minutes followed by aminophylline infusion 500 µg/kg/hr—in patients not on oral theophylline

Indication of Mechanical Ventilation

- Progressive decline in PEFR
- Progressive hypoxia
- Feeble respiration
- Respiratory arrest

Monitoring of Treatment

- PEF recording every 15-30 minutes
- ABG analysis and blood pH—repeatedly in 1-2 hours
- Continuous monitoring of oxygen saturation by pulse oximetry.

Chronic Obstructive Pulmonary Disease (COPD)

This includes chronic bronchitis and emphysema (Table 5.7 and 5.8).

Chronic Bronchitis

This is a condition associated with excessive tracheobronchial mucous production, sufficient to cause cough with expectoration on most days for at least three months a year for more than two consecutive years.

Emphysema

This is defined as dilatation and destruction of air spaces distal to terminal bronchiole. The part distal to terminal bronchiole is known as acini.

Types of Emphysema

- Proximal acinar
- Distal acinar—paraseptal emphysema
- Centriacinar
- Panacinar

Etiopathogenesis of COPD

Predisposing factors
- Smoking, environmental pollution
- β_1 antitrypsin deficiency
- Infection
- Genetic predisposition
- Low birth weight and bronchial hyper responsiveness.

Pathological Changes

- Airway inflammation, hypertrophy of mucous secreting gland, increase in the number of Goblet cells, increased ciliary cells.
- Airway obstruction and decreased mucociliary action
- Centriacinar emphysema → bullae and blebs
- Remodeling of pulmonary vascular system → Pulmonary hypertension → RVH → RVF

Clinical Features

- *Cough with expectoration:* Mucoid tenacious sputum, purulent sputum if infection present.
- Progressive exertional dyspnea.

Signs

- Resting dyspnea ±
- Central cyanosis ±
- Pursed lip breathing
- Tracheal descend during inspiration
- Flap, high volume pulse
- Barrel shaped chest and bilateral reduced chest movement
- Hyper resonant note, bilateral reduced breath sound
- Rhonchi—expiratory and inspiratory
- Crepitations—if infection present
- Elevated JVP, tender hepatomegaly, peripheral edema.

Table 5.7: Difference between emphysema and chronic bronchitis.

Features	Predominant emphysema—pink puffer	Predominant chronic bronchitis—blue bloater
Dyspnea	Severe	Mild
Sputum	Scanty	More
Infections	Less common	Common
Cyanosis	Less	More
Edema	Absent	Present
Respiratory insufficiency	Late and terminal	Repeated attacks usually with respiratory infection
Cor pulmonale	Late and terminal	Common
ABG— Hypercapnea Hypoxia	Absent Present—mild	Present Present—moderate to severe

Table 5.8: Spirometric classification of COPD based on post-bronchodilator FEV_1.

Stage	Severity	FEV_1
I	Mild	$FEV_1/FVC < 0.70$ $FEV_1 >/= 80\%$ predicted
II	Moderate	$FEV_1/FVC < 0.70$ FEV_1 50—79% predicted
III	Severe	$FEV_1/FVC < 0.70$ FEV_1 30—49% predicted
IV	Very severe	$FEV_1/FVC < 0.70$ $FEV_1 < 30\%$ predicted or $FEV_1 < 50\%$ predicted if respiratory failure present

Mild COPD should not be diagnosed on lung function alone if the patient is asymptomatic.

Complications

Chronic respiratory failure—Type 2, cor pulmonale and pneumothorax.

Investigations

- CXR
  - Features of emphysema
    - Squaring of the chest wall
    - Horizontally placed ribs
    - Hypertranslucency—lung field
    - Tubular heart
    - Low flat diaphragm
    - Bullae ±
  - Prominence of bronchovascular marking
- PFT—FEV_1 and VC show obstructive pattern - ↓ FEV_1/VC
- ABG—Hypoxia, hypercapnea ±
- CT chest
  - To quantify the extend and distribution of emphysema
  - To detect bullous emphysema

Management

- Reduction of bronchial irritant—smoking, atmospheric dust and smoke.
- Prevention and treatment of respiratory infection—Vaccination against *H. influenzae* and Pneumococci.
- Bronchodilators—short acting β_2 agonist, inhaled anticholinergic.

Recommendation of Bronchodilator Therapy of COPD (Table 5.9)

Table 5.9: Bronchodilator therapy of COPD therapy.

Stage	FEV1 %	Drugs
1	> 50	β_2 agonist
2	35–49	β_2 agonist + anticholinergic
3	< 35	Above + Sustained release Theophylline, oral corticosteroid

- Anti-inflammatory drugs—inhaled steroid/systemic corticosteroid—moderate to severe COPD.
- Oxygen therapy
- Administration of α_1 antitrypsin—if deficient
- Chest physiotherapy and rehabilitation
- Mechanical ventilation—Indication
  - Altered sensorium
  - Tachypnea > 35/minute
  - Severe hypoxia: PaO_2 < 50 mm of Hg
  - Blood pH < 7.25
  - Hypercapnea: $PaCO_2$ >60 mm of HG

Respiratory Failure

Defined as the inadequate lung function for the oxygenation of blood for the metabolic need of body.

The ABG value to define respiratory failure is PaO_2 <60 mm Hg ± $PaCO_2$ > 50 mm Hg.

Types of Respiratory Failure

- Type 1: Hypoxia and normocapnia—acute and chronic
- Type 2: Hypoxia and hypercapnia—acute and chronic

Blood Gas Abnormality in Various Types of Respiratory Failure (Table 5.10)

Table 5.10: Blood gas abnormality in various types of respiratory failure.

	Type 1		Type 2	
	Acute	Chronic	Acute	Chronic
PaO_2	↓↓	↓	↓	↓
$PaCO_2$	↔ or ↓	↔	↑	↑
pH	↔ or ↑	↔	↓	↓ or ↔
HCO_3	↔	↔	↔	↑

Features of Respiratory Failure (Table 5.11)

- Features of primary respiratory disease
- Features of hypoxia—cyanosis, tachycardia, altered sensorium
- Seizure, permanent brain damage
- Bradycardia and hypotension in severe
- Hypoxia
- Features of hypercapnea - headache—vasodilatation -
  - Elevated CSF pressure and papilledema
  - Flapping tremor
  - Slurred speech

Management

Measures of therapy

- Treatment of underlying cause
- O_2 therapy
  - Long term O_2 therapy in c/c respiratory failure
  - High concentration of O_2 - a/c type 1
- **Indications for mechanical ventilation**
  - Severe dyspnea with use of accessory muscles and paradoxical abdominal motion
  - Respiratory rate >35 breaths/min
  - Life threatening hypoxemia : PaO_2 < 50 mm of Hg or PaO_2/FiO_2 < 200 mm of Hg
  - Severe acidosis (PH < 7.25) and hypercapnia ($PaCO_2$ > 60 mm of Hg)
  - Respiratory arrest
  - Somnolence, impaired mental status
  - Cardiovascular complications (hypotension, shock, heart failure)
  - Non- invasive positive pressure ventilation failure.
- **Indications for non-invasive ventilation**
  - Moderate to severe dyspnoea with use of accessory muscles and paradoxical abdominal motion

Table 5.11: Causes of respiratory failure.

Type 1		Type 2	
Acute	Chronic	Acute	Chronic
Pneumonia - Multilobar	C/c parenchymal disease	Upper respiratory Epiglottitis	C/c ventilatory defect
Pulmonary edema	ILD, Diffuse PT	Laryngeal	COPD
ARDS	Pneumoconiosis	Obstruction	Bronchial asthma
Pulmonary embolism	Cystic disease	Foreign body	

Acute severe asthma	Diffuse bronchiectasis	Respiratory center
		Depression
		Brainstem damage
		Narcotic poisoning
		Chest wall lesions
		  Injury
		  Flail chest
		  Muscle paralysis
		    – GBS, OP poisoning
		    – Snake bite
			Ankylosing spondylitis
			Kyphoscoliosis

- Moderate to severe acidosis (PH >/= 7.35) and hypercapnia ($PaCO_2$ > 45 mm of Hg)
- Respiratory frequency >25 breaths/min

Pneumothorax

Presence of air in the pleural space.

Types of Pneumothorax

- Closed: Spontaneous closure of the communication between the lung and pleural cavity.
- Open: Presence of bronchopleural fistula.
- Tension: Communication act as a check valve, allowing air to enter the pleura during inspiration.

Source of air for pneumothorax
- From lung
- From mediastinum
- From outside

Etiology

Spontaneous, traumatic and iatrogenic

Spontaneous
- Primary
- Secondary

Primary: Subpleural bleb

Secondary
- Emphysematous bullae
- Subpleural tuberculous lesion pneumatocele
- Cavitary lesion—PT
- Cystic disease
- Cystic bronchiectasis
- Pneumoconiosis
- Honey comb lung
- Lung abscess
- Rare causes
  - Tuberous sclerosis
  - Marfan's syndrome
  - Histiocytosis
  - Catamenial pneumothorax

Cause of recurrent pneumothorax
- Tuberous sclerosis
- Marfan's syndrome
- Emphysematous bullae
- Sub pleural bleb.

Clinical Features

- Usually sudden in onset
- Pleuritic pain, acute dyspnea
- Progressive dyspnea and cyanosis—tension pneumothorax
- Mediastinal shift to opposite side
- Hyper resonant note
- VF, VR and breath sounds diminished
- Amphoric breathing in open pneumothorax
- Clicking sound is heard in mild left sided pneumothorax called noisy pneumothorax
- Catamenial pneumothorax—in women of child bearing age developing right sided pneumothorax with menstruation
- Mediastinal emphysema → mediastinal crunching sound with each cardiac cycle—Hamman's sign.

Investigations

- CXR
  - Pneumothorax is evidenced by hypertranslucent area without lung marking, peripheral to the collapsed lung
  - Less than 20% collapse lung—Mantle pneumothorax
  - To find out the etiology.

Management

- Small pneumothorax with less than 20% collapse lung—no active treatment, breathing exercise and follow up
- Pneumothorax with more than 1/3rd collapse and tension pneumothorax—active treatment is required Percutaneous aspiration or intercostal tube drainage. Thoracoscopy and stapling of bleb, pleural abrasion if above measures fail
- Treatment of etiology.

Hydropneumothorax (Fig. 5.15)

Presence of fluid and air in the pleural cavity.

Causes
- Peripheral cavity rupture, lung abscess
- Cystic disease of the lung
- Pneumatocele
- Lung malignancy
- Persistent pneumothorax with fluid collection
- After aspiration of pleural effusion.

Signs—3 'S'
- Straight line dullness (horizontal level of dullness)
- Shifting dullness
- Succussion splash.

Management

- Intercostal drainage
- Treatment of the primary disease.

Pleural Effusion

It is the accumulation of fluid in the pleural cavity.

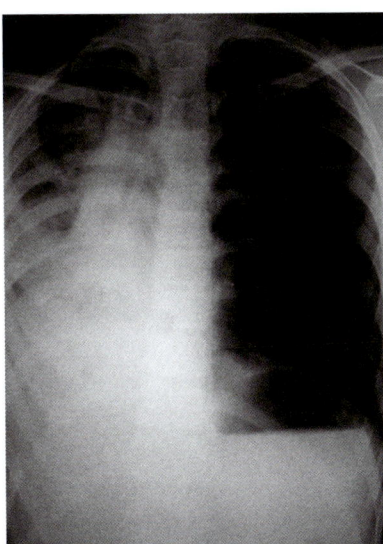

Fig. 5.15: Chest X-ray showing left side hydropneumothorax.

Etiology (Exudative Effusion)

- Infectious
  - Viral—coxsackie—Bornholm's disease
  - Bacterial-Synpneumonic
    - Tuberculosis
    - Subphrenic abscess
  - Parasitic—
    - Amoebic, hydatid disease
  - Rare infections—
    - Nocardia, actinomycosis
- Noninfectious—
  - Malignancy—
    - Primary—mesothelioma
    - Secondary—from lung and other sites
  - Pulmonary infarction
  - Collagen vascular disease
  - Chylothorax, esophageal diseases
  - Acute pancreatitis
  - Meige's syndrome, yellow nail syndrome
  - Uremia, asbestosis
  - Radiation, Drugs—procainamide, amiodarone.

Causes of Hydrothorax—Transudate

- Congestive heart failure syndrome
- Cirrhosis liver
- Hypoproteinemia
- SVC obstruction
- Rarely in hypothyroidism.

Causes of Right Sided Pleural Effusion

- Hepatopulmonary amebiasis
- Meige's syndrome
- Chylothorax—lower thoracic duct damage
- Hydrothorax

Causes of Left Sided Pleural Effusion

- Acute pancreatitis
- Esophageal diseases
- Left subphrenic abscess
- Chylothorax—upper thoracic duct damage

Clinical Features

- Fever, pleuritic pain, dyspnea
- Trepopnea—dyspnea on a particular posture
- In pleural effusion, breathing difficulty on lying on the normal side
- Clubbing—malignant pleural effusion and empyema
- Yellow nail in yellow nail syndrome
- Lymph node enlargement—tuberculosis, lung malignancy, lymphoma, AIDS, etc.

Chest Signs

- Mediastinal shift to opposite side
- Stony dullness—high in the axilla
- VF, VR breath sounds reduced
- Pleural rub ± above the level of effusion
- Traube's space obliteration in left pleural effusion
- For clinical detection—500 mL of pleural fluid.

Encysted Pleural Effusion (Figs 5.16 and 5.29)

- Sites—apical, parietal, subpulmonic
- Mediastinal and Interlobar—phantom tumor of lung
- Cause—TB, pyogenic and CHF—(interlobar).

Pleural Effusion without Mediastinal Shift to Opposite Side

- Mild pleural effusion
- Pleural effusion with fibrosis or collapse of lung
- Encysted pleural effusion.

Pleural Effusion with Mediastinal Shift to Same Side

- Pleural effusion with fibrosis or active collapse of lung.

Investigations

- CXR
  - For radiological detection, 300 mL of pleural fluid is required
  - Homogenous opacity—with obliteration of cardiophrenic and costophrenic angles with concave medial border
  - Mediastinal shift to the opposite side (> 1500 mL of pleural fluid)
- USG of chest—can detect amount and site of pleural collection, also encysted pleural effusion
- Pleural fluid study.

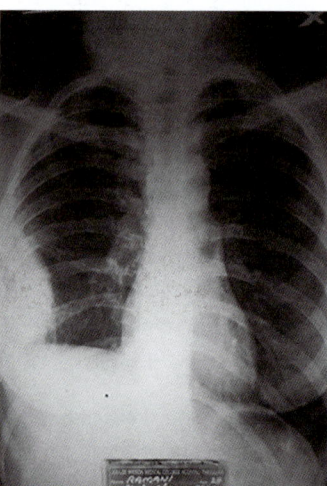

Fig. 5.16: Chest X-ray showing encysted effusion.

Indication for Pleural Fluid Aspiration

- Diagnostic and therapeutic
- Cardiorespiratory embarrassment
- Bilateral pleural effusion
- Pleural effusion with pulmonary edema
- Introduction of intrapleural drug for pleurodesis

Macroscopically

- Clear, straw colored—TB
- Pus—empyema
- Anchovy sauce—amebiasis
- Chylous—thoracic duct damage
- Chyliform—chronic tuberculous effusion and malignancy
- Hemorrhagic—
  - Malignancy—
    - Primary
    - Secondary
  - Pulmonary infarct
  - TB
  - Hemorrhagic pancreatitis
  - Bleeding diathesis
  - Traumatic
- Blood stained fluid—5000–10,000 RBCs/mL
- Frank hemorrhagic fluid - > 1 lakh RBCs/mL

Cytology of Pleural Fluid

- Neutrophilic—synpneumonic, subphrenic abscess
- Lymphocytic—TB, viral, lymphoma, rheumatoid arthritis
- Eosinophilic—with blood eosinophilia—(> 20% eosinophils in pleural fluid)
  - Hydatid disease
  - Tropical pulmonary eosinophilia
  - PAN
  - Hodgkin's disease
- Without blood eosinophilia
  - Pulmonary infarct
  - Synpneumonic effusion
- Malignant cells—malignant pleural effusion
- Plasma cells—plasma cell leukemia

Biochemistry of Pleural Fluid

- Glucose level
  - Normal—same as plasma level
  - < 50 mg—rheumatoid pleural effusion empyema
- Protein
  - Normal 1–2 g%
  - Exudate > 3 g%
  - Transudate < 3 g%
- Amylase level—Increased in pancreatic pleural effusion and esophageal rupture

- LDH—Increased in exudates, > 200 or > 2/3rd of serum LDH
- Adenosine deaminase (ADA)—increased in TB
- pH < 7.2 s/o empyema
- Culture of pleural fluid for—bacteria (pyogenic) and tubercle bacilli
- PCR study—to detect organisms including tubercle bacilli
- RT - PCR—to detect viable bacilli
- Pleural biopsy—in malignancy and TB
- CBC and ESR
- Mantoux test.

Tuberculous Pleural Effusion

- Most common cause of pleural effusion is TB
- Mechanism
  - Allergic to primary focus
  - Subpleural focus spreading to pleura
  - Peripheral cavity rupturing to pleura
  - Part of miliary TB
  - Mediastinal TB lymph node → caseating to pleura
  - TB spine → pleura
  - Rarely TB rib to pleura
- Among these, most common mechanism is—allergic to primary focus.

Clinical Features

Insidious onset, fever with symptoms and signs of pleural effusion.
- Pleural fluid
  - Clear, straw colored, lymphocytic exudates
  - ADA elevated
  - Tubercle bacilli—from fluid—culture/PCR
- ESR elevated
- Mantoux test—positive (Fig. 5.17)
- Pleural biopsy—chronic inflammation, tubercle ±

Complications

- Cardiorespiratory embarrassment—massive pleural effusion
- Pleural thickening
- Pleural fibrosis (fibrothorax)—in untreated cases

Management of TB Pleural Effusion (Figs. 5.18 to 5.29)

- Aspiration and study of fluid
- Anti TB drugs—initial intensive phase and continuation phase
- Systemic corticosteroid—6–8 weeks.

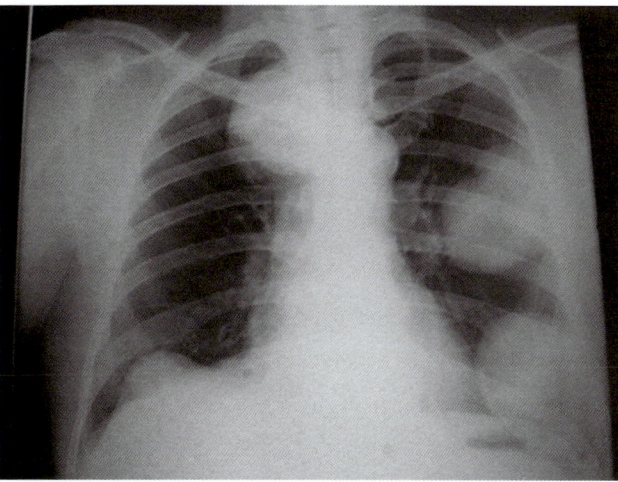

Fig. 5.18: X-ray chest showing multiple hydatid cyst.

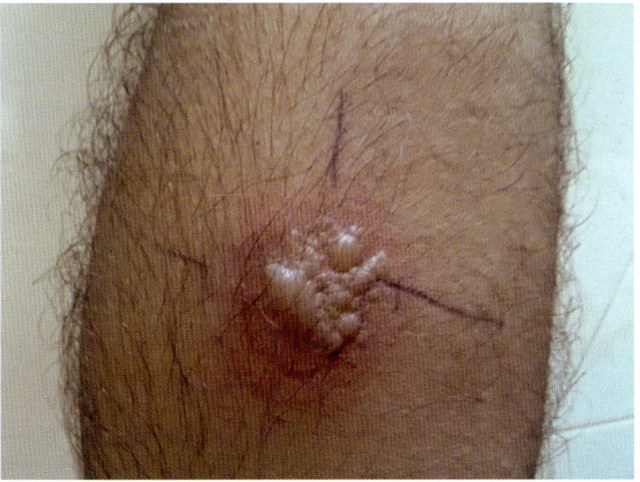

Fig. 5.17: Strongly positive Mantoux test.

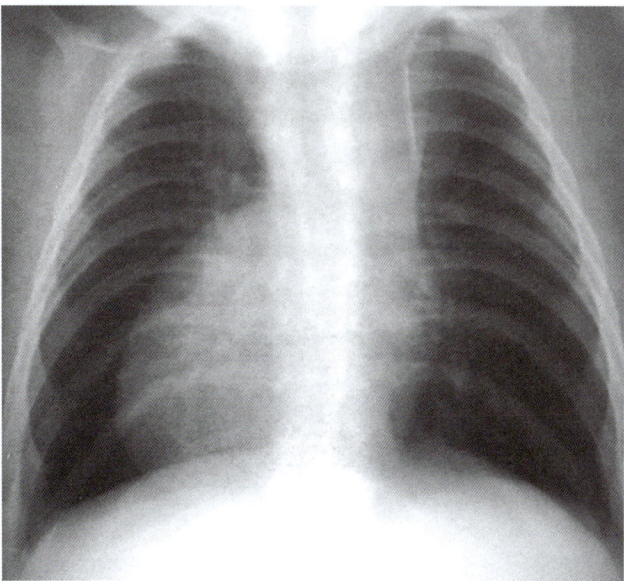

Fig. 5.19: X-ray showing mass lesion–bronchial adenoma.

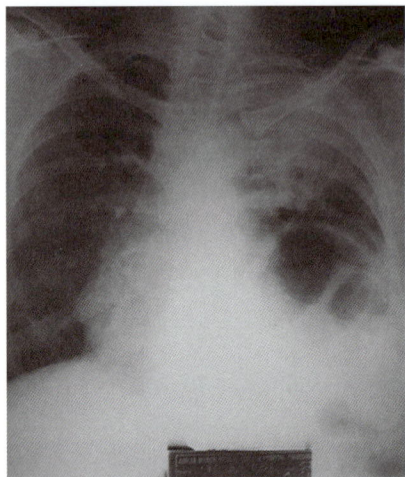

Fig. 5.20: X-ray showing eventration of left diaphragm.

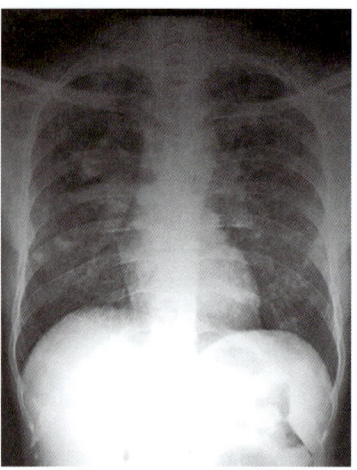

Fig. 5.23: Chest X-ray showing bilateral hilar adenopathy and nodular lesion of the lung.

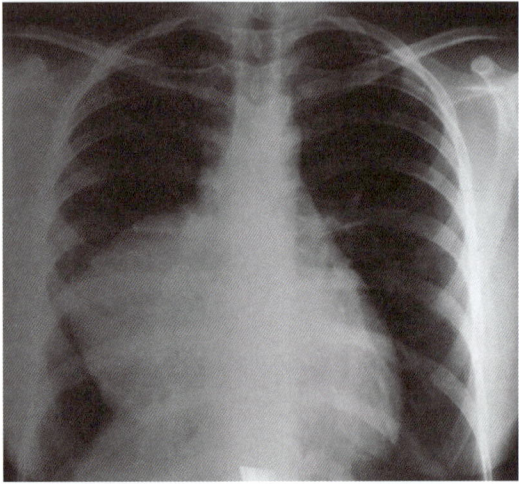

Fig. 5.21: X-ray showing anterior mediastinal mass–teratoma.

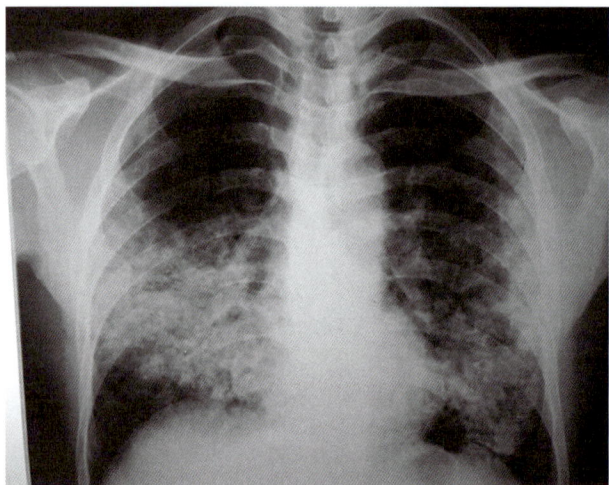

Fig. 5.24: X-ray chest showing bilateral midzone and lower zone alveolar shadows in a patient with *Pneumocystis* pneumonia.

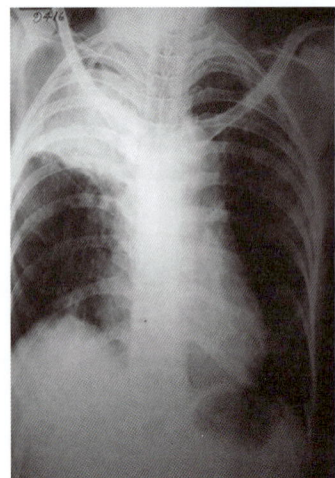

Fig. 5.22: X-ray showing right upper lobe fibrosis with mediastinal shift.

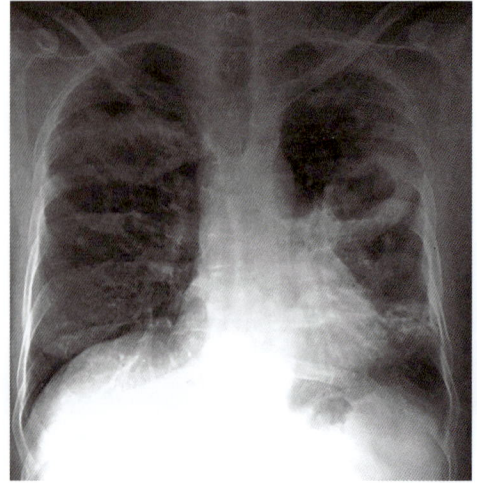

Fig. 5.25: X-ray chest showing tuberculous cavity left side.

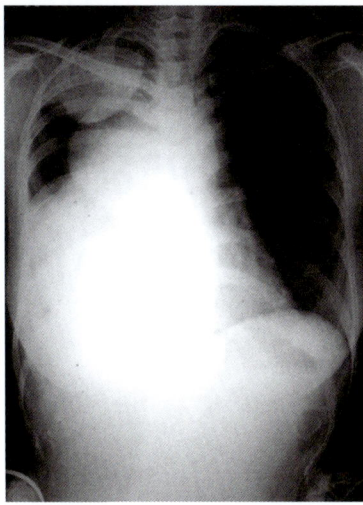

Fig. 5.26: Chest X-ray thymic mass.

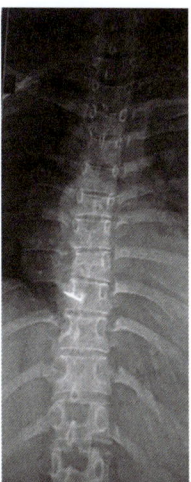

Fig. 5.27: X-ray showing paraspinal abscess right side with left side pulmonary tuberculosis.

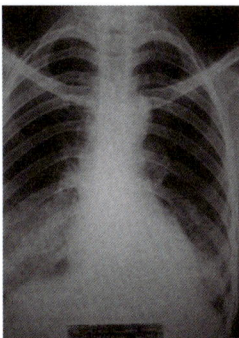

Fig. 5.28: X-ray showing cystic lesion on the 9th rib right side due to tuberculosis of rib.

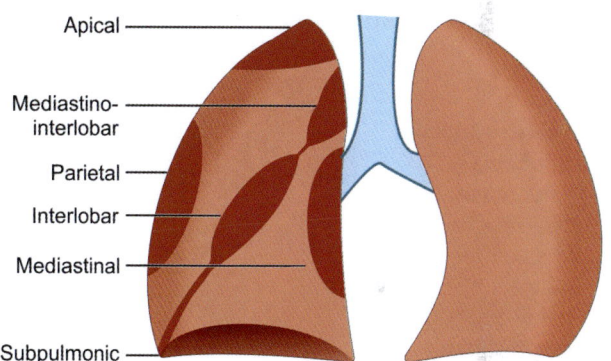

Fig. 5.29: Encysted pleural effusion.

CHAPTER 6

Examination of Alimentary System

SYMPTOMATOLOGY

Upper GI (Gastrointestinal) Symptoms

- Anorexia
- Pica
- Excessive appetite
- Sitophobia
- Water brash
- Ptyalism
- Xerostomia
- Halitosis
- Globus pharyngeus
- Bleeding gum
- Fur on the tongue
- Vomiting
- Heartburn (pyrosis)
- Acid eructation
- Dysphagia
- Flatulence
- Hematemesis

Lower GI (Gastrointestinal) Symptoms

- Abnormal stool
- Hematochezia
- Constipation
- Melena
- Diarrhea
- Abnormal stool

Symptoms of Hepatobiliary Disease

- Jaundice (refer to General examination)
- Dark urine
- Pruritus
- Pale stool
- Pain—right hypochondrium—congestive hepatomegaly
- Biliary colic (refer to Abdominal pain)
- Anorexia
- Upper GI bleeding
- Fever, lethargy, loss of weight

Symptoms of Pancreatic Disease

- Pain—abdomen—due to inflammation/stone (refer to Abdominal pain)
- Distention of abdomen
- Pleuritic pain—left
- Tetany
- In chronic disease—ascites, steatorrhea and IDDM

UPPER GI SYMPTOMS

Anorexia

- Means loss of appetite
- Appetite → pleasurable desire to eat
- Hunger → is the unpleasant sensation produced by the empty stomach and its peristaltic contraction.
- Satiety → is the feeling of satisfaction after the intake of food.
- Early satiety → is the feeling of fullness of stomach even before the required quantity of food is taken.

Causes of Anorexia

Alimentary causes
- Upper GI:
  - Gastritis,
  - Ca stomach,
  - Dyspepsia, etc.
- Hepatic:
  - Acute hepatocellular disease
    - Viral hepatitis

- Chronic hepatocellular disease
    - Cirrhosis liver
    - Hepatocellular failure

Extra-alimentary Causes
- Congestive heart failure
- Uremia
- Chronic respiratory diseases
- *Endocrine:* Hypothyroidism, Addison's disease
- *Infections:* TB, other febrile illnesses
- *Psychological:* Anorexia nervosa, depression, anxiety
- *Drugs:* Antiobesity drugs
    - Fenfluramine
- Side effects of other drugs

Pica

Means perverted appetite, compulsive desire to eat uncommon substances, like sand, clay, uncooked rice, hair, etc.

Causes

- Iron-deficiency anemia
- Pregnancy
- Psychogenic

Excessive Appetite

Excessive appetite is present in:
- Diabetes mellitus
- Thyrotoxicosis
- Hypothalamic disorder
- Depressive psychosis
- Bulimia nervosa

Bulimia nervosa is characterized by recurrent bouts of overeating, lack of self-control on overeating with spontaneous or self-induced vomiting, seen in women of late adolescence or early adulthood.

Sitophobia is the fear of eating.

Water Brash

Sudden filling of mouth with watery fluid. It is of reflex origin in upper GI disorder.

Ptyalism

This is increased flow of saliva. Seen in:
- Painful and inflammatory conditions of mouth
- Preceding nausea and vomiting
- Peptic ulcer disease
- Parkinsonism (parasympathetic overactivity)
- Rabies.

Xerostomia

Xerostomia means dryness of mouth.

Causes
- Dehydration, diabetes mellitus (loss of body fluid)
- Diseases of salivary gland—Sjogren's syndrome
- Postradiation
- *Drugs:* Atropine

Halitosis

Halitosis is bad odor of breath.

Causes
- Oropharyngeal:
    - Poor oral hygiene
    - Caries tooth
    - Pyorrhea alveolaris
    - Ulcerative gingivitis
    - Ca oral cavity
- Suppurative lung disease
- Smoking
- Food, garlic and fish oil
- *Hepatocellular failure:* Fishy odor (fetor hepaticus)
- *Azotemia:* Ammoniacal or urinary odor
- *Diabetic ketoacidosis:* Sweet or fruity odor.

Globus Pharyngeus is the sensation of lump in the throat.

Bleeding Gum

Causes are:
- Local injury
- Gingivitis
- Bleeding diathesis
- Acute leukemia.

Fur on the Tongue

Normal coating of tongue is by a thin whitish film made up of epithelium, food debris and organisms.

Excessive coating of tongue is seen in dehydration and febrile illnesses like enteric fever.

Vomiting (Emesis)

- Means forceful oral expulsion of gastric content by reflex mechanism.
- Nausea means feeling of desire to vomit.
- Retching denotes labored rhythmic contraction of respiratory and abdominal musculature, which precedes or follows vomiting.
- Regurgitation appearance of previously swallowed food in the mouth without vomiting—bringing out esophageal content.
- Vomiting is a complex reflex involving vomiting center which is situated in the medulla, autonomic and somatic neural pathways.

- **Phases of vomiting**

  Phase of nausea
  ↓
  Hypersalivation, sweating
  ↓
  Retching
  ↓
  Expulsion of gastric content

Mechanism of Vomiting

- Synchronous contraction of the diaphragm, intercostal muscles and abdominal muscles → increases the intra-abdominal pressure.
- This is combined with relaxation of the lower esophageal sphincter resulting in forcible ejection of gastric content.
- Vomiting without preceding nausea is called projectile vomiting, seen in CNS disorders with increased intracranial pressure.

Causes of Vomiting

Alimentary Causes
- *Gastritis:* Food, alcohol, drugs
- *Gastroenteritis:* Cholera, viral, food poisoning
- Gastroesophageal reflux disease (GERD), gastroparesis, carcinoma stomach
- Acid peptic disease
- Obstruction of gastric outlet, small intestine
- *Inflammatory lesions:* Cholecystitis, pancreatitis, appendicitis, hepatitis.

Extra-alimentary Causes

- *Renal:* Renal colic, uremia
- *Central nervous system (CNS):* Increased intracranial pressure, cerebrovascular accident (CVA), migraine, meningitis
- *Labyrinthine:* Labyrinthitis, motion sickness
- *Cardiovascular system (CVS):* Inferior wall myocardial infarction (MI)
- Endocrine
  - Addison's disease
  - Diabetic ketoacidosis
- *Pregnancy:* Morning sickness, hyperemesis gravidarum
- *Drugs:* Morphine, digitalis, antimalignant drugs
- *Psychogenic:* Bulimia nervosa, depression, cyclic vomiting syndrome.

Features to be noted in Vomiting

- *Absence of nausea:* CNS disorder, hysteria
- *Other upper GI symptoms:* Colic, distention of abdomen
- *Examination of other systems:* CNS, renal, endocrine, etc.

Examination of Vomitus

- Food material, quantity—large in gastric outlet obstruction
- Blood, coffee ground vomitus
- Bilious vomitus absent in → pyloric stenosis
- Bilious vomitus increased in → intestinal obstruction
- Time of day—in pyloric stenosis, later part of day when large quantity of food has accumulated.
- Mucus—(jelly-like appearance) present in small quantity in most vomitus → large quantity of mucus in catarrhal inflammation of stomach.

Odor

- Sour odor due to acid presence.
- *Offensiveness:* Feculant odor in intestinal obstruction and increased fermentation of food in pyloric obstruction.

Heartburn (Pyrosis)

- It is the sensation of warmth or burning located substernally or high in the epigastrium with often radiation to neck, occasionally to arms.
- Seen in lower esophageal disease—GERD.

Acid Eructation

- Means eructation of small amount of acid gastric contents along with flatus.
- Seen both in functional and organic diseases of the stomach.

Dysphagia

- It is the difficulty in swallowing, better defined as a sensation of sticking or obstruction of the passage of food through the oropharynx or esophagus.
- Aphagia → signifies complete esophageal obstruction, usually due to bolus impaction
- Odynophagia → means painful swallowing
- Phagophobia → means fear of swallowing
- Refusal to swallow → seen in hysteria, tetanus, rabies, pharyngeal paralysis and odynophagia.

Physiology of Swallowing

- *Voluntary phase:* Oral bolus of food pushed to pharynx by the contraction of tongue.
- *Involuntary phase:* Pharyngeal and esophageal phase by deglutition reflex.

Anatomically Two Types of Dysphagia

Oropharyngeal and esophageal.
- *Oropharyngeal disorder:* Results from neuromuscular dysfunction affecting the initiation of swallowing by the pharynx and upper esophageal sphincter, also have nasal regurgitation and choking due to tracheal aspiration.
- *Esophageal disorder:* Results from structural or motility disorder producing the feel of food sticking after swallowing.

Etiologically Two Groups of Dysphagia

1. Mechanical or obstructive
2. Motor dysphagia or paralytic dysphagia

Causes of Mechanical Dysphagia

Esophageal lumen in adult can distend to 4 cm.
 Dysphagia starts for solid food if the lumen is not more than 2.5 cm. If the lumen is less than 1.3 cm, dysphagia always presents.

- **Luminal:** Foreign body, large bolus
- **Intrinsic lesions**
    - Inflammatory conditions: Edema and swelling
        - Pharyngitis
        - Epiglotitis
        - Esophagitis
            - Candidal
            - Viral—herpes
        - Chemical, thermal injury
    - Webs and rings
        - Pharyngeal web (Plummer-Vinson)
        - Lower esophageal mucosal ring (Schatzki ring)
    - Benign strictures
        - Peptic, inflammatory
        - Pill-induced
        - Postoperative
    - Malignant tumors
        - Squamous cell Ca
        - Adenocarcinoma
        - Metastatic Ca
    - Benign tumors
        - Leiomyoma
        - Inflammatory polyp
        - Epithelial papilloma
- **Extrinsic lesions**
    - Retropharyngeal abscess or mass
    - Vertebral osteophytes
    - Vascular compression
        - Aberrant right—subclavian artery (dysphagia lusoria)
        - Right—sided aorta
        - Aortic aneurysm
    - Posterior mediastinal masses

Causes of Motor Dysphagia (Paralytic Dysphagia)

- Difficulty in initiating swallowing
    - Paralysis of the tongue
    - Lesions of the vagus and glossopharyngeal
- Disorders of pharyngeal and esophageal striate muscles
    - Muscle weakness
        - Upper motor neuron (UMN): Pseudobulbar palsy
        - Lower motor neuron (LMN): Motor neuron disease (MND), guillain-barré syndrome (GBS), Polio

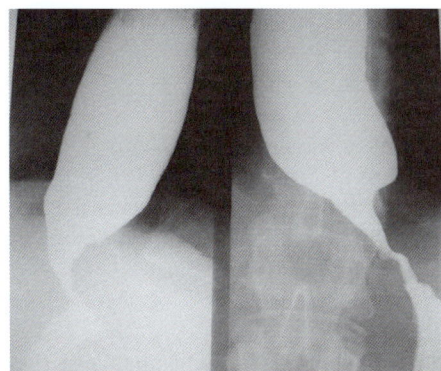

Fig. 6.1: Barium swallow showing achalasia cardia.

   - Neuromuscular: Myasthenia
   - Myopathy
       - Polymyositis
       - Oculopharyngeal myopathy
       - Myotonic dystrophy
- Disorders of esophageal smooth muscles
    - Scleroderma
    - Achalasia cardia (Fig. 6.1)
    - Diffuse esophageal spasm
    - Autonomic neuropathy

Features to Note in Dysphagia

- **Type of food**
  Obstructive lesions: Solid > liquid
  Achalasia cardia: Liquid > solid
  Paralytic lesions: Both for solid and liquid food.
  Force of swallowing is more for solid food; speed of swallowing is more for liquid food.
- **Duration of dysphagia**
  Transient: Inflammatory lesions
  For weeks to months: Carcinoma esophagus
  Episodic: For years – lower esophageal ring
- **Site of dysphagia**
  High: Carcinoma pharynx/esophagus, cervical tumors
   Bulbar palsy
   Iron-deficiency anemia
   Diverticulum
  Middle: Carcinoma esophagus, mediastinal tumors
  Low: Carcinoma esophagus
   Carcinoma fundus of stomach
   Achalasia
   Stricture
   Hiatus hernia
- **Associated symptoms**
    - Nasal regurgitation
        - Palatopharyngeal paralysis
    - Tracheobronchial aspiration
        - Paralysis of pharynx and larynx
        - Tracheoesophageal fistula

- Tracheobronchial aspiration unrelated to swallowing
    - Achalasia
    - Diverticulum
    - GERD
- Weight loss—carcinoma esophagus
- Hoarseness of voice
    - Preceding dysphagia means laryngeal tumors
    - Following dysphagia carcinoma esophagus → Recurrent laryngeal nerve palsy
    - Dysphagia and hoarseness together → Neuromuscular disorder
- Unilateral wheezing and dysphagia → intrathoracic mass lesion
- Presence of chest pain—esophageal spasm, obstruction by large bolus
- Heartburn—GERD, peptic stricture
- Odynophagia (painful dysphagia)
    - Esophagitis—candidiasis, herpes and pill-induced
    - AIDS—opportunistic infection
    - Tumors—lymphoma
- Dysarthria and dysphonia
    - Neuromuscular disorder
- *Also look for*
    - Goiter
    - Spine deformity
    - Skin changes of progressive systemic sclerosis
    - Lymph nodes—malignancy
    - Lungs—aspiration pneumonia.

Common Causes of Motor Dysphagia

- Motor neuron disease—progressive bulbar palsy
- Pseudobulbar palsy
- Myasthenia gravis
- Myotonic dystrophy
- Polymyositis
- Oculopharyngeal myopathy.

Dyspepsia

Dyspepsia is a term to denote a variety of alimentary symptoms arising from upper GI tract, which includes:
1. Upper abdominal pain ± related to food
2. Heartburn, regurgitation, water brash
3. Anorexia, nausea, vomiting
4. Early repletion and satiety after meals
5. Flatulence, belching and bloating.

- **Organic causes**
    - Peptic: Esophagitis, peptic ulcer
    - Upper GI malignancy
    - Hepatobiliary disease
    - Chronic pancreatitis
    - Other system disorders—chronic renal failure (CRF), congestive heart failure (CHF), etc.
    - Drugs—nonsteroidal anti-inflammatory drugs (NSAIDs), corticosteroids
    - Alcoholism
    - Pregnancy
- **Functional dyspepsia (nonulcer dyspepsia):** It is due to motor dysfunction of upper GI mediated by neurohumoral mechanism
- **Alarming features in dyspepsia**
    - Weight loss
    - Anemia
    - Vomiting
    - Hematemesis, melena
    - Dysphagia
    - Palpable abdominal mass

Flatulence

The stomach or intestines may be distended with gas. The patient then complains of wind or flatulence. The wind may be belched through the mouth or passed per rectum; the former is gastric flatulence, the latter intestinal.

The cause of flatulence is various types of digestive disorders, more functional than organic. The gas in the stomach is often swallowed air.

Hematemesis

Means vomiting of blood, due to upper GI bleeding proximal to ligament of Trietz.

Spurious hematemesis: Vomiting of swallowed blood from upper respiratory tract.

Upper GI Bleeding—Source of Blood

Etiologically
　　Variceal and nonvariceal.
Anatomically

- **Esophagus**
    - Varices (10% of UGI bleed)
    - Peptic esophagitis
    - Ulcer esophagus
    - Hiatus hernia
    - Mallory-Weiss syndrome
- **Stomach**
    - Gastric ulcer
    - Erosive gastritis
    - Gastric varices
    - Carcinoma stomach
    - Polyp
    - Leiomyoma
    - Congestive gastropathy—portal HTN
    - Angioma
    - Hereditary hemorrhagic telangiectasia

- Watermelon stomach—gastric antral vascular ectasia (GAVE) syndrome
- Dieulafoy's lesion—mucosal aberrant vessel which bleeds due to pin-point defect in mucosa.
- **Duodenal:** Duodenal ulcer acute and chronic (40% of UGI bleed)

Causes of UGI Bleed Depend on— Order of Frequency

- Most common
  - Duodenal ulcer—40%
  - Gastric ulcer—20%
  - Erosive gastritis—20%
  - Esophagitis
  - Varices—10%
  - Mallory-Weiss tear
- Common
  - Carcinoma stomach
  - Bleeding diathesis
  - Leiomyoma
- Uncommon
  - Angioma—upper GI
  - Hereditary hemorrhagic telangiectasia
  - Watermelon stomach
  - Dieulafoy's lesion
  - Hemobilia
  - Ehlers-Danlos syndrome

Differences between Hematemesis and Hemoptysis

Hematemesis	Hemoptysis
Nausea, vomiting precedes	Cough precedes
Froth – absent	Froth – present
pH – acidic	pH – alkaline
Food particles present	Food particles absent
Coffee-colored	Bright red
Melena – present	Melena – absent
H/o Upper GI disease	H/o Respiratory disease

LOWER GI SYMPTOMS

Diarrhea

Defined as increase in frequency of passage of liquid stool weighing more than 200 g/day, usually more than 3 bowel movements per day.

Pseudodiarrhea: Frequent passage of small volumes of formed stool usually associated with anorectal disorders.

Mechanism

- *Secretory diarrhea:*
  - Increased secretion of electrolytes
  - Enterotoxins—*V. cholerae, E. coli*
  - Vipoma - Pancreatic cholera
  - Villous adenoma
- *Osmotic diarrhea:*
  - Poorly absorbed solutes – $MgSO_4$, laxatives
  - Maldigestion
  - Disaccharidase deficiency
  - Lactose intolerance
- *Exudative diarrhea:*
  - *Inflammatory bowel disease (IBD):* Ulcerative colitis
  - *Infections: Shigella, Entamoeba histolytica*
- *Malabsorption diarrhea:* Small bowel diarrhea [Tropical sprue]
- *Motility disorder:* IBS, thyrotoxicosis
- Acute diarrhea → 7–14 days
- Persistent diarrhea → 2–4 weeks
- Chronic diarrhea → > 4 weeks

Differences between Small Bowel and Large Bowel Diarrhea

Features	Small bowel diarrhea	Large bowel diarrhea
Volume of stool	Large	Small
Type of stool	Watery	Mucoid
Blood in stool	Rare	Common
Nature of stool	Soupy/Greasy	Mucinous/jelly like
Tenesmus	Absent	Present
Abdominal pain	Central	Left iliac fossa

Causes of Acute Diarrhea

Two groups:
1. Infectious
2. Noninfectious

- **Infectious**
  - *Viral:* Rotavirus, adenovirus
  - *Bacterial:* Noninvasive
    - Enterotoxin → increases secretion
    - *V. cholerae*
    - Eltor vibrio
    - *Clostridium*
    - *Staphylococcus aureus*
  - *Bacterial:* Invasive
    - Cytotoxin → mucosal damage
    - *Shigella*
    - *Salmonella*
    - *Campylobacter*
    - *Clostridium difficile*
    - *E. coli*—0157
  - *Protozoal: Entamoeba, Giardia, B. coli, Cryptosporidium*

- **Noninfectious**
  - *Drugs:* Antacids, ampicillin, β-blocker, NSAIDs
  - *IBD:* Acute ulcerative colitis
  - Diverticulitis
  - Ischemic colitis
  - Polyposis of colon
  - Henoch-Schonlein purpura
  - Intussusception

Causes of Chronic Diarrhea

- Infections
  - HIV infection
  - *Entameba histolytica*
  - Intestinal TB
- *Maldigestion:* Lactose intolerance
- *Malabsorption:* Small intestinal/pancreatic
- *IBD:* Ulcerative colitis, Crohn's disease
- Diverticulosis, polyposis, villous adenoma
- *Motility disorder:* IBS
- *Postgastrectomy:* Dumping syndrome
- Endocrine diarrhea
  - Thyrotoxicosis
  - Hypoparathyroidism
  - Diabetes mellitus
  - Addison's disease
  - Zollinger-Ellison syndrome
  - Medullary carcinoma of thyroid
  - Carcinoid syndrome
  - *Vipoma:* Pancreatic cholera

Constipation

It is defined as infrequent passage of hard stools—less than 3 bowel movements per week. It may be a manifestation of many GI and medical disorders.

Features to be noted

- Onset—neonatal—Hirschsprung's disease
- Presence of other lower GI symptoms—bleeding
- Excessive straining—motility disorder
- Symptoms of other system involvement:
  - Hypothyroidism
  - Spinal cord disease

Causes

Gastrointestinal and nongastrointestinal.

Gastrointestinal
- *Dietary:* Lack of fiber diet/fluid intake
  - Colonic
    - Motility disorder, tumor, stricture, megacolon
    - Intestinal obstruction/pseudo-obstruction
  - Anorectal disorder
    - Hemorrhoids, fissure in ano, rectocele
  - Megarectum

Nongastrointestinal
- Drugs
  - Aluminum-containing antacids
  - Opiates
  - Anticholinergic
  - Fe supplements
- Metabolic/endocrine
  - Hypothyroidism
  - Diabetes mellitus
  - Hypercalcemia
  - Hypokalemia
  - Porphyria
  - Pregnancy
- Neuromuscular
  Peripheral
  - Hirschsprung's disease
  - Intestinal pseudo-obstruction
  Central
  - Parkinsonism
  - Spinal cord disease
  - CVA
  - Cauda equina lesion
  - Immobilization
- Elderly people
  - Motility decreased, access to toilet decreased, drugs
  - Neurological disorder
- Psychogenic
  - Depressive illness

Melena

Means passage of tarry black stool due to the presence of altered blood.
- 60 mL or more of upper GI bleed → melena
- One episode of upper GI bleed → 5–7 days of melena
- Blood should remain in the gut for 14 hours or more → melena
- Upper GI bleed and lower GI bleed proximal to middle of transverse colon → melena

Hematochezia

Means passage of red blood per rectum.
- Due to bleeding from lower GI
- Massive bleed from upper GI (transit time is reduced)

Causes of lower GI bleed: This may be due to bleed from small intestine, colon, or anal canal.

Small Intestine

- Mainly vascular ectasia and tumors
- Adenocarcinoma, lymphoma
- Leiomyoma, Meckel's diverticulum
- Benign polyp

- Ischemic, Crohn's disease
- *NSAIDs:* Erosion/ulcer

Colon/Anal Canal

- Hemorrhoids, fissure in ano
- Angiodysplasia
- Polyposis, diverticulosis
- IBD, ischemic colitis
- Ca colon, solitary rectal ulcer

Abnormal Stool

- Melena, hematochezia
- Steatorrhea—malabsorption of fat
- Toothpaste stool—stricture/Hirschsprung's disease
- Rice water stool—cholera
- Pea soup stool—typhoid
- Clay-colored stool—obstructive jaundice
- Red currant jelly stool—intussusception

GENERAL SYMPTOMS

Abdominal pain

This is the most important and commonest alimentary symptom.

Mechanism

- Spasm or stretch of the smooth muscles of hollow viscus
- Ischemia of viscera—spleen, intestine, etc.
- Stretch of the capsule—hepatic **stretch** of Glisson's capsule
- Pain from parietal peritoneum—inflammation, malignancy, irritation, etc.
- Referred pain to abdomen
- Psychogenic—depression, somatization disorder.

Types of Abdominal Pain

- Colicky pain—tubular organ
- Dull aching type of pain—from capsules of viscera—liver
- Sharp well-localized pain—parietal peritoneum
- Referred pain

Colicky pain: Upper GI, lower GI, biliary, renal, uterine.
- Upper GI colic
  - Upper abdominal pain
  - Intermittent
  - Related with food intake, and other upper GI symptom—nausea, vomiting, hematemesis
- Lower GI colic
  - Small intestine—central abdominal pain
  - Large intestine—loin pain
  - Other symptoms like diarrhea, constipation, bleeding PR

- Biliary colic
  - *Pain:* Right hypochondrium and epigastrium
  - Referred to angle of right scapula
  - Related to fatty food
  - Associated with jaundice and fever
  - Virchow's intermittent biliary fever (intermittent colic, jaundice and fever)
- Renal colic
  - Pain from loin to groin, testes and thigh
  - Associated with vomiting, sweating, oliguria, hematuria

Referred pain: Pain arising from lesions outside abdomen and referred to abdomen.
- Acute MI—inferior wall MI → epigastrium
- Diaphragmatic pleurisy → upper abdomen
- Basal pneumonia → upper abdomen
- Radicular pain → D_7 - L_1, bilateral radicular pain encircles the abdomen called girdle pain
- Herpes zoster—preherpetic and postherpetic neuralgia

Site of Abdominal Pain

- Upper abdominal pain—pain from upper GI, biliary tract, pancreas, liver
- Central abdominal pain—pain from small intestine, appendix, proximal colon
- Lower abdominal pain—pain from distal colon, urinary bladder, uterus
- Lateral abdominal pain—pain from spleen, kidney, colon
- Pain in the perineal area—pain form rectum, anus, prostate, urethra.

Features to note with Abdominal Pain

- Site and radiation
- Duration
- Severity
- Precipitating and relieving factors—food, vomiting, defecation, drugs
- Nature—colicky, dull aching
- Pattern—continuous, intermittent
- Associated symptoms—organ-related

Causes of Acute Abdominal Pain

- Inflammatory conditions
  - Appendicitis
  - Cholecystitis
  - Pancreatitis
  - Diverticulitis
  - Salpingitis
- Perforations
  - Peptic ulcer
  - Diverticular disease
  - Malignancy—colonic

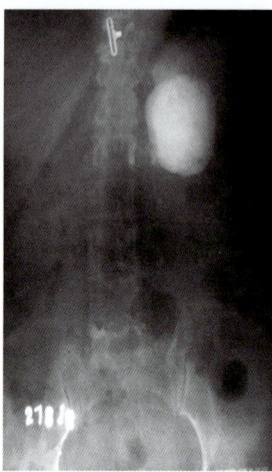

Fig. 6.2: X-ray showing calcified retroperitoneal tumor.

- Vascular
  - Mesenteric occlusion
  - Torsion testes
  - Dissecting aneurysm
  - Ruptured aortic aneurysm
- Obstruction
  - Intestinal obstruction
  - Biliary colic
  - Ureteric colic
- Peritonitis
  - Bacterial—spontaneous
  - Perforation
  - Chemical—pancreatitis
  - Ulcer perforation

Causes of Chronic Abdominal Pain

- Chronic acid peptic disease
- Neurological
  - Herpes zoster
  - Tabes dorsalis
  - Radiculopathy
- Retroperitoneal
  - Malignancy (Fig. 6.2)
  - Lymphadenopathy
  - Abscess
- Metabolic/endocrine
  - Diabetic ketoacidosis
  - Intermittent porphyria
  - Hypercalcemia
  - Dyslipidemia
- Hematological
  - Henoch-Schonlein purpura
  - Sickle-cell disease
  - Bleeding diathesis
- Drugs—corticosteroid, NSAIDs
- Psychogenic
  - Depression
  - Somatization disorder
  - Hypochondriasis
- Chronic inflammation of
  - Appendix, gallbladder
  - Peritoneum, pancreas
- Acid peptic disease

Medical Disorders Producing Abdominal Pain

- Endocrine
  - Diabetic ketoacidosis
  - Addisonian crisis
- Metabolic
  - Intermittent porphyria
  - Hypercalcemia
  - Familial hyperlipidemia
- Hematological
  - HS purpura
  - Sickle-cell anemia
  - Bleeding diathesis
- Neurological
  - Tabes dorsalis
  - Radiculopathy
  - Herpes zoster
  - Abdominal migraine
- Infection/infestation
  - Helminthiasis
  - Basal pneumonia
  - Diaphragmatic pleurisy
  - Spontaneous bacterial peritonitis
  - Tetanus
- Vascular
  - Myocardial infarction
  - Dissecting aneurysm of aorta
  - Mesenteric artery thrombosis
- Others
  - Hereditary angioedema (C_1 esterase deficiency)
  - Lead poisoning

Loss of Weight

- GI disorders
- Malabsorption syndrome
- Internal malignancy—carcinoma esophagus, carcinoma stomach
- Abdominal TB
- Anorexia nervosa
- Chronic liver disease

Distension of Abdomen

This is also a common complaint of patient, caused by the **"5Fs"–fat, flatus, fluid, feces, fetus"**:
- Fat—obesity
- Flatus—obstruction/ileus
- Fluid—ascites
- Feces—constipation
- Fetus—pregnancy

Causes

- Obesity—fat deposition in intra-abdominal and abdominal walls.
- Ascites
    - Peritoneal disease
    - Portal HTN
    - Hypoalbuminemia
- Intestinal obstruction
    - Gastric
    - Small intestinal
    - Large intestinal
- Marked organomegaly
    - Massive hepatomegaly
    - Massive splenomegaly
    - Hydronephrosis
- Mass lesions
    - Neuroblastoma
    - Wilms' tumor
    - Abdominal lymphadenopathy—TB, lymphoma
    - Mesenteric cyst
    - Ovarian tumors
- Uterus—in pregnancy

Feeling of fullness of abdomen without any of the above-mentioned conditions is postprandial fullness in dyspepsia, hepatobiliary disease, etc.

Fever in Alimentary Disorders

- Alimentary infection
    - Infective diarrhea, AIDS
    - Appendicitis, cholecystitis
    - Peritonitis, pancreatitis
    - Abdominal TB
- Inflammatory bowel disease
    - Ulcerative colitis
    - Crohn's disease
- GI malignancy
- Liver disease:
    - Hepatic amebiasis
    - Liver abscess—amebic, pyogenic
    - Cirrhosis liver—spontaneous bacterial peritonitis (SBP), Gram-negative septicemia
    - Liver malignancy
    - Granulomatous hepatitis.

Alimentary Symptoms Depending on the Anatomical Site

Site of disorder	Common symptoms
Esophagus	Dysphagia, odynophagia, heartburn, chest pain, hematemesis/melena
Stomach	Nausea, vomiting, epigastric pain, hematemesis/melena, early satiety, distention
Small intestine	
Duodenum	Pain, nausea, vomiting, hematemesis, melena
Jejunum	Pain, diarrhea, distention
Ileum	Pain, diarrhea, distention
Colon	Pain, diarrhea, constipation, bleeding per rectum (PR), distention
Rectum/anus	Pain, pruritus, constipation, incontinence, tenesmus, bleeding PR
Hepatobiliary	Jaundice, dark urine, pruritus, pale stool, pain, hematemesis/melena, distention
Pancreas	Pain, distension, steatorrhea, diabetes mellitus

HISTORY TAKING IN ALIMENTARY SYSTEM

- Presenting complaints—in chronological order:
    - Symptoms of upper GI, lower GI, hepatobiliary, pancreatic and other disorders.
- History of presenting Symptoms – detailing the symptoms (Refer to Symptomatology)
- Past history
    - Similar illness—peptic ulcer
    - Colitis—postdysenteric irritable bowel syndrome (IBS)
    - Hepatitis, blood transfusion, injections
    - Abdominal surgery—biliary, GI
- Family history
    - Similar illness—acute diarrheal disease
    - Food poisoning
    - Viral hepatitis
    - Genetic liver disease
        - Hemochromatosis
        - Wilson's disease
        - α-1 antitrypsin deficiency
    - Ca colon, IBD
    - Familial polyposis colon
    - Celiac disease
- Personal history
    - Alcoholism (details of quantity, duration)
    - Smoking
    - IV drug abuse
    - Overseas travel
- Treatment history
    - Aspirin, NSAID, corticosteroid
    - Anti-TB drugs
    - Other hepatotoxic drugs
    - Oral contraceptives
- Occupation—farming—leptospirosis, sewage disposal.

GENERAL EXAMINATION IN ALIMENTARY SYSTEM

- **Jaundice**—hepatobiliary disease, septicemia
- **Cachexia/wasting**—malabsorption, GI malignancy, chronic liver disease, abdominal tuberculosis
- **Anemia**
  - GI bleeding—occult/overt
  - Malnutrition, malabsorption
- **Edema**—malnutrition, malabsorption, cirrhosis liver, protein-losing enteropathy
- **Central cyanosis**
  - Cirrhosis of liver due to pulmonary arteriovenous fistula, portopulmonary shunt, tidal volume decreased→ called cirrhotic orthodeoxia
- **Nail:**
  - Clubbing—ulcerative colitis, cirrhosis of liver, malabsorption
  - Cirrhosis of liver—leukonychia, glassy nail, half-half nail
  - Azure lunulae—Wilson's disease—bluish discoloration of base of nail.
- **Pigmentation**
  - Hemochromatosis, cirrhosis of liver
  - Malabsorption syndrome—"Sun-kissed pigmentation" (Addisonian type)
- **Hand**—palmar erythema, Dupuytren's contracture, flapping tremor
- **Eye**
  - Jaundice, anemia, Kayser-Fleischer ring
  - Iritis—inflammatory bowel disease (IBD)
  - Xanthelasma—yellowish plaques or nodules in the subcutaneous tissue in the periorbital region due to deposits of lipids, usually seen in primary biliary cirrhosis, hyperlipidemia.
- **Skin**
  - Jaundice, pigmentation, easy bruisability
  - Petechiae, purpura, ecchymosis
  - Scratch marks—obstructive jaundice
  - *Spider naevi*
    - Consists of central arteriole from which radiate numerous small vessels which look like spider legs.
    - Size is just visible to 5 mm, seen in the area of SVC drainage.
    - Pressure applied with a pointed object to the central arteriole causes blanching of the whole lesion.
    - Presence of two or more always significant
    - Also seen in pregnancy, 2nd to 5th months, and disappear within 8 weeks of delivery.
  - *Paper money skin*
    - This consists of numerous small vessels scattered randomly throughout the skin.
    - These resemble the silk threads in American Dollar notes which accounts for the name.
    - This may be seen in similar distribution to Spider naevi.
  - Acanthosis nigricans—GI malignancy
  - Dermatomyositis—GI malignancy, colonic
  - Scleroderma—dysphagia, esophageal dysmotility.
  - Erythema nodosum—IBD
  - Pyoderma gangrenosum—ulcerative colitis
  - Palmar tylosis—Ca esophagus
- Parotid: Parotidomegaly—alcoholic liver disease, chronic calcific pancreatitis
- Lymph nodes
  - Left supraclavicular—Virchow's lymph node
  - Troisier's sign in upper GI malignancy, testicular tumors
  - Generalized lymphadenopathy—TB, lymphoma, AIDS
- Gynecomastia—cirrhosis liver, chronic alcoholism
- Groin—hernia, lymph node enlargement.

Stigmas of Chronic Liver Disease

In Compensated Liver Disease (from above down) (Figs 6.3 and 6.4)

- Parotidomegaly
- Telangiectasia, spider naevi
- Gynecomastia
- *Palmar erythema:* Reddening of palms of the hands affecting the thenar and hypothenar eminences
- Clubbing, leukonychia (Fig. 6.5)
- *Dupuytren's contracture:* This is a visible and palpable thickening of the palmar aponeurosis, most often of the ring finger, usually bilateral, occasionally affect the soles of the feet.
- *Loss of hair:* Axillary and pubic
- Muscle wasting
- Testicular atrophy

In Decompensated Liver Disease (Fig. 6.4)

With the above features:
- Altered sensorium
- Inversion of sleep rhythm

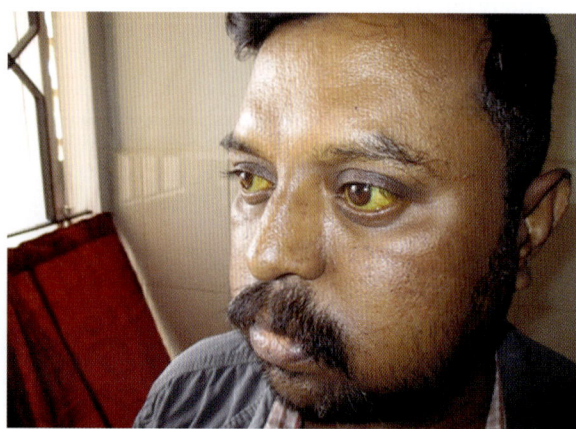

Fig. 6.3: Jaundice and parotidomegaly.

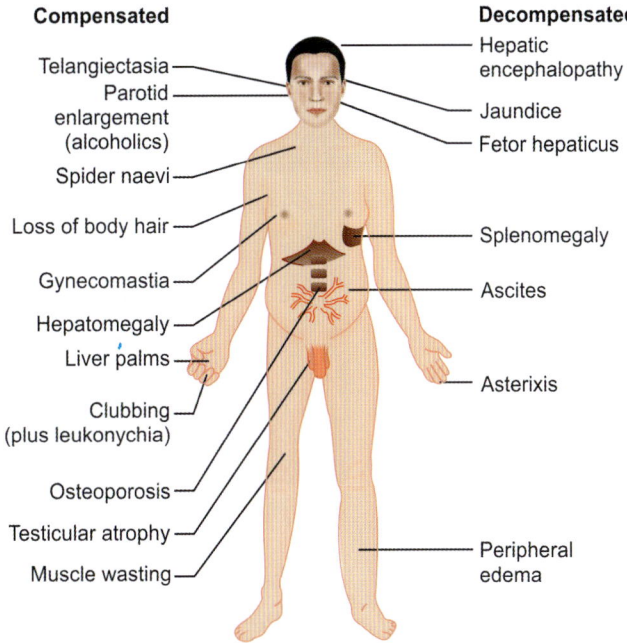

Fig. 6.4: Signs of chronic liver disease.

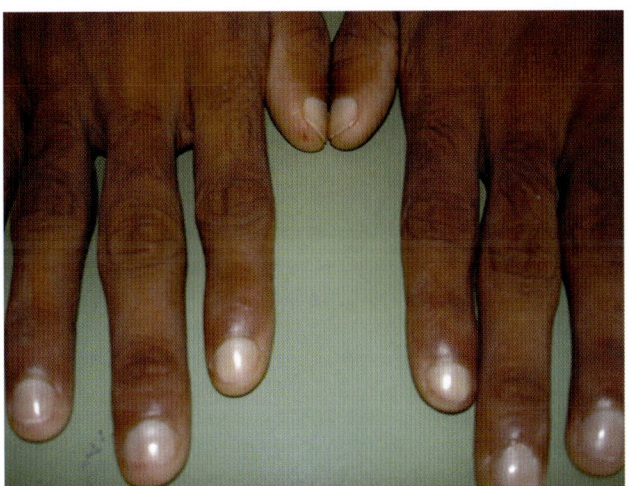

Fig. 6.5: Clubbing and shiny nails in cirrhosis.

- Jaundice
- Fetor hepaticus
- *Flapping tremor:* Ask the patient to stretch out his arms, separate the fingers and extend the wrist. Jerky irregular flexion extension movements at the wrist and metacarpophalangeal joints. This tremor is absent when coma supervenes.
  This also occurs in respiratory, renal failure, occasionally in hypoglycemia and barbiturate intoxication.
- Constructional apraxia, myoclonus
- Ascites, edema
- Hyperreflexia, extensor plantar.

ALIMENTARY SYSTEM EXAMINATION

Consists of:
- Examination of mouth and throat
- Examination of esophagus
- Examination of abdomen

Examination of Mouth and Throat

The very beginning of the GIT is, like the very end of the tract, accessible to examination without elaborate equipment.

Method

Position of the patient—sitting up either in a bed or chair with the head resting comfortably back on pillows.

A bright torch, tongue depressor, a pair of gloves are essential.

The lips, teeth, gums, tongue, palate, fauces and oropharynx are then visualized systematically.

Finally, palpation of the sides of the tongue, floor of the mouth and tonsillar region is carried out.

Lips

Features to be noted:
- Angular stomatitis
  - Cracks or fissures at the corners of the mouth
- Perleche
  - Angular cheilitis with maceration and fissuring of the oral commisures

- Cheilitis
  - Inflammation of the lips
  - Riboflavin deficiency and Fe-deficiency anemia
- Herpes simplex labialis
  - Grouped vesicles on the lips on a red base
  - Seen in febrile illness—pneumonia, malaria, viral fever
  - Uncommon in enteric fever.
- Ulcer lips
  - Aphthous ulcer
  - Ca lip—epithelioma, pyogenic granuloma
  - Chancre of primary syphilis
- Rhagades
  - Radiating scars diverging from the angle of the mouth and nose in congenital syphilis
- Circumoral pigmentation
  - Multiple small brown or black spots on the skin around the mouth
- Telangiectasia
  - Visible vascular lesion formed by dilatation of cutaneous blood vessels—can be a part of hereditary hemorrhagic telangiectasia.
- Retention cyst of mucous gland
  - Round translucent swellings with a white or bluish appearance.

Differential Diagnosis of Pigmented Lesions in the Mouth

- Addison's disease—blotches of dark brown pigment anywhere in the mouth.
- Peutz-Jeghers syndrome—pigmentation of lips, buccal mucosa or palate.
- Hemochromatosis—blue gray pigmentation of hard palate (Fig. 6.6).
- Heavy metals—lead—blue-black line on the gingival margin
- Malignant melanoma—raised painless black lesions anywhere in the mouth.

Teeth

Method: Using a tongue depressor to retract first the lips and then the cheeks, note the number of teeth and look for the following features:
- **Caries teeth**
- **Color of teeth**
  - Tartar—precipitated calcium salt of saliva over the lingual aspect of the lower incisor and canine
  - Reddish brown—chewing beetle nuts
  - Staining of teeth—both deciduous and permanent teeth showing horizontal bands of yellow or grey discoloration due to tetracycline therapy during antenatal period after the 14th week of pregnancy or in children up to the age of 8 years

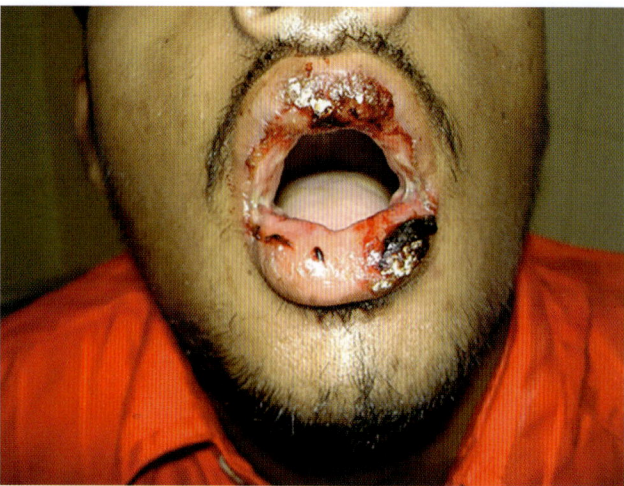

Fig. 6.6: Mouth ulcers—hand-foot and mouth disease.

  - Chalk white patches—in endemic fluorosis—dull englazed appearance sometimes with pitting and brown-staining.
  - Erythrodontia—reddish discoloration in porphyria.
- **Shape of teeth**
  - Ill-formed hypoplastic teeth—ectodermal dysplasia
  - Notched teeth—due to persistent cotton-biting
  - Pegshaped—central upper permanent incisors rounded in section and notched at the biting edge, seen in congenital syphilis—Hutchinson's teeth
  - Transverse ridging of teeth—in scurvy and rickets
  - Separation of teeth—enlarged jaw in acromegaly
  - Loss of upper central incisors—leprosy
  - Mulberry molars—molars with multiple, poorly developed cusps—in congenital syphilis.

Gum

Healthy gum is pink in color, adheres closely to the necks of the teeth and has a sharp border.

Features to Note

- *Gingival recession:* Teeth appear longer and exposing the cementum with increasing age
- *Gingivitis:* Swelling, redness and pain of gum
- *Pyorrhea alveolaris:* Recession of gingiva, presence of pus in the gingival margin or exudation of pus on pressure, indicates periodontal sepsis
- Stippled blue line of gum margin—lead poisoning—Burtonian line
- Red spongy swollen gum—scurvy
- Bleeding from gum—gingivitis, scurvy, immune thrombocytopenic purpura (ITP), acute leukemia

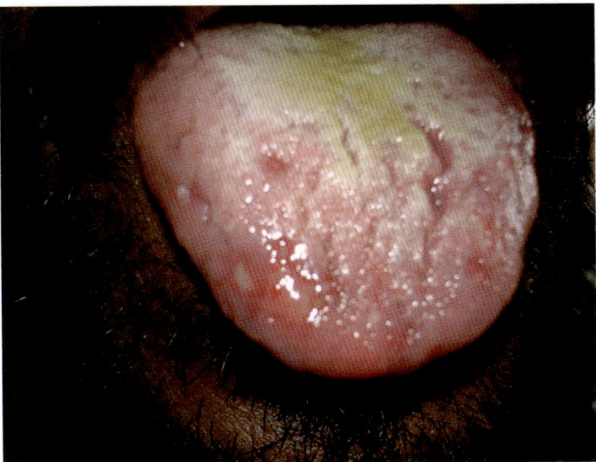

Fig. 6.7: Herpetic gingivostomatitis.

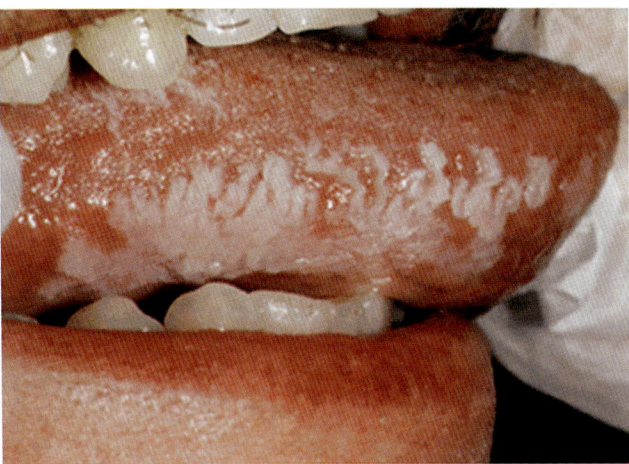

Fig. 6.8: Hairy leukoplakia in an HIV patient.

- Acute herpetic gingivostomatitis (Fig. 6.7)
  - Herpes simplex virus
  - Small vesicles on gum, cheek and palate
- Gum hypertrophy
  - Drug-induced—phenytoin, nifedipine
  - Cyclosporine
  - Pregnancy
  - Scurvy
  - Acute leukemia—monocytic
  - Gingivitis
- *Epulis:* Swelling arising in the gum from the periosteum of maxilla or mandible.

Tongue

Note the Following Features

- **Ankyloglossia**—inability to protrude the tongue.
  Causes—
  - Tongue tie—congenital short frenula
  - Malignancy of tongue
  - Bilateral LMN 12th nerve palsy with wasting and atrophy
- **Size of the tongue**
  - Macroglossia—acromegaly, cretinism, myxedema, amyloidosis, lymphangioma
- **Coating of tongue**
  - Normal—whitish fur—composed of epithelial debris, food materials and oral microbial flora
  - Excessive coating—typhoid fever and other febrile illness (Typhoid V tongue)
  - Moniliasis—thick curdy coating on the tongue.
- **Color of tongue**
  - Pale—anemia
  - Red—glossitis—beefy tongue—vitamin B_{12} deficiency
  - Magenta tongue—vitamin B_2 deficiency
  - Discoloration due to colored food
  - Yellowish—underneath jaundice
  - Bluish—cyanosis
  - Strawberry tongue—scarlet fever—enlarged papillae on a bright red surface
  - Lingua nigra—black tongue—due to elongation of the papillae over the posterior part of the tongue which appears dark brown due to accumulation of keratin
  - Moistness—indicates the state of hydration of body
  - Dryness—dehydration, diabetes mellitus, anticholinergic drug
  - Dry brown tongue—uremia, acute intestinal obstruction
  - Leukoplakia—whitish opaque areas of thickened epithelium (Fig. 6.8)
  - Hairy leukoplakia—pathognomonic feature of HIV infection—corrugated white plaques running vertically on the sides of the tongue— etiology is associated with EB virus
  - Chronic superficial glossitis—designated with 5 Ss—smoking, spirit, sepsis, spices and syphilis
  - Smooth or balded tongue—vitamin B_{12} deficiency, Fe-deficiency anemia.
  - Fissuring of tongue—congenital—horizontal - papillae normal, syphilitic—longitudinal with superficial glossitis
  - Median rhomboid glossitis—Lozenge-shaped area of loss of papillae and fissuring anterior to the foramen
  - Geographical tongue—localized irregular red areas of desquamated epithelium and filiform papillae surrounded by whitish yellow border.
- **Sides and underneath of tongue**
  - Ulcer of tongue—5 types—dental, aphthous, tuberculous, gumma and malignant
  - Calculi in the duct of sublingual salivary gland
  - Ulcer frenulum—in whooping cough
  - Sublingual varicosities
  - Cyst—dermoid cyst and ranula—bluish white swelling due to blockage of the duct of mucous gland.

- **Precancerous lesions of tongue—5 causes:**
  - Chronic superficial glossitis
  - Dental ulcer
  - Sessile papilloma
  - Syphilis
  - Plummer Vinson's syndrome
- **Pigmentation of tongue:**
  - Addison's disease
  - Peutz-Jeghers syndrome
  - Oral Lichen Planus
  - Acanthosis nigricans

Buccal Mucosa

Method: Retract the cheek with a spatula, inspect the buccal mucosa and note the following features:
- Opening of the parotid gland
- Koplik's spots—small bluish white spot surrounded by red areola opposite molar teeth—catarrhal stage of measles
- Pigmentation—causes as described above—in tongue and gum
- Aphthous ulcer, mucous retention cyst, papilloma, leukoplakia
- Monilial stomatitis—white patch seen in:
  - Debilitated children
  - Broad spectrum antibiotic therapy
  - HIV infection
  - Immunosuppressive drugs
  - Diabetes mellitus
  - Hypoparathyroidism—HAM syndrome
    - Hypoparathyroidism
    - Addison's disease
    - Mucocutaneous candidiasis
- Ulcers—causes:
  - Aphthous, traumatic
  - GI diseases—Crohn's disease, ulcerative colitis, celiac disease.
  - Rheumatological—SLE, Behcet's syndrome, Reiter's disease
  - Erythema multiforme
  - Infections:
    - Viral—herpes simplex, coxsackie
    - Bacterial—syphilis—primary chancre, secondary snail track ulcer
  - TB ulcer
  - Malignancy.

The Palate, Fauces and Pharynx

Position of the patient: Patient in the sitting position, keeping the head back, ask the patient to open his mouth wide and inspect the hard palate, soft palate and position of the uvula.

Make the patient to say 'Ah', which raises the soft palate, increases the visibility of the fauces, tonsils and oropharynx. If there is no good view of these structures, introduce a spatula to depress the base of the tongue for better visualization.

- Look for ulcers:
  - Erythema
  - Vesicles of the palate—herpes zoster—maxillary division of 5th
  - Vesicles of the pharynx—herpes zoster of 9th
  - Malignant ulcer—hard palate
  - Hole of the hard palate
  - Imperfect closure of cleft palate
  - Gumma, radionecrosis on treatment of Ca. palate.
- White patch on tonsillar region—causes are:
  - Diphtheria
  - Acute follicular tonsillitis
  - Thrush
  - Infections myonecrosis (IMN)
  - Agranulocytosis
- Rash—oropharynx
  - Exanthematous fevers
  - Herpangina
- Swelling of oropharynx—retropharyngeal abscess.

Palpation of the mouth, oral cavity and tongue for ulcer, swelling and calculi in submandibular duct.

EXAMINATION OF ESOPHAGUS

Esophagus is inaccessible for clinical examination.

Look for the symptoms related to the act of swallowing—dysphagia.

Investigate to reveal the structural and functional abnormalities of esophagus if symptoms present.
- Barium swallow
- Endoscopy
- Motility study—manometry, isotope Tc99 with solid or liquid food.

EXAMINATION OF ABDOMEN

Examination of gastrointestinal system consists of clinical evaluation of the entire length of the gut, the liver, the exocrine pancreas and the peripheral effect of the alimentary diseases.

Functional Anatomy

For purposes of description, abdomen is conveniently divided into 9 regions by the intersection of imaginary planes, 2 horizontal and 2 sagittal. The upper horizontal plane (transpyloric) lies at a level midway between the suprasternal notch and the symphysis pubis. The lower plane passes through the upper borders of the iliac crests. The sagittal planes are indicated on the surface by lines drawn vertically midway between the pubis and anterior superior iliac planes.

Regions over the Abdomen and its Contents (Fig. 6.9)

- Right hypochondrium—right lobe of liver, gallbladder, hepatic flexure of colon.

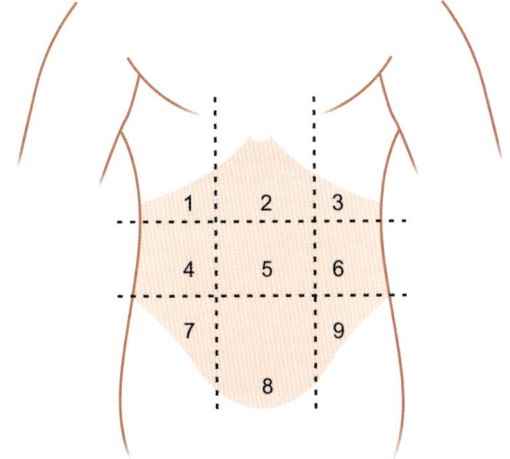

1. Right hypochondrium, 2. Epigastrium, 3. Left hypochondrium, 4. Right lumbar, 5. Umbilical, 6. Left lumbar, 7. Right iliac, 8. Hypogastrium, 9. Left iliac

Fig. 6.9: Regions over the abdomen.

- Epigastrium—left lobe of liver, stomach, transverse colon, lower end of esophagus and esophagogastric junction.
- Left hypochondrium—fundus of stomach, spleen, tail of pancreas, splenic flexure of colon.
- Right lumbar region—right kidney and its suprarenal gland, right ureter, ascending colon.
- Umbilical region—aorta, IVC, portions of stomach, head and body of the pancreas, duodenal loop, mesentery, small intestinal loops, lymph nodes.
- Left lumbar region—left kidney and its suprarenal gland, left ureter and descending colon, spleen if it enlarges grossly.
- Right iliac fossa—cecum, appendix, part of ascending colon, lymph nodes, right ovary and fallopian tube.
- Hypogastrium—urinary bladder, uterus in females, sigmoid colon and rectum.
- Left iliac fossa—part of the descending colon, part of sigmoid colon, left ovary and fallopian tube, lymph nodes.

Surface Marking of Abdominal Organs

Liver
- *Upper border*
  - 5th right intercostal space—midclavicular line
  - 7th right intercostal space—midaxillary line
  - 9th right intercostal space—scapular line—inferior angle of scapula.
- *Lower border:* Follows the right costal margin, in the epigastrium, it is from the tip of the 9th right costal cartilage to the tip of the 8th costal cartilage on the left by an oblique line midway between the xiphisternum and umbilicus.

Spleen
- Related to 9th, 10th and 11th ribs on the left side, long axis along the line of the 10th rib.

- Surface marking can be done by joining 3 points:
  - 9th left intercostal space—midclavicular line.
  - 1.5" to the left of 10th spine
  - 3.5" to the left of 1st lumbar spine.

Gallbladder
- Situated at the junction of 9th costal cartilage and outer border of right rectus abdominis.

Kidney
By drawing the *Morris parallelogram:*
- Two parallel horizontal lines are drawn on the back at the levels of 11th dorsal and 3rd lumbar spines.
- They are intercepted by 2 vertical lines drawn 3.75 cm and 8.75 cm respectively from midline.

INSPECTION OF ABDOMEN

Method: Patient should lie flat with one pillow under the head and the abdomen is exposed from the xiphisternum to the pubic symphysis. Start inspecting the abdomen and note the following features.

Shape of Abdomen
- *Normal:* Scaphoid shape in supine position, moves freely with respiration in vertical direction. No visible mass, no visible peristalsis except in a thin individual.
- Distention of abdomen
  - *Generalized fullness:* All the causes of this will start with the letter 'F'—Fat, Flatus, Fluid, Fetus and Feces.
  - *Localized fullness:* Around umbilicus—mesenteric cyst, small intestinal obstruction.
  - *Asymmetrical fullness:* Massive hepatomegaly, splenomegaly and ovarian tumor.
  - *Hernia:* It is a protrusion of viscus through an abnormal opening → incisional hernia, umbilical hernia, inguinal hernia.
- Sunken abdomen
  - Advanced stage of starvation
  - Upper GI malignancy

Umbilicus
Look at the shape and position of umbilicus.
- *Normal:* Slightly retracted and inverted, midway between xiphisternum and symphysis pubis.
- *Everted:* Umbilical hernia, impulse on cough present
- Slit of umbilicus
  - *Vertical*—Ovarian tumor
  - *Horizontal*—Ascites
- *Omphalolith:* Inspissated desquamated epithelium and other debris.
- Umbilicus buried in fat in obesity.
- Increase in distance between umbilicus and xiphisternum—in upper abdominal mass and ascites.

- Increase in distance between umbilicus and symphysis pubis—lower abdominal mass.
- Shift of umbilicus to opposite side—masses of lumbar and iliac fossa.
- Metastatic deposit in the umbilicus—Sister Mary Joseph nodule.

Scar

- Old scar
- Recent scar—pink—presence of vascularity
- Pigmentation of scar—Addison's disease

Skin over the Abdomen

- Vesicle of herpes zoster—produces abdominal pain which mimic acute abdomen.
- *Striae:* Stretching of the abdominal wall severe enough to cause rupture of the elastic fibers in the skin produces pink linear marks with a wrinkled appearance called striae seen in:
  - Cushing's syndrome—purple-colored striae
  - Ascites, pregnancy and recent loss of weight
- *Erythema Ab Igne:* It is a brown mottled pigmentation produced by constant application of heat.
- Pigmentation of midline below the umbilicus—linea nigra in pregnancy.
- Bruising over the periumbilicus and flanks—in hemorrhagic pancreatitis (Cullen's sign and Grey Turner's sign respectively).

Hair over the Abdomen

Secondary sexual hair—seen in male after puberty and adults.
- Absence—indicates hypogonadism
- Presence—in female, these indicate virilizing tumors

Movement of Abdominal Wall

To surprise the patient and to impress the examiners, squat down beside the bed so that the patient's abdomen is at eye level. Ask him to take slow deep breaths through the mouth and watch for the movement of the abdomen.

Normal—gentle rise in inspiration and fall in expiration.

Markedly decreased or absent—in peritonitis—still silent abdomen.

Visible Peristalsis

Tangential inspection is the best method.

Normal—no visible peristalsis except in thin individual where small intestinal peristalsis is visible.

Gastric visible peristalsis: Gastric outlet obstruction—pyloric stenosis.

Show waves of gastric peristalsis passing from left hypochondrium across the midline and subsiding beneath the right upper rectus.

Small intestinal visible peristalsis: Ladder pattern of peristalsis in the umbilical region.

Large bowel visible peristalsis—in large bowel obstruction, peristaltic waves seen in the upper abdomen moving from right to left (Fig. 6.10).

Veins over the Abdomen

- Normal direction of flow of blood in the veins over the abdomen is:
  - Above the umbilicus—upwards
  - Below the umbilicus—downwards
- Thin veins over the subcostal margin are normal.

Dilated Veins Over the Abdomen

Inferior vena cava obstruction
- Dilated veins seen over the abdomen and chest.
- Direction of flow is from below upwards and look for the direction below the umbilicus.
- These represent dilated anastomotic channels between the superficial epigastric and circumflex iliac veins below, and the lateral thoracic veins above, conveying the diverted blood from long saphenous vein to axillary vein.

Superior vena cava obstruction
- Dilated veins seen over the abdomen and chest.
- Direction of flow is from above downwards.
- Look for the direction above the umbilicus

Portal hypertension
- Portosystemic anastomosis occurs between the paraumbilical vein of the left branch of portal vein to the anterior abdominal wall veins.
- Dilated veins are seen radiating from the umbilicus.
- The direction of flow is away from the umbilicus.
- Because of their engorged appearance, they resemble Medusa's hair after Minerva had turned it into snakes and this sign is called *Caput medusae.*

Demonstration of Direction of Venous Flow

A finger is used to occlude the vein and blood is then emptied from the vein below the occluding finger with a second finger.

The second finger is removed and, if the vein refills, the flow is occurring towards the occluding finger. Repeat the same and remove the occluding finger, if the vein refills, the flow is occurring towards the second finger.

Note: The segment of the vein without tributaries is selected for the demonstration.

Pulsations of the Abdomen

- Visible pulsation of abdominal aorta in thin persons
- Epigastric pulsation—aortic aneurysm, right ventricular enlargement and vascular tumors of the liver.

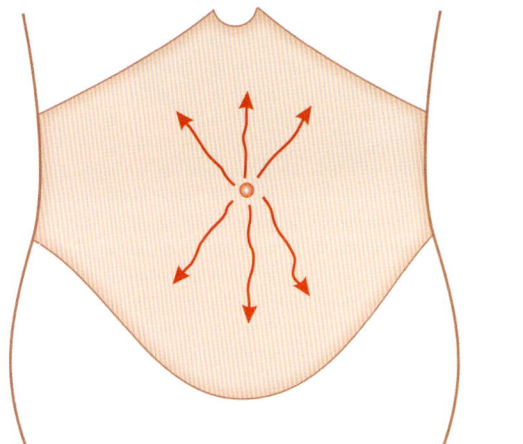

Normal
Direction of blood flow is away from the umbilicus.
Above the umbilicus upward, below the umbilicus downward

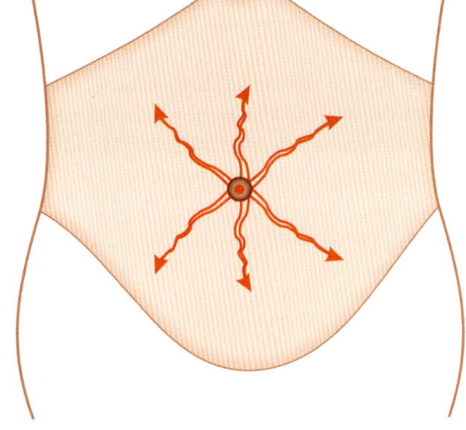

Portal hypertension
Direction of flow away from the umbilicus as normal veins are dilated and tortuous, radiating from the umbilicus
– Caput medusae

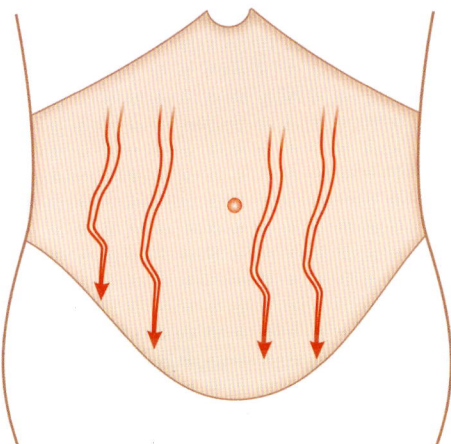

Superior venacaval obstruction
Above and below the umbilicus, the direction of blood flow
– Above downwards

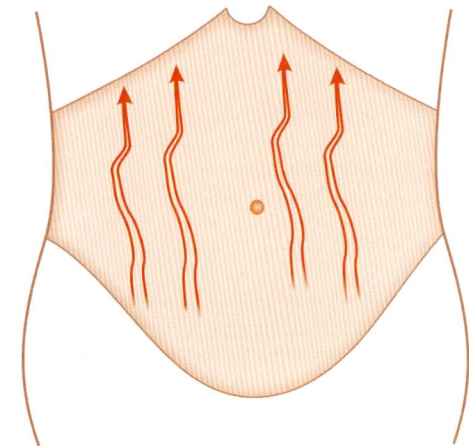

Inferior venacaval obstruction
Above and below the umbilicus, the direction of blood flow
– Below upwards

Fig. 6.10: Veins of the abdominal wall.

Inspection of Groin and External Genitalia

For hernia, lymph node enlargement, size of the penis and scrotal swelling.

PALPATION OF THE ABDOMEN

This part of the examination often reveals the most of the information. Successful palpation needs much practice.

Position of the Patient

Patient is lying flat on his back with head slightly raised with one pillow, the arms to the side.

The thigh flexed to 45° and the knees well drawn up. In palpation of the lower abdomen, it may be helpful to have the legs fully extended.

The examiner's hand should be warm to equalize the temperature of the skin of the anterior abdominal wall.

Successful palpation requires relaxed abdominal muscles. Ask the patient if any particular area is tender and examine this area last.

The art of palpation is to mould the relaxed right hand of the examiner to the abdominal wall of the patient, the best movement is gentle, but with firm pressure with the fingers held almost straight with slight flexion of the metacarpophalangeal joints.

The examiner should have a mental picture of the anatomical structures in each area.

Note the Following Features

- Local rise of temperature
- Guarding—resistance to palpation due to reflex contraction of the abdominal wall muscles. This may be due to tenderness or anxiety.
    - *Localized guarding:* Suggest localized peritonitis.
    - *Generalized guarding* may be due to anxiety.
- *Rigidity*—constant contraction of the abdominal wall muscles, always associated with tenderness, indicative of peritonitis.
- Rebound tenderness is said to be present when the abdominal wall, having been compressed slowly, is released rapidly and a sudden stab of pain results.
    This may make the patient wince and the face should be watched while this maneuver is performed.
    It strongly suggests the presence of peritonitis.
- Rovsing's sign
    - Crossed tenderness
    - Pressure applied over the descending colon may produce pain over right iliac fossa in appendicitis.

Structures Normally Palpable Are

- Lower border of liver in the epigastrium
- Aorta, lower pole of right kidney
- Rectus abdominis and digitations
- Colon in left iliac fossa
- Cecum—right iliac
- Loaded colon with feces—usually intended with examiner's finger
- Distended bladder.

Palpation of Liver (Figs 6.11 and 6.12)

A satisfactory position of the hands can usually be achieved if the examiner sits on the edge of the bed or kneels beside it.

The flat of one or both hands should be placed on the abdomen lateral to the rectus muscle, with the tips of the fingers pointing upwards.

The hands should be pressed firmly inwards and upwards, kept steady while on inspiration and advanced upwards during expiation by 1 or 2 cm.

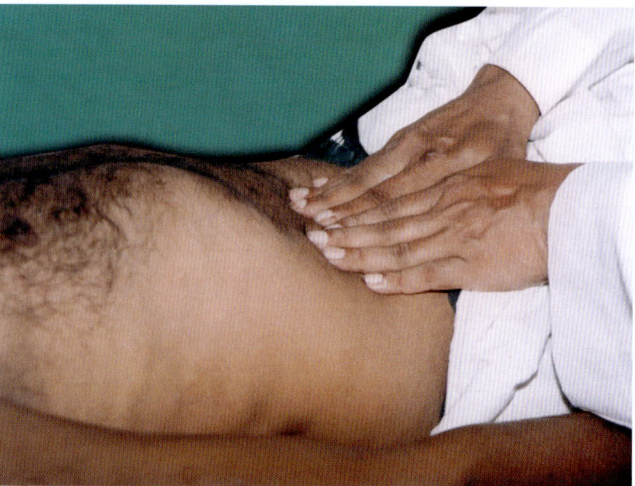

Fig. 6.11: Palpating of the liver—preferred method.

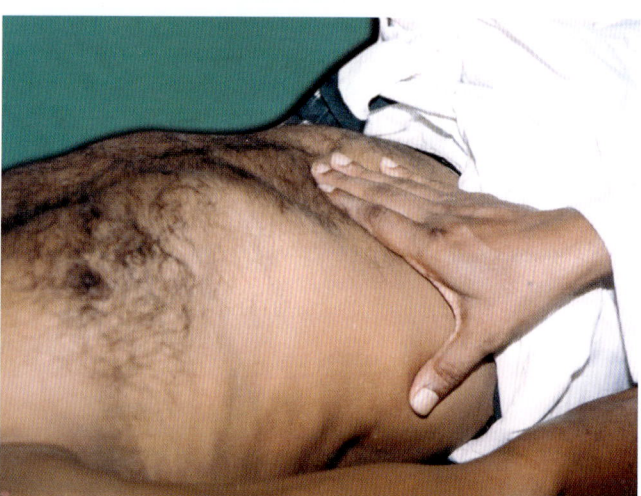

Fig. 6.12: Palpating of the liver—alternative method.

To avoid overlooking gross enlargement, it is advisable to palpate from right iliac fossa, gradually upwards.

By this upward movement, the tip of the fingers will slip over the edge of a palpable liver.

An alternative method of palpation is to place the right hand across the abdomen with the index finger parallel to the lower border of liver. The edge of the enlarged liver will touch the radial border of the index finger while moving up.

Pulsation of the liver is palpated by bimanual method, keeping the left hand behind the costal margin, the right hand over the enlarged liver and apply firm pressure to appreciate the pulsation.

Features to Note

- Measure the enlargement in right midclavicular line.
- Edge of the liver—sharp, round

- Consistency—soft, firm, hard
- Tenderness
- Surface—smooth or uneven/lobulated
- Pulsations of the liver
- *Riedel's lobe of liver:* It is a congenital variant of right lobe, a tongue-like projection from the inferior surface of the right lobe.
  It can be palpated and confused with an enlarged gallbladder or right kidney.

Palpation of Gallbladder

Normally gallbladder is not palpable. When it is enlarged, it is felt as a firm smooth globular swelling with distinct borders just lateral to the edge of the right rectus near the tip of the 9th costal cartilage. It moves well with respiration.

Causes of Palpable Gallbladder

With jaundice: Carcinoma triad.
- Carcinoma head of pancreas
- Carcinoma ampulla of Vater
- Carcinoma bile duct

Without jaundice: Mucocele of gallbladder.
- Cystic duct obstruction by stone
- Carcinoma of gallbladder

Courvoisier's law: In cholelithiasis, the gallbladder is thickened, contracted and not palpable due to repeated cholecystitis.
  Gallbladder is distended and palpable in carcinoma head of pancreas.

Murphy's sign: Ask the patient to breath deeply and palpate for gallbladder, at the height of inspiration, breath is arrested with pain in acute cholecystitis called Murphy's sign.

Palpation of Spleen (Figs 6.13 and 6.14)

- The spleen should enlarge more than 2 times to become palpable.
- For palpation, 2-handed technique is recommended.
- The patient is in supine position.
- The left hand is placed posterolaterally over the left lower ribs.
- The right hand is placed on the abdomen with fingertips directing to left hypochondrium.
- Start palpating from the right iliac fossa towards left hypochondrium.
- Do not start palpating too close to the costal margin, a large spleen will be missed.
- As the right hand is advanced closer to the left costal margin, the left hand compresses firmly over the rib cage so as to

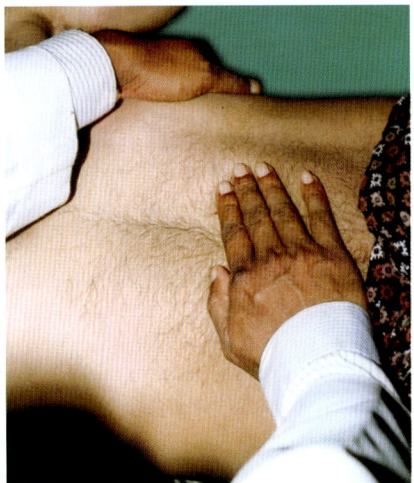

Fig. 6.13: Palpating of the spleen in the supine position.

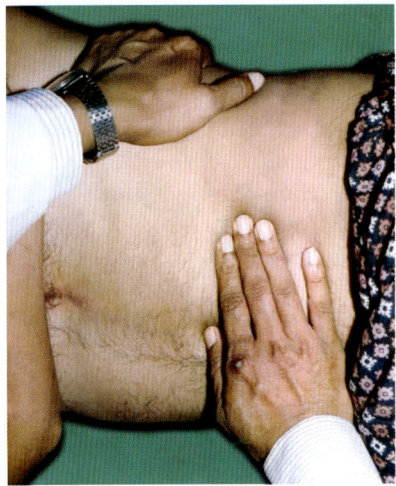

Fig. 6.14: Palpating of the spleen in the right lateral position.

  enable a slightly enlarged soft spleen to be felt as it moves downwards at the end of inspiration.
- If the spleen is not palpable in the supine position, the patient must be rolled onto the right side towards the examiner and palpation repeated. Here one begins to palpate close to the left costal margin.

Note the following features:
- Measure the enlargement from the tip of the 10th costal cartilage on the left side towards the right iliac fossa (10th rib is in line with the long axis of the spleen)
- Movement with respiration—well moving with respiration
- Consistency—soft/firm
- Tenderness
- Notch
- Insinuation of the fingers between the mass and the costal margin is not possible.
- Not bimanually palpable and upper border cannot be felt.

Grading of enlargement:
- *Mild:* 1–2 cm
- *Moderate:* 3–7 cm
- *Massive* > 7 cm

Huge spleen can be bimanually palpable and becomes ballotable if ascites is present with splenomegaly.

Palpation of Kidneys

- Lower pole of right kidney is normally palpable, left kidney is usually not palpable unless either low in position or enlarged.
- Use bimanual technique to palpate the kidneys.
- The patient lies flat on his back.
- The examiner's left hand slides underneath the back to rest with the palm of the hand under the right loin.
- The fingers remain free to flex at the metacarpophalangeal joints in the area of renal angle.
- The examiners right hand is placed over the right upper quadrant.
- Flexing the fingers of the left hand can push the contents of the abdomen anteriorly.
- Firm pressure is exerted by both hands at the height of inspiration to trap the palpable kidney between the two hands, otherwise it will prevent the descent of kidney by the diaphragm.
- Assess the size, surface and consistency of the palpable kidney.
- It is more often possible to feel a kidney by balloting.
- In this case, the renal angle is pressed sharply by the flexing fingers of the posterior hand.
- The kidney can be felt to float upwards and strike the anterior hand. Left kidney is also palpated in the same manner.
- Palpate the renal angle for tenderness.

Though kidney is retroperitoneal, it moves with respiration since it is related to the crus of the diaphragm posteriorly, the movement of the diaphragm is reflected to kidney producing restricted movement during respiration.

Causes of Palpable Kidney
- **Unilateral**
  - Normal right kidney
  - Hypernephroma
  - Hydronephrosis/pyonephrosis
- **Bilateral**
  - Polycystic kidneys
  - Bilateral hydronephrosis/pyonephrosis

Dipping Palpation

When significant ascites is present, the abdominal masses may be difficult to feel by direct palpation. Using the hand placed flat on the abdomen, mould the hand according to the shape of the abdomen, the fingers are flexed at the metacarpophalangeal joints so as to displace the underlying fluid. This enables the fingers to reach a mass covered in ascitic fluid. This method should be attended to palpate an enlarged liver or spleen with ascites.

Palpation of Urinary Bladder

Normally, urinary bladder is not palpable. When there is retention of urine, a smooth firm regular oval-shaped swelling will be palpated in the suprapubic region and its dome may reach as high as the umbilicus. The lateral and upper borders can be readily made out but it is not possible to feel its lower border. In females, however, the palpable bladder has to be differentiated from a gravid uterus, fibroid uterus and an ovarian cyst.

Palpation of Aorta and Femoral Arteries

Normally the aorta is not readily palpable, but with practice it can be felt by deep palpation a little above and to the left of the umbilicus. Palpation of the aorta is done by means of finger tips. Press the extended fingers of both hands held side by side deeply into the abdominal wall to make out the left wall of aorta and its pulsation. Remove both hands repeat the maneuver a few cm to the right. In this way the pulsation and width of aorta can be detected.

The femoral artery is felt just below the inguinal ligament at the midpoint between the anterior superior iliac spine and pubic symphysis. Place the pulps of the right index, middle and ring fingers over this site and palpate the wall of the vessel, strength and character of pulsation. Compare it with the opposite femoral pulse.

Clinical difference between splenomegaly and palpable left kidney.		
Features	Spleen	Left kidney
Movement with respiration	Well moving (2–3 cm)	Restricted movement (1 cm or less)
Notch	Present	Absent
Insinuation of the fingers between costal margin and the organ	Not possible	Possible
Direction of enlargement	Towards RIF	Towards lumbar region
Band of colonic resonance	Absent	Present
Bimanual palpation	Not palpable	Palpable
Ballotability	Not ballotable	Ballotable
Midline crossing	Crosses	Does not cross

Palpation of an abdominal mass

Descriptive features of intra-abdominal masses.
For any abdominal mass, the following should be assessed:
- *Site:* The region involved.
- *Size* (which must be measured) and *shape*
- *Surface:* Regular/irregular.
- *Edge:* Regular/irregular.
- *Consistency:* Soft/firm/hard
- Mobility and movement with inspiration:
  - Free movement
  - Restricted movement
  - No movement
- Whether it is pulsatile or not
- Whether one can get above/below the mass
- Bimanually palpable and ballotable

Causes of Abdominal Masses

Right Iliac Fossa
- Appendicular mass
- Ileocecal tuberculosis
- Amebiasis cecum
- Ca cecum
- Crohn's disease
- Psoas abscess
- Pelvic kidney
- Ovarian tumor/cyst

Left Iliac Fossa
- Loaded colon with feces
- Ca sigmoid or descending colon
- Diverticulitis
- Psoas abscess
- Ovarian tumor/cyst

Upper Abdomen
- Ca stomach
- Pseudopancreatic cyst
- Retroperitoneal lymphadenopathy
- Abdominal aortic aneurysm
- Pyloric stenosis
- Ca transverse colon

Pelvis
- Ovarian tumor/cyst
- *Uterus:* Pregnancy/fibroid
- Distended urinary bladder

Causes of Anterior Abdominal Wall Masses

- Lipoma, sebaceous cyst
- Dermoid, fibroma
- Malignant deposit
- *Hernia:* Epigastric, incisional, umbilical
- Hematoma

Causes of Cystic Masses in the Abdomen

- Epigastrium—pseudopancreatic cyst
- Right hypochondrium—hydatid cyst—liver
- Lumbar regions—hydronephrosis and renal cyst
- Umbilical region—mesenteric cyst
- Iliac fossae—ovarian cyst

Measurements of Abdomen

- Abdominal girth should be measured at umbilical level. Periodic measurement is done to assess prognosis in ascites, paralytic ileus.
- Measure the distance between lower end of xiphisternum to umbilicus and from umbilicus to symphysis pubis. Normally, umbilicus is in mid-position, displaced down in ascites, upper abdominal mass, displaced up in ovarian or pelvic tumors.
- Spinoumbilical measurement—distance between umbilicus and anterosuperior iliac spines. Normally, they are equidistant. Shift of umbilicus to one-side will occur in case of tumors originating from the other side of the abdomen.

PERCUSSION OF ABDOMEN

The aim is:
- Percuss all the quadrants of the abdomen
  - Usually light percussion is done, normally resonant note (tympanitic) over the abdomen, except the liver area.
- To detect fluid in peritonial cavity
  - Shifting dullness
  - Puddle's sign (to detect the presence of minimal fluid).
- To define the border and size of an organ or mass
- When palpation is uninformative, owing to the rigidity of the abdominal wall muscles.

Percussion of Liver

Upper border is defined by tidal percussion—5th right intercostal space in mid-clavicular line.
Lower border is percussed from right iliac fossa to the right costal margin until dullness is encountered.

Liver span
- It is the measurement of liver size from the upper border to the lower border in the midclavicular line.
- Normal liver span is 12.5 cm (12–15 cm)

Liver dullness is obliterated in:
- Severe emphysema
- Right pneumothorax

- Gas under the diaphragm (perforation of a viscus)
- *Shrunken liver:* Massive hepatic necrosis in fulminant hepatocellular failure
- Advanced cirrhosis liver.

Percussion of Spleen

If the spleen seems impalpable, occasionally percussion under the left costal margin may detect the enlargement. With patient supine, a dull percussion note, on full inspiration over the lowest intercostal spaces [8th and 9th] in the anterior axillary line suggests splenomegaly—Castell's method.

Percussion of Kidneys

Percussion over right or left subcostal mass will help to distinguish hepatic or splenic from renal masses due to the presence of colonic resonance.

Percussion of Bladder

An area of suprapubic dullness may indicate the upper border of an enlarged bladder.

Detection of Ascites

Shifting Dullness

With the patient lying supine, percuss the midline to verify resonance (tympanitic).

Now percuss laterally from the midline towards the flank, keeping the fingers in the longitudinal axis until dullness is detected.

This point should be noted and the patient is rolled to the opposite side and allow the fluid to move inside the abdominal cavity and the loops of intestine to float up by keeping the patient for one minute in that position.

Then percussion is repeated over the dull area noted. If shifting dullness is present, the area of dullness has changed to resonant.

Proceed the percussion in the opposite direction to get dullness due to the shifted fluid in the opposite flank.

The amount of peritoneal fluid should be 1.5–2 liters to demonstrate shifting dullness.

Presence of ascites without shifting dullness may occur in loculated ascites, fibrosis of mesentery, occasionally in massive tense ascites.

Fluid Thrill

Patient lies on his back, place the left hand of the examiner over the left lumbar region of the patient.

Get an assistant or the patient himself to put the side of his hand firmly in the midline of the abdomen and then flick or tap gently the right lumbar region with the right hand.

A fluid thrill or a pulsation is felt by the hand placed on the opposite lumbar region.

The purpose of keeping the assistant's hand is to dampen any impulse that may be transmitted **through** the fat of the abdominal wall.

Fluid thrill is present when fluid collection in the peritoneal cavity is >2 liters.

Puddle's Sign

This sign is elicited to detect the presence of minimal fluid when flanks are resonant.

It can detect as little as less than 200 mL of fluid.

Keep the patient in the knee arm position for five minutes so that the umbilical region of the abdomen is the most dependent part.

Now percuss around the umbilicus for dullness. Previously, resonant umbilical region becomes dull if minimal fluid is present.

Clinical Differentiation of Ascites from Ovarian Cyst and Intestinal Obstruction

Ascites
- Umbilicus transverse
- Dullness in the flanks
- Shifting dullness positive
- Fluid thrill positive

Large Ovarian Cyst
- Umbilicus vertical
- Resonance in the flanks
- Mass arising from pelvis
- One cannot get below the mass

Intestinal Obstruction
- Colicky pain
- Vomiting
- Constipation
- Resonant throughout
- Increased bowel sounds

AUSCULTATION OF ABDOMEN

Unfortunately, the sounds produced in the abdominal cavity are not as varied or as interesting as those one hears in the chest, but they are important.

Bowel Sounds

Bowel sounds are produced by the movement of fluid, feces and flatus within the bowel due to peristalsis.

They have a soft gurgling character and occur only intermittently every 5–10 seconds.

Bowel sounds can be heard over most parts of the abdomen in normal healthy people.

Increased Bowel Sounds

- In diarrhea, due to intestinal hurry, loud gurgling sound is produced, also called Borborygmi.
- Intestinal obstruction—bowel sounds are increased in intensity and frequency, high-pitched and tinkling quality due to the presence of air and fluid.
- Severe GI bleeding
- Carcinoid syndrome

Decreased Bowel Sounds

Complete absence of bowel sounds over a 3-minute period of auscultation is suggestive of paralytic ileus in peritonitis.

Friction Rub

A rough creaking or grating noise is heard as the patient breathes due to the rubbing of the inflamed parietal and visceral peritoneum. This may be audible over the liver—hepatic rub, over the spleen—splenic rub.

Causes of Hepatic Rub

- Liver abscess
- Malignancy liver
- After aspiration and biopsy
- Perihepatitis—gonococcal (Fitz-Hugh-Curtis syndrome).

Causes of Splenic Rub

Splenic infarct.

Venous Hum

It is typically heard between the xiphisternum and umbilicus in cases of portal hypertension.
It is due to the large volume of blood flowing through the paraumbilical vein in the falciform ligament to the epigastric or the internal mammary veins in the abdominal wall called Cruveilhier-Baumgarten murmur.
The association of the venous hum and the Caput medusae suggest the site of portal obstruction is intrahepatic.

Hepatic Bruit

Systolic bruit over the liver:
- Hepatocellular carcinoma
- Hemangioma of the liver
- Acute alcoholic hepatitis.

Vascular Bruit

Arterial systolic bruit can be heard over the abdomen:
- *Renal bruit:* Renal artery stenosis—best heard just above the umbilicus about 2 cm to the left or right of the midline.
- Abdominal aortoarteritis
- Abdominal aortic aneurysm
- Celiac axis, superior mesenteric artery narrowing.

Succussion Splash

Patient in the supine position, place the diaphragm of the stethoscope over the epigastrium, then roll the patient from side to side to agitate any fluid and gas in the stomach.
A splashing sound will be heard if the stomach is distended with fluid.
It can be heard normally for 2-3 hours **after food**. If it is present beyond 3 hours, it indicates gastric outlet obstruction in pyloric stenosis and also in advanced intestinal obstruction with grossly distended loops of bowel containing fluid and air.

EXAMINATION OF GROINS

For hernia, femoral pulsation and lymph nodes.

Hernias

Patient should be examined in the lying and standing positions. A strangulated hernia must be excluded in a patient with acute abdomen.

Inguinal Hernia

It lies medial to and above the pubic tubercle.
- Indirect inguinal hernia—passes through the internal inguinal ring which lies 1 cm over the femoral pulse at the mid-inguinal point.
- Direct inguinal hernia protrudes through the Hesselbach's inguinal triangle.
- *Femoral hernia:* This occurs lateral to and below the pubic tubercle, 2 cm medial to the femoral pulse.

Differential Diagnosis of a Groin Lump

Hernia, hydrocele of the tunica vaginalis, cyst of the epididymis, undescended testis, hydrocele of the cord, lipoma, lymph node, femoral aneurysm [pulsatile], saphena varix [disappear on lying down, nonpulsatile], psoas abscess.

Examination of External Genitalia

Examination of the male genitalia consists of inspection of penis and scrotum, palpation of testis, epididymis and vas deferens. Look for hypospadiasis, small testis, absence of testis, scrotal swelling.

Note the following features of the scrotal swelling:
- Get above the swelling
- Swelling—cystic/solid
- Transillumination [hydrocele of Tunica vaginalis, spermatocele]
- Visible only on standing—varicocele

Differential Diagnosis of Scrotal Swelling

- Hydrocele of TV
- Spermatocele [cyst of epididymis]

- Epididymitis—TB
- Varicocele
- Orchitis—mumps
- Tumors of the testes
- Torsion testes

EXAMINATION OF ANUS AND RECTUM

Abdominal examination is not complete without the performance of a rectal examination. The patient lies on his left side with the knees drawn-up—left lateral position. The examiner begins the inspection of anus and perianal area by separating the buttocks. The following must be looked for:
- Rectal prolapse, fistula in ano
- Skin tags, anal fissure
- Condylomata accuminata, thrombosed external piles
- Ca of the anus, pruritus ani

Next, ask the patient to strain: Incontinence and leakage of feces or mucus, abnormal descend of the perineum, presence of patulous anus. The tip of the gloved index is lubricated and placed over the anus. The patient is asked to breathe in and out through the mouth to distract and relax him. Slowly increasing pressure is applied with the pulp of the finger until the sphincter is felt. At this stage, the finger is advanced into the rectum slowly.

Palpate the anterior wall of the rectum for the prostate gland in the male and for the cervix in the female. The finger is then rotated clockwise so that the right lateral wall, posterior wall and left lateral wall of the rectum can be palpated in turn.

The finger is advanced as high as possible into the rectum and slowly withdrawn along the rectal wall. A soft lesion, such as small Ca rectum or polyp, is more likely to be felt in this way.

After the finger has been withdrawn, the gloved finger is inspected for blood, mucus, pus and the color of the feces. Occurrence of pain during the examination suggests anal fissure, ischiorectal abscess, thrombosed external piles and proctitis.

Causes of Palpable Mass in the Rectum

- Ca rectum, rectal polyp, Ca sigmoid colon
- Metastatic deposits in the pelvis [Blumer's shelf]
- Uterine/ovarian malignancy
- Prostatic/cervical malignancy
- Endometriosis, amebic granuloma
- Loaded colon with feces [intend on pressure].

EXAMINATION OF ACUTE ABDOMEN

The acute abdomen is a term which is applied to disorders of sudden onset, with dramatic severity and often requiring prompt surgical treatment. The most common examples are:

- Inflammations
  - Acute appendicitis
  - Acute pancreatitis
  - Acute cholecystitis
- Infections—peritonitis
- Perforation of viscus
- Intestinal obstruction
- Vascular occlusion
- Rupture of ectopic pregnancy

Features to Note

- History
- Pain—*Site*
- Upper abdomen
  - perforation of a gastric/duodenal ulcer
  - cholecystitis
  - pancreatitis
- Midabdomen
  - Small bowel disease
- Right iliac fossa—appendicitis
- Left iliac fossa—diverticulitis
- Lower abdomen—salpingitis, rupture—ectopic pregnancy
- Back pain—pancreatitis, dissecting aneurysm
- *Radiation*
  - Gallbladder pain—from right hypochondrium to right shoulder and interscapular region
  - Renal colic—loin to groin
  - Appendicitis—umbilicus to right iliac fossa
  - Pancreatitis—central upper abdominal pain to back
- *Character of pain*
  Colicky—small bowel
  Lasting for hours—inflammation and infection
- Onset—acute/slow
- Relation with food, drug, alcohol and trauma
- Other features—vomiting, dysuria, hematuria and menstrual irregularity.

Examination

General

- Fever—infective process
- Hypotension/shock—perforation, pancreatitis, rupture aneurysm, rupture—ectopic pregnancy
- Restless—biliary and renal colic
- Lie still—peritonitis
- Hippocratic facies—peritonitis
- Flexion of right hip—acute appendicitis—iliopsoas spasm.

Abdomen—Inspection

- Distension—localized/generalized
- Visible peristalsis—obstruction
- Bruising—trauma, pancreatitis.
- Scar of previous operation.

Palpation

- Guarding, rigidity
- Rebound pain, tenderness
- Obstructed hernia.

Percussion

- Obliteration of hepatic dullness—perforation
- Tympanitic note—intestinal obstruction
- Flank dullness—peritonitis.

Auscultation

- Increased bowel sounds—intestinal obstruction
- Decreased bowel sounds—paralytic ileus—peritonitis.

Conditions Mimicking Acute Abdomen

- Basal pneumonia
- Inferior wall MI
- Herpes zoster—preherpetic neuralgia
- Localized tetanus—anterior abdominal wall muscle
- Diabetic ketoacidosis, porphyria.
  Confirm acute abdomen by X-ray abdomen, USG abdomen and other appropriate laboratory investigations.

OTHER SYSTEM EXAMINATIONS IN ALIMENTARY DISORDERS

Nervous System

- Neuropsychiatric manifestations of hepatic encephalopathy.
- Neurological manifestation of alcoholism—tremor, peripheral neuropathy, Wernicke's encephalopathy.
- Wilson's disease—tremor, extrapyramidal signs, cerebellar signs.
- Autonomic neuropathy.
- Porphyria, tabes dorsalis, herpes zoster.
- Radiculopathy - D_7 to L_1.

Cardiovascular System

- CHF—congestive hepatomegaly, ascites
- Infective endocarditis—visceral infarct, mesenteric occlusion, splenomegaly
- Dissecting aneurysm—abdominal pain, shock
- Acute MI—inferior wall myocardial infarction (IWMI)—upper abdominal pain.

Respiratory System

- Basal pneumonia and diaphragmatic pleurisy → upper abdominal pain.
- Pulmonary TB—dissiminated TB → [TB peritonitis, hepatosplenomegaly, intestinal TB]
- Chronic obstructive pulmonary disease (COPD) and chronic liver disease—$\alpha 1$ antitrypsin deficiency
- Chronic suppurative lung disease → amyloidosis → hepatosplenomegaly
- Anti-TB drugs → hepatitis
- Bronchiectasis and cirrhosis liver—mucoviscidosis.

Rheumatological Disorders

- Inflammatory bowel disease—seronegative spondyloarthritis.
- HS purpura—polyarthritis, abdominal pain, bloody diarrhea.
- Whipple's disease—polyarthritis
- Vasculitis of viscera—rheumatoid arthritis
- Progressive systemic sclerosis—dysphagia, GERD
- SLE—hepatosplenomegaly.
- Analgesic—NSAIDs → gastric and intestinal ulcers

Hematological Disorders

- Sickle-cell disease—abdominal pain
- HS purpura—abdominal pain, bloody diarrhea
- Anemia—malabsorption
- Pernicious anemia—atrophic gastritis, achlorhydria
- Bleeding diathesis—intra-abdominal bleed
- Anticoagulant therapy—intra-abdominal bleed
- Hematological malignancy—hepatosplenomegaly.

Metabolic Disorders

- Diabetic ketoacidosis—upper abdominal pain
- Dyslipidemia—upper abdominal pain
- Acute intermittent porphyria—abdominal pain
- Hypercalcemia—abdominal pain, constipation
- Diabets mellitus—autonomic neuropathy
- Hemochromatosis—Cirrhosis liver.

Internal Malignancy

Secondary liver.

DIFFERENTIAL DIAGNOSIS OF COMMON CLINICAL SIGNS OF ABDOMEN

Differential Diagnosis of Splenomegaly

Mechanism

- Infection—enteric fever
- Proliferation—hemolytic anemia
- Congestion—portal hypertension
- Infiltration—gaucher's disease
- Neoplasm—leukemia.

Causes

Mild Splenomegaly (up to 2 cm)

Infections
- Viral—IMN, viral hepatitis, HIV, CMV, etc.
- Bacterial—enteric fever, miliary TB, infective endocarditis, septicemia, brucellosis
- Parasitic—early malaria, kala-azar.

Noninfections
- Hematological—chronic Fe-deficiency anemia, megaloblastic anemia, multiple myeloma, polycythemia vera
- Rheumatological—SLE, stills disease + causes of moderate and massive splenomegaly.

Moderate Splenomegaly (3–7 cm)
- Hemolytic anemia
- Acute leukemia, lymphoma
- Cirrhosis with portal hypertension + causes of massive splenomegaly.

Massive Splenomegaly (>7 cm)
- Chronic myeloid leukemia
- Chronic malaria
- Myelofibrosis
- Extrahepatic portal hypertension
- Gaucher's disease
- Kala-azar.

Differential Diagnosis of Hepatomegaly

Pathogenesis of Hepatomegaly

- Infection, congestion, infiltration, neoplasm
- Hematological disorder, biliary diseases, etc.

a. *Infections*
   - Viral—viral hepatitis, IMN, HIV
   - Bacterial—enteric fever, septicemia, miliary TB, brucellosis, leptospirosis
   - Protozoal—malaria, kala-azar
   - Parasitic—hydatid disease, schistosomiasis
   - Fungal—histoplasmosis, actinomycosis

b. *Congestion:* CHF, pericardial disease, IVC obstruction, Budd-Chiari syndrome.

c. *Alcoholic liver disease:* Fatty liver, Acute hepatitis, chronic hepatitis, cirrhosis.

d. *Cirrhosis liver:* Macronodular – posthepatic.

e. *Infiltration:* Glycogen storage disease, amyloidosis, Gaucher's disease, fatty infiltration [NASH—non-alcoholic steatohepatitis]

f. *Hematological:*
   - Extramedullary hemopoiesis
   - Hemolytic anemia, myelofibrosis
   - Osteopetrosis, anemia → fatty liver.

g. *Biliary disease:* Primary biliary cirrhosis, obstructive jaundice.

h. *Neoplasms:*
   - Primary: Hepatocellular Ca
   - Secondary: Hematological malignancy—leukemia, lymphoma

i. *Miscellaneous:* SLE, Still's disease.

Differential Diagnosis of Mild Hepatomegaly (Up to 4 cm)

- *Hepatitis:* Viral, bacterial, granulomatous, amebic
- CHF
- Fatty liver, leukemia, lymphoma
- Early malaria, kala-azar.

Differential Diagnosis of Moderate Hepatomegaly (4–8 cm)

- Malaria, kala-azar
- Liver abscess
- Severe CHF
- Macronodular cirrhosis
- Metabolic—glycogen storage disease
- Gaucher's disease
- Malignancy liver
- Hematological—myelofibrosis, osteopetrosis.

Differential Diagnosis of Massive Hepatomegaly (>8 cm)

- Cystic disease—polycystic liver, hydatid disease
- Neoplasms—primary and secondary
- Metabolic—glycogen storage disease
- Gaucher disease
- Congestive hepatomegaly—pericardial disease
- Right ventricular endomyocardial fibrosis (RVEMF).

Differential Diagnosis of Irregular Hepatomegaly

- Macronodular cirrhosis
- Malignancy liver
- Polycystic liver
- Hydatid cyst of liver
- Hepar lobatum.

Causes of Tender Hepatomegaly

- Congestive hepatomegaly—no jaundice
- Amebic liver abscess—no jaundice
- Pyemic liver abscess—jaundice ±
- Hepatitis—Viral—jaundice +
- Toxic hepatitis—jaundice ±
- Hepatic amebiasis—no jaundice
- Cholangitis—jaundice +
- Malignancy—jaundice ±.

Palpable Liver without Hepatomegaly

- Emphysema
- Right-sided pneumothorax

- Right-sided pleural effusion
- Subphrenic abscess
- Visceroptosis.

Causes of Hepatic Calcification

- Hydatid cyst
- TB
- Histoplasmosis
- Hemangioma
- Intrahepatic biliary calculi
- Gumma.

Based on Consistency of Liver

- Soft
  - Acute congestive heart failure
  - Acute infection—viral, enteric, septicemia
- Firm
  - Chronic congestive heart failure
  - Chronic infection
  - Hematological, infiltrative
- Hard
  - Primary tumors—hepatocellular carcinoma
  - Secondaries.

Differential Diagnosis of Hepatosplenomegaly

- *Infections:*
  - *Viral:* IMN, viral hepatitis, HIV
  - *Bacterial:* Enteric fever, miliary TB, septicemia, brucellosis, infective endocarditis
  - *Parasitic:* Malaria, kala azar and hydatid disease
- *Congestive:* CHF, pericardial disease, Budd-Chiari syndrome
- Cirrhosis with portal HTN
- Hematological
  - Hemolytic anemia
  - Osteopetrosis
  - Chronic deficiency anemia (Iron + vit. B_{12})
- Neoplasm
  - Leukemia
  - Lymphoma
  - *Metabolic:* Glycogen storage disease, amyloidosis, Gaucher's disease
  - *Miscellaneous:* SLE, Still's disease.

Causes of Hepatosplenomegaly with Ascites

- Cirrhosis, portal HTN with ascites
- Lymphoma
- Disseminated TB
- Malignancy liver with splenomegaly and peritoneal dissemination.

Causes of Hepatosplenomegaly with Fever

- *Infections:*
  - *Viral:* IMN, HIV, CMV, viral hepatitis
  - *Bacterial:* Enteric fever, miliary TB, septicemia, brucellosis
  - *Parasitic:* Malaria, kala-azar
- *Noninfections:*
  - Leukemia, lymphoma
  - SLE, Still's disease.

Causes of Hepatosplenomegaly with Anemia

- Chronic nutritional anemia, hemolytic anemia, myelofibrosis
- Leukemia, lymphoma
- *Infections:* Septicemia, miliary TB, infective endocarditis
- Chronic malaria, kala-azar
- Cirrhosis with portal HTN, and hypersplenism.

Causes of Hepatosplenomegaly with Lymphadenopathy

- IMN, HIV, miliary TB
- Leukemia, lymphoma
- SLE, Still's disease.

Causes of Hepatosplenomegaly with Jaundice

- *Infections:*
  - *Viral:* Viral hepatitis, IMN, mumps
  - *Bacterial:* Enteric fever, septicemia, leptospirosis
  - *Parasitic:* Malaria
- *Noninfectious:*
  - Cirrhosis liver—decompensated
  - Hemolytic anemia
  - Malignancy liver.

Causes of Hepatosplenomegaly with leeding Tendency

- Septicemia
- Miliary TB
- Cirrhosis liver
- Myelofibrosis
- Systemic lupus erythematosus (SLE)
- Acute leukemia.

Splenomegaly in Malignancy of Liver

- Hepatocellular carcinoma developing in cirrhotic patients
- Portal vein thrombosis
- Disseminated malignancy with portal hypertension.

CLINICAL EVALUATION OF ASCITES

Ascites means fluid collection in the peritoneal cavity.

Symptoms

- Fullness and distension of abdomen
- Abdominal pain
- Respiratory distress—tense ascites.

Signs

- Flanks full, umbilicus everted, umbilical hernia
- Striae
- Scrotal edema
- Pleural effusion—right side
- Shifting dullness, fluid thrill.

Etiology

Divided into two groups:
1. With peritoneal disease
2. Without peritoneal disease.

With Peritoneal Disease

- *Bacterial peritonitis:* Spontaneous/secondary— perforation viscus
- Tuberculosis, granulomatous, Whipple's disease
- Malignancy.

Without Peritoneal Disease

With portal hypertension [refer to topic on portal hypertension]

With hypoalbuminemia
- Cirrhosis liver
- Nephrotic syndrome
- Malnutrition
- Protein-losing enteropathy
- *Endocrine disorders:* Myxedema, Meige syndrome, Struma ovarii
- *Visceral leakage:* Pancreatitis, biliary, chylous, nephrogenic—urine ascites

Etiology Depending on the Nature of Ascites Fluid

Transudates

- Cirrhosis liver (Fig. 6.15)
- Nephrotic syndrome
- Hypoalbuminemia
- CHF
- Pericardial disease
- Budd-Chiari syndrome.

Exudates

- Bacterial peritonitis
- Tuberculosis
- Neoplasm
- Pancreatitis
- Chylous ascites (Fig. 6.16).

Common Causes of Ascites

- Cirrhosis liver
- Nephrotic syndrome
- CHF
- Bacterial peritonitis

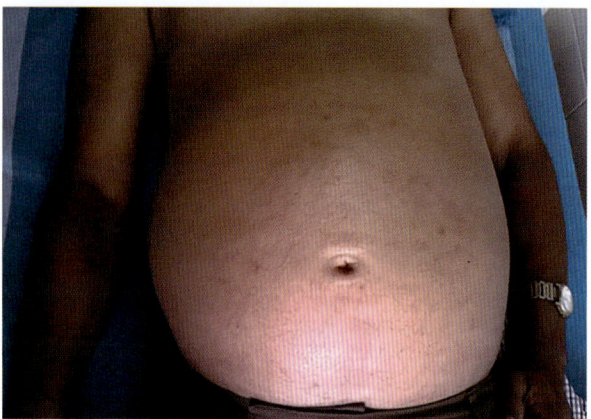

Fig. 6.15: Ascites in a patient with cirrhosis of liver.

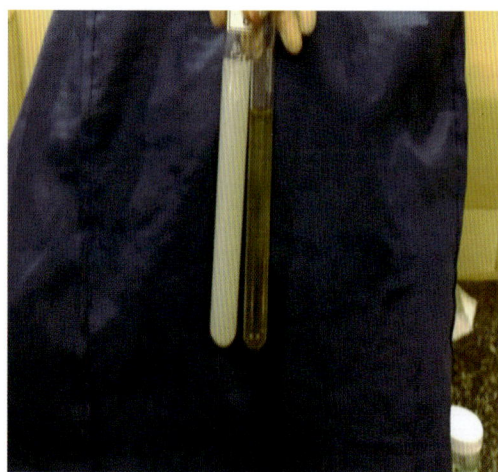

Fig. 6.16: Milky fluid of chylous ascites.

- Tuberculosis
- Malignancy.

Causes of Hemorrhagic Ascites

- *Malignancy:* Mesothelioma of peritoneum
- Secondaries—peritoneum
- Acute hemorrhagic pancreatitis
- Infarction of gut and spleen.

Mechanism of Ascites in Cirrhosis Liver

Primary Factors

- Hypoalbuminemia
- Portal hypertension
- Secondary hyperaldosteronism
- Peritoneal lymphatic obstruction.

Aggravating Factors

- Upper GI bleed
- Portal vein thrombosis

- *Cirrhotic activity:* Alcohol, hepatotoxic drugs
- Malignancy liver
- Spontaneous bacterial peritonitis.

Differential Diagnosis of Ascites

- Mesenteric cyst
- Hydronephrosis
- Ovarian cyst.

Clinical Clues to Ascites

1. Onset
   - Acute → Budd-Chiari syndrome, bacterial peritonitis
   - Subacute → congestive heart failure, nephrotic syndrome
   - Insidious → tuberculosis, malignancy
2. Ascites with fever
   - Infection/malignancy
3. Ascites with pain: Peritoneal diseases
4. Ascites without pain
   - Cirrhosis,
   - Nephrotic syndrome,
   - CHF
5. Ascites with pedal edema
   - Cirrhosis,
   - Nephrotic syndrome
6. Ascites without pedal edema: Peritoneal diseases
7. Ascites with jaundice: Chronic liver disease
8. Ascites without jaundice
   - CHF
   - Nephrotic syndrome
9. Ascites with dyspnea
   - CHF
   - Corpulmonale
   - Tense ascites
10. Ascites without dyspnea—early ascites of any etiology
11. Ascites with bleeding manifestations: Liver disease
12. Ascites without bleeding manifestations: Peritoneal diseases
13. Ascites with hepatosplenomegaly
    - Cirrhosis
    - TB
    - Lymphoma
    - Malignancy liver with portal vein thrombosis
14. Ascites of cardiac cause
    - Constrictive pericarditis
    - RVEMF.

Investigations in Ascites

Ascites Fluid Study

Cytology
- RBCs—hemorrhagic
- WBC > 500—increase in polymorphs—acute infection increase in lymphocytes—chronic infection—TB
- Malignant cells.

Protein
- >3 g—exudates
- <3 g—transudates

SAAG < 1.1—exudates
LDH > 200—exudates
CEA [carcinoembryogenic antigen]—Ca colon
AFP - Hepatocellular Ca
Culture of the fluid

USG abdomen

CT abdomen

Spontaneous Bacterial Peritonitis

Seen in:
- Cirrhosis liver
- Nephrotic syndrome with ascites decreased immunological status.

Spread of organism
- Hematogenous
- Lymphatic and
- Through bowel wall.

Organism
- E. coli
- Pneumococci
- H. influenzae.

Clinical features
- Fever,
- Pain in abdomen,
- Tender ascites,
- Precipitation of hepatic encephalopathy
- Hypotensions
- Septicemia.

Diagnosis
- Ascites fluid > 500 WBC/mL, >50% polymorphs
- Isolation of organism from ascites fluid.

Diagnostic Criteria of Types of Ascitic Fluid Infection

Monomicrobial

Spontaneous bacterial peritonitis—polymorph > 250, culture +ve.
  Monomicrobial non-neutrocytic bacterascites—polymorphs < 250, culture +ve {MNB}.
  Culture negative neutrocytic ascites [CNNA]—polymorphs > 250, culture –ve.

Polymicrobial

Secondary bacterial peritonitis—polymorphs > 250, culture +ve, multiple [Perforation viscus] organism.
  Polymicrobial bacterascites—polymorphs < 250, culture +ve, multiple organisms.

Management of Spontaneous Bacterial Peritonitis (SBP)

- *Drug treatment:* Antibiotic, depends on culture and sensitivity

- New generation cephalosporin
- Newer quinolones
- Metronidazole
- Other supportive measures
- Treatment of ascites and liver disease.

MALABSORPTION SYNDROME

It refers to defective absorption of essential nutrients, vitamins, minerals, and electrolytes.

Pathogenesis

- Luminal defect
  - Maldigestion—exocrine pancreatic abnormality
- Mucosal defect
  - Mucosal damage—tropical sprue
  - Mucosal reduction of absorption surface— intestinal resection
- Postmucosal defect
  - Lymphatic obstruction—TB, lymphoma.

Etiology

Digestive Disorders

- Pancreatic disease
- Gastric surgery
- Abnormal bile salt metabolism—liver disease
- Distal ileopathy—small intestine-bacterial overgrowth [Blind loop syndrome]

Absorption Disorders

Mucosal abnormality—may be global defect or isolated defect

- Tropical sprue
- Hartnup disease
- Coeliac disease
- A β lipoproteinemia
- Whipple's disease
- Congenital megaloblastic anemia
- Lymphoma
- Disaccharidase deficiency
- Intestinal tuberculosis
- Radiation enteritis
- Crohn's disease.

Reduced Absorption Surface

- Short bowel syndrome—intestinal resection
- Ileojejunal bypass.

Infections

- Tropical sprue
- Acute enteritis
- Parasites—*Giardia, Strongyloides.*

Drugs

- Neomycin
- Colchicine
- Biguanides
- Phenindione.

Lymphatic Obstruction

Tuberculosis, lymphoma.

Chronic Venous Congestion of Intestine

- Chronic CCF
- Pericardial disease.

Clinical Features

Main features are:
- Diarrhea
- Malnutrition
- Weight loss.

Malabsorbed Substance

Clinical features
- Fat:
  - Steatorrhea: Bulky, greasy, malodorous stool.
  - Weight loss
- Protein: Muscle wasting, edema, leukonychia.
- Carbohydrates:
  - *Fullness of abdomen*, watery diarrhea, flatus, borborygmi.
- *Vitamin A:* Follicular hyperkeratosis, night blindness.
- *Vitamin D:* Rickets, osteomalacia, proximal myopathy.
- *Vitamin K:* Bleeding tendency.
- *Vitamin B_{12} and folic acid:* Anemia, neuropathy, angular stomatitis, glossitis.
- *Vitamin C:* Scurvy—bleeding gum.
- *Iron:* Anemia, cheilitis, glossitis, koilonychia.
- Zinc:
  - Acrodermatitis enteropathica
  - Calcium and magnesium
  - Paresthesia, tetany
- Bile salt
  Steatorrhea, deficiency of fat soluble vitamin.

Investigations

Stool

- Macroscopy: Steatorrhea
- Microscopy:
  - Fat globules stool fat estimation (normal <7 g/day)
- Fecal nitrogen: Normal—2.5 g/day.

Blood Examination

- Serum protein, serum Fe, S –B_{12}
- Serum folate, serum calcium, serum magnesium
- Prothrombin time
- Peripheral smear.

Specific Tests

- *D-xylose test:* Carbohydrate absorption—25 g given orally and urinary excretion for the next 5 hours, more than 4.5 g is normal
- Shilling test for vitamin B_{12} absorption
- *Lundh test:* For pancreatic function
- *Imaging*
  - Barium meal follow through
  - Tropical sprue: Flocculation and segmentation
  - Anatomical abnormality: Ulceration, stricture, fistula, diverticula, blind loop.
- *Culture of small intestinal content:* Normal < 10^5 organism/mL
- *Biopsy of small intestine*
  Mucosa: Villous pattern, crypts, inflammatory cell infiltration
  Celiac disease: Subtotal/partial villous atrophy
  Tropical sprue: Partial villous atrophy
  Whipple's disease: PAS positive macrophage
  Lymphoma: Infiltration of abnormal lymphoid cells
  Tuberculosis: Characteristic granulomatous lesions
  - Breath test
    - Hydrogen breath test—in lactase deficiency
    - C-xylose test—(C^{14} labelled)—bacterial overgrowth indicates $\uparrow {}^{14}CO_2$ production.

Management

- Fat and carbohydrate intake is ↓ if diarrhea present.
- Supplementation of substance malabsorbed.
- Parenteral support of nutrients, if needed.
- Treatment of primary cause.

INFLAMMATORY BOWEL DISEASE

Consists of ulcerative colitis and Crohn's disease, denotes idiopathic chronic inflammatory disease of intestine.

Ulcerative colitis (UC) is an inflammatory disorder of the colonic mucosa with remission and relapse, rectal mucosa is always involved with variable extension proximally.

Crohn's disease is an inflammatory disorder affecting any part of the GI tract, of unknown etiology, most commonly affects the terminal ileum or the ileocecal region.

Etiology

- Genetic factors
  - Inflammatory modulating gene,
  - Chromosome 16 in Crohn's disease
  - Chromosome 12 in UC
  - HLA – DR 103 – severe UC
- Environmental factors
  - Nonsmokers—UC
  - Smokers—Crohn's disease
- Appendicectomy protects from ulcerative colitis.
- *Diet:* Low residue high refined sugar diet—Crohn's disease.
- *Immunological:* Humoral and cellular immune response to a variety of antigens have been described. Cytokines—TNF α and IL_1 → fever and systemic symptoms.

Pathology

Ulcerative Colitis

- Most common site—proctosigmoid—40%
- Histologically mucosal inflammation—acute and chronic inflammatory cell infiltration of lamina propria and crypts—cryptitis and crypt abscess
- Distortion and disappearance of Goblet cells
- Dysplasia and ↑ mitotic rate → Ca colon.

Crohn's Disease

- Most common site—distal ileum and right side of colon
- Entire wall is affected, edema, thickening, deep ulcers, fistula to bowel, bladder, vagina
- More than one segment of the bowel with normal intestine between skip lesions
- Mesenteric lymph node enlargement and mesenteric thickening
- Chronic inflammation—all layers of the wall with focal aggregation of epithelioid cells and lymphocytes—granuloma formation
- Mucosa—tiny aphthous ulcer.

Clinical features—Ulcerative colitis

Intestinal Manifestation

- Bloody diarrhea, rectal bleeding, constipation, abdominal pain
- Gradual onset, first attack is severe
- Systemic features—anorexia, weight loss, anemia and fever
- Distension of abdomen—toxic megacolon.

Extraintestinal Manifestation (Seen with Pan Colitis)

- Related to activity
  - Aphthous ulcer
  - Erythema nodosum
  - Episcleritis
  - Pyoderma gangrenosum,
  - Arthritis—large joint
- Unrelated to activity
  - Sacroiliitis,
  - Primary sclerosing cholangitis

- Ankylosing spondylitis
- Sweet's syndrome.

Clinical features—Crohn's disease

Intestinal Manifestations
- Diarrhea, abdominal pain, weight loss, fever, rectal bleeding,
- Anal lesion—fistula
- Ileal lesions—pain, obstructive symptom, malabsorption, inflam: mass - RIF
- Colonic lesion—rectal bleeding, perianal lesion, extra-intestinal feature
- Rectal lesions—bleeding PR.

Extraintestinal manifestations
- Related to activity
  - Aphthous ulcer
  - Pyoderma gangrenosum
  - Arthritis - large joints
  - Episcleitis
  - Uveitis
- Unrelated to activity
  - Sacroiliitis
  - Ankylosing spondylitis—HLA - B_{27} positive.

Severity of Ulcerative Colitis (UC)

Severity of UC			
Feature	Mild	Moderate	Severe
Motions per day	<4	Four to six	>6
Rectal bleeding	Little	Moderate	Large amounts
Temperature	Apyrexial	Intermediate	>37.8° C on 2 of 4 days
Pulse rate	Normal	Intermediate	>90 beats/minute
Hemoglobin	Normal	Intermediate	<10.5 g/dL
ESR	Normal	Intermediate	>30 mm/hr

Liver Disease with Inflammatory Bowel Disease

- Primary sclerosing cholangitis in ulcerative colitis.
- Gallstones in Crohn's disease.
- Fatty change, amyloidosis, granuloma.

Complications of IBD

- Toxic megacolon—ulcerative colitis and Crohn's disease
- Perforation of small intestine and colon
- Lower GI bleeding
  - Small intestinal stricture—Crohn's disease
  - Perianal lesions and fistulas—Crohn's disease
  - Perianal lesions—fissure, fistula, abscess and fleshy skin tag
  - Fistulas—enteroenteric, enterovaginal, enterovesical
- Ca colon—UC
- Extraintestinal complications
  - Primary sclerosing cholangitis
  - Gallstones
  - Amyloidosis
  - Right ureteric stricture
  - Pyelonephritis.

Differential Features of Ulcerative Colitis and Crohn's Disease

Features	Ulcerative colitis	Crohn's disease
Clinical features		
Bloody diarrhea	Common	Less common
Abdominal mass	Rare	Common
Perianal disease	Less common	Common
Signs of malabsorption	None	Common [small bowel disease]
Radiological features		
Rectal involvement	Invariable	Uncommon
Distribution	Continuous	Segmental, discontinuous
Mucosa	Fine ulceration 'Double contour'	'Rose thorn' ulcers
Strictures	Rare	Common
Fistulas	Very rare	May occur
Histological features		
Distribution	Mucosal	Transmural
Cellular infiltrate	Neutrophils, plasma cells, eosinophils	Lymphocytes, plasma cells macrophages
Glands	Mucin depletion Gland destruction Crypt abscesses	Gland preservation
Special features	None	Granulomas Aphthoid ulcers Histiocyte- lined fissures

Differential Diagnosis of Inflammatory Bowel Disease

Infective
- Viral: Herpes simplex proctitis, *Chlamydia proctitis*
- Bacterial: *Salmonella, Shigella, Campylobacter jejuni, E. coli*, Pseudomembraneous colitis, TB
- Protozoal: Amebiasis.

Noninfective
- Ischemic colitis, microscopic colitis [collagenous colitis]
- *Drugs:* NSAIDs, Colonic Ca, diverticulitis, lymphoma, dysmotility diarrhea.

DD of Small Bowel Crohn's Disease
- Appendicular mass
- Ileocecal tuberculosis
- Mesenteric adenitis.

Investigations

Aim–To confirm diagnosis, disease distribution, activity and identify complications.
- Blood test:
  - S albumin, Fe, Folic acid, vitamin B_{12}
  - Erythrocyte sedimentation rate (ESR)
  - c-reactive protein (CRP)
- *Bacteriology:* Stool culture—to rule out enteric infection
- *Endoscopy*
  - Sigmoidoscopy/colonoscopy
  - To visualize nature of lesions, its extend, skip lesions, pseudopolyp, carcinoma.
- Biopsy and histopathological study
- Barium studies
- Barium enema—less sensitive investigation.
  - UC—shortening of colon, loss of haustration and pseudopolyp
  - Crohn's disease—skip lesions, strictures, deep ulcers.
- Plain radiograph
  - In toxic megacolon–dilatation of colon > 6 cm- ↑ perforation.
  - Mucosal edema—thumb printing appearance
  - Evidence of perforation/obstruction
- Radionuclide scans
  - Radio labelled white cell scan reveal active inflammation.
- MRI scan
  - Accurate in delineating pelvic or perineal lesions of Crohn's disease
- Antineutrophil cytoplasmic antibody (ANCA) studies
  - Perinuclear (p)-ANCA >70% positive in ulcerative colitis
- Anti-Saccharomyces cerevisiae antibodies (ASCA)
  - 60-70% positive in Crohn's disease
  - 10-15% positive in ulcerative colitis.

Management

Principles are treat acute attack, prevent relapse.
- Detect carcinoma at early stage
- Select patients for surgery

Drug Treatment of Ulcerative Colitis

Active colitis: Corticosteroid is the drug of choice.
- Steroid foam or liquid retention enemas → poor response → oral prednisolone 40 mg/day.
- IV methyl prednisolone - 60 mg/day in severe active colitis.

Immunosuppressant drugs: Relapse after steroid/requiring maintenance steroid therapy.
- Azathioprine—1.5-2 mg/kg daily
- 6 MP—1.5-2 mg/day
- Methotrexate—10 mg/week
- Cyclosporine

Maintenance therapy: 5 amino salicylic acid [5 ASA].
- Mesalazine 4 g daily or Osalazine [dimer of 5 ASA].

Drug Treatment of Small Bowel Crohn's Disease

Corticosteroid: Prednisolone 30-40 mg/day for 2 weeks and reducing over 6-8 weeks.
  Relapse or steroid dependent immunosuppressants
- Azathioprine—1.5-2 mg/kg/day
- Methotrexate—15-25 mg/week

Budesonide: Synthetic corticosteroid 9 mg/day.

Immunotherapy: Antibody to TNF α [Infliximab] - in healing fistulas of Crohn's disease.

Indications for Surgery

Ulcerative colitis
- Failure of medical therapy
- Fulminant colitis
- Disease complications unresponsive to medical therapy
- Arthritis, pyoderma gangrenosum
- Perforation, Ca colon, severe dysplasia.

Procedure: Pan colectomy with ileostomy.

Crohn's disease
- Perforations, abscess, fistula unrelieved obstruction, failure of medical therapy.

Prognosis

- 90% of UC patients have intermittent disease activity
- 10% continuous disease activity
- 1/3rd require surgical treatment
- Clinical recurrence following resectional surgery is 50% by 10 years.

CLINICAL EVALUATION OF JAUNDICE

Types of Jaundice

- Hemolytic jaundice
- Hepatocellular jaundice
- *Cholestatic jaundice:* Obstructive jaundice.

Pathogenesis of Jaundice

- Increased production of bilirubin—hemolysis
- Impaired excretion of bilirubin
- Congenital nonhemolytic hyperbilirubinemia
  - Gilbert's syndrome
  - Crigler-Najjar type 1 and type 2
  - Dubin-Johnson syndrome
  - Rotor's syndrome.

Hepatocellular Jaundice

- Acute parenchymal liver disease
  - Viral hepatitis
  - Nonviral hepatitis
    - Leptospirosis
    - Toxoplasmosis
    - Septicemia
    - Toxic hepatitis
  - Drugs
    - INH
    - Rifampicin
    - Paracetamol
    - Alchoholism
  - Toxins
    - Mushroom, carbontetrachloride
  - Metabolic-Wilson's disease, α1 antitrypsin deficiency
- Chronic paranchymal liver disease
  - Chronic hepatitis
  - Cirrhosis liver.

Cholestatic Jaundice

- Intrahepatic cholestasis
  - Viral hepatitis
  - Alchoholism
  - Drugs
  - Chronic hepatitis
  - Postoperative jaundice
  - Cholestatic jaundice of pregnancy
  - Benign recurrent intrahepatic cholestatis (BRIC)
  - Primary biliary cirrhosis
- Extrahepatic cholestasis
  - Biliary stones
  - Carcinoma triad
    - Ca pancreas
    - Ampullary Ca
    - Ca biliary duct
  - Stricture bile duct
  - Lymph node—porta hepatis
  - Choledochal cyst.

Isolated Hyperbilirubinemia

- Unconjugated hyperbilirubinemia
  - Hemolytic disorders
  - Ineffective erythropoiesis
  - Crigler-Najjar
  - Gilbert's syndrome
- Conjugated hyperbilirubinemia
  - Dubin Johnson syndrome
  - Rotor's syndrome.

Biochemical Types of Jaundice

- Unconjugated hyperbilirubinemia
- Conjugated hyperbilirubinemia
- Mixed hyperbilirubinemia.

History Taking in Jaundice

A complete medical history is perhaps the most important part of the evaluation of the patient with jaundice.
- Age of onset
  - Neonetal—physiological, biliary atresia, Caroli's disease
  - Old age—malignancy—pancreas, hepatobiliary.
  - Febrile jaundice—Hepatisis A virus, leptospirosis, malaria, septicemia, biliary infection, Ca liver.
- Past history
  - Details of drug intake prior to jaundice—hepatotoxic drugs
  - H/o blood transfusion, surgery, IV injection, IV drug abuse.
- Family H/o viral hepatitis, congenital nonhemolytic jaundice, hereditary hemolytic disease—spherocytosis.
- Personal history
  - H/o alcoholism in detail.
  - Recurrence of jaundice
    - Hemolytic jaundice
    - Biliary stone
    - Congenital nonhemolytic jaundice-
    - Benign recurrent intrahepatic cholestasis
  - Recent travel history
    - Tropical infection
    - Schistosomiasis
    - Hydatid disease
- Associated symptoms
  - Myalgia, rash → leptospirosis, IMN
  - Pruritus, pale stool, steatorrhea → cholestasis
  - Fever, rigor, pain RHC → cholecystitis, cholangitis
  - Weight loss → Ca liver, Ca pancreas, cirrhosis liver

Examination of Jaundiced Patient

- Wasting, cachexia → malignancy liver, cirrhosis liver.
- Anemia with jaundice → hemolytic anemia
- Anemia with pedal edema and ascites → chronic liver disease
- Stigmas of chronic liver disease
  - Spider naevi
  - Palmar erythema
  - Parotid enlargement,
  - Gynecomastia
  - Testicular atrophy
- Left supraclavicular lymph node enlargement → upper GI malignancy, testicular malignancy.
- Periumbilical nodule → Sister Joseph nodule—suggestive of intra-abdominal malignancy.
- Pruritus, scratch marks → cholestasis
- Kayser-Fleischer ring → Wilson's disease
- Palpable liver—tender hepatomegaly→hepatitis, liver abscess, CHF
- Irregular hepatomegaly → malignancy liver
  - Primary and secondary
  - Cyst of liver→hydatid cyst, congenital polycystic

- Murphy's sign – a/c cholecystitis
- Shrunken liver→fulminant hepatocellular failure, late stage of cirrhosis liver
- Hepatic bruit→hepatocellular carcinoma, a/c alcoholic hepatitis.
- Ascites→decompensated cirrhosis liver, malignancy liver with peritoneal spread.
- Palpable gallbladder→carcinoma triad, mucocele of gallbladder, Ca gallbladder.
- Splenomegaly→portal hypertension, hemolytic anemia, pancreatic tumor with splenic vein obstruction
- Raised JVP→CHF with tender hepatomegaly.
- Cardiomegaly, cirrhosis liver→hemochromatosis.
- Peripheral neuropathy→alcoholic liver disease.
- Tremor, extrapyramidal signs and cerebellar signs→Wilson's disease.
- COPD and cirrhosis liver→α1 antitrypsin deficiency.
- Bronchiectasis and cirrhosis liver→mucoviscidosis.

DIFFERENTIATING FEATURES OF VARIOUS TYPES OF JAUNDICE

Features	Hemolytic	Hepatocellular	Cholestatic
Mechanism	↑ Bilirubin production	Hepatocellular disease	Biliary obstruction
Cause	Hemolysis	Virus, drugs, alcohol metabolic	Gallstone, Ca pancreas, etc.
Symptoms	Anemia, jaundice	Anorexia, nausea, vomiting, jaundice	Biliary colic, fluctuating jaundice
Splenomegaly	+	+/–	–
Palpable gallbladder	–	–	+
Bradycardia	–	–	+
Pruritus	–	+/–	+
Serum bilirubin	Unconju-gated	Mixed	Mainly conjugated
Transaminase	Normal	Increased	Slightly increased
Serum alkaline phosphatase	Normal	Slightly increased	Grossly increased
Urine	Colorless acholuric jaundice	High colored	High colored
Urobilinogen	++	+	–
Pale stool	–	+/–	+
Reticulocytosis	+	–	–

Etiology

Viral hepatitis is caused by one of the specific hepatitis viruses, hepatitis due to other viruses accounts for 1–2% of the cases.

VIRAL HEPATITIS

- Hepatitis A virus (HAV)
- Hepatitis B virus (HBV)
- Hepatitis C virus (HCV)
- Hepatitis D virus (HDV)
- Hepatitis E virus (HEV)
- Hepatitis G virus (HGV)
- Non A –E virus
  - Cytomegalovirus
  - Epstein-Barr virus
  - Herpes simplex virus
  - Yellow fever virus
  - Mumps virus.

HBV Susceptible Group

Medical and nursing staff, lab staff handling blood, IV drug abusers, homosexuals, chronic hemodialysis.

Clinical Features

- Pre icteric symptoms—Fatigue, malaise, anorexia, nausea, vomiting, fever, upper abdominal pain, bowel disorder
- Jaundice—deepening for 5–10 days, prodromal symptoms disappear
- In HBV—arthralgia, urticaria also present.
- Signs—tender hepatomegaly, splenomegaly - (5–10%), lymph node enlargement ±
- Course: 3–6 weeks - Jaundice ↓, urine color ↓, GI symptoms↓, appetite ↓

Investigation

- Serum bilirubin ↑—mixed hyperbilirubinemia
- Enzymes—SGPT, SGOT ↑
- CBC, Hb—normal, S. protien—normal, prothrombin time-normal
- Serological markers for virus
  - HAV—IgM anti HAV
  - HBV—HBs Ag, IgM anti HBc
  - HCV—Anti HCV
  - HDV - HDAg, IgM anti HDV

Complications

Hepatic complications

- Fulminant hepatocellular failure, relapsing hepatitis, cholestatic hepatitis
- Chronic hepatitis, cirrhosis liver, posthepatitis hyperbilirubinemia, posthepatitis syndrome, hepatocellular carcinoma, Gilbert's syndrome:
- Hepatitis.

Nonhepatic complications
- Polyarthritis, polyarteritis, immune complex glomerulonephritis
- Henoch–Schonlein purpura, aplastic anemia, GB syndrome

Differential Diagnosis
- Leptospirosis, drug induced hepatitis, alchoholic hepatitis, toxic hepatitis.

Management
- Bed rest, diet—2000–3000 cal/day, fruits and glucose.
- Drugs—no specific drug, avoid hepatotoxic drug, alcohol, etc.
- In severe HBV infection
  - Lamivudine 100 mg/day (trial).
  - Interferon trial in HCV.

Bad Prognostic Indicators
- Serum bilirubin > 20 mg/dL, marked ↑ in transaminase
- Protrombin time ↑ by 4–5 secs, shrunken liver
- HBV < HCV and HDV infection—variable prognosis.

CHRONIC HEPATITIS

Definition: Hepatic inflammation for more than six months with characteristic pathological features.

Etiology
- Primary autoimmune
- HBV, HDV and HCV
- Alchohol related
- Drugs—INH, rifampicin, α-methyl dopa
- Metabolic - Wilson's disease, α1 antitrypsin deficiency.

Pathological Types
- Chronic persistent hepatitis—portal tract infiltration by mono nuclear and plasma cells. It is seen with HBV, recovering acute alcoholic hepatitis, schistosomiasis.
- Chronic lobular hepatitis—portal zone infiltration and spotty necrosis (single cell necrosis). It occurs with hepatitis HBV, autoimmune liver disease.
- Chronic active hepatitis—severe form of chronic hepatitis, can lead to cirrhosis and hepatocellular failure. Pathological features are portal zone infiltration, piece meal necrosis, bridging necrosis, regenerating nodule, fibrosis and lobular collapse.

Histopathology
Ground glass hepatocytes that stains positive for HBsAg is found in chronic hepatitis B infection.

The histologic triad of C/c hepatitis C infection is:
1. Dense lymphoid aggregation
2. Inflammatory bile duct damage in portal tracts
3. Micro- and macrovesicular steatosis.

Clinical Features of Chronic Active Hepatitis
- Insidious onset, fatigue, anorexia, jaundice, hepatomegaly ±, stigmas of chronic liver disease like spider naevi, palmar erythema.
- Features of complications like ascites, coagulopathy, encephalopathy, bleeding varices
- Extrahepatic manifestation
  - In HBV c/c hepatitis—arthritis, vasculitis and glomerulonephritis.
  - In autoimmune chronic hepatitis—arthritis, vasculitis (PAN), fibrosing alveolitis, thyroiditis, peripheral neuropathy, etc.

Investigations
- Routine hematology – ESR ↑, Hb ↓
- LFT—S bilirubin ↑, transaminase ↑, S ALP N/↑, S. albumin—normal/decreased, prothrombin time ↑.
- Viral markers (Antigen and antibody)
  - HBV—HBsAg, HBeAg, IgG anti-HBc, HBV DNA
  - HCV—HCV RNA, anti-HCV, anti-LKM1
  - HDV—HDV RNA and anti-HDV, anti-LKM3
- Autoantibody in autoimmune hepatitis
  - Type 1—ANA, ASMA (antismooth muscle antibody)
  - Type 2—anti-LKM1 (antibody to liver kidney microsome)
  - Type 3—anti-SLA (antibody to soluble liver antigen)
  - Type 4—no detectable antibody
- Drug induced chronic hepatitis—anti-LKM2
- Immunoglobulin—IgG↑, IgM and IgA normal
- Copper kinetics—S copper, urine copper and S ceruloplasmin—Wilson's
- KF ring—Wilson's disease
- S. α1 antitrypsin.

Management of Chronic Hepatitis
Specific Measures

Aim of treatment:
- To prevent progression to cirrhosis and hepatocellular carcinoma
- To eliminate the cause
- To improve the survival
- **HBV chronic hepatitis:**
  - Interferon alpha - 5 million units daily S/C or 10 million units thrice weekly for 4 months.
  - Lamivudine 100 mg OD until HBeAg becomes negative
  - A positive response to treatment is defined by loss of viral replication markers (HBeAg and S HBV DNA by non-PCR

assays) within 12 months of initiation of treatment which can be achieved in 30-40% of patients.
- Adefovir and Tenofovir are the other drugs.
- Adefovir 10 mg daily or Tenofovir 300 mg daily-
  - Till HbeAg conversion to Anti HbeAg,
  - HBV DNA undetectable,
  - SGPT < 30 units in males and < 90 units in females
- **HCV chronic hepatitis:**
  - Combination of interferone and ribavirin.
  - α Interferon—3 million units thrice weekly S/C
  - Ribavirin 1000 mg/day for 1 year
- **Autoimmune chronic hepatitis:**
  Immuno suppressive therapy
  - Prednesolone 30-40 mg/day for 2-3/12 maintenance dose at least for 2 years
  - Azathioprine 50-100 mg/day with prednesolone to reduce the dose of it to 10 mg/day, to reduce the side effect.

General Measures

- Avoid hepatotoxic drugs, alcohol, good nutrition
- Prompt management of complications like encephalopathy and upper GI bleed.

Liver transplantation: Failure of medical therapy in chronic hepatitis, before developing encephalopathy.

CIRRHOSIS LIVER

Definition: Diffuse fibrosis with nodular regeneration of liver.

Macroscopic Types

- Micronodular—alcoholic cirrhosis
- Macronodular—posthepatitis
- Mixed nodular—biliary cirrhosis.

Pathological Process

Necrosis → Degeneration → Fibrosis → Regeneration → Nodule formation and loss of architecture.

Pathogenesis

Injured hepatocytes and other cells of liver → Cytokines and various growth factors (IGF, TGFα, TGFβ1 and PDGF) → Quiescent fat storing cell → Hepatic stellate cell → Activated myofibroblast like cell → Collagen synthesis → Fibrosis.

Etiology

- Alcoholic liver disease, viral hepatitis
- *Drugs:* INH, rifampicin, α methyl dopa, oxyphenisatin
- Metabolic
  - Wilson's disease
  - α1 anti-trypsin deficiency
  - Hemochromatosis
  - Mucoviscidosis
  - Glycogen storage disease
- *Biliary disease:* Primary biliary cirrhosis, obstructive jaundice.
- Cardiac cirrhosis
- Autoimmune liver disease
- Cryptogenic cirrhosis.

Clinical Features

Are due to:
- Hepatocellular dysfunction
- Portal hypertension.

General Features

- Jaundice
- Pedal edema (Fig. 6.17)
- Clubbing

Differentiating features of hepatitis viruses.

Features	HAV	HBV	HCV	HDV	HEV	HGV
Genome	RNA	DNA	RNA	RNA	RNA	RNA
Family	Picorna	Hepadna	Flavi	Viroid	Calci	Flavi
Size (nm)	27	42	30–38	35	27	-
Incubation period (days)	15–45	30–180	15–150	30–180	15–60	14–35
Transmission	Feco-oral	Blood, saliva, sexually	Blood	Blood, sexually	Feco-oral	Percutaneous
Fulminant course	0.1%	0.1–1%	0.1%	5–20%	1–2%	Unknown
Chronicity	None	1–10%	50%	Common	None	Yes
Prevention Active →	Inactivated vaccine	Recombinant vaccine	No	Prevention of HBV infection	No	No
Passive →	Immunoglobulin	Hyperimmune globulin	No	No	No	No

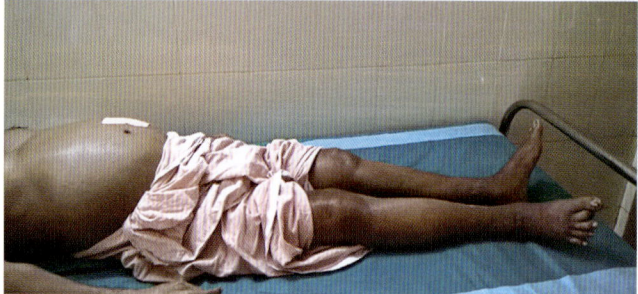

Fig. 6.17: Ascites and pedal edema in a patient with cirrhosis of liver

- Leuconychia
- Hepatomegaly
- Ascites (Fig. 6.17)
- Parotid enlargement

Mechanism of Ascites

- Hypoalbuminemia, portal hypertension, secondary hyper aldosteronism and peritoneal lymphatic obstruction.
- Aggravating factors
    - Upper GI bleed
    - Portal vein thrombosis,
    - Cirrhotic activity (further hepatic necrosis)
    - Hepatocellular Ca,
    - Spontaneous bacterial peritonitis (SBP).

Circulatory Features

- Palmar erythema
- Spider naevi
- Cyanosis
- Hyperdynamic circulatory state
- Hemic murmur
- Cardiomegaly.

Hematological Feaures

- Coagulation failure, bleeding tendency, epistaxis, purpura, menorrhagia
- Bleeding tendency in cirrhosis are due to
    - Coagulation failure—vitamin K dependent and independent factors
    - Thrombocytopenia—hypersplenism
    - Porto systemic connection—varices
    - Disseminated intravascular coagulation (DIC)

Endocrine Features

- Gynecomastia
- Testicular atrophy
- Loss of libido
- Hair loss (Fig. 6.19)
- Impotence
- Breast atrophy
- Irregular menstruation.

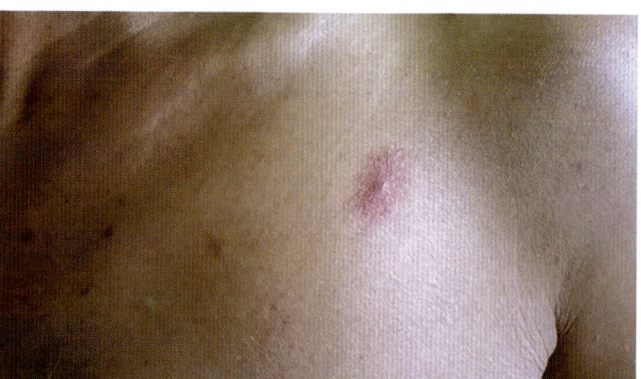

Fig. 6.18: Spider naevi in a patient with cirrhosis of liver

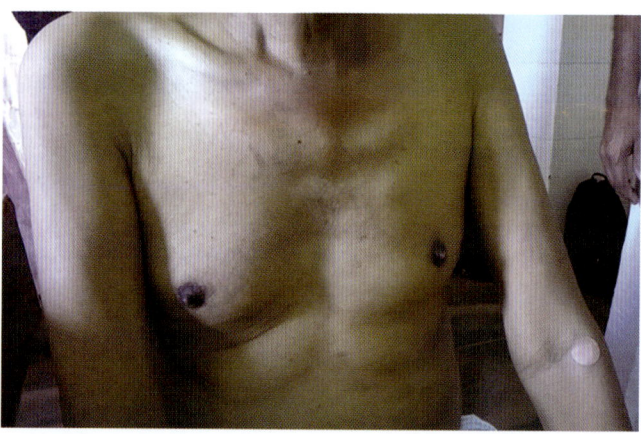

Fig. 6.19: Jaundice over the body and loss of hair in a patient with cirrhosis of liver

- Silver Streni Corda syndrome → Gynecomastia and testicular atrophy in cirrhosis liver.

Respiratory Features

- Tidal volume↓, pulmonary arteriovenous fistula, central cyanosis.

Neuropsychiatric Features

- Encephalopathy
- Inversion of sleep rhythm
- Flapping tremor
- Constructional apraxia
- Myoclonus
- Hyperreflexia
- Extensor plantar
- Porto systemic myelopathy
- Extrapyramidal signs (Wilson's disease)
- Peripheral neuropathy (alcoholic cirrhosis).

Features due to Portal Hypertension

- Congestive splenomegaly
- Caput medusa

- Hypersplenism
- Congestive gastropathy
- Favoring
  - Ascites, hepatic encephalopathy, hepatorenal syndrome, gram-negative septicemia.

Mechanism of Portal Hypertension in Cirrhosis

Reduced number of sinusoids due to nodular degeneration and fibrosis, pressure of regenerating nodule, arteriovenous collaterals in portal tract, neovascularity in the septa.

Features of Compensated Cirrhosis

- Spider naevi (Fig. 6.18)
- Telengiectasia
- Parotid enlargement
- Gynecomastia
- Palmar erythema
- Clubbing
- Leuconychia
- Loss of hair (Fig. 6.19)
- Hepatosplenomegaly
- Dialated veins
- Testicular atrophy
- Wasting of muscles.

Features of Decompensated Cirrhosis

- Altered sensorium, inversion of sleep rhythm
- Jaundice, foetor hepaticus
- Flapping tremor, constructional apraxia, myoclonus
- Ascites, pedal edema
- Hyperreflexia, extensor plantar.

Complications of Cirrhosis Liver

- Upper GI bleed
  - Vericeal and
  - Nonvericeal-Erosive gastritis
  - Congestive gastropathy
  - Peptic ulcer
- Encephalopathy - (acute on chronic and chronic)
- Portal hypertension, ascites, hypersplenism
- Hepatorenal syndrome
- Gram negative septicemia
- Spontaneous bacterial peritonitis
- Portosystemic mylopathy
- Hepatocellular carcinoma
  - Maximum incidence of hepatocellular carcinoma is seen with cirrhosis due to α1 antitrypsin deficiency, least with Wilson's disease, never with cardiac cirrhosis.

Precipitating Factors for Hepatic Encephalopathy

- Upper GI bleed, hepatotoxins—alcohol and drugs.
- Sedatives and diuretics (injudicious use)
- *Infection:* Alimentary and extra-alimentary
- Increased dietary protein, constipation
- Electrolyte disturbance—hypokalemia
- Paracentesis abdominis.

Investigations in Cirrhosis Liver

Two groups:
1. Investigations to establish cirrhosis
2. Investigations for the cause of cirrhosis
   - Urine and blood routine
   - Blood sugar, S electrolyte, RFT
   - LFT—S protein—reversal of albumin globulin ratio (Alb <3 g/dL and Glob > 4 g/dL).
     - S. bilirubin
     - Enzymes—SGPT, SGOT, GGT.
     - BSP excretion test.
   - Platelet count, prothrombin time.
   - EEG
   - Liver biopsy—for tissue diagnostics
     - Contraindicated—deep jaundice, coagulation failure, HC failure, ascites.
   - Viral markers for HBV, HCV, HDV
   - Copper kinetic study, S ceruloplasmin—Wilson's disease.
     - Iron kinetic study—hemochromatosis.
   - α1 antitrypsin estimation
   - Radiological study—barium swallow—esophageal varices
     - USG study—echo texture, focal lesions.
     - Isotope scan of liver
   - Upper GI endoscopy—esophageal varices
     - Source for nonvariceal bleed.

Management

- Compensated cirrhosis
- Cirrhosis with ascites and pedal edema
- Cirrhosis with encephalopathy.

Compensated Cirrhosis

- Avoid all hepatotoxins and drugs
- Abstinence of alcohol
- Adequate nutrition and vitamins
- Treatment of primary cause, if any—viruses—HBV, HCV
- Wilson's disease, hemochromatosis
- Periodic evaluation—clinical, LFT and others.

Cirrhosis with Ascites and Pedal Edema

- Besides the above measures
- Bed rest, salt restriction—20-40 mEq of sodium/day, I/O chart
- Fluid restriction 500-1000 mL/day (rate of reabsorption of ascitic fluid is 700-900 mL/day)
- Diuretics—spironolactone—50-400 mg/day
  - ± Frusemide 40-160 mg/day
- Adequate response means—loss of 0.75 kg of body weight/day, if ascites alone
  - Loss of 1.5 kg of body weight/day if ascites + pedal edema.
- Daily weight recording and abdominal girth measurement
- In refractory ascites (failure of drug therapy)
  - Paracenteses abdominis 2-5 liters
  - Infusion of salt poor albumin
  - Peritoneovenous shunt-Leveen shunt.

Cirrhosis with Encephalopathy

(Refer Hepatic Encephalopathy).

Prognosis of Cirrhosis Liver

Cirrhosis carries a high mortality. Overall, only 25% patients survive 5 years from diagnosis. Cirrhosis with good liver function, 50% survive for 5 years, 25% survive for 10 years.

Bad Prognostic Signs

- Encephalopathy
- Ascites
- Increasing bilirubin,
- Falling S. albumin < 3 g
- Hyponatremia < 120 mEq
- Rise in prothrombin time.

Child Pugh classification of prognosis in cirrhosis.			
Score	1	2	3
Encephalopathy	None	Mild	Marked
Ascites	None	Mild	Marked
Bilirubin(μmol/L)	<34	34–50	>50
Albumin(g/L)	>35	28–35	<28
PT – Prolonged in sec	<4	4–6	>6

Inference
Child's A = < 7
Child's B = 7–9
Child's C = >9

PORTAL HYPERTENSION

Normal pressure: 2-5 mm Hg
Portal hypertension: >12 mm Hg

Branches and tributaries of portal vein:
Splenic vein and superior mesenteric vein → portal vein.
Left gastric [from portal vein], right gastric, cystic vein, paraumbilical vein [form left branch of portal vein].

Etiology of Portal Hypertension (Fig. 6.20)

Divided into 3 groups:
1. **Presinusoidal**
   - Extrahepatic
     - Portal vein thrombosis
     - Cavernous malformation
     - Portal vein atresia
     - Obstructionat porta hepatis
   - Intrahepatic
     - Infiltrative lesions—fatty infiltration, lymphoma
     - Schistosomiasis
     - Congenital hepatic fibrosis
     - Noncirrhotic portal fibrosis (NCPF)
     - Sarcoidosis
2. **Sinusoidal**
   - Cirrhosis liver
3. **Postsinusoidal**
   - Intrahepatic
     - Cirrhosis liver
     - Veno-occlusive diseases
   - Extrahepatic
     - Budd-Chiari syndrome
     - Congenital atresia of hepatic vein
     - Thrombosis of IVC
     - Tumor pressing on IVC
     - Pericardial disease
     - Right sided cardiac failure.

Causes of Portal Vein Thrombosis

Umbilical sepsis, pregnancy, oral contraceptive, polycythemia, CML, cirrhosis liver [10%].

Hyperkinetic Portal Hypertension (↑ Portal Vein Blood Flow without Obstruction)

- Hepatic artery portal vein fistula
- Splenic arteriovenous fistula
- Massive splenomegaly.

Major Sites of Porto Systemic Anastomosis

- Lower end of esophagus—azygos vein with left gastric vein-varices
- Around the umbilicus—paraumbilical vein with superficial veins of the anterior abdominal wall

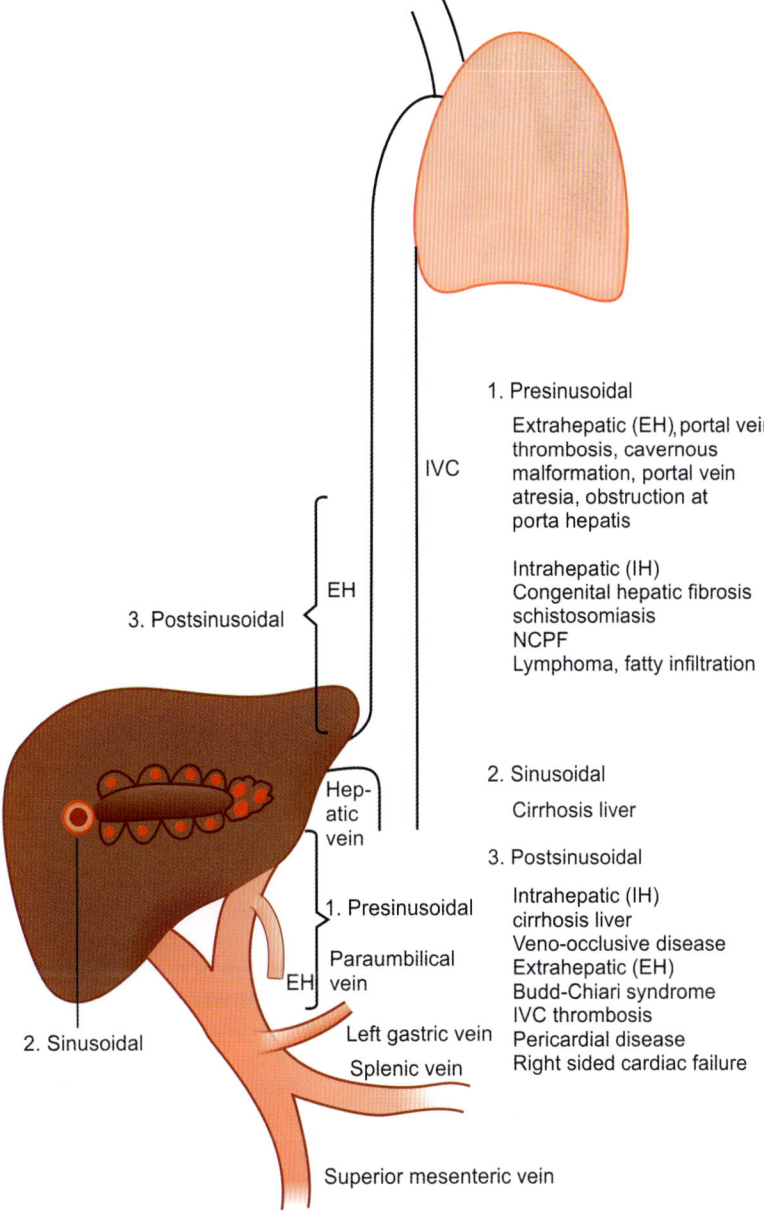

Fig. 6.20: Etiology of portal hypertension.

- Superior hemorrhoidal with inferior and middle hemorrhoidal veins
- Varices:
  - Up hill varices—in portal hypertension
  - Down hill varices—in Preazygotic SVC obstruction.

Clinical Features of Portal Hypertension

- Dilated veins over the abdomen—Caput medusae
- Venous hum around the umbilicus
- Congestive splenomegaly
- Varices and hematemesis.

Complications

- Hematemesis
- Hypersplenism
- Congestive gastropathy
- Ascites
- Hepatic encephalopathy
- Hepatorenal syndrome
- Gram-negative septicemia.

Investigations

- Endoscopy and barium swallow—for demonstration of varices
- LFT, Liver biopsy—to rule out primary liver disease
- USG—dilated portal vein and its collaterals
- CT abdomen, isotope scan of liver
- Hepatic vein catheterization: Wedge hepatic venous pressure
  - Normal - 5-6 mm Hg
  - In portal hypertension >20 mm Hg
- Selective visceral angiography
- Splenoportovenography—to delineate with the anatomy of portal system.

UPPER GI BLEED

Manifests as
- Hematemesis
- Melena
- Hematochezia
- Anemia
- Hypotension and shock.

Etiology

Refer: Hematemesis-symptomatology
- Duodenal ulcer—40%
- Gastric ulcer—20%
- Erosive gastritis—20%
- Varices—10%
- Others—10%

Assessment of Blood Loss

- Clinical
  - No symptoms except in anemic and elderly patients upto 500 mL of blood loss
  - Tachycardia, postural hypotension, syncope—1000 mL blood loss
  - Hypotension and profound shock—2000 mL or more of blood loss
  - Signs of shock—pulse rate >100, SBP <100, urine output < 30 mL/mt
  - Signs of impaired tissue perfusion
- Laboratory
  - Hemoglobin : < 10 g
  - PCV - ↓
  - Motion occult blood
- Upper GI endoscopy—variceal and nonvariceal bleeding
- Selective angiography—to detect the site of bleeding >0.5 mL or >/mt.
- Radiolabelled RBC—to detect very low grade bleeding from GI tract—0.1 mL or >/mt.

Differentiation between upper GI and lower GI bleed.

Features	Upper GI bleed	Lower GI bleed
Site	Above the ligament of Treitz	Below the ligament of Treitz
Presentation	Hematemesis/melaena	Hematochezia/melena
Bowel sounds	Hyperactive	Normal
Nasogastric aspiration	Blood	Clear fluid

Management of Variceal Bleed and Portal Hypertension

- **Establish IV line and CVP**
- **Resuscitation** with blood transfusion, clotting factors with fresh frozen plasma [blood transfusion if SBP <100, heart rate >100 and Hb <10 g]
- **Measures to reduce the portal venous pressure**
  - Drugs
    - Vasopressin—20 units in 100 mL in 20 minutes
    - Telipressin—2 mg QID → 1 mg QID
    - Somatostatin—250 μg IV bolus, IV infusion 250 μg per hr till bleeding stops
    - Octreotide—50 μg IV bolus, IV infusion 50 μg hourly till bleeding stops
  - TIPSS and shunt surgery [described below]
- **Local measures**
  - Emergency endoscopy—sclerotherapy/banding
  - Balloon tamponade—[if sclerotherapy is difficult due to active bleeding]—Sengstaken-Blakemore tube or Minnesota tube is used
  - Esophageal transection—with a stapling gun
- **Prevention of recurrence of bleeding**
  - Sclerotherapy/endoscopic banding
  - Drugs—propranolol/nitrates
  - TIPSS—Transjugular intrahepatic portosystemic shunt
  - Portosystemic shunt surgery
- **Liver transplantation**.

Management of Nonvariceal Bleed

- Establish IV line and CVP
- Introduce nasogastric tube
- Blood transfusion [SBP < 100, heart rate >100, Hb <10 g]
- IV H2 receptor antagonist/PPI, liquid antacids
- Endoscopic procedures—heater probe, electrocoagulation, sclerotherapy with ethanol/epinephrine, laser therapy
- Selective angiography and microembolization
- Surgery—uncontrolled bleed in gastroduodenal ulcers.

Poor Prognostic Signs in UGI Bleed

- Variceal bleeding
- Severe initial bleeding
- Continuous bleeding
- Recurrence of bleeding
- Age >60 years

- Presence of liver disease—jaundice, ascites, hypo-albuminemia and encephalopathy
- Presence of cardiac, respiratory and renal disease.

HEPATIC ENCEPHALOPATHY

Definition

Neuropsychiatric syndrome developing in patients with hepatocellular failure, with or without portosystemic collaterals.

Types of Hepatic Encephalopathy

- Chronic hepatic encephalopathy
- Acute on chronic hepatic encephalopathy
- Fulminant hepatocellular failure—hepatic encephalopathy with coagulopathy occurring in patients with liver disease of <8 weeks.

Subtypes:
- Hyperacute hepatocellular failure within 7 days.
- Acute hepatocellular failure—8-28 days.
- Subacute hepatocellular failure—5-12 weeks.
- Subfulminant hepatocellular failure—hepatic encephalopathy occurring in patients with liver disease of > 8 weeks to 6 months, usually with ascites
- Subclinical hepatic encephalopathy (SHE)—this is the state of early hepatocellular failure before the clinical manifestation of signs of hepatic encephalopathy, detected by tests like number connection test.

Etiology

Chronic Hepatic Encephalopathy

- Chronic liver disease— cirrhosis, chronic hepatitis

Acute on Chronic Hepatic Encephalopathy

- Chronic liver disease with a precipitating factor—UGI bleeding, high protein intake—constipation, diuretics, sedatives, hepatotoxins and alcohol, infection, paracentesis abdominis, electrolyte imbalance—hypokalemia

Fulminant Hepatocellular Failure

- **Infections**
  - Hepatitis viruses[A, B, C, D]
  - Leptospirosis, CMV
- **Metabolic**
  - Wilson's disease
  - Acute (a/c) fatty liver of pregnancy
  - Reye's syndrome
  - Galactosemia
- **Drugs**
  - Acetaminophin
  - INH
  - Methyldopa
  - Tetracycline
  - Sodium valproate
  - Halothane
  - Diphenylhydantoin
- **Miscellaneous**
  - Mushroom poisoning
  - Autoimmune hepatitis
  - Budd-Chiari syndrome
  - Veno-occlusive disease
  - Partial hepatectomy.

Pathogenesis

- ↑ blood ammonia level → encephalopathy
- *False neurotransmitters:* Octopamine and β hydroxyphenyl ethanolamine [competing with dopamine]
- *Amino acids:*
  - ↑ in aromatic amino acids—tyrosine, phenylalanine, tryptophan → increased serotonin formation
  - ↓ branched chain amino acids—leucine, isoleucine and valine
- Plasma free fatty acid (FFA) ↑
- Gamma-aminobutyric acid (GABA) activity increase.

Mechanism (Fig. 6.21)

- Neurotrophic factors ↓ - cytidine and uridine
- Neurotoxic substances ↑ - due to hepatocellular dysfunction and portosystemic shunt.

Clinical features

- **Psychiatric symptoms:** Due to initial stimulation and later depression of renin-angiotensin system (RAS) of brainstem
  - Altered sensorium
  - Personality changes
  - Intellectual decline
  - Reversal of sleep rhythm
- **Neurological features**
  - Flapping tremor
  - Constructional apraxia
  - Myoclonus
  - Hyperreflexia
  - Extensor plantar
  - Failure to do number connection test
  - Seizure
  - Cerebral edema and ↑ intracranial pressure (ICP) in fulminant hepatocellular failure
- **Features of liver disease**
  - Jaundice
  - Fetor hepaticus
  - Ascites,
  - Hepatosplenomegaly
  - Shrunken liver in fulminant hepatocellular failure
  - Pedal edema
  - Stigmas of chronic liver disease

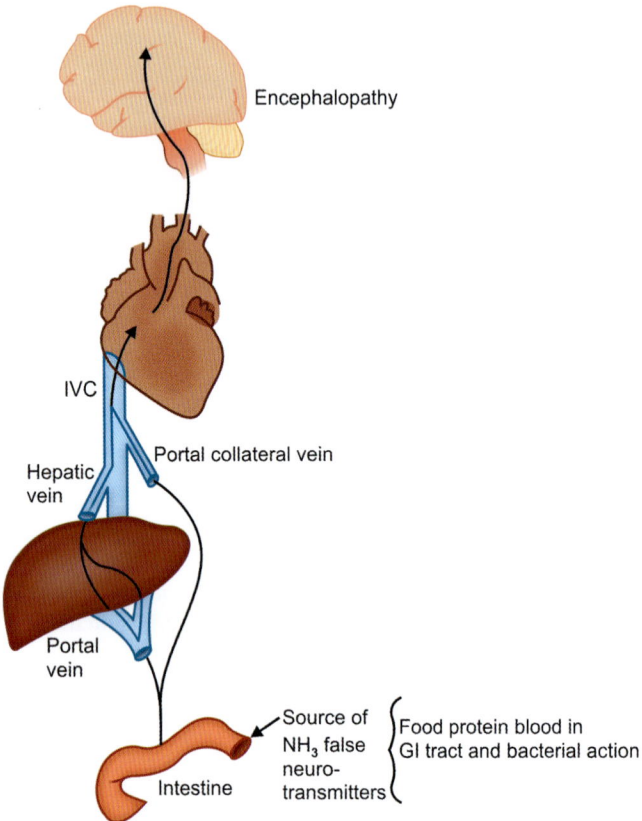

Fig. 6.21: Mechanism of hepatic encephalopathy.

- Palmar erythema
- Spider naevi

Parotidomegaly, etc.

Differential Diagnosis of Acute and Chronic Encephalopathy

Chronic encephalopathy
- Long duration of liver disease
- Spider nevi, hepatosplenomegaly

Acute encephalopathy
- Impalpable shrunken liver.

Differential Diagnosis of Hepatic Encephalopathy

- Subdural hematoma
- Alcohol intoxication
- Delirium tremens
- Wernicke's encephalopathy
- Hypoglycemia
- Alcoholism with head injury.

Grading of Hepatic Encephalopathy

Grade 1: Poor concentration, slurred speech and altered sleep rhythm.
Grade 2: Drowsy, lethargic, but easily rousable
Grade 3: Stuporous, responds to pain
Grade 4: Poor response to external stimuli, unconscious.

Complications of Fulminant Hepatocellular Failure

- Cerebral edema and ↑ Intracranial pressure
- Respiratory failure—infection, acute respiratory distress syndrome (ARDS)
- Renal failure—functional, acute tubular necrosis (ATN)
- Coagulation failure
- Systemic infection, pancreatitis, hypotension
- Hypoglycemia, electrolyte imbalance.

Investigations

- *Hematological:* Total count (TC), differential count (DC), hemoglobin (Hb), platelet count, prothrombin time, erythrocyte sedimentation rate (ESR), blood grouping
- *Biochemical:* Blood (B) Glucose, B urea, serum (S) creatinine, S electrolyte, S proteins, S enzymes—transaminase, alkaline phosphatase, amylase
- S. calcium
- Viral markers—for hepatitis viruses
- Autoantibodies—Antinuclear antibodies (ANA), anti-smooth muscle antibodies (ASMA), antimitochondrial antibodies (AMA), liver kidney microsomal (LKM) antibodies
- Blood culture, urine culture and sputum culture
- USG—abdomen
- Copper kinetics—Wilson's disease.

Diagnosis of Hepatic Encephalopathy

- Evidence of acute or chronic liver disease ± extensive porto systemic anastomosis
- Altered sensorium
- *Neurological signs:* Flap, hyper-reflexia and extensor plantar
- Characteristic electroencephalography (EEG) changes.

Management

Principles:
- Reduce neurotoxic substances
- Induce regeneration of liver
- Remove precipitating factors.

General measures:
- Protein restriction to < 20 g/day, glucose 300 g/day
- Prevention and prompt treatment of UGI bleeding
- High bowel wash
- Gut sterilization Rifaximin/Ampicillin/Neomycin—to destroy the urea splitting organism
- Oral lactulose - ↓ the bowel pH, induce diarrhea and prevent ammonia absorption by inhibiting nonionic ammonia formation, 30 mL, 2–3 times daily

- Lactobacillus—inhibit the growth of urea splitting organisms.

Treatment of Precipitating Factors

UGI bleed, avoid hepatotoxic drugs, alcohol, injudicious use of diuretics and sedatives, high protein intake, prompt treatment of infections, and correction of electrolyte imbalance.

Measures in Fulminant Hepatocellular Failure

- IV mannitol—cerebral edema
- IV glucose—blood glucose <100 mg
- Renal failure—dialysis and other supportive measures
- Respiratory failure—intubation and ventilation
- Infection—specific antibiotics
- Bleeding—vitamin K, coagulation factors and platelet
- H_2 receptor antagonist/PPI—to keep upper GI pH >5
- N acetyl cysteine in acetaminophen poisoning.

Measures in Chronic Hepatocellular Failure

- Bromocriptine
- L-dopa orally or rectally
- Infusion of branched chain amino acids.

Artificial Liver Support

- Exchange transfusion
- Charcoal hemoperfusion
- Extracorporeal liver perfusion—Pig or cadaveric
- Extracorporeal liver assist device—cultured human/porcine hepatocyte
- Liver transplantation.

King's college hospital prognostic criteria of Fulminant hepatocellular failure

Fulminant Hepatocellular Failure (FHF)—Nonparacetamol Induced

Prothrombin time >100 sec (INR > 6.5)

or

- The coexistence of
  - Age <10 or >40
  - Jaundice >7 days before encephalopathy
  - Sero negative hepatitis
  - Prothrombin time >50 seconds
  - Serum bilirubin >17.5 mg.

Fulminant Hepatocellular Failure (FHF)—Paracetamol Induced

- pH <7.3

or

- The coexistence of
  - Prothrombin time >100 (INR >6.5)
  - Creatinine >300 µ mol/L
  - Grade 3 or more encephalopathy.

CHAPTER 7

Examination of Musculoskeletal System

COMMONLY USED TERMS IN RHEUMATOLOGY

Arthralgia: Pain arising in joints.

Arthritis: Objective joint abnormality due to inflammation:
- *Monoarthritis*: Arthritis affecting only one joint.
- *Oligoarthritis/Pauciarticular disease*: Arthritis affecting 2–4 joints or joint groups.
- *Polyarthritis*: Arthritis affecting more than 4 joints or joint groups.

Synovitis: Clinically apparent inflammation of synovial membrane.

Tenosynovitis: Tendon sheath inflammation.

Tendinitis: Inflammation of a tendon.

Bursitis: Inflammation of a bursa.

Enthesopathy/Enthesitis: Inflammation or abnormality of an enthesis (the site of ligament, tendon or capsule insertion into periosteum or bone).

Myopathy: Disease or abnormality of muscle.

Myositis: Inflammatory disease of muscle.

Serositis: Inflammation of pleura, pericardium or peritoneum.

SYMPTOMATOLOGY

Locomotor Symptoms and General Symptoms

Locomotor Symptoms

Pain:
- *Onset*: Acute, subacute and insidious.
- Site of maximum intensity and radiation of pain.
- *Rest pain*: Inflammatory pain (improves with activity)
- *Night pain*:
  - Destructive pain
  - Avascular necrosis
  - Mutilating arthritis
  - Malignancy.
- *Movement pain*: Use increases the pain and rest decreases the pain.
- *Persistent pain*: Bone pain.

Stiffness:
- Sensation of tightness.
- Fluid distension of capsule, tenosynovium or bursa.
- In the morning, stiffness increases and activity decreases due to clearing of fluid.
- Duration of morning stiffness.

Swelling: Soft tissue, bony and fluid.

Deformity: Malalignment, subluxation or dislocation.

Disability: Inadequate function.

Pattern of joint involvement: Number of joints affected.

Pattern of development: Episodic/simultaneous/migratory symmetrical/asymmetrical small/large joints.

Precipitating factors for joint involvement:
- Trauma
- Infection—Sore throat, urethritis, dysentery
- Sexually transmitted diseases
- Contact with infectious disease.

Aggravating and relieving factors: Rest, exercise, activity, immobility and drugs.

General Symptoms

Fever, sweating, weight loss, fatigability.

Extra-articular: Alopecia, rashes, ocular symptoms.

Neurological: Symptoms of neuropathy, myelopathy, myositis and myopathy.

GIT: Symptoms of inflammatory bowel disease (IBD).

Genitourinary system: Symptoms of urethritis, hematuria, glomerulonephritis and chronic renal failure (CRF).

Cardiorespiratory system: Dyspnea, asthma, fibrosing alveolitis, pleuropericardial involvement.

HISTORY TAKING

Presenting symptoms
- Articular and extra-articular symptoms
- History of presenting complaints (refer symptomatology).

Past history
- Trauma
- Infection—urethritis, dysentery
- Similar illness—rheumatic fever, gout, palindromic rheumatism
- H/o sexually transmitted disease—secondary syphilis, Charcot's joint.

Treatment history
Aspirin, NSAID, steroids, DMARD, surgery.

Family history
- Rheumatoid arthritis
- Osteoarthrosis, gout
- Seronegative spondyloarthropathies.

Social history
- Domestic setup, occupation
- Marital status.

EXAMINATION

General Examination

Skin

- *Erythema* - joint → septic arthritis, crystal arthropathy, palindromic rheumatism
- *Rash* → SLE, vasculitis, drugs, Still's disease
- Psoriasis
- *Keratoderma blenorrhagica* – Reiter's syndrome
- *Mucosal ulcers* – Behcet's syndrome, SLE
- *Pyoderma gangrenosum* – IBD
- *Palmar erythema* – Rheumatoid arthritis
- *Photosensitivity* – Development of rash on exposure to sunlight of less than 30 minutes – SLE

Subcutaneous Nodules

- Rheumatoid arthritis
- Rheumatic fever
- Gout
- Sarcoidosis
- SLE
- Hyperlipidemia.

Nail Changes

- *Clubbing*: Fibrosing alveolitis, hypertrophic osteoarthropathy
- *Pitting and onycholysis*: Psoriasis
- *Splinter hemorrhage*: Small vessel vasculitis, infective endocarditis.

Mucous Membrane Lesions

- Reactive arthropathy, Reiter's syndrome, Behçet's syndrome, SLE, IBD.
- *Dryness*: Sjögren's syndrome.

Eye Changes

- *Episcleritis and scleritis*: Rheumatoid arthritis
- *Iritis*: Ankylosing spondylitis
- *Iridocyclitis*: Juvenile chronic arthritis
- *Conjunctivitis*: Reiter's syndrome.

Sclerosing Tenosynovitis of Superior Oblique Tendon

Brown's syndrome in rheumatoid arthritis.

Lymphadenopathy

Still's disease, SLE.

Locomotor System Examination

- **Examination of joints:**
  - Number → Mono, Oligo and Poly
  - Attitude → Swelling, deformity and muscle wasting
  - Swelling:
    - Soft in consistency
      - Fluid – joint, bursae, tenosynovium
    - Soft to firm in consistency
      - Soft tissue
    - Hard in consistency
      - Bony swelling
  - Warmth: Inflammatory arthropathy.
  - Tenderness
    - Capsular – Arthropathy
    - Periarticular – Bursitis or enthesopathy
    - Joint line – Intracapsular arthropathy
- **Assessment of joint tenderness**
  - *Grade 1* – The patient says the joint is tender
  - *Grade 2* – The patient winces
  - *Grade 3* – The patient winces and withdraws the affected part
  - *Grade 4* – The patient will not allow the joint to be touched

- **Crepitus**
  - Fine – Synovitis, tenosynovitis, bursitis
  - Coarse – Cartilage or bony damage
- **Movement of joint**
  - *Active movement*→Range, pain, crepitus, stability, correctable deformities.
  - *Passive movement*→Range, pain, crepitus, other abnormalities.
- **Soft tissues**
  - *Muscles:* Power, wasting, tenderness.
  - *Tendons:* Thickening, tenderness, crepitus, rupture.
  - *Bursae:* Swelling, tenderness, signs of inflammation.
  - *Ligaments:* Tenderness, stability.
  - *Tenosynovium:* Swelling, tenderness.

Examination of Individual Joints

Hands and Wrist

Wrist joint, metacarpophalangeal joint, proximal and distal interphalangeal joint, carpometacarpal joint of thumb.

Normal Range of Movement
- Wrist—70° flexion and extension, 30° side flexion.
- MCP—45° extension, 90° flexion.
- PIP—120° flexion.
- DIP—90° flexion, 10° extension.

Look for
Skin, swelling, deformity, attitude, crepitus, trigger finger, muscle wasting.

Hand function: By grip strength, key grip, opposition strength.

Deformities of Hand (Refer: Rheumatoid Arthritis)
- Swan neck deformity
- Boutonniere deformity
- Z deformity
- Haygarth nodosities
- Opera glass hand.

Heberden's node: Osteoarthrosis of DIP.

Bouchard's node: Osteoarthrosis of PIP.

Elbow Joints

Movement: Flexion – 160°, Extension 5°

Examine for: Joint effusion

Epicondyle tenderness: Medial – Golfer's elbow

Lateral: Tennis elbow

Wrist extension ↑ lateral epicondylar pain.

Wrist flexion ↑ medial epicondylar pain.

   Subcutaneous swellings over olecranon rheumatoid nodule and tophi.

Olecranon bursitis: Fluctuant tender swelling over olecranon.

Shoulder Joint

- Movements
  - Abduction 175°
  - Adduction 50°
  - Flexion 160°
  - Extension 60°
  - Rotation (internal and external) – 70°
- Painful limitation of movement in all direction → intra-articular lesion
- Tendinitis → limitation of movement in one direction
- Bicipital tendinitis → localized pain over the bicipital groove
- Tenderness over the acromioclavicular joint
- Examine the rotator cuff → supraspinatus, infraspinatus, subscapularis and teres minor
- Periarticular lesions of shoulder joint
  - Rotator cuff lesions
  - Subacromial bursitis
  - Bicipital tendinitis

Temporomandibular Joint

- Look for swelling in front of the ear
- Feel the head of the mandible by placing a finger in front of the ear while the patient opens and closes his mouth. Temporomandibular joint is affected by rheumatoid arthritis and neuropathic joint.

Hip Joint

- Movements
  - Flexion–110°
  - Extension–30°
  - Abduction–30°
  - Adduction–30°
  - Rotation – internal and external – 45°
- Examine for flexion deformity
  - Trendelenburg test – The patient stands on one leg and then on the other. Normally the nonweight bearing hip rises. But with proximal myopathy, or hip joint disease, the nonweight bearing hip sags.
  - Measure the true leg length from the anterior superior iliac spine to the medial malleolus and apparent leg length from the umbilicus to the medial malleolus for each leg.
  - A difference in true leg length indicates hip disease on the shorter side, while apparent leg length is due to tilting of the pelvis.
- Tendinitis
  - Adductor tendinitis – tenderness over the adductor region, by resisted adduction.
  - Gluteal tendinitis – lateral pain worsened by resisted abduction.
- Periarticular lesions at the hip
  - Trochanteric bursitis → Tender over greater trochanter
  - Gluteal enthesopathy → Tender over greater trochanter and pain aggravated by resisted abduction

- Adductor tendinitis → Tenderness over the adductor origin and pain aggravated by resisted adduction
- Ischiogluteal bursitis → Tenderness over ischial prominence worsened on sitting
- Iliopectineal bursitis → Tenderness - anterior groin-lateral to femoral pulse, not worsened by internal rotation of hip.

Knee Joint

Movements - Flexion - 130°
Note the following:
- Deformity
  - Genu varum/Genu valgus
  - Position of patella
  - Wasting of quadriceps
  - Tenderness - joint line
- Swelling
  - Patellar tap—to confirm presence of large effusions. One hand rests over the lower part of the quadriceps muscle and compresses the suprapatellar bursa. The other hand pushes the patella downwards. The sign is positive if the patella is felt sink and then comes to rest with a tap as it touches the underlying femur.
  - Bulge sign—in which the medial parapatellar fossa is emptied by pressure of the flat of the hand sweeping proximally. It is seen to refill (the bulge) as the suprapatellar area is emptied by the pressure from the flat of the hand. Feel the popliteal fossa for a Becker's cyst which is a pressure diverticulum of the synovial membrane occurring through a hiatus in the knee capsule.

Ankle and Foot

- Movements
  - Ankle joint → 40° dorsiflexion, 50° plantar flexion
  - Subtalar joint → 5° inversion, 5° eversion
  - Midtarsal joint → 30° inversion—30° eversion

Look for
- Swelling
- Deformity
  - Hallux valgus and varus
  - Clawing of foot—fixed flexion deformity due to small muscle wasting
  - Crowding of toes
  - Sausage deformity of the toes
  - Psoriatic arthritis
  - Ankylosing spondylitis
  - Reiter's disease
- Callosities-On points of abnormal pressures
- Day light sign-Abnormal spreads of 2 adjacent toes
- Palpate tendo-Achilles for tendinitis, Rheumatoid nodule
- Heel tenderness in plantar fascitis
- Tendinitis-Tendo-Achilles, peroneal tendon and tibialis posterior tendon

- Bursitis-Pre-Achilles and retro-Achilles
- Causes of heel pain
  - Achilles enthesitis
  - Achilles tendinitis
  - Achilles bursitis
  - Plantar fasciitis and calcaneal spur
  - Heel pad fat atrophy.

Spine

Normal curvature: Cervical lordosis, thoracic kyphosis and lumbar lordosis.

Deformities (Fig. 7.1)
- Anterior curvature - Lordosis
- Posterior curvature - Kyphosis
- Lateral curvature - Scoliosis
- Knuckle deformity - Prominence of one spinous process due to collapse of one vertebra
- Gibbus deformity (angular deformity) - Due to 2 or 3 vertebral collapse - tuberculosis, trauma, secondaries.

Movement of spine
- *Cervical spine*
  - Rotation (ask the patient to look over one, then the other shoulder)
  - Flexion (ask the patient to touch chin to chest)
  - Extension (ask the patient to look up to the ceiling)
  - Lateral bending (ask the patient to bend the neck sideways and try to touch the shoulder with the ear without raising the shoulder).
- *Thoracolumbar spine*
  - Flexion (ask the patient to try to touch toes, without bending at the knees)
  - Extension (ask the patient to bend backwards)
  - Lateral bending (ask the patient to run the hand down the side of the thigh as far as possible)
  - Thoracic rotation (ask the seated patient, with arms closed, to twist round to the left and right as far as possible)

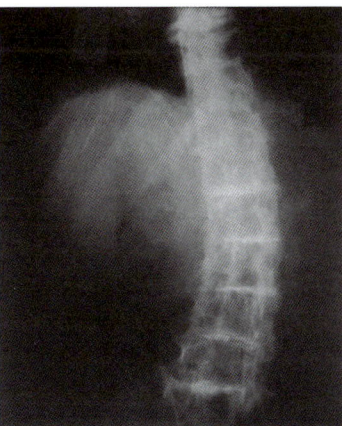

Fig. 7.1: X-ray showing intervertebral disk calcification in a patient with alkaptonuria

- *Swelling*
  - Meningocele – sacral or occipital region
  - Cold abscess – paravertebral region
- **Schober's test:** For the flexion movement of the lumbar spine—mark the midpoint of a line connecting the two posterior superior iliac spine. Draw a vertical line from there, upwards 10 cm long. Ask the patient to touch his toes. An increase of less than 5 cm length of the line indicates the limitation of flexion as in ankylosing spondylitis.
- **Straight leg raising test:** Patient lies supine on the examining table and is asked to raise one lower limb keeping the knee straight. If the pain is evoked under 40° rise, suggest pressure on a nerve root by the protruded intervertebral disk.
- **Lassegue's sign:** When the patient experiences pain on straight leg raising, the ankle is passively dorsiflexed. This causes aggravation of pain due to additional traction to the sciatic nerve.
- **Femoral nerve stretch test:** Patient lies on his abdomen and flex the knee of the affected side. Patient complains of pain in front of the thigh suggest protruding disk L2, L3 which is irritating the femoral nerve.

Sacroiliac Joint

Examination
- Direct pressure over each sacroiliac joint
- Firm pressure with the side of the hand over the sacrum
- Bilateral compression of anterior iliac crests towards midline
- Patrick's test
- Gaenslen's sign.

GALS Screen (Gait, Arms, Legs and Spine)

This is a quick reliable screen of the locomotor system and indicates more detailed examination of the sites of locomotor disease.

Method: With patient undressed, observe them from the front, back and sides looking for any asymmetry or deformity such as unequal leg length, flexion deformity at hip or knee or abnormality of spinal curvature—kyphosis, scoliosis, loss of lordosis.

Gait

Ask patients to walk and observe whether they swing their arms and move their legs symmetrically. The normal gait is distorted when a patient has pain, because persistent muscle contractions splints the painful part. In an antalgic gait, patient avoid bearing weight on the painful leg or foot and spend most of the gait cycle on the unaffected leg (Table 7.1).

Table 7.1: Gait abnormalities in rheumatological disorders.

Site of lesion	Clinical abnormality
Back pain	Decreased swing phase and difficulty turning; stiff backed
Hip arthropathy	Antalgic gait (reduced stance phase on painful side)
Abnormality of hip abduction	Trendelenburg gait (Pelvic drop on contralateral side to affected leg during stance phase)
Knee	Antalgic gait, stiffness of leg during stance phase
Hindfoot	Antalgic gait; decreased heel strike, walking on toes
Midfoot	Antalgic gait; worse on uneven surfaces
Forefoot	Antalgic gait, walking on heels, reduced toe – off phase
Footdrop	Slapping, high – stepping gait; scuffing of toes, tripping

Arms

- Ask the patients to hold out their hands, palms down, inspect the arms for obvious abnormalities (e.g. swelling, deformity, nodules). Inspect the hands for skin or nail changes that may be associated with arthritis (e.g. the scaly rash or onycholysis of psoriasis, the digital vasculitis of SLE, the color changes of Raynaud's disease).
- Ask the patients to turn their hands over. This assess the radioulnar joint, which is commonly affected in rheumatoid arthritis (RA). Inspect the palms, looking for signs of Dupuytren's contracture and thenar wasting.
- Ask the patients to make a tight fist with each hand and check that the fingers flex fully into the palms. Power of grip can be assessed by offering the index and middle fingers of your hands asking patients to grip your fingers tightly.
- Ask the patients to place the tip of each finger, in turn, onto the tip of the thumb. This assesses the opposition of the thumb and fine movements, which are often limited in RA.
- Squeeze across the hand from the second to the fifth metacarpophalageal joints, to assess tenderness.
- Ask the patients to put their hands behind the head, pressing the elbows back. This movement assess abduction and external rotation of the shoulders and flexion at the elbows, and is of functional importance in combing the hair.

Legs

- With the patient lying supine on the couch, inspect the flexion deformity at the hip or knee, then passively flex the hip and knee with a hand placed over the knee. Assess knee flexion while feeling for crepitus and assessing hip flexion.
- Passively internally rotate the hip with the knee and hip still flexed. Internal rotation is the first movement to become restricted in hip disease.

- Ask the patients to flex, extend, invert and evert the ankle to assess tibiotalar movement (affected by osteoarthritis) and subtalar movement (affected by TA).
- Squeeze across the foot at the level of the metatarsophalangeal joints, looking for tenderness.

Spine

- With the patient standing, ask them to put their ear on his shoulder on the same side, keeping the shoulder still. This assesses the lateral flexion of the cervical spine, which is the first movement to become restricted in degenerative or inflammatory disease.
- Place two of your fingers over adjacent spinous process in the lumbar region and ask the patient to bend over and touch his toes. Your fingers should move apart. This is an essential part of the assessment of the lumbar spine because patients with a rigid spine caused by ankylosing spondylitis may be able to touch their toes if they have supple hips.

Hypermobility of Joint (Fig. 7.2)

- In 10% of normal people, Marfan syndrome, Ehlers-Danlos syndrome
- Hypermobility is assessed by modified Beighton score' (Table 7.2).

Examination of Other Systems

CVS

- Pericarditis – rheumatoid arthritis, progressive systemic sclerosis
- Pancarditis – rheumatic fever, SLE
- Conducting system lesion – rheumatoid arthritis
- Aortitis – psoriasis, reiter's, rheumatoid arthritis, ankylosing spondylitis

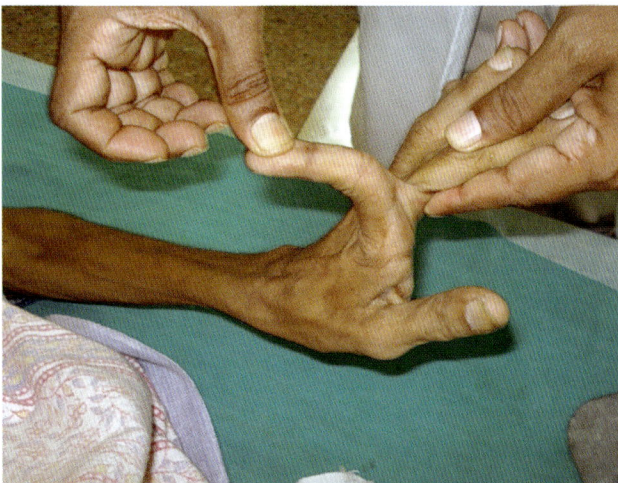

Fig. 7.2: Hyperextensibility of the joints

Table 7.2: Beighton score.

Beighton scores	Score
Extend little finger > 90°	1 point for each finger
Bring thumb back parallel or to touching forearm	1 point for each thumb
Extend elbow > 10°	1 point for each elbow
Extend knee > 10°	1 point for each knee
Touch floor with palms of hand, keeping the legs straight	1 point
A score of 6 or more indicates hypermobility	

Nervous System

- Myelopathy – Atlantoaxial dislocation – Rheumatoid arthritis
- Neuropathy – Entrapment neuropathy – Rheumatoid arthritis
- Mononeuritis multiplex – Rheumatoid arthritis, Polyarteritis nodosa
- Peripheral neuropathy – Churg-Strauss syndrome, SLE
- Proximal myopathy – Polymyositis, dermatomyositis
- Arthrogenic wasting of muscles.

Respiratory System

- Upper respiratory tract lesion – Wegener's granulomatosis
- Pleural lesion – Rheumatoid arthritis, SLE, progressive systemic sclerosis (PSS)
- Lung fibrosis – SLE, rheumatoid arthritis, PSS
- Lung nodules and cavity – rheumatoid arthritis
- Caplan's syndrome—rheumatoid nodule with pneumoconiosis
- Alveolar hemorrhage – Microscopic polyangitis and SLE
- Bronchiolitis – Rheumatoid arthritis
- Hemoptysis – Wegener's granulomatosis, microscopic polyangitis, SLE
- Asthma – Churg-Strauss syndrome
- Chest expansion < 2 cm – ankylosing spondylitis

GIT

- *Oropharyngeal ulcer*: SLE, Behçet's syndrome.
- *IBD*: Seronegative spondyloarthritis.
- *Vasculitis*: Rheumatoid arthritis.
- *Hepatosplenomegaly*: Still's disease, SLE.
- *Abdominal pain and bleeding PR*: HS purpura.
- *Gastric and intestinal ulcer*: NSAID in rheumatological disorder.
- *Pancreatitis:* Arthritis of knee and ankle joint, panniculitis.

Genitourinary System

- *Renal rickets, renal osteodystrophy:* Bone pain.
- *Nephritis:* SLE, HS purpura, vasculitis – Wegener's granulomatosis, microscopic polyangitis and Churg-Strauss syndrome

- *Urethritis:* Reactive arthropathy
- *Analgesic nephropathy:* Rheumatoid arthritis
- Renal vasculitis:
  - Wegener's granulomatosis
  - Microscopic polyangitis
  - PSS-renal crisis.

Endocrine System

- *Hypothyroidism and acromegaly:* Rheumatic symptoms
- *Acromegaly:* Secondary osteoarthrosis
- *Hyperparathyroidism:* Bone pain
- *Diabetes mellitus:* Cheiroarthropathy, periarthritis shoulder
- *Pseudo Cushing's syndrome:* Steroid therapy in rheumatological disorders.

Metabolic

- Gout, pseudogout, ochronosis: Spine involvement
- Hemochromatosis: Hand arthropathy

Internal Malignancy

- *Polyarthritis:* A/c leukemia, Ca breast
- *Hypertrophic osteoarthropathy:* Bronchogenic Ca
- *Amyloid arthropathy:* Multiple myeloma
- *Secondary gout:* Myeloproliferative disorders

DIFFERENTIAL DIAGNOSIS OF ARTHRITIS

Depending on Etiology

Arthritis in Adult

- *Infections*
  - Viral–HBV, Parvovirus, HIV, chikungunya (Fig. 7.3)
  - Bacterial – Gonococci
  - Infective endocarditis
  - Hansen's disease, syphilis, tuberculosis

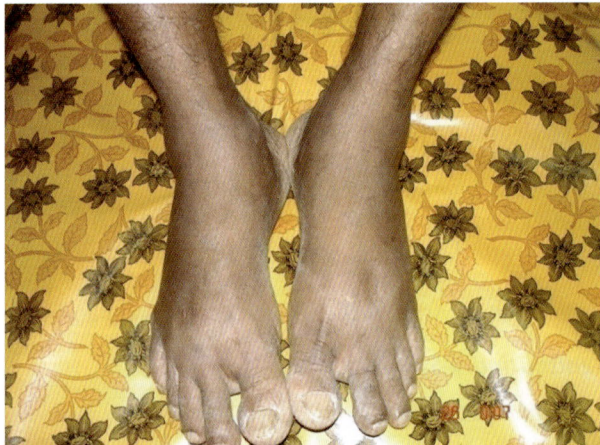

Fig. 7.3: Arthritis and subcutaneous edema in a patient with chikungunya

- *Postinfectious*
  - Rheumatic fever
  - Poncet's disease
  - Reactive arthropathy
- *Immune mediated*
  - Rheumatoid arthritis
  - Seronegative spondyloarthropathy
  - Collagen vascular disease
- *Degenerative arthropathy*
  - Osteoarthrosis
- Metabolic arthropathy
  - Gout, pseudogout, alkaptonuria, hemochromatosis
- *Endocrine*
  - Diabetes mellitus
  - Hypothyroidism
  - Acromegaly
- *Hematological*
  - HS purpura
  - A/c leukemia
  - Sickle cell anemia
  - Hemophilia
  - Poncet's disease (polyarthritis as an allergic manifestation to primary TB)

Arthritis in Children

- Juvenile chronic arthritis
- Infections – Same as above
- Post infectious – Same as above
- Hematological - Same as above
- Endocrine
  - Diabetes mellitus
  - Cretinism
  - Gigantism
- Metabolic – Same as above.

Depending on the Duration and Number of Joints Involved

Acute

- Monoarthritis
  - Inflammatory: Septic arthritis, gout, palindromic
  - Noninflammatory: Trauma, torn meniscus, hemochromatosis, hemophilic
- Polyarthritis
  - Infections: Viral, Gonococcal
  - Reactive arthritis
  - HS purpura
  - Rheumatic fever
  - Erythema nodosum

Chronic

- Monoarthritis
  - Inflammatory: Tuberculosis
  - Noninflammatory: Osteoarthrosis, hemophilic

- Polyarthritis
  - Inflammatory: Rheumatoid arthritis, seronegative spondyloarthropathy, Polyarticular gout, Collagen vascular disease
  - Noninflammatory: Polyarticular generalized osteoarthropathy.

Differential Diagnosis of Polyarthritis

Symmetrical

- *Rheumatoid arthritis*: PIP joint. MTP joint, wrist and elbow
- Juvenile chronic arthritis
- SLE, polyarteritis nodosa
- Hypertrophic osteoarthropathy
- Polymyalgia rheumatica
- Hemochromatosis
- Primary generalized osteoarthrosis
- Remitting seronegative symmetrical synovitis with pitting edema (RS3PE)

Asymmetrical

- Seronegative spondyloarthropathy
- Infections
- Postinfective
- Rheumatic fever
- Reactive arthropathy
- Poncet's disease
- Gout, pseudogout
- Osteoarthrosis
- Collagen vascular disease
- Oligoarticular juvenile chronic arthritis

Differential Diagnosis of Oligoarthritis

- Seronegative spondyloarthritis
- Juvenile chronic arthritis
- Rheumatic fever
- Oligoarticular presentation of polyarthritis
- Erythema nodosum
- Infections
- Osteoarthrosis

Differential Diagnosis of Monoarthritis

- Septic arthritis
- Tuberculosis
- Gout (Fig. 7.4)
- Pseudogout
- Osteoarthrosis
- Traumatic
- Hemophilic
- *Monoarticular*: Rheumatoid arthritis, reactive arthritis

Differential Diagnosis of Deforming Polyarthropathy

- Rheumatoid arthritis
- Seronegative spondyloarthritis—psoriatic arthritis

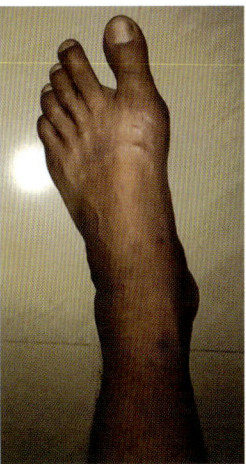

Fig. 7.4: Gouty arthritis—1st metatarsophalangeal joint.

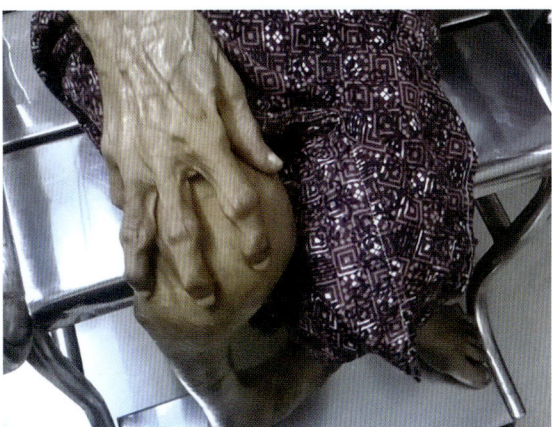

Fig. 7.5: Primary generalized osteoarthritis involving small joints of hand including DIP and knee joint.

- Reiter's arthritis
- Chronic tophaceous arthritis
- Primary generalized osteoarthritis (Fig. 7.5).

Differential Diagnosis of Symmetrical Deforming Polyarthritis

- Rheumatoid arthritis
- Jaccoud's arthritis
- Juvenile chronic arthritis
- Primary generalized osteoarthritis
- Post chickengunya chronic arthritis

Differential Diagnosis of Arthritis with Subcutaneous Nodules

- Rheumatoid arthritis
- Rheumatic fever
- Gout
- Sarcoidosis
- SLE (rare)

Differential Diagnosis of Fleeting Arthritis

- Rheumatic fever
- Gonococcal arthritis

Overnight Joint Swelling

- Gonococcal
- Hemophilic
- Traumatic

Multisystem Diseases with Arthritis

With Positive Serology

- Rheumatoid factor
  - Rheumatoid arthritis
  - Primary Sjogren's syndrome
  - Mixed cryoglobulinemia
- Antinuclear antibody
  - SLE (DNA, Sm, RNP, Ro)
  - Primary Sjogren's syndrome (Ro, La)
  - Antiphospholipid antibody syndrome (Anticardiolipin)
  - Polymyositis (PM, Jo-1 – Lung diseases)
  - Scleroderma (Scl 70 – diffuse, anticentromere– local)
  - Mixed connective tissue disease (ribonucleoprotein antibody)
  - Wegener's vasculitis (cANCA)
  - Vasculitis (pANCA)
  - Microscopic polyangiitis

With Negative Serology

- Sarcoidosis
- Behçet's syndrome
- Amyloidosis
- Familial mediterranean fever
- Polyarteritis nodosa
- Paraneoplasia.

Polyarthritis and Infection

Viral: HBV, HIV, parvovirus, rubella, chikungunya.
Bacterial: Gonococcal, infective endocarditis, Hansen's disease—ENL.
Syphilis, tuberculosis, brucellosis, Lyme arthritis: Borrelia burgdorferi.
Fungal: Aspergillosis, candidiasis, actinomycosis.
Parasitic: Giardiasis, stongyloidiasis.
Postinfectious: Rheumatic fever, reactive arthritis, Poncet's disease.

COMMON RHEUMATOLOGICAL DISORDERS

RHEUMATOID ARTHRITIS (RA)

First described by Archibald Garrod in 1876.

Definition

Chronic inflammatory disease of autoimmune origin affecting the synovial joint and a variety of extra-articular structures.

Etiology

Multifactorial: Genetic—HLA DR4 and 1.
Triggering stimuli: Viral antigen with cross reactivity due to molecular mimicry.

Immunopathology

Synovial microvascular injury → proliferation of synovial cells → infiltration by inflammatory cells → CD4 T cell, macrophage, plasma cells, fibroblast cytokines → IL, TNF-α, IFN, GMCSF, TGF
B cell activation → Rheumatoid factor → Immune complex
Villous like proliferation of synovial tissue – pannus

All these lead onto
- Articular damage
- Vascular damage
- Systemic damage

Clinical Features

Articular and extra-articular
- *Female to male ratio*: 3:1
- *Age*: 4th and 5th decade.

Articular Manifestation

- *Onset*: Insidious—70%
- *Acute*: 15%
- *Systemic onset*: 10%
- *Palindromic*: 5%
- Polymyalgic onset.

Pattern of Joint Involvement
- *Polyarticular, symmetrical*: 35%
- *Oligoarticular*: 44%
- *Monoarticular*: 21%.

Joints Affected
PIP, MCP, wrist, elbow, knee, ankle, MTP sparing DIP.
Swelling: Fluid, synovial hypertrophy, capsule thickening, warmth, morning stiffness, limitation of movement.
Spine: Atlantoaxial joint, mid cervical joint, acromioclavicular, emporomandibular and sternoclavicular joint.
  Persistent inflammation → deformity due to laxity of tissue, destruction of ligament and joint capsule, cartilage and bony damage, muscle weakness.

Hand in Rheumatoid Arthritis

Deformities
Spindling of joint: PIP—Hegarthes nodosity.

Swan neck deformity:
- Flexion of MCP
- Extension of PIP
- Flexion of DIP

Boutonniere deformity:
- Extension of MCP
- Flexion of PIP
- Extension of DIP
- Ulnar subluxation.

Opera glass hand appearance: Mutilating arthropathy.
- Insinuation of distal phalanx into the destroyed proximal phalanx.
- Palmar erythema, digital vasculitis.
- Nail fold infarct and ulcer.
- Carpal tunnel syndrome, arthrogenic wasting of muscles.

Extra-articular Manifestation

- *Systemic*: Fever, loss of weight, fatigue
- *Rheumatoid nodule*: Nontender subcutaneous nodule – extensor aspect around tendons, also seen in lung, pleura and sclera.
- *Vasculitis* (Two types)
  1. Leucocytoclastic vasculitis: Small vessel vasculitis
  2. Severe necrotizing vasculitis
     - Cutaneous ulcer and infarct
     - Digital gangrene and visceral infarct
     - Mononeuritis and mononeuritis multiplex
     - Large ischemic ulcer and digital gangrene due to necrotizing vasculitis called malignant rheumatoid disease
- *Respiratory system:* Pleurisy, pleural effusion, pulmonary nodule and cavitation, fibrosing alveolitis, obliterative bronchiolitis, Caplan's syndrome.
- *Cardiovascular system*: Pericarditis, conducting system abnormality, granulomatous aortitis and aortic regurgitation.
- *Nervous system*
  - Peripheral neuropathy
  - Mononeuritis and mononeuritis multiplex
  - Carpal Tunnel syndrome
  - Spinal cord – Atlantoaxial dislocation and myelopathy
  - Myopathy—Arthrogenic and drug induced- chloroquine/steroids
- *Eye*
  - Episcleritis, scleritis, scleromalacia perforans
  - Brown's syndrome
  - *Keratoconjunctivitis sicca*: Secondary Sjögren's syndrome.
- *Hematological*
  - Anemia—Chronic inflammation, iron deficiency – bleeding
  - Platelet count—Thrombocytosis
  - WBC count—Normal/increased/decreased
  - Leucopenia
  - Lymphadenopathy, splenomegaly—Still's disease/Felty's syndrome
- *Renal*
  - *Vasculitis, amyloidosis*: Nephrotic syndrome
  - *Drug-induced (NSAID)*: Analgesic nephropathy
  - *Gold and pencillamine*: Proteinuria.
- *Nonarticular rheumatic features*: Tenosynovitis, bursitis, plantar fascitis, osteoporosis.
- *Skin*
  - Subcutaneous nodule, palmar erythema
  - *Cutaneous vasculitis*: Ulcer, necrosis, infarct.

Diagnostic Criteria–American College of Rheumatology (Table 7.3)

- Morning stiffness > 1 hour
- Arthritis of 3 or more joints—14 joint areas—proximal interphalangeal (PIP), metacarpophalangeal (MCP), wrist, elbow, knee, ankle
- Arthritis of hand joints—PIP, MCP and wrist
- Symmetrical arthritis
- Rheumatoid nodule
- Rheumatoid factor
- Radiological changes—erosion/juxta-articular osteopenia.
  - *Four or more features diagnostic of rheumatoid arthritis*
  - *1 to 4 criteria should be present for 6 weeks or more.*

Table 7.3: European League Against Rheumatism (EULAR)/ACR 2010 Criteria.

Criteria	Score
Joints affected	
1 large joint	0
2–10 large joints	1
1–3 small joints	2
4–10 small joints	5
Serology	
Negative RF and ACPA	0
Low positive RF or ACPA	2
High positive RF or ACPA	3
Duration of symptoms	
< 6 weeks	0
>6 weeks	1
Acute phase reactants	
Normal CRP and ESR	0
Abnormal CRP or ESR	1

Abbrevations: RF-rheumatoid factor, ANCA-antineutrophil cytoplasmic antibodies, CRP-C reactive proteins, ESR: erythrocyte sedimentation rate

Patients with a score ≥ 6 are considered to have definite RA.

The following features go against the diagnosis of rheumatoid arthritis:
- Inflammatory backache
- *Persistent asymmetric arthritis*: Large joints
- High fever
- Active urinary sediment
- Mucocutaneous lesion
- Psoriatic skin lesions
- Balanitis

Disease Evaluation

Categorization

- Early disease—>6 weeks and <6 months duration
- Established disease—>6 months duration
- Advanced disease—>3 years duration.

Disease Activity

- Number of tender joint
- Number of swollen joint—swelling due to synovial proliferation or effusion and not bony
- Duration of morning stiffness
- Pain assessed by the patient on visual analogue scale
- Physicians and Patient's global assessment with reference to fatigue, appetite, weight loss and well being—erythrocyte sedimentation rate (ESR) or C-reactive protein (CRP)
- Platelet count, hemoglobin
- Damage—joint erosion and joint space narrowing
- Disability—health assessment questionnaire (HAQ)
- Extra-articular manifestation.

Clinical Variants

- Mono/oligoarticular type
- *Juvenile rheumatoid arthritis*: 10% of juvenile C/c arthritis
- *Felty's syndrome*: Chronic rheumatoid arthritis, splenomegaly, neutropenia
- *Caplan's syndrome*: Rheumatoid nodule in lung with pneumoconiosis
- Mutilating arthropathy
- *Malignant rheumatoid disease*: Rheumatoid arthritis with severe vasculitis
- Secondary Sjögren's syndrome.

Differential Diagnosis

- Rheumatic fever
- Infections with arthritis
- Seronegative spondyloarthritis
- Collagen vascular disease
- Polyarticular gout
- Primary generalized osteoarthosis.

Investigations

- To establish the diagnosis
- To assess the disease activity
- To monitor the safety of drugs.

To establish the diagnosis
- Markers of inflammation
  - ESR, CRP, alkaline phosphatase, platelet count, albumin, hemoglobin
- Serology
  - Rheumatoid factor
    - IgM, IgG, IgA and IgE
    - 20 or more IU/ml – Positive
    - 75 % RF positive
    - 25 % RF negative
  - ANA positive in 30%
- Radiology
  - X-ray of hands and other joints
  - Soft tissue swelling
  - Juxta—articular osteopenia
  - Narrowing of joint space—loss of cartilage
  - Erosion of joint margin
  - Deformities and subluxation
- Synovial fluid analysis
  - To differentiate infection, bleeding, crystal arthropathy and degenerative arthropathy
  - Protein is increased
  - WBC increased
  - Turbid
  - Globulin decreased
  - C3, C4 decreased
  - WBC > 2000/mm^3, > 75 % polymorphs
- Arthrography, USG, CT, MRI (early assessment) – To know the pathological extend
- Arthroscopy

To Assess the Disease Activity

ESR, CRP and hemoglobin.

To Monitor the Safety of Drugs

Complete blood count, urine analysis, renal function test (RFT) and liver function test (LFT).

Disease with Positive Rheumatoid Factor

Articular
Rheumatoid arthritis, mixed connective tissue disease (MCTD), Primary Sjögren's syndrome (PSS), SLE.

Nonarticular
- Fibrosing alveolitis
- Chronic active hepatitis
- Infective endocarditis
- Myeloma
- Kala azar
- Hansen's disease
- *Normal people*: 5%.

Poor Prognostic Factors

- Insidious onset
- > 20 joints inflammation
- Rheumatoid nodule
- Vasculitis
- Bony erosion
- Extra-articular manifestation
- High ESR
- High rheumatoid factor titer
- HLA DR4 positive

Complications

- *Septic arthritis*: Staphylococcal
- Ruptured tendon and joint capsule
- Amyloidosis, atlantoaxial dislocation
- *Drugs*: GI bleeding, nephropathy, marrow failure.

Management of RA

Goals of Therapy

- Relief of pain
- Reduction of inflammation
- Conservation of function of joints
- Control of systemic involvement

Measures

- Medical
  - Rest
  - Drugs
  - NSAID
  - DMARD
  - Corticosteroids
  - Biological agents
- Physiotherapy
- Surgical therapy

NSAID

- Nonselective Cox inhibitors
  - Indomethacin: 25–75 mg/day
- Selective Cox-2 inhibitors
  - Etoricoxib: 60,90 to 120 mg/day
- Side effects of NSAID
  - Anaphylaxis, drug rash, asthma
  - GI side effect–ulcer and bleed
  - Renal side effect – Interstitial nephritis, papillitis necroticans.

DMARD (Table 7.4)

- Chloroquine
- Methotrexate
- Sulphasalazine
- D-penicillamine
- Gold injection
- Gold oral
- Leflunomide
- Response to DMARD
  - Leflunomide → 2-4 weeks
  - Methotrexate and sulfasalazine → 1-2 months
  - Others → 3-6 months for its effects

Table 7.4: Disease modifying antirheumatic drugs (DMARDs).

Name	Dose	Side effects	Monitoring	Onset of action
Chloroquine	250 mg od for 3 months then alternate days	Skin Pigmentation, Retinopathy, Nausea, Psychosis, Myopathy	Fundoscopy and perimetry 6 monthly	2–4 months
Methotrexate	7.5–15 mg once a week orally	Bone marrow suppression, Hepatotoxicity, Pulmonary fibrosis, Mucositis, Nausea	Blood counts, LFT every 2 weeks for 3 months, then monthly	1–2 months
Sulphasalazine	2 g daily orally	Rash myelosuppression	CBC, LFT monthly	1–2 months
D-penicillamine	250–500 mg po daily	Rash, cytopenias, proteinuria, autoimmune disease	Blood counts, urine analysis	3–6 months
Gold injection	10–50 mg weekly	Rash, stomatitis, cytopenias, nephropathy	Blood counts, urine analysis	3–6 months
Gold oral	3 mg bd orally	Rash, stomatitis, cytopenias, nephropathy. GI effects more common	Blood counts, urine analysis	3–6 months
Leflunomide	20 mg/day	GI side effect, rash, alopecia, hepatitis, HTN	Blood count, LFT every 2 weeks for 3 months, then monthly	2–4 weeks

- Combination of DMARD
  - Methotrexate and sulphasalazine
  - Methotrexate and cyclosporine
  - Methotrexate and leflunomide

Corticosteroids
- Intra-articular injections to relieve pain
- Bridge therapy given for the period of onset of action of DMARDs
- Therapeutic failure with NSAID and DMARD → 5–7.5 mg of Prednisolone/day (oral background therapy). Rheumatic flare—to suppress the inflammation
- Extra-articular involvement – ocular, pericarditis
- Vasculitis and interstitial lung disease.

Biological Agents
Biological response modifiers
- Anticytokine treatment (Table 7.5)
- Gene therapy
- Antilymphocyte therapy – against CD4 T cell.

Surgical Therapy
- Soft tissue resection: Carpal or tarsal tunnel syndrome
- Tendon repair: Rupture tendon
- Synovectomy: For recalcitrant monoarthritis
- Arthroplasty: Subluxation
- Arthrodesis: Improve hand function
- Joint replacement

Rehabilitation
- Prevention of disability by appliances
- Job retraining
- Domestic adaptation

Remission Criteria
1. Morning stiffness < 15 months
2. No fatigue
3. No joint pain
4. No joint tenderness or pain on movement
5. No soft tissue swelling
6. ESR < 20 in males, < 30 in female
   → Remission means 5 out of 6

SYSTEMIC LUPUS ERYTHEMATOSUS

Definition: Multisystem inflammatory disease of unknown etiology characterized by the presence of numerous autoantibodies.

Etiology

Multifactorial disorder
- Immune factors – Defect in suppressor T cell, activation of polyclonal B lymphocytes producing uncontrolled autoantibodies
- Genetic factors – HLA, B8 and DR3
- Environmental factors
- Provocation by sunlight
- Induction by drugs

Clinical Features

- *General:* Fever, Fatigue, Anorexia
- *Musculoskeletal*
  - Arthralgia
  - Myalgia
  - Symmetrical nondeforming arthritis
  - Hand deformity due to capsule and tendon contracture
  - Ischemic necrosis of bone
  - Myositis and myopathy
  - Drug-induced myopathy (steroid and chloroquine)
- *Skin*
  - Malar butterfly rash (Fig. 7.6)
  - Discoid rash (Fig. 7.7)
  - Photosensitivity
  - Oropharyngeal ulcers
  - Alopecia
  - Lupus hair
  - Vasculitis
  - Panniculitis
  - Livedo reticularis
  - Raynaud's phenomenon
  - Purpura
- *Hematological*
  - Hemolytic anemia
  - Leucopenia

Table 7.5: Anticytokine treatment.

Drug	Nature	Dose	ROA
Etanercept	Dimeric fusion protein against TNF α	25 mg twice weekly	Subcutaneous
Infliximab	Chimeric monoclonal Ab against TNF α	3 mg/kg at 0, 2 6 weeks and every 8 weeks thereafter	Intravenous
Adalimumab	Fully humanized monoclonal Ab against TNF α	40 mg every 2 weeks	Subcutaneous
Anakinra	Recombinant human IL-1 receptor antagonist	100 mg/day	Subcutaneous
Rituximab	Ab against CD20 of B cells	1000 mg; repeated after 2 weeks	Intravenous

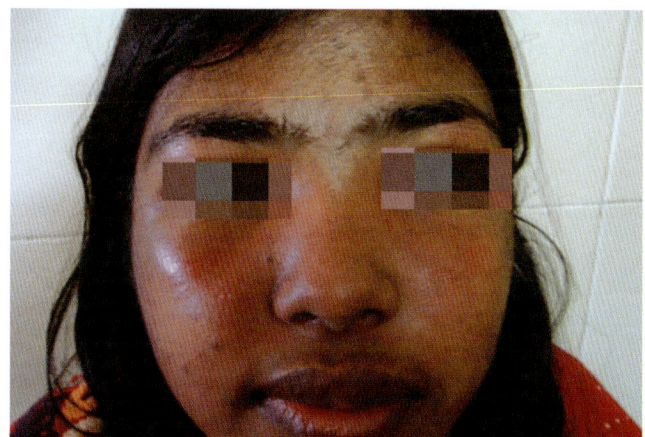

Fig. 7.6: Butterfly rash in SLE.

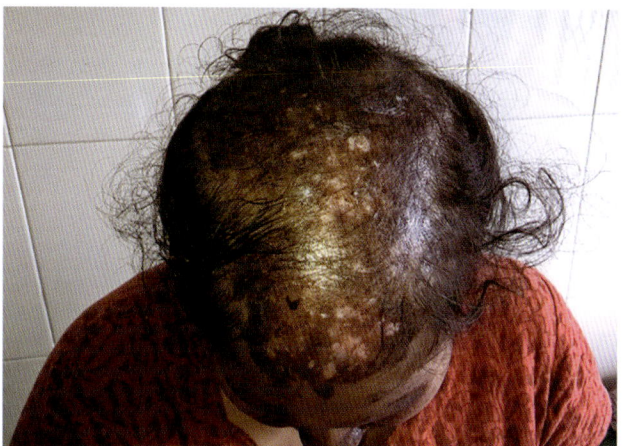

Fig. 7.7: Discoid lesion in SLE.

- Thrombocytopenia
- Pancytopenia
- Lymphadenopathy
- Splenomegaly
- Circulating anticoagulants (Ab to factor VIII and IX),
- Antiphospholipid syndrome
- **Neurological**
  - Psychosis
  - Seizure
  - Cognitive dysfunction
  - Stroke
  - Cerebellar lesion
  - Chorea
  - BIH
  - Aseptic meningitis
  - Optic neuropathy
  - Cranial nerve palsy
  - Peripheral neuropathy
  - Sneddon's syndrome (livedo reticularis, cerebral thrombosis and APL Ab)
- **Cardiopulmonary**
  - Pleurisy
  - Pleural effusion
  - Lupus pneumonitis
  - Interstitial fibrosis
  - Pulmonary arterial hypertension
  - Small lung syndrome (B/L weakening and elevation of diaphragm)
  - Intra-alveolar hemorrhage
  - Pericarditis
  - Myocarditis
  - Libman-Sack's endocarditis
  - Valvular heart disease: MR, AR
  - Pulmonary infarct: Secondary APL syndrome
- **GIT**
  - Anorexia
  - Vomiting

- Vasculitis of GIT
- Perforations
- Ascites
- Hepatomegaly
- Pancreatitis
- Drug-induced ulcers and bleed
- Budd-Chiari syndrome
- **Renal**
  - Criteria for lupus nephropathy proteinuria of more than 0.5 gm/day or cellular cast
  - Manifestation
    - Asymptomatic proteinuria
    - Symptomatic proteinuria
    - Nephrotic syndrome
    - Proliferative glomerulonephritis
    - Progressive renal failure
  - **WHO classification of lupus nephropathy**
    - Class I – Normal kidney
    - Class II – Mesangial
      IIa – Mesangial deposit
      11b – Mesangial hypercellularity
    - Class III – Focal glomerulonephritis
    - Class IV – Diffuse glomerulonephritis
    - Class V – Membranous glomerulonephritis
    - Class VI – Chronic glomerulosclerosis

Ocular: Conjunctivitis, episcleritis, sicca syndrome, retinal vasculitis, cystoid body (superficial nerve fiber infarct).

Disease Subsets

- *Subacute cutaneous lupus*: Features limited to skin
- DLE
- Lupus panniculitis
- *Neonatal and Juvenile*: Rash, photosensitivity and congenital heart block
- Antiphospholipid syndrome
- MCTD
- Drug-induced lupus.

Diagnostic Criteria

American College of Rheumatology, revised criteria in 1982
1. Malar erythema
2. Discoid lesion
3. Photosensitivity
4. Oropharyngeal ulcer
5. Nonerosive polyarthritis
6. Serositis – pleurisy, pericarditis
7. Renal – proteinuria > 0.5 gm in 24 hrs/cellular cast
8. CNS – psychosis/seizure
9. Hematological–hemolytic anemia/leucopenia/thrombocytopenia/lymphopenia
10. Immunological–Positive LE cell/anti DNA/anti-Sm/ biological false positive serological test for syphilis
11. ANA

Diagnostic requirement—4 or more criteria serially or simultaneously suggest SLE (Table 7.6).

DD of SLE

- MCTD
- Rheumatoid arthritis
- Progressive systemic sclerosis
- Primary
- Sjogren's syndrome
- Disseminated sclerosis
- ITP

Clinical Presentations of SLE

- Pyrexia of unknown origin (PUO)
- PUO with mucocutaneous lesions
- PUO with symmetrical arthritis and mucocutaneous lesions
- Seizures with psychosis
- Fever with acute dyspnea—lupus pneumonitis, pulmonary alveolar hemorrhage
- Immune thrombocytopenia with high ESR
- AIHA with high ESR
- Nephropathy
- APLA syndrome-fetal loss
- MCTD

Investigations

- Complete blood count, ESR, hemoglobin, platelet count
- CRP: Normal in SLE
- Elevated in infection in SLE or cardiopulmonary lupus
- Urine analysis, RFT, 24 hours urinary protein
- ANA, anti ds-DNA, antiphospholipid antibody, VDRL
- Antibody to extractable nuclear antigen (ENA)
- Anti-Ro, anti-La, anti-Sm, anti-RNP
- Complement C3, C4
- Renal biopsy, skin biopsy
- EEG, CT, MRI, SPECT scan

Diseases with ANA Positivity

- *Fluorescent ANA*: Homogenous, nonspecific
- *Rim*: SLE
- *Speckled*: SLE/MCTD
- *Nucleolar*: Progressive systemic sclerosis
- *Diseases*: SLE, MCTD, Progressive systemic sclerosis, Rheumatoid arthritis, Sjögren's syndrome
- Polymyositis, fibrosing alveolitis, C/c active hepatitis
- Hansen's disease, IMN, thyroiditis

Autoantibodies in SLE and Disease Pattern (Table 7.7)

- *ANA*—in 98% of SLE.
- *Anti-ds DNA—in 70%*: Lupus nephritis
- *Anti-Sm—in 30%*: Specific for SLE
- *Anti RNP*: MCTD (PSS, SLE, polymyositis)
- Anti Ro-Sjogren's syndrome, ANA negative lupus, neonatal lupus, SCLE
- *Anti-La*: Sjögren's syndrome
- *Anti-histone*: Drug induced SLE
- *Antiphospholipids (lupus anticoagulant/anti-cardiolipin)*: APL syndrome and SLE
- *Antineuronal antibody*: CNS lupus

Tanble 7.6: SLICC Classification Criteria for SLE.

Clinical criteria	Immunologic criteria
1. Acute cutaneous lupus 2. Chronic cutaneous lupus 3. Oral or nasal ulcers 4. Nonscarring alopecia 5. Arthritis 6. Serositis 7. Renal involvement 8. Neurologic involvement 9. Hemolytic anemia 10. Leukopenia 11. Thrombocytopenia	1. ANA 2. Anti-DNA 3. Anti-Smith 4. Antiphopholipid Ab 5. Low complement (C3, C4, CH50) 6. Direct Coomb's test 7. Do not count in the presence of hemolytic anemia

SLICC : Systemic Lupus International Collaborating Clinics

Requirements: >/= 4 criteria (at least 1 clinical and 1 laboratory criteria or biopsy-proven lupus nephritis with positive ANA or Anti-DNA)

Table 7.7: Assessing disease activity.

Clinical	Laboratory
Fatigue	Anemia
Weight loss	Leucopenia
Pallor	Thrombocytopenia
Fever	Hematuria/proteinuria/cellular cast
Arthritis	ESR increase
Seizure	Anti-dsDNA increase
Oral ulcer	Decrease in complement C3, C4
Edema/oliguria	Complement split product

- *Antiribosomal P antibody*: CNS lupus—psychosis and depression.
  - Absence of other organ inflammation.

Management

Preventive Measures

- Avoid offending drugs which induce lupus
- Avoid exposure to sunlight to reduce photosensitivity.

3 Groups

1. Mild
   - Skin and joint involvement
   - Absence of other organ inflammation
2. Moderate
   - Inflammatory involvement of other organs also
   - Class II lupus nephropathy
3. Severe
   - Severe inflammatory involvement of vital organs
   - Class III or more lupus nephropathy
   - CNS lupus
   - Cardiopulmonary involvement

Treatment

Mild

- Hydroxychloroquine
- NSAID ± low dose steroid for arthritis
- Sun screening agent
- Topical steroid
- Intralesional steroid
- Hydroxylchloroquine – skin lesions
- Hydroxychloroquine – oral ulcers and SCLE

Moderate

- Prednisolone – 0.5 mg/kg daily till remission. Tapering to 10 mg/day, (1 mg/month reduction) for several months
- Azathioprine – 2.5 mg/kg/day

Severe

1. Prednisolone –1 mg/kg/day or
2. Methylprednisolone 1 gm IV for 3 days and pulse cyclophosphamide oral/IV (750–1000 mg IV, if RFT normal, 500–750 mg; if RFT is abnormal)
   - Monthly for 6 months than 3 monthly for 2 years.

Bad Prognostic Signs

- Renal involvement with renal failure
- CNS lupus
- Hypertension
- Presence of infection.

SERONEGATIVE SPONDYLOARTHROPATHY (TABLE 7.8)

Common Features

- Sacroilitis
- Peripheral arthropathy – asymmetrical oligoarthritis
- Absence of rheumatoid factor
- Enthesopathy
- Ocular involvement – anterior uveitis
- Involvement of heart, lung and skin
- Familial association
- Overlap of various spondyloarthropathies
- High prevalence of HLA B27
  - 95% in ankylosing spondylitis
  - 50% in psoriatic/enteropathic

Disease Include

- Ankylosing spondylitis
- Reiter's arthropathy/Reactive arthropathy
  - EARA (enteric acquired reactive arthropathy)
  - SARA (sexually acquired reactive arthropathy)
- Enteropathic arthropathy—Crohn's/ulcerative colitis
- Psoriatic arthropathy
- SEA syndrome (seronegative enthesopathic arthropathy)
- Pustulotic arthro-osteitis – SAPHO (Synovitis, Acne, Pustulosis – palmoplantar, hyperosteosis of spine and osteitis)
- Undifferentiated seronegative spondyloarthropathy

DIAGNOSTIC CRITERIAS OF RHEUMATOLOGICAL DISORDERS (TABLE 7.9)

Rheumatoid Arthritis (Refer Rheumatoid Arthritis)

SLE (Refer SLE)

Rheumatic Fever (Jones Criteria)

- *Major criteria*
  - Carditis
  - Polyarthritis (Fig. 7.8)

Table 7.8: Juvenile chronic arthritis.		
Classification	Immunological profile	Prognosis
Oligoarticular (mainly girls)	80% ANA positive	Good
Polyarticular	Negative auto Ab	Progressive damage
Systemic onset	Negative auto Ab, High serum ferritin	Variable outcome
Juvenile rheumatoid arthritis	IgM RF positive	Poor articular prognosis
Juvenile ankylosing spondylitis	HLA B 27 positive	Sacroilitis and spondyliitis may develop

Table 7.9: Vasculitic disorders.

Clinical syndrome	Vessels involved	Clinical features
Large vessel vasculitis		
• Giant cell arteritis	Large arteries	• Age > 50 years • Female to male = 4:1 • Unilateral headache, fever, scalp tenderness, visual loss due to ischemic optic neuritis • Thickened tender superficial temporal artery • ESR > 50 • Biopsy of artery – granulomatous lesion • Treatment: Prednisolone → 40–60 mg/day
• Takayasu's disease (Aortic arch arteritis)	Large artery – Aorta	• Young female • Panarteritis before the age of 40 • Fever, loss of upper limb pulsation, HTN, CAD, AR • Diagnosed by Ishikava diagnostic criteria (refer criteria for diagnosis) • Treatment – High dose corticosteroid, immunosuppressants and reconstructive surgery
Medium vessel vasculitis		
• Polyarteritis nodosa	Medium sized arteries	• Hepatitis B virus related • Fever, weight loss, renal vasculitis, hypertension, mononeuritis multiplex, visceral infarct, pericarditis, stroke • Biopsy of vessel – necrotizing vasculitis • Treatment – corticosteroids, immunosuppressants, HBV antiviral
• Kawasaki disease	Medium sized arteries	• Systemic disease of childhood • Age < 5, boys > girls • Fever, conjunctival congestion, erythema of lips, nonsuppurative lymphadenitis, coronary dilatation and aneurysm, myocardial infarction • High ESR, ANCA positive, coronary angiogram for coronary lesion • Treatment – Aspirin, IV immunoglobulin
Small vessel vasculitis		
• Wegener's granulomatosis	Arteries, venules, capillaries	• Upper respiratory tract lesion • Pulmonary lesion – Pulmonary nodule, cavitatory lesion, hemoptysis • Necrotising glomerulonephritis, purpura • High ESR, C-ANCA positive • Treatment – high dose corticosteroid, immunosuppressants
• Churg-Strauss syndrome	Small arteries and veins	• Allergic asthma – pulmonary infiltrate, eosinophilia > 1500/mm^3, multisystem necrotizing vasculitis – purpura, neuropathy, glomerulonephritis • Nerve biopsy – vasculitis with eosinophilic infiltration, ANCA positive • Treatment – high dose corticosteroid
• Microscopic polyangiitis	Capillaries and venules	• Fever, palpable purpura, hematuria, necrotizing glomerulonephritis, alveolar hemorrhage, hemoptysis • p–ANCA and c–ANCA positive GBM Ab negative • Treatment – high dose corticosteroid and immunosuppressants

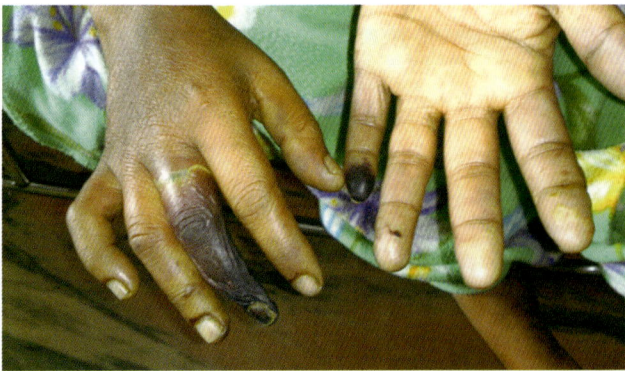

Fig. 7.8: Digital gangrene in cutaneous polyarteritis nodosa.

- Chorea
- Erythema marginatum
- Subcutaneous nodule

• *Minor criteria*
- Fever
- Arthralgia
- Previous rheumatic fever
- Raised ESR or C-reactive protein
- Leucocytosis
- First degree or second degree AV block
- Evidence of recent streptococcal infection
    - Positive throat swab culture
    - Antistreptococcal antibody
    - ASO, anti-DNAase, Antihyaluronidase

- Diagnosis is by
  - Two major criteria or
  - One major and two minor criteria in the presence of an evidence for recent streptococcal infection

Mixed Connective Tissue Disease (Figs. 7.9 and 7.10)

- Common symptoms: Raynaud's phenomenon, swollen fingers/sclerodactyly
- Anti-U1RNP antibody
- Mixed finding
  a. *SLE like*
     - Polyarthritis
     - Facial erythema
     - Pleuropericarditis
     - Leucopenia/thrombocytopenia
     - Lymphadenopathy

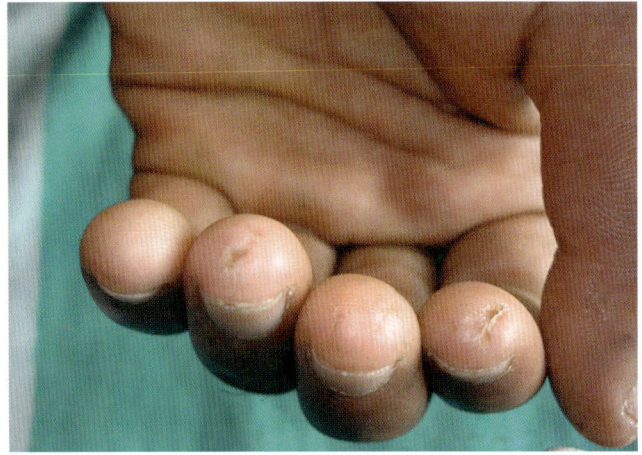

Fig. 7.11: Pitted scar of scleroderma

  b. *Scleroderma like*
     - Sclerodactyly (Fig. 7.11)
     - Pulmonary fibrosis
     - Esophageal dysmotility
  c. *Polymyositis like*
     - Muscle weakness
     - Raised CPK
     - Myogenic pattern of EMG
- *Requirement for diagnosis*
  - Positive in either of the 2 common symptoms
  - Positive anti-U1RNP antibody
  - Positive in one or more findings of two or three disease

Takayasu's Disease

Ishikawa diagnostic criteria

- Obligatory criteria: Age < 40 years
- Two major criteria
  - Left midsubclavian artery lesion
  - Right midsubclavian artery lesion
- Nine minor criterias
  - High ESR
  - Hypertension
  - Aortic regurgitation
  - Carotid artery tenderness
  - Lt. midcommon carotid artery lesion
  - Distal brachiocephalic lesion
  - Pulmonary artery lesion
  - Descending thoracic aorta lesion
  - Abdominal aorta lesion
- *Requirement for diagnosis*
  - Obligatory criteria + 2 major criteria
  - Obligatory criteria + 1 major + 2 or more minor
  - Obligatory criteria + 4 or more minor criteria

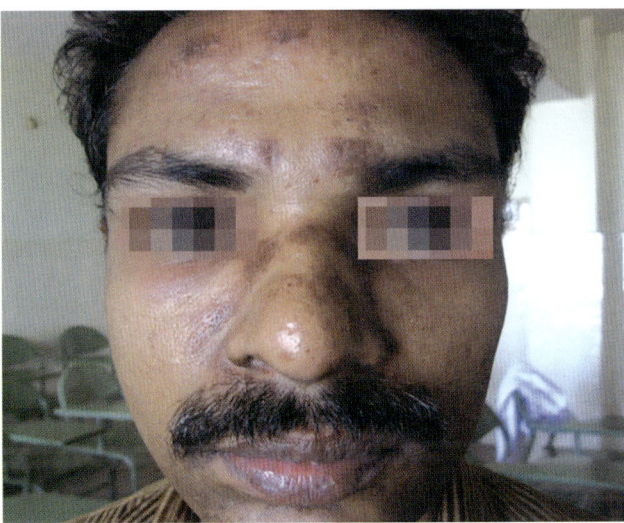

Fig. 7.9: Heliotropic rash—violaceous discoloration over periorbital area and nose seen in dermatomyositis

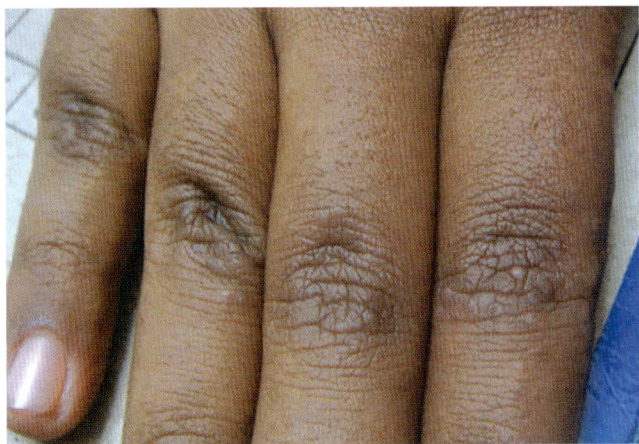

Fig. 7.10: Gattron's papules of dermatomyositis

Progressive Systemic Sclerosis

- Major
  - Proximal scleroderma – proximal to MCP or MTP joint
- Minor
  - Sclerodactyly (Cutaneous sclerosis distal to MCP or MTP joint)
  - Digital pitting scars (Fig. 7.11)
  - Interstitial lung disease
- Diagnosis – by one major or two minor

Ankylosing Spondylitis

- New York criteria for diagnosis
  - H/o inflammatory back pain
  - Decreased movement of lumbar spine in more than one plane, anterior and lateral
  - Chest expansion < 2.5 cm
  - Radiographic evidence of sacroilitis
- *Diagnosis* – by presence of radiographic sacroilitis + one of the other criteria

Reactive Arthropathy

American rheumatic association criteria
- Peripheral arthritis of more than one month with urethritis/cervicitis

Sjogren's Syndrome

SanFrancisco Criteria or Sandiego criteria
- Keratoconjunctivitis sicca
- Xerostomia
- Presence of auto-antibody- Ro/La
- Histological evidence of minor salivary gland involvement

Diagnosis-Presence of 3 or more features to diagnose Sjogren's syndrome

CHAPTER 8

Examination of Endocrine System

SYMPTOMATOLOGY

Symptoms of endocrine disorders are referable to any systems in the body and imitate diseases of the other system.

Lethargy

Feeling of unwell:
- Hypothyroidism
- Diabetes mellitus (DM)
- Hyperparathyroidism
- Addison's disease
- Cushing's syndrome
- Syndrome of inappropriate antidiuretic hormone (SIADH)

Loss of Weight

- Hyperthyroidism
- Type 1 diabetes mellitus
- Addison's disease
- Anorexia nervosa.

Obesity and Weight Gain

- Hypothyroidism
- Cushing's syndrome
- Pseudohypoparathyroidism
- *Primary hypothalamic disorder:* Fröhlich syndrome (adipose genital dystrophy)
- Primary obesity.

Short Stature

- Hypopituitarism
- Cretinism
- Juvenile Cushing's syndrome
- Pseudohypoparathyroidism
- Turner's syndrome.

Tall Stature

- Gigantism
- Klinefelter syndrome
- Eunuchoidism.

Polyuria and Polydipsia

- Diabetes mellitus
- Diabetes insipidus
- Thyrotoxicosis
- Hyperparathyroidism
- Conn's syndrome
- Hypercalcemia.

Temperature Intolerance

- *Cold intolerance:* Hypothyroidism
- *Heat intolerance:* Hyperthyroidism, menopause.

Excessive Sweating

- Hyperthyroidism
- Hypoglycemia
- *Pheochromocytoma:* Paroxysmal sweating
- *Acromegaly:* Increase in the size of sweat gland
  - Gustatory hyperhidrosis—autonomic neuropathy in DM.

Flushing

Menopause, carcinoid syndrome.

Hypertrichosis

Acromegaly.

Hirsutism

Isolated development of sex hair in female.
- Polycystic ovarian disease (PCOD)
- Congenital adrenal hyperplasia
- Androgen secreting ovarian and adrenal tumors

- Cushing's syndrome
- *Drugs:* Phenytoin, minoxidil.

Loss of Hair

- Hypopituitarism
- Hypothyroidism [especially after treatment—Telogen effluvium]
- Hypoparathyroidism
- Thyrotoxicosis.

Pallor

- Hypopituitarism
- Hypothyroidism
- Primary testicular failure.

Vitiligo (Fig. 8.1)

- *Autoimmune endocrine disease:* Graves' disease
- Hashimoto's thyroiditis, Addison's disease.

Pigmentation

- Addison's disease
- Nelson's syndrome
- Adrenocorticotropic hormone (ACTH) dependent Cushing's syndrome.

Coarsening of Features

- Acromegaly
- Hypothyroidism.

CVS Symptoms

Palpitation

- Thyrotoxicosis
- Pheochromocytoma
- Hypoglycemia.

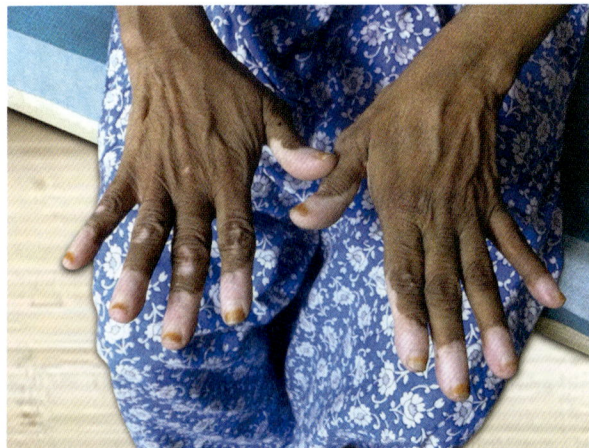

Fig. 8.1: Vitiligo of the fingers.

Dyspnea

- Inspiratory dyspnea: Retrosternal goiter
- Exertional dyspnea:
  - Secondary hypertension
  - Pericardial effusion in hypothyroidism.
  - Catecholamine induced cardiomyopathy in pheochromocytoma.

Edema

Hypothyroidism, obesity.

Respiratory Symptoms

Hoarseness of Voice

- Myxedema, recurrent laryngeal nerve palsy after thyroid surgery
- Retrosternal goiter.

Stridor

Retrosternal goiter, hypoparathyroidism.

Gastrointestinal symptoms

- Appetite:
  - Diabetes mellitus
  - Thyrotoxicosis.
- Anorexia:
  - Hypothyroidism
  - Addison's disease.
- Vomiting:
  - Diabetic ketoacidosis (DKA)
  - Addison's disease
  - Pituitary tumor
  - Hyperparathyroidism
  - Hypercalcemia.
- Diarrhea:
  - Thyrotoxicosis
  - Hypoparathyroidism
  - Carcinoid syndrome
  - VIPoma
  - Zollinger-Ellison syndrome
  - Medullary carcinoma thyroid.
- Constipation:
  - Hypothyroidism
  - Hyperparathyroidism.
- Dysphagia:
  - Retrosternal goiter
  - Thyrotoxic bulbar myopathy.

Nervous System Symptoms

Headache

- Secondary hypertension
- Migraine headache in pheochromocytoma

- Increased intracranial pressure in hypothalamic pituitary tumors.

Convulsion

- Hypoglycemia
- Hypertensive encephalopathy in pheochromocytoma
- Increased intracranial pressure
- Hyperosmolar nonketotic coma
- Hypocalcemia
- Hypoparathyroidism.

Tetany

- Hypoparathyroidism
- Hypocalcemia
- Hypomagnesemia.

Tremor

- Thyrotoxicosis
- Hypoglycemia.

Altered Sensorium

- Coma related to diabetes
  - Hypoglycemia
  - DKA
  - Hyperosmolar
  - Lactic acidosis.
- Myxedema coma
- Addison's with encephalopathy
- Pituitary insufficiency—SIADH, hyponatremia

Speech Disturbance

- Hypothyroidism
- Hypoglycemia.

Paresthesia

- Neuropathy of diabetes mellitus
- Entrapment neuropathy of hypothyroidism, acromegaly.

Muscle Weakness

Proximal muscle weakness
- Painless:
  - Thyrotoxicosis
  - Acromegaly
  - Cushing syndrome
  - Steroid therapy.
- Painful:
  - Diabetic amyotrophy
  - Osteomalacia
  - Hypothyroidism (Rhabdomyolysis)
  - Hypokalemic weakness
  - Conn syndrome
  - Hypokalemic periodic paralysis with thyrotoxicosis.

Generalized muscle weakness
- Hypogonadism
- Myasthenic weakness with thyrotoxicosis.

Hypertrophy of muscle
- Hypothyroidism—Hoffmann's syndrome

Muscle Cramps

- Hypokalemia
- Hypocalcemia
- Hypoparathyroidism.

Renal Symptoms

- *Polyuria and nocturia:* Diabetes mellitus, diabetes insipidus and hypercalcemia
- *Colic:* Hyperparathyroidism with renal stone
- *Chronic renal failure (CRF) symptoms:* Diabetic nephropathy.

Ocular Symptoms

- Prominence of eyes: Exophthalmos [Graves' disease]
- Visual disturbance: Pituitary tumor
- Ophthalmoplegia:
  - Ophthalmoplegic exophthalmos
  - Pituitary apoplexy.
- Periorbital edema: Exophthalmos (Graves' disease)
- Ptosis: Myasthenia with thyrotoxicosis
- Puffy eyelid: Myxedema.

Symptoms of Thyroid Gland

- *Goiter:* Diffuse/nodular
- *Pain:* Viral thyroiditis, hemorrhage into the nodule
- *Rapid enlargement:* Anaplastic carcinoma of thyroid.

Symptoms Referable to Breast

Gynecomastia: Glandular proliferation of male breast (Fig. 8.2)
- Klinefelter's syndrome
- Cirrhosis liver
- Estrogen producing tumors of testis
- Bronchogenic carcinoma
- *Drugs:* Digoxin, spironolactone, cimetidine.

Galactorrhea: Inappropriate lactation
- *Idiopathic:* ↑sensitivity to normal prolactin
  - Prolactinoma
- *Hypothyroidism:* ↑TRH → ↑Prolactin
- *Acromegaly:* ↑Prolactin and lactogenic effect of growth hormone
- *Drugs:* Metoclopramide, digoxin, chlorpromazine
- Estrogen producing tumors of adrenal and testis

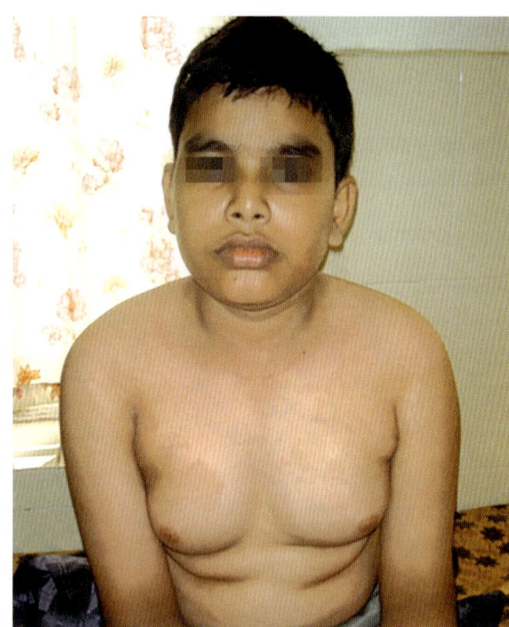

Fig. 8.2: Gynecomastia in a boy—physiological.

- *Premature thelarche:* Isolated breast development without other signs of precocious puberty. Breast buds usually appear as early as 8 years. In premature thelarche, it may appear in the age of 1.5–4 years.

Reproductive Symptoms

Amenorrhea

Primary
- Physiological delay of puberty
- Hypothalamic-pituitary dysfunction
- Hypothyroidism
- *Gonadal dysgenesis:* Turner's syndrome
- Congenital adrenal hyperplasia
- Autoimmune ovarian failure.

Secondary
- *Physiological:* Pregnancy, lactation, menopause
- Prolactinoma
- Cushing's syndrome
- PCOD.

Impotence

- *Decreased erectile potency reduced blood supply to penis:* Atherosclerosis
- *Neural dysfunction:* Autonomic neuropathy
- Diabetes mellitus
- *Testosterone deficiency:* Pituitary and testicular failure
- *Drugs:*
  - β-blocker
  - Psychological.

Precocious Puberty

Male: Pubertal changes before the age of 10
- Congenital adrenal hyperplasia (CAH), hypothalamic tumors (Hamartoma)
- Hypothyroidism
- McCune-Albright's syndrome
- Hepatoblastoma [↑ hCG].

Female: Pubertal changes before the age of 8.
- CAH
- Ovarian and adrenal tumors
- Hypothyroidism
- McCune-Albright's syndrome
- Hepatoblastoma.

Delayed Puberty

Male: Normally puberty occurs at age of 10–16 years.
- Delayed puberty means, pubertal changes beyond the age of 16.
  - Constitutional delay
  - *Testicular disease:* Development and chromosomal
  - Hypothalamic-pituitary disease.

Female: Puberty—9–15 years of age, menstruation 10–17 years of age.
- Constitutional delay
- Hypothalamic-pituitary disease
- Ovarian disease.

HISTORY TAKING IN ENDOCRINE DISORDERS

- *Presenting symptoms:* In chronological order
- *History of presenting complaints:* Detailing each symptom (Refer to symptomatology).

Past history
- History of meningitis/encephalitis → hypothalamic-pituitary disease
- History of mumps → orchitis/oophoritis → hypogonadism
- *History of surgery on endocrine gland:* Thyroid, pituitary tumor, adrenal tumor, etc.
- History of snake bite → hypopituitarism
  - History of APH/PPH → hypopituitarism—Sheehan's syndrome
- *Endocrine milestones:* Puberty, secondary sexual character, menarche, pregnancy, menopause, growth delay.

Family history
History of goiter, diabetes mellitus, multiple endocrine neoplasia, etc.

Personal history
Impotence.

Menstrual history
Detailing menstrual cycle.

Treatment history
- Iodine, thyroid hormone, antithyroid drugs
- Insulin, oral hypoglycemic agents (OHA)
- Steroids, oral contraceptives
- Digoxin, phenothiazine, metoclopramide, spironolactone.

EXAMINATION OF ENDOCRINE SYSTEM

General Examination
- Anemia and pallor:
  - Hypopituitarism
  - Hypothyroidism
  - Hypogonadism.
- Body habitus *(Refer to General Examination)*
  - Acromegaly
  - Gigantism
  - Cushing's syndrome
  - Addison's disease
  - Myxedema
  - Hyperthyroidism
  - Cretinism
  - Rickets.
- Facies *(Refer to General Examination)*
  - Acromegaly
  - Cushing's syndrome
  - Myxedema
  - Cretinism
  - Hyperthyroidism.
- Hand *(Refer to General Examination)*
  - Acromegaly → large spade hand
  - Pseudohypoparathyroidism → short fourth metacarpal
- Anthropometry *(Refer to General Examination)*
  - Short stature, tall stature
- Skin *(Refer to General Examination)*
- Cushing's syndrome → striae, acne, hirsutism, purpura, acanthosis nigricans
- Acromegaly → thick hyperpigmented skin on acral parts of the body, Acanthosis nigricans
- Addison's disease → hyperpigmentation of skin of axillae, groin, areola of nipple and palmar creases
- Hyperthyroidism → warm moist skin; pretibial myxedema
- Myxoedema → dry rough cold skin; non-pitting edema
- Hypopituitarism → pale complexion
- Dyslipidemia
  - Xanthoma—yellowish-orange papule or nodule of skin due to lipid loaded cells
  - Xanthelasma
  - Xanthoma tuberosum
  - Xanthoma tendinosum
  - Eruptive xanthoma.
- Diabetes mellitus
  - Necrobiosis lipoidica diabeticorum → papular/nodular, brownish-yellow with waxy surface and telangiectasia → ulceration → scar formation due to microangiopathy
  - Diabetic rubeosis → flushed skin over the face
  - Diabetic dermopathy → pigmented pretibial dermatosis/shin spots/spotted leg syndrome–pigmented macules and dull red flat topped papules - microangiopathic lesion
  - Scleredema diabeticorum → diffuse waxy nonpitting induration of skin—on the back of the neck and upper trunk
  - Earlobe crease → diagonal earlobe crease
  - Skin infection—bacterial and fungal infection.

Pulse
- *Sinus tachycardia:* Thyrotoxicosis, pheochromocytoma
- *Sinus bradycardia:* Hypothyroidism, ↑ intracranial pressure
- *Irregular pulse:* Atrial fibrillation-thyrotoxicosis.

Blood Pressure
- *Hypertension:* Cushing's syndrome, pheochromocytoma, Conn's syndrome
- *Hypotension:* Acute adrenal, pituitary insufficiency
  - *Postural hypotension:* Diabetic autonomic neuropathy.

Edema
Hypothyroidism and obesity: Chronic venous insufficiency.

Lymph Node Enlargement
- *Generalized:* Hyperthyroidism
- *Localized:* Carcinoma thyroid with secondaries.

Neck
- *Webbing of neck:* Turner's syndrome
- *Buffalo hump:* Cushing's syndrome
  - Accumulation of fat on the dorsal aspect of lower neck and upper thorax.

Breast
- Gynecomastia (Refer Fig. 8.2)
- Galactorrhea.

Hair
- Hirsutism
- Loss of hair
- Virilization
- *Loss of lateral part of eyebrow (Madarosis):* Myxedema
- *Premature pubarche:* Refers to isolated development of sex hair most commonly pubic, occasionally axillary with no other sexual maturation of precocious puberty.

Eye
- Conjunctival congestion, periorbital edema, proptosis—Graves' disease
- *Puffy eyelid:* Hypothyroidism.
- *Infrequent blinking:* Graves' disease (normal blinking 3–5/mt)
- *Stare:* Thyrotoxicosis, pheochromocytoma (↑sympathetic activity)

- *Band keratopathy:* Hyperparathyroidism
- *Cataract:* Hypoparathyroidism, dibetes mellitus
- Defective field of vision
- *Bitemporal hemianopia and superior quadrantanopia:* Pituitary tumors
- *Papilledema:* Hypothalamic-pituitary tumors, hypoparathyroidism and Addison's disease (cellular overhydration)
- *Optic atrophy:* Pressure effect by tumors
- *Retinopathy:* Diabetic and hypertensive
- Ocular signs of Graves' disease (Refer to hyperthyroidism).

Systemic Examination

Cardiovascular System

- *Thyrotoxicosis:* Sinus tachycardia, AF, high output CHF
- *Hypothyroidism:* Sinus bradycardia, cardiomegaly, pericardial effusion—acromegaly—cardiomegaly, cardiomyopathy and CHF
- *Secondary hypertension:* Cushing's syndrome, Conn's syndrome, pheochromocytoma
- *Catecholamine cardiomyopathy:* Pheochromocytoma.

Nervous System

- *Altered sensorium*
  - Coma related to diabetes
  - Myxedema
  - Hypopituitarism
  - Addison's disease.
- *Optic nerve:*
  - Compression by pituitary tumors
  - Malignant exophthalmos.
- *Ophthalmoplegia:* Pituitary apoplexy, exophthalmic ophthalmoplegia
- *Cerebellar ataxia:* Hypothyroidism
- *Bulbar myopathy:* Thyrotoxicosis
- *Myeloradiculopathy:* Change in spinal canal in acromegaly
- Neuropathy:
  - Peripheral neuropathy, mononeuritis multiplex → diabetes mellitus
  - *Autonomic neuropathy:* Diabetes mellitus
  - *Entrapment neuropathy:* Acromegaly, hypothyroidism (carpal tunnel syndrome)
- *Proximal myopathy:* Hypothyroidism, acromegaly, Cushing's syndrome, osteomalacia, thyrotoxicosis
- *Tremor:* Thyrotoxicosis
- *Tetany:* Hypoparathyroidism, hypocalcemia, hypomagnesemia
- *Hypertrophy of muscle:* Hypothyroidism (Hoffmann's syndrome)
- *Deep tendon reflexes:* Delayed relaxation—hypothyroidism (Wottman's sign)
- *Areflexia:* Conn's syndrome
- *Muscle weakness:* Periodic paralysis, thyrotoxicosis, myasthenia gravis—thyrotoxicosis

- *Hypokalemia:* Conn's syndrome
- *Depressive illness:* Hypothyroidism, Addison's disease.

Gastrointestinal Tract

- Lips—Increase in size—acromegaly, MEN 2b—mucosal neuroma
- *Macroglossia:* Acromegaly, cretinism and myxedema
- Teeth
  - *Delayed dentition:* Hypopituitarism and cretinism
  - *Resorption of lamina dura:* Hyperparathyroidism
  - *Loose teeth:* Hyperparathyroidism and striations
  - Hypoparathyroidism
  - *Separation of teeth:* Dental diastasis—acromegaly (enlargement of jaw)
- *Organomegaly:* Acromegaly
- *Ascites:* Myxedema
- Suprarenal mass, ovarian mass
- Myxedema megacolon.

Respiratory System

- *Hoarseness of voice:* Acromegaly, retrosternal goiter
- *Defective hearing:* Hypothyroidism
- *Sleep apneas syndrome:* Acromegaly, Hypothyroidism
- *Pleural effusion:* Hypothyroidism
- *Pemberton's sign:* Thoracic outlet obstruction by retrosternal goiter—make the patient to lift both arms as high as possible, ask him to take a deep breath through mouth. Watch for congestion, cyanosis of face, respiratory distress and inspiratory stridor.

Examination of Thyroid Gland

Examination of thyroid gland is easy since the gland has been placed conveniently in front of the neck.

Inspection

- Normally only the isthmus is visible as a diffuse central swelling
- Enlarged thyroid is visible on inspection
- Look whether the swelling is diffuse or localized
- Watch the movement while swallowing sips of water
- Thyroid gland will move up during swallowing because of attachment to the larynx
- Note whether the inferior border is visible as the gland rises
- Look for any scar of thyroidectomy, dilated veins over the thyroid
- Dilated veins over the upper chest suggest reterosternal extension of goiter.

Palpation

Procedure

Palpation is best begun from behind. Both hands are placed with the pulps of the fingers over the gland. Neck should be slightly flexed so as to relax the sternomastoid muscles.

Feel both the lobes of the gland and it is isthmus. Then move to the front and palpate again using the thumbs for the better feel of localized swelling. Note the position of the trachea.

Consider the Following:
Normal thyroid: Soft movable mass readily moving on swallowing.
- Size of the gland
- Shape of the gland
- Consistency
- *Soft:* Normal
- *Firm:* Simple goiter, Hashimoto's thyroiditis
- *Stony hard:* Carcinoma thyroid
- *Woody consistency:* Riedel thyroiditis
- *Tenderness:* Thyroiditis, bleed into cyst
- Mobility
- Absence of mobility—carcinoma thyroid with infiltration
- *Lower margin:* Impalpable in reterosternal extension
- *Pulsation and bruit:* Thyrotoxicosis
- *Cervical lymph nodes:* Carcinoma thyroid with secondaries.

Percussion

Dull upper part of manubrium in retrosternal extension.

Auscultation

Bruit—systolic/continuous: Sign of increased blood supply in hyperthyroidism.

Examination of Breast

Inspection: Note the following:
Swellings, dimples, discoloration, eczema nipple, nipple retraction, discharge from nipple, prominent veins.

Palpation:
Palpate the whole of each breast with flat of the palm and fingers both in the sitting and supine positions.

Normal breast tissue: Soft to firm, nontender.

Tenderness: Mastitis
Milk the nipple to detect any discharge.

Palpable mass: Position, size, consistency, tenderness, regional lymph nodes.

Examination of Male Reproductive System

Testis

- *Normal adult testis:* Size 3.5–5.5 cm
- <2.5 cm is small
- Volume is 15–25 mL
- Look for - Absence - Cryptorchidism
- *Small testis:* Hypogonadism
- *Tenderness:* Orchitis—mumps, filariasis

- *Tumors:* Seminoma
- Hydrocele, varicocele and inguinal hernia

Penis

- Adult penis is 8–12 cm long
- *Palpate:* Glans penis, penile urethra, corpora cavernosa, corpus spongiosum
- Look for urethral discharge
- Enquire about erection and ejaculation
- In hypogonadism the penis size is less than 2.5 cm.

Examination of Female Reproductive System

- Look for the pubic hair, labia majora and minora, clitoris, vaginal opening and hymen
- Enquire about menarche, development of secondary sexual character, menstrual period, menopause
- For further information digital and colposcopic examination is done.

EXAMINATION OF A DIABETIC PATIENT

General Examination

Weight

- *Under weight:* Type 1 diabetes mellitus
- *Obesity:* Type 2 diabetes mellitus.

Hydration: Dehydration—DKA, hyperosmolar state

Skin: Refer general examination.

Systemic Examination

Cardiovascular System

Look for:
- *Peripheral vessels:* Macrovascular disease
- Systemic hypertension
- Hypertensive heart disease
- Coronary artery disease (CAD)
- Cardiomyopathy and congestive heart failure (CHF).

Respiratory System

For evidence of respiratory infection/tuberculosis.

Gastrointestinal Tract

Mouth
- Monilial infection
- Dental infection
- Pyorrhea alveolaris
- Monilial esophagitis.

Gastroparesis

Motility disorder: Diarrhea/constipation

Hepatomegaly: Fatty liver

Ascites: Diabetic nephropathy and TB peritonitis.

Nervous System

Altered sensorium:
- Coma related to diabetes
- Coma due to cardiovascular accident (CVA), chronic renal failure (CRF)

Neuropathy:
- *Peripheral neuropathy:* Sensory/motor/mixed
- Autonomic neuropathy
- Mononeuritis multiplex
- *Mononeuritis:* Peripheral—femoral neuritis
- *Cranial:* Facial palsy, ophthalmoplegia
- Truncal neuropathy
- *Diabetic pseudotabes:* Posterior radiculopathy
- Diabetes insipidus diabetes mellitus optic atrophy and deafness (DIDMOAD) syndrome (Wolfram's syndrome)
- *Optic fundi:* Retinopathy of diabetes and hypertension
- *Mucormycosis:* Ophthalmoplegia and visual defect—optic nerve involvement.

Kidney and Urinary System

- Diabetic nephropathy
- Urinary tract infection (UTI) upper and lower, renal abscess.

Rheumatological Features

- Trigger finger
- Diabetic hand syndrome—Cheiroarthropathy
  - Stenosing tenosynovitis → Inability to extend the metacarpophalangeal or interphalangeal joints of at least one finger bilaterally. This can be demonstrated in the Salam's sign or prayer sign.
- Dupuytren's contracture
- *Neuroarthropathy:* Charcot's joint
- Gout and pseudogout
- *Periarthritis shoulder:* Adhesive capsulitis
- *Shoulder hand syndrome:* Adhesive capsulitis of shoulder, pain, swelling, tenderness, dystrophic skin and vasomotor instability in the hand
- Diabetic foot due to neuropathy, angiopathy–macro- and microinfection and trauma.
  - Features are → Paresthesia, ulcers—painless/painful, digital gangrene, callous, cracks, fissures, neuropathic joint, muscle wasting, clawing of foot and edema, osteolysis of forefoot.

Infections

- Skin and systemic infections
- *Mucormycosis:* Involving paranasal sinuses and orbit
- Malignant external otitis.

Treatment and Follow-up of Diabetic Patient

Selection of Treatment

Type 1 diabetes: Insulin is the only treatment that should be tried in this condition WHO Goal-FBS <110, PPBS <160.

Type 2 diabetes:
- Oral hypoglycemics of different groups are available.
- Primary management is done using
  - Sulfonylureas [Glibenclamide, glipizide, gliclazide and glimepiride] in nonobese patient while metformin for obese subjects.
  - Inadequate control nonobese with either agent alone may necessitate adding of other group of drug to the treatment regimen.
- Thiazolidinedione
  - Working in the nucleus activating peroxisome proliferator activated receptors (PPAR) by facilitating transcription of mRNA coding for enzymes involved in glucose and fat metabolism is a novel approach in the treatment of diabetes
  - Pioglitazone and rosiglitazone belong to this group
  - The drugs, which are useful, should be used with caution as it can cause significant water retention, weight gain and cardiac failure in some patients
  - Hepatotoxicity, a side effect of earlier thiazolidinediones does not occur with newer agents.
- Non-sulfonylurea insulin secretagogues like
  - Repaglinide and nateglinide can also be
  - Used when meal timing of the individual is irregular. Starch blockers like acarbose help in the disease control by preventing digestion and absorption of carbohydrates in proximal intestine.
- Alpha-glucosidase inhibitors
  - Prevents the breaking down of polysaccharide
  - Prevents digestion and absorption of carbohydrates in proximal intestine
  - Acarbose, miglitol, voglibose are used with food
  - Side effect: Dyspepsia and flatulence
  - This group is used for the control postprandial hyperglycemia.
- **Incretins**

Gut hormones:
- GLP 1 (glucogan like peptide 1)
- GIP (Glucose dependent insulinotropic peptide).

Two groups of drugs:
1. GLP-1 receptor agonist (Incretin mimetics)
   - Liraglutide and exenatide
   - Both are given subcutaneously
   - Promote glucose dependent insulin production
   - Inhibit glucagon production.
2. DPP4 inhibitors (Gliptins)
   - Inhibit degradation of incretins and numerous other substances

- Add on therapy to insulin sensitizers, insulin secretogogues and insulin
- Vildagliptin, sitagliptin, linogliptin
- Teneligliptin
- This will reduce both fasting and postprandial hyperglycemia.
- **Latest group of oral antidiabetic drugs**
  - SGLT 2 inhibitors (Sodium glucose co-transporter type 2)
  - This group is known as Gliflozin
  - Urine glucose excretion is increased thus reducing the hyperglycemia in T2DM
  - Canagliflozin and empagliflozin.

Insulins Presently in Use

- Recombinant human insulin
  - Short-acting/regular insulin
  - Intermediate acting insulin
  - Premixed insulins—short-acting and intermediate acting insulins mixed in 30/70, 25/75, 50/50 proportions.
- Insulin analogues
  - Rapid acting analogues
  - Long-acting analogues

Rapid Acting Analogues

- Lyspro insulin (e.g. Humalog)
  - Normally, B chain has- 28th proline, 29th lysine
  - In Lyspro, reciprocal change of position 28th lysine and 29th proline.
- Insulin aspart (e.g. NovoRapid)
  - 28th proline is replaced by aspartic acid
- Insulin glulisine (e.g. Apidra)
  - 29th lysine is replaced by glutamic acid.

Long Acting Analogues

- Insulin glargine (e.g. Lantus)
  - A chain 21st position asparagine is replaced by glycine
  - Two moles of arginine are added to B chain 30th position.
- Insulin detemir (e.g. Levemir)
  - In this insulin, to the lysine 29th position of B chain, a 14 carbon atom fatty acid (myristic acid) is attached
  - Threonine from 30th position is removed.
- Insulin degludec (e.g. Tresiba): To the lysine 29th position of B chain, a 16 carbon atom fatty acid is attached through glutamic acid.
- Premixed analogues: Protaminised rapid acting insulin (with intermediate duration of action), is mixed with rapid acting insulin in definite proportion 25/75 or 30/70.

Use of Insulins in Diabetes Mellitus

- Type I diabetes mellitus
- Type II diabetes mellitus
  - Gestational diabetes mellitus
  - Oral hypoglycemic agents (OHA) failure
  - Diabetic ketoacidosis
- Hyperosmolar hyperglycemia
- Severe infection
- Major surgery
- Organ failure
- Type 2 DM with lean body weight.

Action of insulin preparations			
Insulin	Onset of action	Peak	Duration of action
Rapid acting analogue	10 minutes	1–2 hours	3–4.5 hours
Short-acting (Regular insulin)	30 minutes	3–4 hours	6–8 hours
Intermediate (Insulin NPH)	1–3 hours	3–8 hours	7–14 hours
Long-acting analogue	1–2 hours	None (Peakless)	18–24 hours

Laboratory Evaluation and Follow-up

- Daily urine sugar test
- *Blood sugar test:* Done periodically till the disease is controlled. Further frequency of blood sugar test is decided by the severity and brittleness of the disease. Usually monthly blood sugar test is done once the disease is under control.
- *Renal function test:* Blood urea and serum creatinine is done at the time of diagnosis and yearly thereafter
- *Lipid profile:* Done initially and yearly if values are normal. If abnormal, patient is treated for dyslipidemia and more frequent measurements are indicated.
- *Microalbuminuria:* Is an early indicator of endothelial damage and predictor of cardiac outcome. It is measured initially and thereafter yearly. Normal albumin excretion is < 30 mg/24 hours
- *Electrocardiogram:* In all patients with Type 2 diabetes mellitus at the time of diagnosis and yearly thereafter. In Type 1 ECG is done if there is any clinical marker of cardiac involvement
- Yearly ophthalmic check-up
- *Doppler study for arterial patency:* When limb ischemia is suspected
- *Feet examination:* Sensory assessment clinically and bioesthesiometer, also for signs of diabetic foot.
- HbA1c estimation is done once in 3 months in uncontrolled cases and once in 6 months in controlled cases
- Frequent BP check-up.

EXAMINATION OF A HYPERTENSIVE PATIENT

History

- Duration and Level of high BP
- History of symptoms of target organ involvement

- Symptoms of CAD, PVD and CHF
- Symptoms of cerebrovascular disease
- Symptoms of renal involvement
- History of symptoms suggesting a cause for hypertension like renal disease, endocrine disease—Cushing's syndrome, pheochromocytoma, etc.
- History of risk factors like diabetes mellitus, dyslipidemia, smoking
- Past history of renal disease like acute glomerulonephritis (AGN), pregnancy-induced HTN
- Family history of hypertension, risk factors, renal disease like PKD and cardiovascular disease
- *Dietetic history:* Regarding salt intake and other food habits.
- Socioeconomic and environmental factors.

Physical Examination

- Measurement of BP for detection and confirmation of hypertension
- Measurement of height, weight, waist hip circumference
- CVS examination for—cardiomegaly, heaving apex, accentuation of aortic component of S2, S4, CHF
- Peripheral pulsations—lower limb pulsation to rule out coarctation of aorta, peripheral vascular disease
- Examination of abdomen—for enlarged kidney—PKD, hydronephrosis
- Renal bruit—renal artery stenosis
- Nervous system examination—for cerebrovascular disease
- Optic fundi—hypertensive retinopathy.

Examination of Other Systems for Identifiable Cause for Hypertension

- Endocrine disorders:
  - Cushing's syndrome
  - Pheochromocytoma
  - Conn syndrome
  - Thyroid disease.
- *Renal diseases:* Renal parenchymal disease like
  - AGN
  - CRF
  - PKD
  - Renovascular disease
  - Renal artery stenosis.
- Coarctation of aorta/aortoarteritis.

Follow-up and Monitoring of a Hypertensive Patient

- Once antihypertensive drug therapy is initiated, most patients should return for follow-up and adjustment of medications at approximately monthly intervals until the BP goal is reached
- More frequent visits will be necessary for patients with stage 2 hypertension or with complicating comorbid conditions
- Serum potassium and serum creatinine should be monitored at least one to two times per year
- Even if urine analysis is normal, screen for microalbuminuria once in 6 months
- After the BP at goal and stable, follow-up visits can usually be at 3–6 months interval
- Systemic hypertension require lifelong medication, follow-up and reducing or stopping medications have to be done under very strict supervision
- Comorbidities such as heart failure, associated diseases such as diabetes, chronic kidney disease, cerebrovascular disease, peripheral vascular disease and the need for laboratory tests influence the frequency of visits
- Other cardiovascular risk factors should be treated to their respective goals, and smoking should be strictly stopped
- **Goal of therapy:** According to JNC VIII
  - Antihypertensive therapy should achieve and maintain SBP below 150 mm Hg and DBP below 90 mm Hg in a patient who is < 60 years of age and with no DM and CKD
  - Patient who is >60 years of age or any patient with DM and CKD, maintain SBP below 140 mm Hg and DBP below 90 mm Hg.
- All members of the healthcare team (specialists, general physicians, family physicians, nurses, and the pharmacists) should work together to influence and reinforce instructions to improve patients' lifestyles and BP control.

COMMON CLINICAL DISORDERS OF ENDOCRINE SYSTEM

ACROMEGALY

Acromegaly is caused by excessive growth hormone secretion, usually from a macroadenoma of pituitary.

Growth hormone (GH) exerts direct effect in target tissues, many of its physiologic effects are mediated indirectly through IGF-1.

Incidence

3 million people/year.

Etiology

Macroadenoma of pituitary.

GRH induced, by hypothalamic tumors: Hamartoma ganglion neuroma.

Ectopic GRH from:
- Oat cell carcinoma of lung
- Medullary carcinoma of thyroid

- Islet cell tumor of pancreas
- Bronchial carcinoid.

Ectopic GH: Islet cell tumor of pancreas

Clinical Features

Are due to:
- Excessive growth hormone
- Pressure effect by tumor
- Increased intracranial pressure.

Gigantism: Prepubertal onset, before the fusion of epiphysis → increased linear growth.

Acromegaly: Postpubertal onset, after the fusion of epiphysis except the small bones of hands, feet and flat bones.

General Features

Weight gain, coarse facies, increased sweating and fatigability.

Soft Tissue Changes

Macroglossia with increased fissures, enlargement of lips and nose, skin tag, oily skin, hypertrichosis, acanthosis nigricans, increased depth of soft tissues.

Cardiovascular System

Systemic hypertension, cardiomegaly, cardiomyopathy, CHF.

Respiratory System

Increase in size of sinuses, deep voice, obstructive sleep apnea syndrome.

Nervous System

Neuropathy, carpal tunnel syndrome, proximal myopathy, myeloradiculopathy due to change in the spinal canal.

Skeletal Changes

Acral enlargement—increase in size of hand and feet—spade hand, prognathism, prominent supraorbital ridge, large frontal sinus, wide spacing of teeth, dental diastasis, overgrowth of jaw, kyphosis, osteoarthrosis.

GIT

Organomegaly: Hepatosplenomegaly.

Genitourinary system: Reduced libido, impotence, oligomenorrhea, infertility.

Endocrine Changes

- Goiter with hypo/hyperthyroidism
- Diabetes mellitus, diabetes insipidus
- Multiple endocrine adenoma
- *Galactorrhea:* Disconnection hyperprolactinemia, increased prolactin secretion by the tumor, lactogenic effect of GH
- Hypercalcemia, hyperphosphatemia.

Features of Pressure Effect

- *Visual field defect:* Bitemporal hemianopia
- 3rd, 4th, 6th cranial nerve palsy.
- *Upward pressure on hypothalamus:* Polyphagia, Polydipsia, abnormal thermal regulation.
- Pressure on temporal lobe → Complex partial seizure
- Posterior pituitary dysfunction → Diabetes insipidus.

Features of Increased Intracranial Pressure

- Headache, projectile vomiting, altered sensorium.

Investigations

- *Serum growth hormone estimation:*
  - Normal 5 µg/L
  - Acromegaly >10 µg/L
  - *Multiple estimation is done:* In acromegaly GH always detectable unlike in normal where it is undetectable sometimes.
- *Postglucose suppression:*
  - GH estimation—60–120 minute after giving 75 g of oral glucose
  - Normal - GH <1 µg/L
  - *Acromegaly:* Nonsuppressible, paradoxical GH rise after glucose in 20%
  - *Mechanism:* Glucose → increased insulin → liver → ↑IGF-1 → ↓ GH
- Estimation of IGF-1—increased in acromegaly
- Blood sugar, serum calcium, serum phosphorus
- TRH administration → rise in GH in acromegaly
  - No rise in normal
- Estimation of prolactin, cortisol, thyroid hormone, testosterone (to rule out other organ failure)
- *X-ray skull:* Double flooring and enlargement of sella tursica.
- X-ray hand tufting of distal phalanx
- Heel pad thickness—in acromegaly
  - 18 mm in female
  - 21 mm in male.
- CT and MRI to detect the tumor and its size.

Two laboratory test suggestive of acromegaly are:
- Postglucose nonsuppression of GH
- Increased IGF-1 level.

Complications

Metabolic

- Diabetes mellitus, hypercalcemia and hyperphosphatemia
- *Hyperphosphatemia:* GH increases tubular absorption of phosphate
- GH increases 1α hydroxylase activity →↑ 1,25 dihydroxy cholecalciferol →↑ calcium
- *Endocrine:* Pituitary apoplexy, hypothyroidism, hypoadrenalism, hypogonadism

- *CVS:* Hypertension, cardiomyopathy, CHF
- *Respiratory system:* Obstructive sleep apnea syndrome
- *Nervous system:* Entrapment neuropathy, proximal myopathy
- Pressure effect of tumor on neighboring structures
- ↑ Intracranial pressure—acute ophthalmoplegia in pituitary apoplexy.

Gastrointestinal tract
Colonic polyp and malignancy.

Management

Principles: Normalization of growth hormone.
- Removal of tumor
- Preservation of rest of pituitary
- Replacement of other hormones

Measures of Therapy

- *Surgical:* Trans-sphenoidal surgery
- *Radiotherapy:* Used as second line treatment if acromegaly persist after surgery
  - Conventional teletherapy
  - Yttrium implantation
  - Stereotactic radiosurgery
  - Stereotactic focused radiation (gamma knife).

Medical: If acromegaly persisting after surgery, to lower the GH level to < 5 µg/L.

Drugs used are:
- Bromocriptine 20–60 mg/day.
- Cyproheptadine—4 mg OD

Octreotide: 50 µg subcutaneous tid gradually increased to 1,000 µg/day.

HYPOPITUITARISM

The order of failure of hormone in hypopituitarism is:
Growth hormone (GH) → prolactin → luteinizing hormone (LH) and follicle-stimulating (FSH) → thyroid-stimulating hormone (TSH) → adrenocorticotropic hormone (ACTH).

Isolated hormone deficiency is seen with GH and gonadotropin.

Etiology

- *Isolated hormone deficiency:* Congenital (Fig. 8.3) or acquired
- Tumors:
  - Non-functioning pituitary adenoma
  - Pituitary apoplexy
  - *Hypothalamic tumors:* Craniopharyngioma, glioma, chordoma, etc.
- *Inflammatory disease:* Granulomatous disease—TB, sarcoidosis, histiocytosis

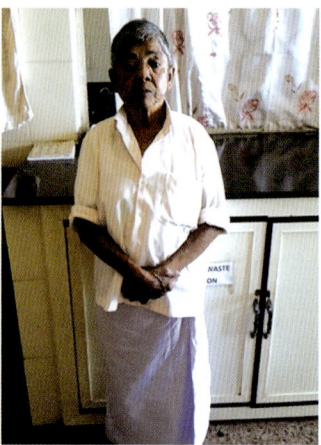

Fig. 8.3: Proportionate dwarfism.

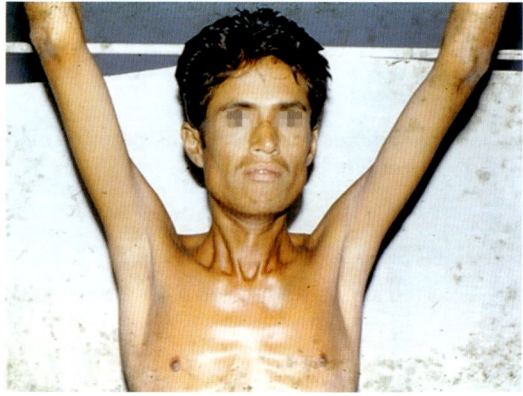

Fig. 8.4: Post-snake bite hypopituitarism showing loss of beard, moustache and axillary hair.

- Lymphocytic hypophysitis
- *Vascular disorders:*
  - Sheehan's postpartum necrosis
  - Diabetic peripartum necrosis
- *Infiltration:* Hemochromatosis, amyloidosis
- *Snake bite:* Viper (Fig. 8.4)
- *Developmental:* Pituitary aplasia, encephalocele
- *Trauma and destruction:* Surgery, radiation
- *Idiopathic:* Autoimmune.

Clinical Features

Due to deficiency of:
- *GH:* Fine wrinkling of the angle of mouth and eyes
  - Growth retardation, atrophic papery skin
- *TSH:* Fatigue, cold intolerance and puffy eyelid, without goiter
  - *ACTH:* Fatigue, loss of weight, reduced pigmentation of skin, pallor, abnormal response to stress.
- *Gonadotropin:*
  - *Female:* Infertility, amenorrhea
  - *Male:* Reduced libido, reduced facial and body hair, impotence.

Altered Sensorium—Multiple Factors

- Insulin sensitivity → hypoglycemia
- Water intoxication → cortisol deficiency
- Hypothyroidism.

Investigations

- *Basal function of pituitary:* Estimation of GH, prolactin, TSH, LH, FSH
- *Estimation of target organ hormones:* T3, T4, cortisol, estrogen, testosterone
- *Dynamic test:* Insulin hypoglycemia and GH estimation
  Insulin: 0.05–0.1 unit/Kg IV → hypoglycemia—blood sugar <40 mg → GH >3 μg/L—normal, cortisol ↑ >3 times of the basal
- *ACTH stimulation test:* Estimation of cortisol
- *Test for pituitary reserve:*
  - GRH → GH
  - GnRH → LH and FSH
  - TRH → TSH
  - CRH → ACTH.

Management

Substitution Therapy

- *Cortisol:* Tablets hydrocortisone→20 mg—0–10 mg OR prednisolone—5 mg morning, 2.5 mg evening
- *Thyroxine:* 100–200 μg/day
- *Sex hormone:* Female.

Premenopausal

- *Estrogen* (1–21 days) and progesterone (14–21 days)
- Postmenopausal—HRT ± for fertility—LH, FSH replacement.
- Hypothalamic dysfunction—GnRH pulsatile infusion.

Male

- Testosterone replacement
- *For fertility:* Gonadotropin replacement
- Hypothalamic damage GnRH pulsatile infusion
- GH replacement.
   For young patients [before completion of linear growth] dose is 25–35 μg/kg/day.
   For adult: 3 μg/kg/day.

HYPOTHYROIDISM

Clinical syndrome produced by deficiency of thyroid hormone leading to cellular hypometabolism and hydrophilic mucopolysaccharide accumulation in tissues.

Etiology

Thyroidal causes 95% (primary hypothyroidism).

Goitrous (Fig. 8.5)

- Dyshormonogenesis
- Iodine deficiency (Iodine intake <25 μg/day)
- *Chronic thyroiditis:* Hashimoto's
- *Drugs:* Lithium, amiodarone
- Iodine excess (>6 mg/day—Wolff-Chaikoff effect).

Non-goitrous (Thyroprivic)

- *Congenital:* Agenesis
- Idiopathic atrophic hypothyroidism [autoimmune]
- *Postablation:* Surgery, radioactive iodine
- *Postradiation:* Radiation to neck in lymphoma, etc.

Suprathyroidal 5% (Secondary hypothyroidism)

- *Pituitary:* Causes of hypopituitarism
- *Hypothalamic:* Tumors.

Subclinical hypothyroidism: Clinically euthyroid with normal T_4 and elevated TSH.

Causes:

- *Primary atrophic:* Autoimmune
- Graves' disease on I^{131} therapy
- Hashimoto's thyroiditis
- Transient hypothyroidism—usually seen in:
  - Subacute thyroiditis
  - Postpartum thyroiditis
  - Following subtotal thyroidectomy.

Clinical Features

Male to female ratio 1:6
Depends on the age of onset

- *Cretinism:*
  - Thyroid deficiency in the last trimester and early postnatal period
  - Dwarf, mental retardation, broad flat nose, protruded tongue and belly, coarse facies, dry skin, constipation.

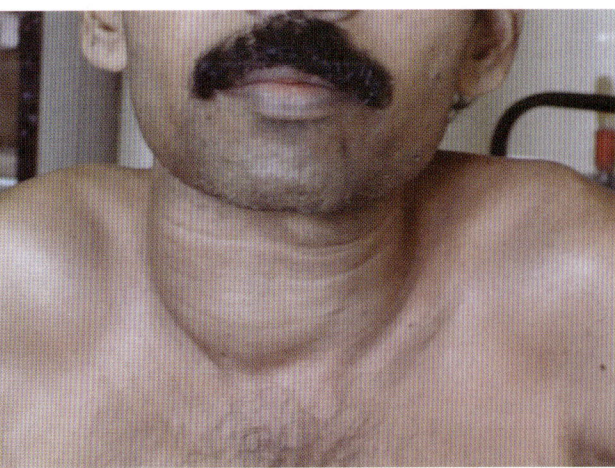

Fig. 8.5: Thyroid swelling: Goiter.

- *In newborn:* Increased physiological jaundice, feeding problem, constipation, hoarse cry.
- *Infantile hypothyroidism:* Acquired deficiency—between the age of 6 months to 3 years.
- *Juvenile hypothyroidism:*
  - Between the age of 3 years and adolescence
  - Short stature, delayed sexual maturation
  - Occasionally precocious puberty
  - Poor scholastic performance.
- *Adult hypothyroidism:* Myxedema.

General Features

- *Fatigability, cold intolerance, weight gain, increased sleep:* Somnolence
- Puffy pale coarse facies, dry skin, loss of hair.

Gastrointestinal Tract

Anorexia, macroglossia (dysarthria-linguals) (Fig. 8.6), constipation, ascites, megacolon.

Respiratory

Hoarseness of voice, obstructive sleep apnea, pleural effusion.

Cardiovascular System

Sinus bradycardia, cardiomegaly, pericardial effusion, dilated cardiomyopathy (DCM).

Nervous System

- *Entrapment neuropathy:* Carpal tunnel syndrome
- Defective hearing
- Cerebellar ataxia
- *Hypertrophy of skeletal muscles:* Hoffman (calf) syndrome (Fig. 8.7)
- Pseudomyotonia
- Myxedema
  - *Delayed relaxation of DTR:* Woltman's sign
  - *Dysarthria:* Due to macroglossia.
- *Myxedema madness:* Elderly with decreased memory and hearing, somnolence, paranoia
- Myxedema coma.

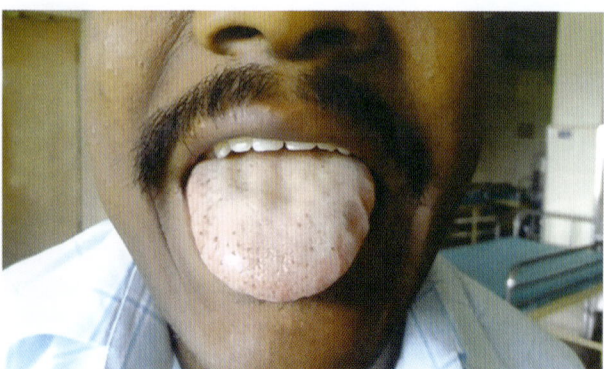

Fig. 8.6: Macroglassia in a patient with hypothyroidism.

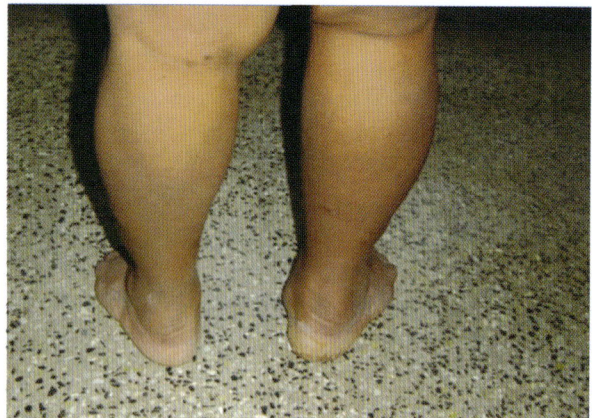

Fig. 8.7: Calf muscle hypertrophy in hypothyroidism.

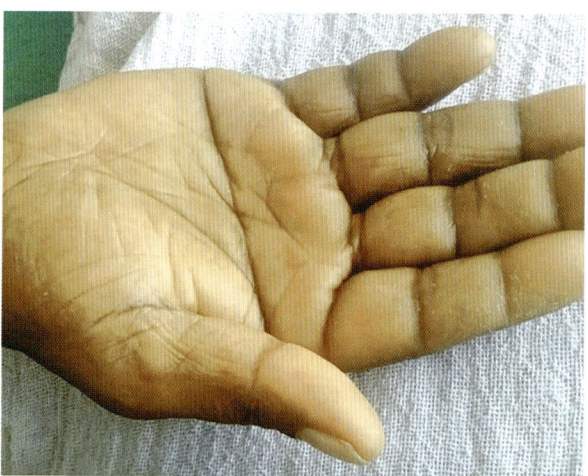

Fig. 8.8: Carotenemia in a patient with hypothyroidism.

Metabolic

Hyponatremia: SIADH, reduced free water clearance.

Skin

Dry, pruritus, alopecia, vitiligo, carotenemia (Fig. 8.8).

Reproductive

Menorrhagia, infertility, galactorrhea, impotence.

Blood

- *Normocytic normochromic anemia, microcytosis—iron deficiency anemia:* Due to menorrhagia
- *Megaloblastic anemia:* Bacterial overgrowth due to hypomotility of intestine.

Presentation of Primary Hypothyroidism

Common Types of Presentations

- Fatigability
- Feeling of unwell

- Obesity and weight gain
- Edema
- Puffiness of face
- Refractory anemia
- Menorrhagia
- Rheumatic symptoms—arthralgia, myalgia
- Hypertrophy of muscle with myotonic deep tendon reflexes.

Uncommon Types of Presentations

- Bilateral or unilateral carpal tunnel syndrome
- Painful proximal myopathy
- Rhabdomyolysis
- Cerebellar ataxia
- Reversible dementia
- Peripheral neuropathy
- Myxedema madness
- Myxedema coma
- Hyponatremia—SIADH
- Lingual dysarthria
- Pseudomyotonia
- True myotonia
- Myxedema.

Investigations

- Thyroid function test
- TSH
  - ↑; Primary hypothyroidism
  - ↓; Secondary hypothyroidism
- Serum T4 and free T4 reduced
- TSH response to TRH increase
- *ECG:* Bradycardia, low voltage QRS complex
- *X-ray:* Epiphyseal dysgenesis, bone age is decreased in cretinism
- Autoantibody against thyroglobulin and microsomal TPO
- Serum cholesterol increased.

Differential Diagnosis of Hypothyroidism

Mongolism, nephrotic syndrome, chronic renal failure (CRF).

The diagnostic index of Billewicz et al. Clinical scoring of signs and symptoms of Hypothyroidism.		
	Diagnostic weight	
	Present	Absent
Symptoms		
Dry skin	+ 3	- 6
Cold intolerance	+ 4	- 5
Hoarseness	+ 5	- 6
Weight gain	+ 5	- 1
Constipation	+ 2	- 1
Decreased sweating	+ 3	- 6
Contd...		
Paresthesia	+ 5	- 4
Decreased hearing	+ 2	0
Signs		
Slow movements	+ 11	- 3
Coarse skin and hair	+ 7	- 7
Cold skin	+ 3	- 2
Periorbital puffiness	+ 4	- 6
Bradycardia	+ 4	- 4
Slow reflex relaxation	+ 15	- 6

In patients with no other illness and receiving no other medication, a total score of >/= 19 indicates hypothyroidism and a score of </- 24 excludes.

Clinical profile of hypothyroid cases.			
Symptom	% of occurrence	Signs	% of occurrence
Lethargy	88.9	Facial puffiness	80.7
Somnolence	79.4	Pallor	61.9
Weight gain	78.3	Delayed reflexes	34.8
Behavioral changes	64.8	Slow movements	30.8
Constipation	63.9	Falling of hair	20.4
Change in voice	62.6	Pericardial effusion	12.6
Paresthesia	62.3	Enlarged tongue	9.3
Muscular pains	58.9	Galactorrhea (F)	5.5
Dyspnea	51.8	Xanthelasma	3.2
Cold intolerance	45.9	Coarse skin	3.1
Reduced appetite	44.7		
Poor memory	37.1		
Decreased sweating	34.1		
Obstructive sleep Apnea	24.6		
Decreased hearing	20.8		

F: Female

Management

- Life long substitution with thyroid hormone
- Levothyroxine 50–200 µg/day.

Monitoring of Therapy

- Serum TSH test is a measure of efficacy of replacement therapy
- The drop in serum TSH lags behind the changes in T_4
- Therefore change in L-thyroxine doses should only be made after 6–8 weeks interval.

Difference between primary and secondary hypothyroidism is given in Table 8.1.

Table 8.1: Difference between primary and secondary hypothyroidism.

Features	Primary	Secondary
Skin	Coarse and dry	Soft and pale
Blood pressure	Normal/hypertension	Normal/hypotension
Heart size	Increased	Normal/decreased
Menstrual cycle	Menorrhagia	Amenorrhea
Serum TSH	Increased	Decreased
Serum cholesterol	Increased	Normal
Deficiency of other pituitary hormones	Absent	Present

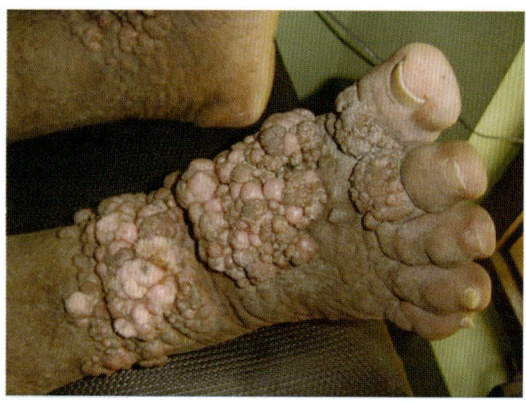

Fig. 8.9: Dermopathy in Graves' disease.

THYROTOXICOSIS

The term thyrotoxicosis refers to biochemical and physiological manifestation of excessive quantities of thyroid hormones, irrespective of source of hormones. The term hyperthyroidism is applied, if there is over production of hormones by thyroid.

Etiology

- Disorders with increased thyroid function
  - Abnormal thyroid stimulation
  - Graves' disease
  - Trophoblastic tumors.
- Increased TSH
  - Pituitary adenoma of thyrotrophs.
- Intrinsic thyroid autonomy
  - Toxic adenoma
  - Toxic multinodular goiter (MNG)
- Disorders without increased thyroid function
  - Subacute thyroditis with thyrotoxicosis
  - Chronic thyroiditis with thyrotoxicosis.
- Extrathyroid source of hormone
  - Thyrotoxicosis facticia
  - *Ectopic thyroid tissue:* Struma ovarii
  - Functioning follicular carcinoma.

GRAVES' DISEASE (BASEDOW'S DISEASE)

- *Characterized by:*
  - Hyperthyroidism with goiter
  - Ophthalmopathy
  - Dermopathy (Fig. 8.9).
- *Prevalence:*
  - 3rd and 4th decade
  - Female to male ratio 7:1.

Etiology

- Autoimmune disease with myasthenia, pernicious anemia
- Association with human leukocyte antigen (HLA)—DR_3
- Thyroid stimulating antibody against TSH receptor (TSI)
- This is a cytostimulant type VI immunological reaction.

Clinical Features Due to thyrotoxicosis

General

Nervousness, insomnia, weight loss, heat intolerance, fatigability.

Skin

Warm, moist, hyperhidrosis, alopecia, pretibial myxedema (Fig. 8.10), vitiligo.

Nail

Acropachy (Fig. 8.11)—a form of clubbing in Graves' associated with dermopathy, in less than 1%.

Cardiovascular System

Sinus tachycardia, high volume pulse, systolic murmur, Cardiomegaly, high output CHF, atrial fibrillation.

Gastrointestinal Tract

Polyphagia, polydipsia, tremor of tongue, diarrhea, hepatomegaly.

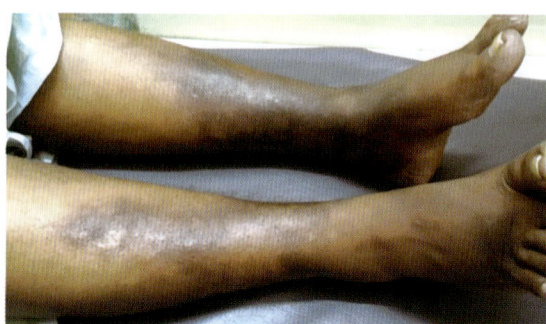

Fig. 8.10: Pretibial myxedema both legs in Graves' disease.

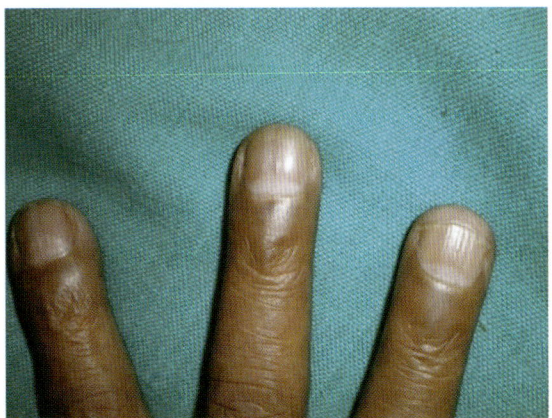

Fig. 8.11: Acropachy in Graves' disease.

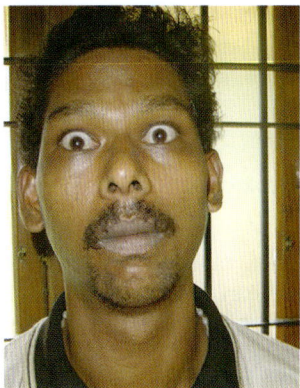

Fig. 8.12: Exophthalmus and diffuse goiter in a patient with Graves' disease.

Nervous

Fine tremor, bulbar myopathy, proximal myopathy, myasthenic weakness, periodic paralysis, chorea, stupor and coma.

Metabolic

Increased serum calcium, decreased serum magnesium raised alkaline phosphatase, hypercalciuria.

Hemopoietic

Anemia, lymphocytosis, lymphadenopathy enlarged thymus, splenomegaly.

Bone

Osteoporosis.

Reproductive

Irregular menstruation, gynecomastia, infertility.

Psychiatric

Restlessness, irritability, anxiety, depression.

Due to Graves' Disease

Diffuse hyperfunctioning goiter with bruit.

Ophthalmopathy

Mechanism:
- Increased sympathetic stimulation
- Infiltrative ophthalmopathy
- Congestive oculopathy.

Manifestation
- Stare, lid lag, wide palpebral fissure (Fig. 8.12)
- Proptosis—unilateral/bilateral, symmetrical/asymmetrical
- Periorbital edema
- Ophthalmoplegia
- Exposure keratitis, corneal ulcer
- *Loss of vision:* Optic nerve involvement (Malignant exophthalmos).

Normal distance from outer bony margin of the orbit to the apex of the cornea is 17 mm using exophthalmometer—asymmetry of proptosis means difference of more than 5 mm distance.

Ocular Signs

- *Von Graefe sign:* Lid lag
- *Joffroy's sign:* Absence of wrinkling of forehead on looking up
- *Dalrymple's sign:* Visibility of sclera around cornea
- *Moebius sign:* Absence of accommodation.

Orbital Changes in Graves'—Acronym

NO SPECS
- 0: No signs or symptoms
- 1: Only signs (lid lag or retraction), no symptoms
- 2: Soft tissue involvement (periorbital edema)
- 3: Proptosis (>22 mm)
- 4: Extraocular muscle involvement (diplopia)
- 5: Corneal involvement
- 6: Sight loss.

Dermopathy

- Pretibial myxoedema
- Raised thickened pruritic hyperpigmented, well demarcated lesion of skin (see Fig. 8.9).

Various Types of Presentation of Hyperthyroidism

- Progressive loss of weight
- Chronic diarrhea
- Palpitation and congestive heart failure (CHF)
- Tremor and muscle weakness

- Anxiety, panic disorder
- Thyrotoxic crisis and shock
- *Euthyroid Graves:* Ophthalmopathy/dermopathy.

Investigations

To Establish Thyrotoxicosis

- TSH ↓, FT$_3$/T$_4$ ↑
- Radioactive iodine uptake test (RAIU) study:
  – Increased uptake in hyperthyroidism
  – Decreased uptake in thyroiditis with thyrotoxicosis.

To Establish Graves' Disease

Autoantibody:
- Thyroglobulin antibody
- Microsomal antibody—thyroid peroxidase antibody (TPO Ab)
- TSH receptor antibody, not estimated routinely, due to difficulty in assay.

Differential Diagnosis of Graves' Disease

Anxiety state, pheochromocytoma, hyperparathyroidism.

Management

Three measures:
- Medical
- Surgical
- Radioactive iodine.

Medical

- *Indication:* Children, young adult and pregnant women.
- *Drugs:*
  – Propylthiouracil 100–150 mg, 8th hourly or
  – *Carbimazole:* 40 mg/day till the patient becomes euthyroid, then maintenance dose for 2 years
  – *β-blocker:* Propranolol 40–120 mg/day to reduce the sympathetic overactivity.

Surgical

Subtotal thyroidectomy.

Indication

- Recurrence after drug therapy
- Drug toxicity
- Large goiter
- Age less than 40 years
- Failure to follow medical treatment.

Preparation

- Make euthyroid state with antithyroid and β-blocker
- *Iodides:* KI 60 mg twice daily for 10–14 days, OR
- *Lugol's iodine:* 5 drops/day for 10 days.

Complications

- Hemorrhage, respiratory obstruction
- Recurrent laryngeal nerve palsy
- Hypothyroidism, hypoparathyroidism
- Recurrence of thyrotoxicosis in 15%.

Radioactive Iodine – I^{131}

Indication
- Older patients, refusal of surgery
- Relapse after surgery/drug therapy
- *Systemic disease:* Contraindication for surgery
- Dose 80–160 μc/g of gland
- Discontinue antithyroid several days before I^{131} administration
- Hypothyroidism in 50–70% within 10 years.

Management of Ophthalmopathy

Measures like:
- Mild cases
  – Raise the head end of bed
  – Diuretics
  – 1% solution of methyl cellulose
- Severe cases
  – Prednisolone 120–160 mg/day
  – Orbital radiation
  – Finally orbital decompression.

Other Varieties of Thyrotoxicosis

Thyrotoxicosis in Pregnancy

- Treatment of choice is antithyroid drugs
- Smallest dose of antithyroid to control thyrotoxicosis
- Antithyroid drugs crosses placenta and prevent neonatal hyperthyroidism and may induce fetal hypothyroidism
- No β-blocker or radioactive iodine
- Those requiring high dose of antithyroid, subtotal-thyroidectomy is done in 2nd trimester.

Neonatal and Childhood Thyrotoxicosis

- Usually Graves' disease
- Treatment of choice is antithyroid drugs
- No radioactive iodine because of fear of carcinogenic effect and later hypothyroidism.

TSH Secreting Pituitary Adenoma

- Increased TSH, increased T$_3$ and T$_4$
- Subunits of TSH increase
- TSH response to TRH is poor.

Selective Resistance of Pituitary Thyrotrophs

- Resistance to feedback inhibition by thyroid hormones → increased TSH, no rise in subunits
- TSH response to TRH is normal.

Trophoblastic Tumor → Thyrotoxicosis

Hydatidiform mole/choriocarcinoma → thyroid stimulation by a variant of human chorionic gonadotrophin (hCG).

Thyrotoxicosis Factitia

- Ingestion of supraphysiological doses of thyroid hormone, endogenous thyroid function is reduced radioactive iodine uptake is reduced
- Serum T_3, T_4 increased if T_4 is taken
- Serum T_4 reduced, T_3 increased, if T_3 is taken.

Ectopic Thyroid Tissue-induced Thyrotoxicosis

- Struma ovarii
- Thyroid carcinoma functioning metastasis
- Follicular carcinoma.

Iodine-induced Thyrotoxicosis: Jod Basedow Phenomenon

Iodine administration in endemic goiter with iodine deficiency and nontoxic MNG → increased synthesis of thyroid hormone → thyrotoxicosis. Iodine deficiency favors this phenomenon.

T_3 Toxicosis

- Excessive production of T_3
- T_4 normal/decreased in the absence of deficiency of thyroxine-binding globulin (TBG)
- May be seen in Graves', toxic adenoma, relapse after treatment
- $T_3 > T_4$ in all types of thyrotoxicosis except T_4 toxicosis.

T_4 Toxicosis

Serum T_4 increased, inhibition of T_3 neogenesis → T_3 normal or decreased.

Apathetic Thyrotoxicosis

- Elderly patient usually with toxic MNG
- Features of thyrotoxicosis is less
- CVS manifestation like congestive heart failure (CHF) and arrhythmia
- Anorexia, weakness and wasting of muscles.

Thyroiditis → Thyrotoxicosis

- Subacute thyroiditis, chronic thyroiditis—Hashimoto's thyroiditis
- T_3, T_4 increased, TSH decreased
- Radioactive iodine uptake is decreased.

CUSHING'S SYNDROME

Features produced by hypercortisolism.

Etiology

Two groups: Adrenocorticotropic hormone (ACTH) dependent and ACTH independent.

1. **ACTH dependent**
   - Excessive pituitary ACTH
   - Pituitary macro/microadenoma
   - Hypothalamic dysfunction/tumor →increased CRH
   - Ectopic ACTH
   - Bronchogenic carcinoma—oat cell
   - Islet cell tumor
   - Thymoma
   - Medullary carcinoma thyroid
   - Bronchial carcinoid—usually undetectable
   - Occult ectopic ACTH syndrome.
2. **ACTH independent**
   - Adrenal neoplasm:
     - Adrenal adenoma
     - Adrenal carcinoma
   - Iatrogenic: Prolonged use of supraphysiological dose of corticosteroid.

Incidence

- 2/3—by Cushing's disease (Increased pituitary ACTH)
- 1/3—by ectopic ACTH and adrenal neoplasm.

Clinical features

- Due to hypercortisolism:
  - Deposition of fat in characteristic site
  - Truncal obesity
  - Plethoric round moon face (Fig. 8.13)
  - Buffalo hump
  - Mesenteric bed
  - Sparing the extremities
  - Mobilization of peripheral supportive tissue
  - Proximal myopathy
  - Osteoporosis, collapse vertebra
  - Cutaneous striae (Weakening and rupture of dermal collagen fiber)
  - Easy bruisability

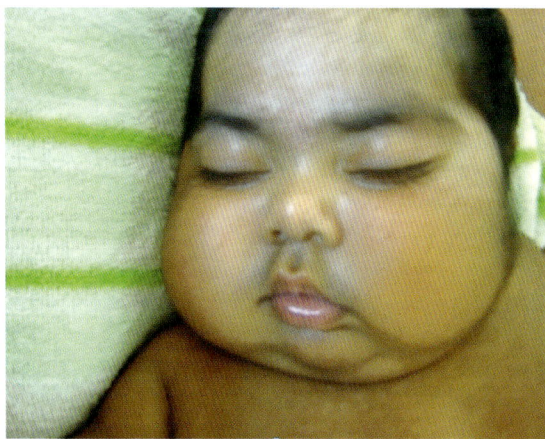

Fig. 8.13: Face showing features of Cushing's syndrome in a baby.

- Hepatic gluconeogenesis and insulin resistance → Diabetes mellitus in 20% cases
- Eye—cataract
- Gastrointestinal tract—Peptic ulcer
- Systemic hypertension.
• Due to excessive androgen.
- Hirsutism
- Oligomenorrhea
- Acne
- Recession of hair of forehead.
• Emotional changes: Depression, psychosis, confusion
• Electrolyte imbalance:
- Hypokalemia
- Metabolic alkalosis.
• Growth retardation in Juvenile Cushing's
• Pigmentation: In ACTH dependent Cushing's syndrome.

Investigations

Diagnosis is by demonstration of
• Increased cortisol production with loss of circadian rhythm
• Failure to suppress endogenous cortisol production by dexamethasone.

Test for Cushing's syndrome
• Urine free Cortisol >100 µg/day
• Serum cortisol is increased
• Overnight dexamethasone suppression test
  - 1 mg dexamethasone orally at midnight
  - Measure the plasma cortisol at 8–9 am
  - Plasma cortisol > 5 µg s/o Cushing
• Diurnal rhythm of plasma cortisol
  - Sample for cortisol at 9:00 hours and 23:00 hours
  - Evening level >75% of the morning level s/o Cushing's syndrome.
• Low dose dexamethasone suppression test
  - 0.5 mg 6th hourly for 48 hours
  - Urine cortisol and plasma cortisol
  - Nonsuppression s/o Cushing's syndrome
• High dose dexamethasone suppression test
  - 2 mg 6th hourly for 48 hours
  - Estimate urine and plasma cortisol
  - Nonsuppressible—adrenal neoplasm and ectopic ACTH
  - Suppressed to < 50% cortisol—pituitary Cushing's syndrome.
• ACTH and high dose DXM suppression
  - ACTH reduced and no suppression: Adrenal neoplasm
  - ACTH increased and No suppression: Ectopic ACTH
  - ACTH increased and partial suppression: Cushing's disease (↑Pituitary ACTH)
• Bilateral inferior petrosal sinus sampling for ACTH
  - In undetectable microadenoma of pituitary < 5 mm size.

Radiological Evaluation
• *CT, MRI of pituitary:* For pituitary adenoma (microadenoma—usually undetectable)
• *CT abdomen:* For adrenal neoplasm >4 cm adrenal Ca < 4 cm adrenal adenoma
• *CT chest:* Source for ectopic ACTH.

Bilateral Inferior Petrosal Sinus Sampling for ACTH
In undetectable microadenoma of pituitary <5 mm size.

Management

Pituitary Adenoma – Cushing's Disease
• Trans-sphenoidal pituitary surgery
• Radiation
• Antiadrenocortical drugs: Metyrapone—2 g/day—four divided dose
• Aminoglutethimide—1 g/day
• Bilateral adrenalectomy.

Adrenal Neoplasm
• Excision of tumor
• Adjuvant therapy in adrenal Ca—Mitotane—8–10 g/day divided dose.

Ectopic ACTH: Resection of responsible tumor if not, bilateral adrenalectomy.

Replacement therapy in all cases after surgical correction. Normal pituitary adrenal axis is suppressed in all cases of Cushing's syndrome.

Nelson's Syndrome

ACTH-secreting pituitary adenoma is progressed after bilateral adrenalectomy in Cushing's disease → hyperpigmentation, local pressure effect and reduced level of other pituitary hormones.

HYPOADRENALISM

Primary: Addison's disease
Secondary: Hypopituitarism (Table 8.2)
Primary Hypoadrenalism (Addison's disease)
Described by Thomas Addison in 1850.

Etiology

• Anatomical destruction of gland
• Autoimmune disease: Autoimmune polyglandular syndromes
• Infections:
  - Tuberculosis, fungal, viral—CMV in AIDS
  - Meningococcemia (Waterhouse-Friderichsen syndrome)
  - Leptospirosis—hemorrhage into adrenal
• Surgical removal

Table 8.2: Difference between primary and secondary adrenal insufficiency.

Features	Primary	Secondary
Skin color	Pigmented	Pallor
Hypopituitarism	Absent	Present
Electrolyte imbalance	Present	Absent
Hypoglycemia	Less	More (ACTH and GH decreased)
Plasma ACTH	Increased	Decreased
Mineralocorticoid	Decreased	Normal

- Infiltration by malignancy
  - Amyloidosis
  - Hemochromatosis
- Failure of hormone synthesis
  - Congenital adrenal hyperplasia.

Autoimmune polyglandular syndromes
- Type 1 polyglandular (HAM syndrome):
  - Hypoparathyroidism
  - Addison's disease
  - Mucocutaneous candidiasis.
- Type II:
  - Type II a → Addison's disease + autoimmune thyroid disease—Schmidt syndrome
  - Type II b → Addison's disease + Type 1DM—Carpenter syndrome.
- Type III:
  - Autoimmune thyroid disease + other autoimmune diseases like gonadal failure, myasthenia, pernicious anemia
  - Type III a → autoimmune thyroid disease + Type 1DM
  - Type III b → autoimmune thyroid disease + pernicious anemia
  - Type III c → autoimmune thyroid disease + any other autoimmune diseases like gonadal failure/myasthenia.

Clinical Features

Clinical features are due to:

Glucocorticoid Deficiency

- Weight loss, fatigability, weakness
- Anorexia, nausea and vomiting
- Postural hypotension
- Hypoglycemia.

Mineralocorticoid Deficiency

- Hypotension
- Syncope.

Increased ACTH

Pigmentation in exposed region, palmar creases, knuckles, mucous membrane, areola of nipple.

Androgen Deficiency

Decreased body hair in females.

Features of Primary Disease

- *Vitiligo:* Autoimmune primary hypoadrenalism
- Abdominal tuberculosis
- Human immunodeficiency virus
- *Features also depend on the onset:* Acute, chronic, acute on chronic.

Investigations

- *Serum electrolyte:* Hyponatremia, hyperkalemia
- *Fasting blood sugar:* Low
- *Serum cortisol level:*
  - Decreased level with normal diurnal rhythm
  - Decreased level with absence of diurnal rhythm
  - Normal level with normal diurnal rhythm.
- *Serum ACTH level:* Increased in primary hypoadrenalism
  - Reduced in secondary hypoadrenalism
- *ACTH stimulation test:* 25 units of ACTH IV/IM for rapid screening test, blood samples at 0, 30 and 60 minutes interval taken
  - *Normal:* Plasma Cortisol increased
  - *Primary:* No change
  - *Secondary:* Subnormal increase.
- *Mineralocorticoid estimation*
  - Plasma renin activity increased, aldosterone reduced/normal
- Human immunodeficiency virus (HIV) screening
- *Detection of antibody to steroid secreting cells:* Autoimmune disease.

MRI abdomen: Small adrenal in autoimmune diseases increased in size in tuberculosis, calcification of adrenal.

Management of Primary Adrenal Insufficiency

- *Replacement therapy:*
  - Hydrocortisone
    - 20 mg in morning
    - 10 mg in evening
  - Or
  - *Prednisolone:*
    - 5 mg in morning
    - 2.5 mg in evening
  - *Mineralocorticoid:*
    - Fludrocortisone
    - 0.05 – 0.1 mg/day
- Treatment of the primary cause.

Acute Adrenal Insufficiency: Adrenal Crisis

Causes

- *Acute on chronic adrenal insufficiency:* Sepsis and surgery
- *Acute adrenal hemorrhage:* Meningococcemia, leptospirosis

- Anticoagulant, pregnancy
- Adrenal vein thrombosis
- Sudden withdrawal of steroid from patient with chronic steroid therapy
- Congenital adrenal hyperplasia with stress.

Features

- Hypotension, shock
- Nausea, vomiting, diarrhea
- Hyponatremia, hypoglycemia and hyperkalemia.

Therapy of Adrenal Crisis

- Rapid replacement of glucocorticoid, saline and glucose
- *Hydrocortisone:* 100 mg 6th hourly for 24 hours—½ the dose every 24 hours for 5 days oral replacement and maintenance dose
- IV glucose and saline to correct hyponatremia and hypoglycemia.

DISORDERS OF CALCIUM HOMEOSTASIS

Calcium Metabolism

- Total body calcium (CA) 1200–1500 g—99% in bones
- Daily intake—0.5–1 g adult
  - 2 g in pregnancy
  - 1–1.5 g children
- Urinary excretion 160 mg/day
- Fecal excretion 600 mg/day
- Through sweat 40 mg/day
- Serum calcium 9–11 mg%.

Diffusable form (60%)
- Ionized Ca 4.5 mg% (50%)
- *Non-ionized Ca 0.5 mg% (10%):* Combined with citrate.

Nondiffusable form: Protein bound (40%).

Factors Regulating Calcium

- Parathormone → Serum Ca increased, PO_4 reduced
- Calcitonin → Serum Ca decreased, PO_4 decreased
- Vitamin D → Serum Ca increase
- Thyroxine → Stimulates osteoclast and decalcification, increased Ca excretion
- Estrogen and androgen →↑ in production of bone matrix
- Glucocorticoid → increased bone breakdown, increased Ca excretion.

Functions of Calcium

- Coagulation of blood
- Bone and teeth formation
- Cardiac rhythmicity
- Neuromuscular activity
- Milk secretion.

Differential Diagnosis of Hypocalcemia

- *Vitamin D deficiency:* Rickets
- Hypoparathyroidism
- Malabsorption syndrome
- Hypomagnesemia
- Chronic renal failure
- Acute pancreatitis
- Nephrotic syndrome.

Hypoparathyroidism

Actions of parathormone: Increased serum calcium—bone resorption, ↑renal reabsorption of Ca→↑ formation of 1,25 $(OH)_2 D_3$ →↑ intestinal absorption of Ca→↑ Serum PO_4— phosphaturic effect at proximal tubule of kidney.

Mechanism of Action

Activation of adenyl cyclase →↑ cAMP ↑ permeability of osteoclast and osteoblast to Ca.

Regulation of parathormone secretion
- Reduced Ca and Mg → increased PTH
- Increased Ca → reduced PTH
- Increased PO_4 → increased PTH.

Causes of Hypoparathyroidism

- *Postoperative:* Thyroid and parathyroid surgery
- *Infantile:* DiGeorge syndrome
- Maternal hyperparathyroidism
- *Idiopathic:* Autoimmune disease ± adrenal, thyroid and ovary
- *Polyglandular deficiency syndrome:* Hypoandrogen metabolic (HAM) syndrome
- Radiation
- Hemochromatosis.

Clinical Features

- Tetany
- Psychosis
- Convulsion
- Alopecia
- Cataract
- Moniliasis
- Aberrant calcification—basal ganglion
- Increased intracranial pressure—papilledema.

Investigation

- Serum Ca reduced, Serum PO_4 increased
- RIA of PTH
- Urinary cyclic AMP response to PTH increase.

Treatment

- Oral Ca 2–3 g/day
- Active vitamin D—1,25$(OH)_2 D_3$ - 0.25–1 µg/day

- 1α OH D₃—1–2 μg/day
- In tetany—10 mL of 10% calcium gluconate slow intravenous (IV).

Pseudohypoparathyroidism

- Failure of end organ response to PTH
- Sex-linked disorder/autosomal dominant
- Features of hypoparathyroidism with distinct developmental and skeletal abnormality
- A short 4th and 5th metacarpals
- Moon face, dwarfism and obesity
- Serum PTH is increased
- Urinary cyclic AMP response to PTH is decreased.

Pseudopseudohypoparathyroidism

Somatic abnormality of pseudohypoparathyroidism + normal serum calcium and phosphorus.

Differential Diagnosis of Hypercalcemia

- Hyperparathyroidism
- Lithium—PTH-mediated
- Familial hypocalciuric hypercalcemia (FHH)
- Malignancy related hypercalcemia
  - PTH like factor
  - Pseudohyperparathyroidism in carcinoma lung and kidney
  - PGE—carcinoma breast
  - OAF (osteoclast activating factor)—myeloma
  - Increased 1,25(OH)₂ D₃—lymphoma
  - Multiple bone secondaries
- Vitamin D intoxication
- Sarcoidosis-↑1,25(OH)₂ D₃—by the macrophage system of the granuloma
- Idiopathic hypercalcemia of infancy—William syndrome
- Hypercalcemia due to increased bone turnover
  - Hyperthyroidism
  - Immobilization
  - Thiazide diuretic
  - Vitamin A intoxication.
- Hypercalcemia with renal failure—severe secondary hyperparathyroidism
- Milk alkali syndrome—Burnett's syndrome (Milk and calcium carbonate antacid).

Hyperparathyroidism

Causes

- Primary:
  - Adenoma—81%
  - Carcinoma—4%
  - Hyperplasia—15%.
- Secondary
  - Chronic renal failure (CRF)
  - Rickets and malabsorption
- Tertiary—autonomous activity in secondary
- Multiple endocrine neoplasia (MEN)
  - *Type I*: Wermer syndrome
    - Pituitary
    - Parathyroid
    - Pancreatic tumors.
  - *Type II a*: Sipple syndrome
    - Medullary carcinoma thyroid (MCT)
    - Pheochromocytoma
    - Hyperparathyroid.
  - *Type II b*
    - MCT
    - Pheochromocytoma
    - Mucosal neuroma +/- Café au lait spots
    - Marfanoid features.
  - *Type III a*
    - Pheochromocytoma
    - Duodenal carcinoid
    - Multiple neurofibromatosis.
  - *Type III b*: Pheochromocytoma + Von Hippel Lindau syndrome + Islet cell tumor.

Clinical Features

- About 50% asymptomatic
- Features due to increased serum calcium
  Fatigue, anorexia, nausea, vomiting, constipation, polyuria
- Renal:
  - Renal parenchymal calcification
  - Nephrocalcinosis
  - Nephrolithiasis
  - Nephrogenic diabetes insipidus
  - Pyelonephritis and renal failure.
- Skeleton:
  - *Osteitis fibrosa cystica*: Von Recklinghausen's disease of bone
  - Resorption of phalangeal tufts
  - Loss of lamina dura of teeth
  - Tiny punched out lesions of skull (salt and pepper appearance)
  - Chondrocalcinosis and pseudogout.
- Central nervous system
  - Depression, confusion and coma
  - *Neuromuscular:* Proximal muscle weakness
  - Easy fatigability.
- *Gastrointestinal tract*: Duodenal ulcer, pancreatitis
- *Eye*: Band keratopathy
- *Skin*: Pruritus
- Serum calcium 11.5–12 mg% → symptoms
  >13 mg% → ectopic calcification—renal, blood vessel
  >15 mg% → severe hypercalcemia
  > 15–18 mg% → encephalopathy.

Investigations

- Serum calcium: Hypercalcemia—sustained/intermittent
- Hypercalciuria, serum PO₄ decreased/normal (If CRF+)
- Serum alkaline phosphatase elevated

- *Radiological:*
  - Resorption of terminal phalanx
  - *Demineralization and subperiosteal erosion of phalanx:* Radial side of middle phalanx
  - *Skull:* Pepper and salt appearance
  - Loss of lamina dura
  - Nephrocalcinosis and nephrolithiasis
- Corticosteroid suppression test
  - Hydrocortisone 100 mg for 10 days → reduced serum calcium in other hypercalcemic conditions
- Urinary cyclic AMP raised
- Radioimmunoassay (RIA) of parathyroid hormone (PTH)
- Localization of parathyroid tumor
- Ultrasonography
- Arteriography
- CT scan
- Differential thallium-technetium imaging.

Treatment

- Surgical:
  - *Solitary adenoma:* Removal
  - *Hyperplasia:* Remove all four glands and transplant some tissue to forearm
  - *Carcinoma:* Wide excision of tissue with tumor
- Medical:
  - Management of hypercalcemia
  - Hydration of the patient
  - Saline infusion and diuretic (furosemide)
  - Phosphate—1–3 g orally
  - IV K dihydroxy PO_4 1500 mg BID (when serum calcium >15 mg%).

Corticosteroid: Prednisolone 10–15 mg QID
- Mithramycin 25 µg/kg body weight
- Calcitonin 2 units S/C 4th hourly.

CHAPTER 9

Examination of the Kidneys and the Urinary System

SYMPTOMATOLOGY

Alteration in the Amount of Urine

Normal → 1.5 L/24 hours [800 mL–2.5 L]. Minimum volume of urine required to excrete the solutes is 500 mL/24 hours.

Oliguria

About <400 mL/24 hours or <20 mL/hour
- Prerenal—hypovolemia, hypotension
- Intrinsic renal disease—acute tubular necrosis (ATN)
- Postrenal—obstructive uropathy.

Anuria

About <50 mL/24 hours
- Obstructive uropathy and urolithiasis
- Rapidly progressive glomerulonephritis (RPGN)
- Renal cortical necrosis
- Cryoglobulinemia
- Renal tubular obstruction—by uric acid, hemoglobin (Hb) and sulfadiazine.

Polyuria

About > 3L/24 hours or >2 mL/min
- Diabetes insipidus—central and nephrogenic
- Diabetes mellitus
- Chronic renal failure—early stage
- Diuretic phase of ATN on recovery
- Thyrotoxicosis
- Hypercalcemia, hypokalemia.

Nocturia

Nocturnal polyuria
- Normal—diurnal and nocturnal volume of urine is 2:1 in healthy adults
- Nocturia means nocturnal volume equalize or exceeds diurnal urine volume—
- Seen in early stage of CRF, benign prostatic hypertrophy, diabetes mellitus, diabetes insipidus.

Alteration in the Urinary Composition

Hematuria

- Presence of excessive amounts of RBCs in urine (>3 RBCs per mm^3 of uncentrifuged urine)
- Normal:
  - Not >3 RBCs/mm^3 of uncentrifuged urine
  - < 1 RBC/hpf of centrifuged urine
- Site of lesion—urethra to glomeruli
- Quantity:
  - Microscopic → glomerular lesion
  - Macroscopic → stone, tumors and glomerular lesion
- Painful hematuria → stone
- Painless hematuria → glomerular lesion, renal TB
- Persistent hematuria → bladder neoplasm
- Intermittent hematuria → IgA nephropathy, Alport's syndrome
- Initial hematuria → urethral disease
- Terminal hematuria → bladder/prostatic disease
- Isolated hematuria—hematuria without significant proteinuria and cast → in urolithiasis, renal TB, tumor, trauma [non-glomerular lesion].

- *Causes of hematuria*
  - Urolithiasis
  - Infections—cystitis, urethritis
  - Renal TB
  - Malignancy—kidney, bladder
  - Glomerular disease—IgA nephropathy, Alport's syndrome
  - Thin basement membrane disease
  - Papillitis necroticans, papilloma
  - Vascular malformations of urinary tract
  - Bleeding diathesis.

- **Glomerular hematuria**
  - Dysmorphic urinary red blood cells (RBCs)
  - Presence of RBC cast
  - Proteinuria (>1 g/day)
- **Nonglomerular hematuria**
  - Isomorphic urinary RBCs
  - Absence of RBC cast
  - No significant proteinuria.
- **Differential diagnoses of hematuria**
  - Hemoglobinuria
  - Myoglobinuria
  - Porphyria
  - Drugs like rifampicin and pyridium.

Pyuria

- Means presence of pus cells in urine
- More than 3 pus cells/mm³ of uncentrifuged urine in adult male is abnormal, more than 10 pus cells/mm³ in adult female is abnormal
- More than 5 pus cells/hpf of centrifuged urine suggestive of pyuria irrespective of sex.
- **Sterile pyuria**
  - Presence of pyuria and the culture is sterile (culture negative pyuria)
  - Causes:
    - Glomerulonephritis, enteric fever, urolithiasis, analgesic
    - Nephropathy, febrile episode, to rule out renal TB.

Proteinuria

- Normal—150 mg/day [75-150 mg/day]
- 10-15 mg albumin/day
- More than 300 mg/day—Frank proteinuria/overt proteinuria
- Normal protein composition of urine (total-150 mg/day)
  - Tamm-Horsfall protein—70 mg
  - Blood group related antigen—35 mg
  - Albumin—15 mg
  - Mucopolysaccharide—15 mg
  - Immunoglobulins—5 mg
  - Rest-hormones and enzymes—10 mg
- Pathophysiological types (Table 9.1)
  - Glomerular proteinuria: Due to glomerular injury usually >1.5 g/day
  - Tubular proteinuria: Due to acute on chronic tubulointerstitial disease, not > 2 g/day
  - Overflow proteinuria
    - Abnormally large amount of small molecular weight protein present in serum whose filtration exceeds the capacity of tubular reabsorption
    - Bence-Jones proteins (Multiple myeloma)
    - Myoglobin (Rhabdomyolysis)
    - Hemoglobin (IV hemolysis).

Table 9.1: Difference between tubular and glomerular proteinuria.

Tubular	Glomerular
Injury to tubulointerstitial region	Injury to glomerulus
Consists of Tamm–Horsfall protein, β2 microglobulin and Enzymes	Predominantly albumin/globulins in nonselective
Proteinuria < 2 g/day	Proteinuria > 2 g/day

- Quantitative assessment of proteinuria
  - Mild—< 1 g/24 hr
  - Moderate—1-3.5 g/24 hr
  - Massive—> 3.5 g/24 hr
- Selective proteinuria
  - Low molecular weight proteins > high molecular weight protein
  - Determined by the ratio of IgG to albumin in urine
  - Ratio less than 0.1 selective seen in minimal change renal disease
- Nonselective proteinuria
  - High molecular weight protein is also filtered
  - Indicates more damage of glomerulus
  - Ratio is more than 0.1 seen in membranous nephropathy
  - Size of albumin—3.6 nm
  - Filtering pore size—5 nm
  - Size of globulin—5.5 nm.
- Microalbuminuria
  - 30-300 mg of albumin/day or albumin excretion rate of 20-200 µ g/min (normal albuminuria <30 mg/day or 20 µg/per min)
  - Causes:
    - Diabetic nephropathy
    - Systemic hypertension
    - SLE, etc.
- Overt albuminuria
  - 300 mg of albumin/day—dipstick positive
- Isolated proteinuria
  - Proteinuria usually less than 2 g/24 hr.
  - Normal urinary sediment
  - Radiologically normal urinary tract
  - Absence of known renal disease.

Clinically proteinuria can be:
- Asymptomatic proteinuria
- Symptomatic proteinuria
- Nephrotic syndrome.

Hemoglobinuria

- Presence of Hb in urine producing reddish discoloration and RBCs absent on microscopy
- Causes:
  - Intravascular hemolysis in—mismatched transfusion
  - G6PD deficiency
  - Snake bite
  - Black water fever
  - Paroxysmal nocturnal hemoglobinuria

Myoglobinuria

- Presence of myoglobin in urine producing reddish discoloration and RBCs absent on microscopy
- Causes—Rhabdomyolysis in:
  - Status epilepticus
  - Sea snake bite
  - Electroconvulsive therapy (ECT)
  - Electric shock
  - Acute alcoholism
  - Drug induced—Gemfibrozil and statins.

Pneumaturia

- Passing air bubbles in urine
- Causes:
  - Vesicocolic fistula
  - Emphysematous pyelonephritis by gas producing organism in diabetes mellitus.

Symptoms of Disorders of Micturition

- *Dysuria:*
  - Refers to pain or burning sensation during urination
  - Due to diseases of lower urinary tract—bladder prostate urethra
- *Frequency:*
  - Frequent voiding of urine due to irritable bladder
  - Normal—About 5 times
  - Causes → Lower urinary tract infection (UTI), prostatitis, benign prostatic hyperplasia (BPH), anxiety state.
- *Polyuria:* Frequency and volume is increased
- *Hesitancy:* Delay in initiation of micturition
- *Urgency and precipitancy:* Sudden uncontrollable urge to pass urine with incontinence before reaching toilet
  - Causes:
    - Local lesions
      - Trigonitis
      - Bladder stone
      - BPH, urethritis
    - Neurogenic bladder
    - Automatic bladder.
- *Incontinence of urine:*
  - Inability to hold urine in the bladder
  - Causes:
    - Lesions of the lower spinal cord involving micturition reflex
    - Incompetent or injured urethral sphincter
    - Fistulous communications—vesicovaginal fistula.
- *True incontinence:* Constant dribbling of urine due to incompetent or injured urethral sphincter or fistulous connection
- *Overflow incontinence (false incontinence):* Due to mechanical obstruction to urethra or bladder neck, overfilling of bladder → intermittent dribbling of urine
- *Stress incontinence:*
  - Involuntary passage of urine due to rise in intra-abdominal pressure as in coughing, laughing, etc.
  - This may occur in female in prolapse of uterus or laxity of the pelvic floor.
- *Enuresis:*
  - Involuntary voiding of urine during sleep
  - Normal till the age of 2–3 years
  - Causes:
    - Anxiety and fear
    - Urinary obstruction and infection
    - Neurological disorders—spina bifida, lower spinal cord lesions
    - Urethral discharge—in urethritis of both sex.
- *Pain in urogenital tract disorders:*
  - Pain of renal disease is felt in the flanks and hypochondrium
  - Acute pyelonephritis, perirenal abscess
  - Ureteric colic (Refer Abdominal pain)
  - Pain of bladder and urethra referred to lower abdomen, perineum and glans penis due to passage of solid material like stone, blood clot and infection
  - Strangury—painful passage of urine drop by drop
  - Pain of prostate is referred to perineum and rectum, as in prostatitis.
- *Edema and puffiness of face is a feature of renal disease (Fig. 9.1)* (refer General examination—edema)
  - Differential diagnosis of puffiness of face
    - Renal edema
    - Generalized edema of any etiology
    - Hypothyroidism
    - Superior vena cava (SVC) obstruction
    - Chronic obstructive pulmonary disease (COPD)
    - Local causes like angioedema and sinusitis
    - Baggy eyelid of old age.

Uremic symptoms

- Symptom complex produced by the accumulation of toxic nitrogenous waste products and due to loss of substances

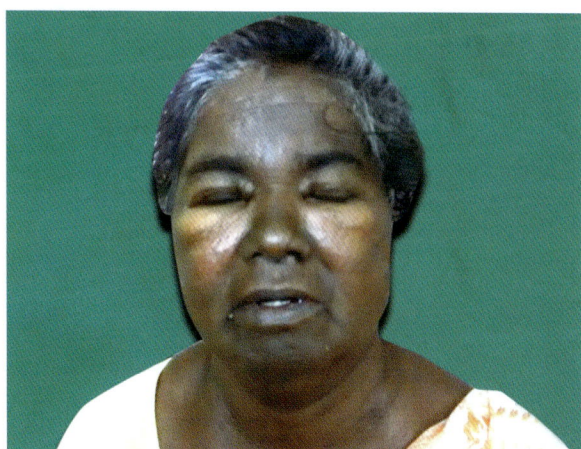

Fig. 9.1: Edema and puffiness of face.

which are normally retained by tubular reabsorption. Symptoms are referable to all systems like anorexia, nausea, loss of weight, dehydration, pallor, hemorrhagic tendency, dyspnea and neuropsychiatric symptoms (refer CRF).

Distention of abdomen
- Generalized—ascites—nephrotic syndrome
- Localized—enlarged kidney in hydronephrosis, polycystic kidney disease (PKD).

Fever in genitourinary disorder
- Fever with rigor and chills → urinary tract infection, renal TB, hypernephroma—renal cell carcinoma
- Septicemia with renal involvement
- Collagen vascular disease with renal involvement.

HISTORY TAKING IN RENAL DISORDERS

Presenting symptoms in chronological order
- Renal symptoms
- Systemic disease with renal involvement like diabetes mellitus, hypertension and collagen vascular disease, etc.

History of presenting illness: Detailing the symptoms (refer Symptomatology)

Past history:
- History of UTI
- Recent skin and upper respiratory tract infection
- Post streptococcal glomerulonephritis
- Other renal symptoms like glomerulonephritis.

Drug history:
- Nonsteroidal anti-inflammatory drug (NSAID) → interstitial nephritis
- Angiotensin-converting-enzyme inhibitor (ACE-I) → renal failure in renal artery stenosis
- Gold and d-penicillamine → glomerular damage
- Analgesic—papillitis necroticans (papillary necrosis)
- Cephalosporin, cisplatin → acute tubular necrosis.

Dietetic history: Details of intake of calorie, protein, fat, sodium, potassium.

Personal history:
- Leptospirosis—farm workers
- Lead nephropathy—welders, painters
- Intravenous drug abuse.

Family history: Polycystic kidney, Alport's syndrome, medullary cystic renal disease, diabetes mellitus, systemic hypertension.

Obstetric history:
- Pregnancy-induced hypertension (PIH)
- Toxemia of pregnancy
- Antiphospholipid syndrome
- Acute renal failure in obstetric accidents.

EXAMINATION OF THE KIDNEYS AND URINARY SYSTEM

General Examination
- Puffiness of face, edema
- *Anemia*: Chronic renal failure
- *Skin:*
  - Dry, scaly, uremic frost—bearded area and skin folds
  - Scratch mark, palpable subcutaneous nodule—dystrophic calcification
  - Sallow complexion—urochrome deposition
  - Rash—connective tissue disease, systemic lupus erythematosus (SLE) drug-induced skin lesions
    - Purpura and striae—corticosteroid therapy
    - Alopecia—cyclophosphamide
    - Hirsutism and discoloration of hair—cyclosporine
  - Skin in systemic disorders
    - SLE
    - Progressive systemic sclerosis
    - Henoch-Schonlein purpura
    - Fabry's disease.
- *Nail:*
  - Half-and-half nail—uremia
  - Transverse parallel white lines (Muehrcke's line)—due to protein loss in nephrotic syndrome
  - Splinter hemorrhage—infective endocarditis and vasculitis.
- *Eye:*
  - Band keratopathy—is a calcium deposition beneath the corneal epithelium in the same plane as the interpalpebral fissure, seen in hypercalcemia, hyperparathyroidism
  - Perilimbal calcification and conjunctival congestion long standing uremia
  - Fundus—retinopathy of diabetes mellitus and hypertension
  - Keratoconus and lenticonus—Alport's syndrome.
- *Gum hyperplasia:* Cyclosporine in post-transplant patient
- *Deafness:* Alport's syndrome
- *State of hydration:*
  - Dehydration—prerenal uremia
  - Over hydration—fluid overload in acute renal failure
  - Acute glomerulonephritis.
- *Mouth:*
  - Uremic fetor—ammoniacal odor due to breakdown of urea into ammonia in the saliva
- *Mucosal ulcer*
- *Growth retardation:*
  - Children with chronic renal failure
  - Renal rickets.

SYSTEMIC EXAMINATION

Examination of Abdomen

- *Inspection*:
  - Nephrectomy scar—in the loin
  - Renal transplant scar—right or left iliac fossa
  - Small scars of peritoneal dialysis—center of the lower abdomen
  - Distension of abdomen:
    - Generalized—ascites
    - Localized—hydronephrosis, polycystic kidney.
- *Palpation*:
  - Palpable renal mass—unilateral or bilateral (refer palpation-kidneys)
  - Distended bladder
  - Renal angle tenderness in—
    - Perinephric abscess
    - Hemorrhage into the cyst
    - Acute pyelonephritis.
- *Percussion*:
  - Evidence of ascites
  - Splenic flexure resonance—to differentiate renal mass from splenomegaly
  - Percuss for an enlarged bladder.
- *Auscultation*:
  - Arterial bruit—renal artery stenosis—just above the umbilicus about 2 cm to the left or right of the midline
  - Abdominal aortoarteritis → aortic bruit
  - Iliofemoral bruit—aortoiliac arteritis.

Examination of External Genitalia

- Mucosal ulcers—Reiter's syndrome, Behcet's syndrome
- Urethral discharge or urethritis
- Testes—impalpable—undescended testis
- Small testes—hypogonadism
- Sinus from the scrotum—tuberculous epidydimo-orchitis
- Penis—pin hole meatus—obstructive uropathy—hydronephrosis
- Phimosis
- Left varicocele—left renal vein thrombosis.

Examination of the Other Systems

Cardiovascular System

- Blood pressure measurement—hypertension in:
  - Renal parenchymal disease
  - Renovascular disease
  - Left ventricular hypertrophy (LVH).
- Pericarditis—hemorrhagic/fibrinous pericarditis
- Uremic cardiomyopathy
- Congestive heart failure due to:
  - Fluid overload
  - Cardiomyopathy
  - Systemic hypertension.
- Infective endocarditis → renal lesions.

Respiratory System

- Pulmonary edema due to:
  - Uremic lung
  - Fluid overload
  - Cardiomyopathy.
- Pleural effusion—in nephrotic syndrome
- Pneumonia
- Acidotic breathing.

Central Nervous System

- Altered sensorium:
  - Uremic encephalopathy
  - Seizure.
- Flapping tremor, myoclonus
- Peripheral neuropathy
- Muscle cramps
- Restless leg syndrome.

NORMAL URINE

- Volume: 1.5 L/day (800–2500 mL)
- Specific gravity: 1.010–1.025 (1.003–1.030)
- Osmolality: 50–1200 mOsmol/L (> 800 mOsmol is normal)
- Color: Pale lemon yellow due to urochrome
- Odor:
  - Fresh urine—odorless
  - Pungent odor—by splitting urea to ammonia by the bacteria producing ammoniacal odor
- Reaction: pH—4.6–8 (5–6)

Chemical Composition

- Protein—75–150 mg/24 h
- Albumin—10–15 mg/24 h
- Inorganic substances—sodium—6 g/day
- Potassium—2 g/day
- Calcium—200 mg/day
- Phosphorous—1.7 g/day
- Urea—20–30 g per day
- Uric acid—600 mg/day
- Creatinine—1200 mg/day.

Microscopy

- RBC: Not more than 3/mm^3 of uncentrifuged urine
- WBC: Not more than 3/mm^3 of uncentrifuged urine
- Hyaline cast: Occasionally [< 15/mL urine]
- Crystals: Triple phosphate crystal—alkaline urine
- Calcium oxalate crystals: Acid urine
- Uric acid crystals: Occasionally.

CLINICAL PRESENTATION OF RENAL DISEASES

1. **Acute nephritic syndrome**—refers to acute onset of:
   - Oliguria
   - Hematuria

- Proteinuria
- Puffiness of face, edema
- Hypertension.

2. **Nephrotic syndrome:**
   - Means massive proteinuria ≥ 3.5 g/24 hr, edema,
   - Hypoalbuminemia, and
   - Hyperlipidemia.
3. **Acute kidney injury (AKI):**
   - Defined as any of the following:
     - Increase in serum creatinine by >0.3 mg/dL (> 26.5 mmol/L) within 48 hours; or
     - Increase in serum creatinine to 1.5 times baseline, which is known or presumed to have occurred within the prior 7 days; or
     - Urine volume < 0.5 mL/kg/h for 6 hours.
4. **Acute kidney disease (AKD):**
   - AKI
     or
   - Glomerular filtration rate (GFR) <60 mL/min per 1.73 m² for <3 months
     or
   - Decrease in GFR by >/= 35%
     or
   - Increase in serum creatinine by > 50% for <3 months
   - Structural criteria: kidney damage for <3 months.
5. **Acute renal failure:** Preferably should be restricted to patients who have AKI and need renal replacement therapy (RRT).
6. **Chronic kidney disease (CKD):**
   - GFR <60 mL/min per 1.73 m² for >3 months
   - Structural criteria: Kidney damage for >3 months.
7. **Chronic renal failure:** Progressive irreversible damage of nephrons leading onto chronic decline in renal function producing the clinical syndrome of uremia of more than 3 months duration.
8. **Azotemia:** Elevation of blood urea nitrogen (BUN) and serum creatinine levels.
9. **Uremia:** Clinical syndrome associated with fluid, electrolyte, and hormone imbalances and metabolic abnormalities, which develop in parallel with deterioration of renal function.
10. **Urinary tract infection:** Microbial colonization of urine, established by the presence of significant number of microorganisms in urine culture of > 105 colonies/mL
11. **Asymptomatic urinary abnormalities:**
    - Microscopic hematuria
    - Non-nephrotic proteinuria
    - Abnormal RFT
12. **Urinary tract obstruction**
13. **Systemic hypertension**
14. **Nephrolithiasis**
15. **Renal tubular defect:**
    - Renal tubular acidosis
    - Renal glycosuria
    - Phosphaturia
    - Aminoaciduria.

PRIMARY GLOMERULAR DISEASES

- Proliferative glomerulonephritis
  - Diffuse proliferative glomerulonephritis
  - Mesangial proliferative glomerulonephritis
  - Focal glomerulonephritis
  - Rapidly progressive glomerulonephritis (RPGN)
  - Membranoproliferative glomerulonephritis (MPGN) (Mesangio capillary glomerulonephritis)
- Minimal change nephropathy
- Membranous nephropathy
- Focal segmental glomerulosclerosis (FSGS)
- Chronic sclerosing glomerulonephritis—in end stage renal disease.

Acute Glomerulonephritis

Definition: Acute onset of oliguria, hematuria and proteinuria with edema, puffiness of face, hypertension, with or without uremia.

Pathogenesis

- Immunologically mediated injury to glomeruli
- Immune complex mediated (Type III reaction)
  - Immune complex
    - Exogenous antigen—streptococci
    - Endogenous antigen—DNA - SLE
- Antiglomerular basement membrane mediated (Type II reaction)
  - Goodpasture's syndrome
  - Renal lesions as a part of systemic disease
  - Henoch-Schonlein (HS) purpura
  - Secondary mechanism of glomerular injury
  - Complement activation
  - Neutrophil dependent inflammation
  - Activation of kinin system.

Pathology of Proliferative Glomerulonephritis

- Diffuse proliferation: Poststreptococcal glomerulonephritis (PSGN)
- Mesangial proliferation: Recovering PSGN
- Focal glomerulonephritis:
  - IgA nephropathy
  - HS purpura
  - Infective endocarditis.
- Rapidly progressive glomerulonephritis
  - Crescentic glomerulonephritis, crescent formation in more than 50% glomerulus, usually >70%
  - Primary RPGN are 3 types
    - Type I → Anti GBM antibody-mediated
    - Type II → Immune complex-mediated
    - Type III → Pauci-immune (non immune) mediated–renal limited ANCA glomerulonephritis

- Secondary RPGN
  - Postinfective
  - Multisystem disease—SLE, HS purpura, Wegener's granulomatosis (WG)
  - Drugs—Rifampicin
  - Idiopathic.
- Membranoprolifeative glomerulonephritis (MPGN)
  - Primary
  - Secondary
  - SLE, Hepatitis B virus, infective endocarditis
  - 3 types:
    - Type I—Subendothelial and mesangial deposit
    - Type II—Intramembranous deposit (dense deposit disease)
    - Type III—Subendothelial, mesangial and subepithelial deposit.

Etiology of Acute Glomerulonephritis (AGN)

- Poststreptococcal GN—strain 1, 3, 4, 5 and 12—throat, 24, 49, 55, 57 and 60—skin
- Non streptococcal infection—virus-HBV, mumps, IMN
- Nonviral—pneumococci, IE
- Toxoplasmosis
- Multisystem disease—SLE, HS purpura, Goodpasture's syndrome
- Vasculitis—microscopic polyangiitis
- Primary glomerular disease—RPGN, IgA nephropathy, MPGN
- Focal glomerulonephritis.

Clinical Features of AGN (Poststreptococcal GN)

- History of upper respiratory tract infection (RTI), skin infection—2-3 weeks prior to the onset
- Age—Children-6-10 years, Adult
- Puffiness of face (Fig. 9.2), edema, oliguria, hematuria
- Smoky urine due to denatured hemoglobin
- Mild to moderate hypertension—due to reduced GFR → Na-H_2O retention
- Features of complications
  - Hypertensive encephalopathy—headache, seizure, altered sensorium with high blood pressure
  - Hypertensive congestive heart failure (CHF)—dyspnea, raised jugular venous pressure (JVP), basal crepitations
  - Acute renal failure—oliguria and features of uremia
  - Hyperkalemia
  - Features of other system involvement in multisystem disease like SLE, HS purpura and Goodpasture's syndrome.

Complications of AGN

- Hypertensive encephalopathy
- Hypertensive CHF
- Acute renal failure-in RPGN
- Hyperkalemia.

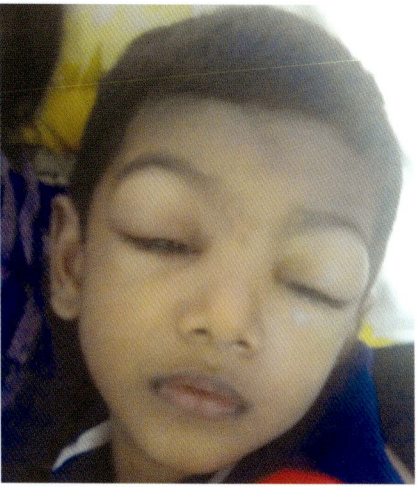

Fig. 9.2: Puffiness of face and facial edema in acute glomerulonephritis.

Investigations

- Urine—oliguria, specific gravity increase, Albumin+, hematuria—micro/macro
- Microscopy—RBC-dysmorphic, WBC +, RBC cast
- Proteinuria—<2 g/24 hours, nonselective
- RFT—blood urea, serum creatinine—normal or increases, GFR—creatinine clearance ↓
- Culture of throat swab/skin lesion—nephritogenic strain
- ASO titer ↑, anti DNAse B ↑, complement C3/C4 ↓ (normal in IgA nephropathy)
- X-ray chest—cardiomegaly ±, evidence of pulmonary edema ±
- Renal imaging—normal
- Renal biopsy—proliferative GN
- Investigation in multisystem disease—ANA, anti dsDNA, Anti Ro, Anti La, ANCA, cryoglobulin, etc.

Prognosis

- In children—70% recovery, adult—50% recovery, the rest will develop chronic glomerular disease, nephrotic syndrome, CRF, RPGN
- Poor prognostic factors—age-adult
  - Proteinuria—nephrotic range
  - Hypertension, renal failure
  - Glomerular sclerosis.

Management

- Bed rest, input/output (I/O) chart
- Salt and fluid restriction (700 mL + amount equal to previous day urine output)
- Antibiotics—for 10 days—penicillin/erythromycin (if infection present)
- Control of hypertension—by-loop diuretics/Ca channel blockers
- Dialysis—If fluid overload, uremia, electrolyte imbalance which cannot be controlled by drugs

- Treatment of complications
  - Hypertensive encephalopathy
    - Rapid reduction of blood pressure—loop diuretic/sublingual nifedipine (2.5 mg) for children and Captopril (12.5 mg) for adults
    - Drugs to reduce cerebral edema
    - Antiepileptic
  - Hypertensive congestive heart failure (CHF)
    - High dose loop diuretic—furosemide
    - Dialysis if needed
  - Acute renal failure
    - Conservative treatment
    - Dialysis if needed.

Course of the Disease

- Urine output starts increasing within 2 weeks time
- Urea, creatinine → normal within 3–4 weeks
- Proteinuria, hematuria can persist to 6/12 to 1 year.

Indications of Renal Biopsy in AGN

- Severe renal failure requiring dialysis
- Abnormal RFT> 4 weeks
- C3 reduction of > 8 weeks (differentiate from MPGN)
- Nephrotic range of proteinuria of >4 weeks
- Abnormal urinary sediment >1 year.

NEPHROTIC SYNDROME

Definition: It is characterized by
- Massive proteinuria >3.5 g/24 h
- Edema
- Hypoalbuminemia
- Hyperlipidemia and
- Lipiduria.

Etiology

- Primary glomerular disease (idiopathic)
  - Minimal change nephropathy
  - Membranous glomerulonephritis
  - MPGN
  - Focal segmental glomerulosclerosis
  - Mesangioproliferative glomerulonephritis
- Secondary glomerular disease—multisystem disease:
  - Diabetes mellitus
  - SLE
  - Amyloidosis
  - HS purpura
  - Goodpasture's syndrome
  - Wegener's granulomatosis.
- Infection:
  - Viral
    - Hepatitis B virus
    - Autoimmune deficiency syndrome
    - Cytomegalovirus
    - Infectious mononucleosis.
  - Bacterial
    - Poststreptococcal glomerulonephritis
    - Infective endocarditis Hansen's disease
    - Syphilis.
  - Parasitic
    - Malaria
    - Filariasis
    - Schistosomiasis.
- Malignancy:
  - Multiple myeloma
  - Hodgkins disease, non-hodgkin's lymphome (NHL)
  - Bronchogenic carcinoma.
- Drugs:
  - Penicillamine
  - NSAID
  - Captopril
  - Primidone.
- Toxins:
  - Gold
  - Mercury
  - Bee stings.
- Heredofamilial disease:
  - Alport's syndrome
  - Fabry's disease
  - Nail-patella syndrome (NPS)
  - Congenital nephrotic syndrome.

Pathogenesis

- *Proteinuria:*
  - About ≥3.5 g/day, due to either change in pore size or decrease in anion barrier (polyanionic lining of foot process of epithelium)
  - Ratio of IgG: Albumin<0.1
    - Selective proteinuria
    - Due to loss of anion barrier
  - Ratio of IgG: Albumin>0.1
    - Non-selective proteinuria
    - Due to increase in size of pore
  - Proteinuria also depends on GFR, serum albumin.
- *Hypoalbuminemia:*
  - It is due to renal catabolism of filtered albumin
  - Compensated increased synthesis of albumin is defective (normal:12–14 g/day).
- *Edema:*
  - Mechanism is hypoalbuminemia (<3 g/dL) →↓ in oncotic pressure →↓ in extracellular fluid →↑ intravascular fluid →↓ renin angiotensin aldosterone—ADH, ↓ atrial natriuretic polypeptide →↑ Na and water retention. Intrarenal factors →↓ GFR →↑ tubular reabsorption of Na → edema
- *Hyperlipidemia*:
  - Increased lipoprotein synthesis by liver triggered by hypoalbuminemia →↑ LDL and total cholesterol

- Hypercoagulability:
  - ↓ antithrombin 3, protein C and S
  - ↑ fibrinogen, ↓ fibrinolysis
  - ↑ platelet aggregation,
  - ↑ factor 5 and 8 spontaneous arterial and venous thrombosis (Renal vein thrombosis and pulmonary embolism).
- Others:
  - Transferrin loss in urine → iron deficiency anemia
  - Cholecalciferol binding protein loss → deficiency of vitamin D
  - Thyroxin binding globulin loss →↓ thyroxin level
  - Loss and increased catabolism of IgG →↑ emergency department (ED) infection

Clinical Features

- In children (2–6 years); M > F
- In adult, seen equally in both sexes
- Puffiness of face, generalized edema
- Oliguria, ± Hematuria ± Uremia ± Hypertension
- Frequent infection + features of primary disease in secondary nephrotic syndrome + features of complications if present like thrombosis

Investigations

- Proteinuria >3.5 g/24 hours or > 40 mg/m² in children
- Urine deposit (depends on the type of lesion) RBC, RBC cast, WBC
- *Serum protein*: Hypoalbuminemia—<3 g/dL—reduced serum complement (normal in minimal change disease)—serum cholesterol ↑ LDL, ↑ total cholesterol
- Renal biopsy, light microscopy, electron microscopy, immunofluorescent study
- In children common cause is minimal change disease, thus renal biopsy is not usually done. Biopsy is done in children who are <1 year and >10 year
- Investigation for primary disease—blood sugar, ANA, antids DNA, ANCA, anti GBM antibody, cryoglobulin, serum electrophoresis in myeloma.

Management

Principles:
1. Control of glomerular damage—to reduce proteinuria
2. Correction of hypoalbuminemia
3. Treatment of edema, hyperlipidemia
4. Treatment of complication—renal failure, hypertension
5. Treatment of primary cause if any

1. ***Control of glomerular damage***
Minimal change in nephrotic syndrome can be taken as a prototype of nephrotic syndrome
 - Corticosteroids- Prednisolone
   - 1 mg/kg body wt. for adult or 60 mg/m² for children per day, to be continued for 4 weeks
   - If good response present (steroid responsive), make the dose alternate days for the next 4 weeks, then taper the dose (5 mg reduction/week) till it is over
   - Steroid resistance—Poor response with full dose of corticosteroid for 8 weeks
   - Frequent relapse >3 relapse/year or >2 relapse per 6 months
   - Steroid sensitive—relapse on tapering or stopping corticosteroid
   - Steroid dependent—high dose of steroid for maintaining remission
   - In case of relapse, repeat the initial course of steroid as mentioned above
   - For frequent relapsers/steroid dependent patients → course of immunosuppressant drug like cyclophosphamide is given
 - Immunosuppressants
   - Cyclophosphamide: 2 mg/kg-8 weeks, 6 months interval between for repeat course
   - Levamisole (T cell stimulant-2.5 mg/kg alternate days)
   - Cyclosporine-6 mg/kg to start with, maintain trough level of 100–200 mg per mL for 8 weeks
   - Mycophenolate mofetil-500 mg bid

2. ***Correction of hypoalbuminemia***
 - Diet: Protein intake 0.6 g/kg + amount of proteinuria in grams
 - Salt poor albumin infusion.

3. ***Treatment of edema***
 - Salt restriction
 - Diuretics: Hydrochlorothiazide 2 mg/kg for children and 25 mg/adult. If necessary loop diuretics like furosemide may also be used. Monitor S. electrolyte, urine output and body weigh.
 - In massive edema, IV albumin with furosemide is used. Albumin 0.25–1 g/kg body weight (20% salt poor albumin)

4. ***Treatment of complications***
 - Uremia
 - Systemic HTN
 - Infection
 - Thrombosis.

5. ***Treatment of primary cause, if any***
 - Diabetes mellitus
 - SLE
 - Amyloidosis
 - Infection (Malaria, leprosy, HBV).

Complications

- Hypercoagulability→thrombosis
  - Arterial and venous
  - Renal and peripheral venous thrombosis
- Infections
- Spontaneous bacterial peritonitis

- Acute renal failure due to:
  - Decreased plasma volume (diuretics, loss of fluid)
  - Interstitial renal edema
  - Drug-induced interstitial nephritis
  - Decreased vasodilator prostaglandin (NSAID)
  - Renal vein thrombosis.
- Vitamin D deficiency→osteomalacia and secondary hyperparathyroidism.

Bad Prognostic Features

- Systemic hypertension
- Decreased complement level
- GFR <30%
- Nonselective proteinuria.

ACUTE RENAL FAILURE

Definition : Acute decline in renal function, usually reversible, with retention of nitrogenous waste products and other substances leading on to uremia (Biochemical definition: *Rise in serum creatinine >200 µmol/dL*).

Types

Depends on the urine output
1. Oliguric: <400 mL/24 hours
2. Nonoliguric: >400 mL/24 hours
3. Anuric: <50 mL/24 hours

Pathogenesis

- Renal hypoperfusion → prerenal (50%)
- Intrinsic renal disease → renal (40%)
- Obstruction to urine flow → postrenal (10%).

Etiology

Prerenal Causes (Table 9.2)

- Renal hypoperfusion → decreased GFR
  - Hypovolemia
  - Cardiogenic shock
  - Septic shock
  - Congestive heart failure.
- • Decreased GFR without hypotension
  - Acute hypercalcemia
  - Marked hyponatremia.
- Renal vasoconstriction
  - Hepatorenal syndrome
  - Septicemia.

Renal Causes

- *Acute tubular necrosis (ATN) (Table 9.2)*
  - Renal ischemia
  - Nephrotoxins
  - Intravascular hemolysis

Table 9.2: Differentiating features between prerenal and renal (ATN) uremia.

Features	Prerenal	ATN
Urinary sodium	>500	<350
Urinary sodium	<20 mEq/L	>40 mEq/L
Urine specific gravity	>1.020	<1.020
Renal failure index (RFI)	<1	>1
Fractional excretion of Sodium (FENa)	<1	>1
Urinary deposit	Hyaline cast	Brown granular cast

*RFI: (Urinary Na/Urinary creatinine) × serum creatinine
*FENa: (Urinary Na/Serum Na) × (Serum creatinine/urinary creatinine) × 100

  - Disseminated intravascular coagulation (DIC)
  - Obstetrics accidents—Septic abortion, eclampsia, APH, PPH
- *Glomerular diseases*
  - RPGN
  - Lupus nephritis
  - Goodpasture's syndrome.
- *Acute interstitial nephritis*
  - Infection
  - Septicemia
  - Drugs.
- *Acute cortical necrosis*
  - Shock
  - Snake venom
  - Nephrotoxins
  - Obstetric accidents.
- *Acute pyelonephritis—bilateral:*
- *Renovascular*
  - Renal vein thrombosis
  - Renal artery occlusion
  - Malignant hypertension
- *Intrarenal obstruction (Renal tubular obstruction)*
  - Hb (Intravascular hemolysis)
  - Myoglobin (Rhabdomyolysis)
  - Sulfa
  - Uric acid crystals

  [Acute tubular necrosis (ATN) = 85%, Acute glomerulonephritis (AGN) = 5%, Acute interstitial nephritis (AIN) = 10%]
- *Anuric renal failure:*
  - Acute cortical necrosis
  - RPGN
  - Paraproteinemia with radio contrast
  - Cryoglobulinemia
- *Nonoliguric renal failure:*
  - Aminoglycosides (gentamicin)
  - Interstitial nephritis
  - Leptospirosis
  - Snake venom

- Hypercatabolic renal failure [Rise in blood urea >100 mg/day, potassium > 0.5 mEq/day, serum creatinine >2 mg/day]
  - Infection
  - Injury
  - Drugs—corticosteroids, tetracycline.

Postrenal (Causes)

- Acute obstruction to the urinary collecting system
- Urethral obstruction
- Ureteric obstruction of single functioning kidney
- Bilateral ureteric obstruction
- Calculus anuria, bladder neck obstruction.

Mechanism of Oliguria in Acute Renal Failure

- Vasoconstriction of afferent arteriole
- Microthrombi in glomerular capillary
- Change in the permeability of glomerular capillary
- Tubular obstruction by epithelial debris
- Back diffusion of fluid.

Pathology (ATN)

- Renal ischemia
  - Loss of tubular epithelium
  - Disruption of tubular BM
  - Patchy involvement.
- Nephrotoxins
  - Loss of tubular epithelium
  - Tubular basement membrane is normal
  - Proximal tubular involvement.

Clinical Features

Due to:
1. Sodium and water retention → (fluid overload) *edema, puffiness and pulmonary edema*
2. Potassium, hydrogen, magnesium, phosphate retention → *Hyperkalemia, acidosis, hypocalcemia*
3. Nitrogenous waste product retention → *Uremia.*

Course of Acute Renal Failure

- Onset phase
  - From precipitating illness to oliguria
  - Features of primary disease—blood urea/serum creatinine normal
- Oliguric phase
  - 2–3 weeks
  - Fluid overload
  - Metabolic acidosis
  - Hyperkalemia
  - Uremic features
    - Gastrointestinal (GI) tract—nausea, vomiting, anorexia, pancreatitis, bleeding
    - Cardiovascular system—pericarditis, CHF
    - Respiratory system—pleurisy, pulmonary edema
    - Central nervous system—encephalopathy, seizure, flap myoclonus.
  - Rise in blood urea/serum creatinine
- Diuretic phase
  - Polyuria, dehydration
  - Hyponatraemia, hypokalemia
  - Fall in blood urea, serum creatinine
  - Poor renal concentration function
- Postdiuretic phase
  - Recovery phase
  - Minimal dysfunction in acidification and concentration
  - Blood urea and serum creatinine normal.

Investigations

1. *Urine:*
   - Volume, specific gravity, osmolality, sodium, urea, deposit, RBC, RBC cast, WBC, WBC cast, eosinophil, hyaline cast, brown granular cast
   - Proteinuria, hemoglobinuria, myoglobinuria, uric acid crystals
2. *Blood biochemistry:* Urea, creatinine, electrolyte, calcium, phosphate, uric acid, serum protein electrophoresis
3. *For primary disease:*
   - ANA, dsDNA antibody, ANCA, complement
   - Viral markers—HBV, HCV, antibody to leptospira
   - Serum ACE inhibitors
   - Serum aminoglycoside.
4. For hypovolemia and hypotension
   - GI bleeding,
   - ADD
   - Septic shock
   - Heart disease
   - Shock and CHF.
5. *Postrenal causes:* Imaging—USG, IVU, CT, Retrograde pyelography
6. *Renal biopsy:* Oliguria >4–6 weeks, glomerular disease → renal failure.

Management

Principles:
- Correction of reversible causes—renal hypoperfusion, obstruction
- Minimize catabolism—Diet with 2000 calorie/day, protein 0.6 g/kg body weight, carbohydrate—50–200 g/day, fat—75–150 g/day
- Supportive therapy
  - Fluid balance 500 ml + amount of urine output (Insensible loss + measurable loss)
  - Acidosis-correct if bicarbonate <15 mEq/L
    - 10% Ca gluconate 10 mL iv bd
    - 50% glucose 50 ml IV bd +10 units insulin bd

Infections: Avoid indwelling catheter/IV cannula
Hypertension: CCB/Diuretics
Anemia: PCV< 20%, Packed cells

- Dialysis - indication
  - Biochemical:
    - Blood urea >200 mg
    - Serum creatinine >5 mg
    - Serum potassium >6.5 mEq
    - Serum bicarb <15 mEq
    - Rise in blood urea > 50 mg/day
    - ECG: Evidence of hyperkalemia.
  - Clinical
    - Anuria >4 days
    - Pericarditis
    - Fluid overload
    - Pulmonary edema
    - Encephalopathy—convulsion.
- *Drugs in ARF:*
  High dose loop diuretic–incipient phase
  Low dose dopamine 3 µg/kg/mt (Dopamine→ renovasodilation)–with hypotension ANP-↓Na and water reabsorption
  Growth factors—IGF1 (↑renal epithelial growth)
- Specific drugs
  - Vasculitis, SLE → Immunosuppressants
  - Hypercalcemia → saline/bisphosphonate
  - A/c interstitial nephritis → steroids
  - Goodpasture's syndrome → plasmapheresis
  - Pigment nephropathy → IV mannitol/frusemide.

Complications

- Hypertension
- Pulmonary edema
- Arrhythmia
- Hyperkalemia
- Metabolic acidosis
- Infection
- Encephalopathy.

Prognosis

- Better in ATN and
- Bad in acute cortical necrosis.

Prevention (ARF)

- Preoperative correction of fluid and electrolyte
- Prompt detection and correction of prerenal causes
- Prompt detection and correction of obstructive uropathy
- Early renal biopsy and immunosuppressants in immune mediated renal disease
- Allopurinol with antimalignant drugs
- Caution with nephrotoxic drugs—NSAID, ACE inhibitor, Aminoglycoside, cisplatin.

CHRONIC RENAL FAILURE

Definition: Progressive irreversible damage to nephrons of more than 3 months duration leading onto chronic decline in renal function producing the clinical syndrome of uremia.

Pathogenesis

- Progressive loss of nephrons
- Hypertrophy of functioning
- ↓ed concentration function→polyuria
- GFR 50 mL/min-blood urea and serum creatinine↑
- GFR 30 mL/min—Features of uremia, phosphate retenstion, ↑in PTH
- GFR 20 mL/min—↓ed bicarb absorption, ↓ed hydrogen and ammonia excretion
- GFR 10 mL/min—Impaired tubular handling of Na and water
- GFR 5 mL/min-end stage renal disease, impaired potassium handling.

Rapidly progressive renal failure—in 2 weeks to 3 months—normal sized kidneys.

Etiology of CRF

- Congenital: Polycystic kidney disease (PKD), Alport's syndrome
- Primary glomerular disease
  - PGN, MPGN, membranous nephropathy.
- Secondary glomerular disease
  - Diabetes mellitus
  - Hypertensive-nephrosclerosis
  - Amyloidosis
  - SLE
  - HS purpura
  - Polyarteritis nodosa (PAN).
- Interstitial renal disease:
  - Chronic pyelonephritis
  - Analgesic nephropathy
  - TB kidney
  - Nephrocalcinosis.
- Obstructive uropathy
- Heavy metals and toxins.

Common causes of CRF
- Diabetes mellitus
- Hypertension
- Chronic glomerulonephritis
- Chronic pyelonephritis
- Obstructive uropathy
- PKD.

Clinical Features of CRF

- General
  - Weakness
  - Fatigability
  - Loss of weight
  - Puffiness of face
  - Pallor
  - Edema.
- Gastrointestinal tract
  - Anorexia
  - Nausea

- Vomiting
- Uremic fetor
- Macroglossia
- Peptic ulcer
- GI bleeding.
- Cardiopulmonary
  - Hypertension
  - CHF
  - Uremic lung
  - Cardiomyopathy
  - Hemorrhagic and fibrinous pericarditis
- Central nervous system (CNS)
  - Fatigue, insomnia, altered sleep rhythm, loss of memory, flap, myoclonus, seizure, coma
  - Peripheral neuropathy
  - Restless leg syndrome
  - Muscle cramps
  - Proximal myopathy
  - Dialysis dementia (Aluminum intoxication)
    - Speech apraxia, dementia, myoclonus and convulsion
  - Dialysis disequilibrium
    - Due to reduction in pH, osmolality of ECF in brain following rapid reduction in blood urea → cerebral edema
    - Features are nausea vomiting, headache drowsiness convulsion and coma.
- Musculoskeletal
  - Renal osteodystrophy: ↓ed 1-25 dihydroxy D_3 ↓→ ed Ca absorption → osteomalacia
  - Phosphate retention → secondary hyper-parathyroidism →↑ed PTH → osteitis fibrosa cystica
  - Osteosclerosis—Rugger jersey spine
  - Osteoporosis—Due to malnutrition, acidosis, aluminum intoxication, iron overload
  - Metastatic calcification—Ca/PO_4 Product is ↑
  - Proximal myopathy.
- *Fluid and electrolyte imbalance*
  - Fluid overload
  - Metabolic acidosis (Wide anion gap)
  - Increase in magnesium
  - Hyponatremia and hypotension
  - Hypokalemia and muscle weakness.
- *Endocrine features*
  - Secondary hyperparathyroidism
  - Impaired glucose tolerance (IGT)
  - Hypogonadism
  - Dwarfism.
- Hematological features
  - Anemia: Normocytic normochromic, due to:
    - Erythropoietin deficiency
    - Increased bone marrow toxins
    - Increased hemolysis
    - Loss by hemorrhage
    - Aluminum toxicity
    - Reduced food intake
    - Malabsorption.
  - Leukocyte dysfunction, neutrophil dysfunction and lymphocytopenia
  - Bleeding diathesis—platelet dysfunction.
- Dermatological features
  - Pallor, pigmentation, pruritus, ecchymosis, uremic frost, sallow yellow color (urochrome).
- Ocular
  - Visual blurring—hypertensive retinopathy, retinal vascular thrombosis
  - Conjunctivitis—calcium deposit at limbus
  - Infections due to reduced cellular and humoral immunity.

Stages of Chronic Kidney Disease (Table 9.3)

Table 9.3: Stages of chronic kidney disease.

Stage	GFR in ml/min/1.73m²
0	>90—with risk factors for CKD
1	≥90—with demonstrated kidney damage
2	60–89
3	30–59
4	15–29
5	<15—ESRD

CKD: Chronic kidney disease; ESRD: End-stage renal disease

Investigation

- Urine—volume, specific gravity-fixed 1.010
  - Osmolality 300 milliosmoles
  - Proteinuria—glomerular damage
  - Sediment—broad hyaline cast.
- Blood biochemistry:
  - Blood urea
  - Serum creatinine, serum Mg, serum Ca, serum Bicarb, serum PO_4
- USG abdomen: For size of kidney
  - Large kidney—PKD, hydronephrosis
  - Amyloidosis, multiple myeloma
- Small kidney:
  - Chronic glomerulonephritis—regular
  - Chronic pyelonephritis—irregular
- Normal sized kidney—diabetic nephropathy PGN.

Management

Principles of management in CRF
- Correct anemia
- Manage hypertension
- Manage osteodystrophy
- Fluid balance
- Electrolyte balance
- Acid base balance
- Infection control
- Removal of obstruction
- Avoid nephrotoxic drugs
- Nutrition

Conservative
- Treatment of uremic complications
  - Correction of fluid imbalance —↓ed fluid intake-edema, CCF, HTN
  - Correction of electrolyte imbalance
    ↓ed Na intake—CCF, edema, HTN
    ↑↑ed Na and fluid intake—polyuria, dehydration
  - Correction of metabolic acidosis
    Sodium bicarbonate 1 g tid or calcium carbonate 3 g/day
  - Diet—Adequate calorie 30 kcal/kg
    Protein 0.6 g/kg in severe uremia 20 g/day
  - Correction of anemia: Recombinant human erythropoietin 25–50 units/kg three times a week, maximum 6000 units/week-iron in Fe deficiency anemia
  - Renal osteodystrophy
    - Diet less in phosphorous
    - Aluminum hydroxide 300–600 g before meal to reduce phosphate absorption
    - Active vitamin D3-0.25–1 µg/day-Ca carbonate 500 tid
  - *Hypertension*:
    - Salt restriction
    - Diuretics
    - Beta blockers
    - CCB
    - Keep BP < 125/75 if proteinuria >1 g/24 hours
  - CHF
    - Diuretics
    - Inotropics
- Treatment of reversible renal factors:
  - UTI, other infections
  - Urinary obstruction
  - Correction of renal perfusion
  - Avoid nephrotoxins
  - Treat reversible renal disease like:
    - Analgesic nephropathy
    - Hypertensive nephropathy
    - Hypercalcemic nephropathy.

Renal replacement therapy (In end-stage renal disease)
- Dialysis-hemodialysis, peritoneal dialysis
- Renal transplantation
  - Cadaveric donor
  - Live donor.

Hemodialysis
- Blood access: AV fistula-Nondominant arm (for CRF)
- Double lumen cannula-in a central vein-femoral, internal jugular, subclavian
- Technique: Blood pumped from patient through a tubing to a dialyzer, a semipermeable membrane separates the patient's blood form a constantly replenished volume of dialysis solution (Dialysate)
- Solutes diffuse across the dialyzer membrane down the concentration gradient
- For example, urea diffuses from patient's blood (high concentration) across the membrane into the dialysis solution.

A standard dialysis solution contains:
- Potassium—2 mEq/L
- Acetate/bicarbonate—35/38 mEq/L
- Calcium—5–6 mg/mL
- Magnesium—1–1.5 mg/mL.

In addition to solutes, plasma water is removed during dialysis. This is called ultrafiltration. Thus by increasing the transmembrane pressure gradient, more plasma water can be removed, especially in situations of pulmonary edema. The risk of hypotension can be minimized by shutting off the flow of dialysate fluid.

This is called selective ultrafiltration.

Newer modalities are:
- SCUF—slow continuous ultrafiltration
- CAVH—continuous arteriovenous hemofiltration
- CVVH—continuous veno-venous hemofiltration
- CVVHD—continuous veno-venous hemodialysis
- CAVHD—continuous arteriovenous hemodialysis.

Peritoneal dialysis: Alternative to hemodialysis, in both acute and chromic renal failure, peritoneal dialysis can be done. Here the solute and water movement occurs across the peritoneal membrane. The dialysis fluid is infused into the peritoneal cavity through a catheter (40 mL/kg body wt.) and allowed to remain for a variable period and is then drained by gravity into a container, placed below the patient. New dialysate is run in after the drainage is complete.

Other forms of peritoneal dialysis:
- CAPD—continuous ambulatory peritoneal dialysis
- CCPD—continuous cyclic peritoneal dialysis
- NIPD—nocturnal intermittent peritoneal dialysis

Duration:
- 12 hours/week in CRF
- Even daily in acute renal failure

Renal transplantation: This offers the possibility of restoring normal kidney function and correcting all the metabolic abnormalities of CRF. The kidney graft is taken from a cadaver donor or from a relative. ABO (blood group) compatibility between donor and recipient is essential, and it is usual to select donor kidneys on the basis of human leukocyte antigen (HLA) matching as this improves the graft survival.

Immune-mediated graft rejection is the main cause of failure. Long term immunosuppressive therapy is required following kidney transplantation. Many therapeutic regimens have been used, but the most common involves a combination of prednisolone, azathioprine and cyclosporin A. The role of newer immunosuppressive agents such as tacrolimus (FK 506), *Mycophenolate mofetil* and rapamycin is currently being established by clinical trials.

COMMON ELECTROLYTE DISTURBANCES

Disorders of Potassium Homeostasis

Physiology

Distribution of Potassium (K)
- Total body K—3500 mEq
- Intracellular K—150-160 mEq/L
- Extracellular K—3.5-5 mEq/L
- Daily intake of K—80-100 mEq/day
- Normal urinary excretion—85% of dietary K
- Normal fecal excretion—10-15% of dietary K
- 45 mEq of K/kg body weight.

Regulation of K
- Internal mechanism at cellular level
  - Na-K ATPase pump—K into the cell
  - Insulin—K into the cell
  - β agonist—K into the cell
  - Aldosterone—K into the cell
  - Acidosis—K out of the cell
  - Alkalosis—K into the cell
  - ECF osmolality—K out of the cell
- External mechanism
  - Renal handling of K
  - Absorption of K by proximal nephron
  - About 85% excreted by distal nephron
  - Renal handling is regulated by
  - Distal tubular delivery of Na
    - Cellular K concentration
    - Blood pH
    - Aldosterone
    - Impermeant anions
    - Tubular flow rate
  - GI handling of K: 10-15% of dietary K is excreted by colon.

Hypokalemia (<3.5 mEq/L)

Causes
- Reduced intake
  - GI loss
  - Vomiting, diarrhea, intestinal obstruction-Ileus, fistulas, villous adenoma.
- Renal loss
  - Extra renal factors
    - Diuretics
    - Conn's syndrome
    - Cushing's syndrome
    - Metabolic alkalosis
    - Liddle's syndrome
    - Drugs
      - Amphotericin-B
      - Acetazolamide
      - Corticosteroid.
- Renal diseases
  - Recovery phase of ATN
  - Relief of obstructive uropathy
  - RTA (renal tubular acidosis)
- ECF to ICF shift of K
  - Hypokalemic periodic paralysis
  - Insulin therapy
  - Alkalosis
  - β agonist.

Clinical Features
- Features are due to skeletal muscle, heart, kidney and GI involvement
- Symptoms will manifest when K level < 2.5 mEq/L
- Neuroparalysis will develop when K level < 2 mEq/L
- Skeletal muscle
  - Hyporeflexic paralysis of limb and respiratory muscles
  - Rhabdomyolysis.
- GIT-Smooth muscle paralysis-Paralytic ileus
  - Heart-↑ excitability producing arrhythmia—PAT with block
  - Kidney
  - ADH insensitivity → diabetes Insipidus
  - Vacuolar nephropathy
    - Metabolic alkalosis, paresthesia.

Diagnosis
- Serum K <3.5 mEq/L
- Urinary K
  - <20-25 mEq/L → Extra renal loss of K
  - >20-25 mEq/L → Renal loss of K.
- ECG
  - When K+ <3 mEq/L
    - Flat T wave
    - Sagging of ST segment
    - Prominence of U wave
    - Prolongation of QT interval
  - When serum K <1 mEq/L: The pattern of prominent U wave combined with depressed ST segment and flattened T wave is known as Roller-Coaster effect.
- Assessment of acid base status.

Treatment of Hypokalemia
- Prevention of hypokalemia: K supplementation on diuretic therapy and corticosteroids-KCl 20-60 mEq as elixir or cap/day
  - Patients on parenteral nutrition-KCl 60-80 mEq/day
- *Correction of hypokalemia:*
  - Total deficit = Half of body weight in kg × (5−SK)
  - For IV therapy, the rate of infusion of KCl should not exceed 20 mEq/hour or 200 mEq/24 hours
  - Concentration of K in IV fluid should not be > 60-80 mEq/L

- For oral therapy, K gluconate or citrate is preferred to avoid gastrointestinal ulceration by KCl.
- *Indication for IV infusion of K:*
  - Diarrheal disease with hypokalemia
  - Hypokalemic paralysis
  - On treatment of diabetic ketoacidosis
  - Forced alkaline diuresis
- Treatment of cause of hypokalemia.

Hyperkalemia (More than 5 mEq/L)

Pathogenesis

Three important factors for development of hyperkalemia are:
- Tissue damage with release of K
- Rapid administration of K by mouth or IV
- Impaired renal excretion of K.

Etiology

- ↑ dietary intake
- *Shift of K from tissue:*
  - Tissue damage—hemolysis, rhabdomyolysis, crush injury, snake bite
  - Acidosis, insulin deficiency, β-adrenergic antagonist
  - Hyperkalemic periodic paralysis
  - Hyperosmolality of extracellular fluid.
- *Impaired renal excretion:*
  - Acute renal failure
  - End-stage renal disease
  - ↓ tubular excretion as in SLE, transplanted kidney, Gordon's syndrome
  - Drugs–K sparing diuretic, ACE inhibitors
- *Abnormalities of renin angiotensin aldosterone system:*
  - Addison's disease
  - Congenital adrenal hyperplasia
  - Primary hypoaldosteronism
- *Hyporeninemic hypoaldosteronism:* Diabetic nephropathy
  - Interstitial nephritis
- Pseudohyperkalemia—*In vitro* release of K from cells in thrombocytosis and leukocytosis
- Artifactual hyperkalemia: Hemolyzed sample and tight application of Tourniquet.

Clinical Features

- Due to alteration of cardiac excitability
- *ECG changes and SK level:*
  - Peaked T-wave: SK+ is 6.5–7 mEq
  - PR↑ and absence of P wave-SK 8 mEq
  - Wide QRS complex: SK 10 mEq
  - Sine wave: SK 11 mEq
  - VF and cardiac arrest: SK 12 mEq
- Flaccid areflexic paralysis of limb muscles
- Acroparesthesia
- Diagnosis by SK estimation and characteristic ECG changes

- Treatment of hyperkalemia
  - Mild hyperkalemia
  - < 6 mEq/L + peaking of T-wave
  - Moderate hyperkalemia: 6–8 mEq/L + peaking of T-wave
  - Severe hyperkalemia: >8 mEq/L + absent P wave, wide QRS, sine wave
  - *Elimination of causes:* Avoid K sparing diuretic, correction of acidosis and hyperosmolality of blood.

Principles of Management

- Reversal of membrane abnormalities
- Redistribution into the intracellular space
- External removal of potassium.

Measures to Antagonize the Physiological Effects of Hyperkalemia

1. *Membrane effect*
   - IV Calcium gluconate 10 mL slowly in 2–5 minutes
   - Immediate onset of action with duration of action of 30 minutes.
2. *Intracellular shift of K^+*
   - IV glucose and insulin—50% glucose, 50 mL IV with 10 units insulin twice daily, action starts within 15–30 minutes and lasts for 2–6 hours
   - $NaHCO_3$ 50 mL IV—action starts within 15–30 minutes and continue for 2–6 hours
   - Salbutamol nebulization-action in 15–30 minutes and duration for 2–6 hours
3. Measures to removal of excess K
   - Cation exchange resins—resin absorb K, given orally or as retention enema — sodium polystyrene sulfonate
   - 70% sorbitol, 25 g in 20 mL TID or QID
   - 100 mL of 35% sorbitol for enema
   - Diuretics—frusemide
   - Hemodialysis/peritoneal dialysis in patients with hyperkalemia and renal failure.

HYPONATREMIC DISORDERS

Physiology of Sodium

- Sodium (Na) intake—8–12 g/day (150–160 mEq)
- Daily requirement 100 mEq/day
- Urinary excretion 20 mEq < the intake (20–1200 mEq/L)
- Salt restricted diet—< 5g/day (70–80 mEq)
- Salt free diet <2 g/day (20–30 mEq).

Distribution of Sodium

- ECF—135–145 mEq/L
- ICF—14 mEq/L
- 58 mEq of Na/Kg body weight—70% exchangeable
- Hypernatremia → >150 meq/L
- Symptoms of hyponatremia → < 25 mEq/L
- Encephalopathy → < 15 mEq/L
- Seizure and coma → <100 mEq/L
- Hyponatremia (135 mEq/L).

Hyponatremia (<135 mEq/L)

Mechanism

- Na loss
- Water excess
- Na sequestration
- Internal dilution—SIADH.

Etiology

- Gastrointestinal loss: Vomiting, diarrhea, nasogastric aspiration, GI fistula
- Renal loss:
  - Recovery of ATN—Polyuric phase
  - Relief of obstructive uropathy
  - Tubulointerstitial renal disease
  - Diuretics.
- Endocrine: Addison's disease, diabetic ketoacidosis, congenital adrenal hyperplasia
  - Na sequestration—intestinal obstruction, Ileus, ascites
  - Skin loss—excessive sweating, scalded skin.

Clinical Types

- With overhydration—CHF, cirrhosis liver, nephrotic syndrome
- With dehydration—GI loss, DKA, Addison's disease, renal loss
- With euhydration—SIADH
- Pseudohyponatremia—hyperlipidemia, paraproteinemia and hyperglycemia
- Essential hyponatremia—sickle cell syndrome
  - Shift of Na into the cells.

Clinical Features

- ECF loss—dry tongue, dry skin, ↓skin turgor, muscle cramps (2 liter)
- IVF loss—tachycardia, orthostatic hypotension, oliguria, syncope (2-4 liter)
- ICF loss—encephalopathy, seizure and coma (> 4 liter).

Correction of Hyponatremia

- **Depletional hyponatremia**
  - Acute diarrheal disease
  - Diabetic ketoacidosis
  - Severe Addison's
  - Requisites
    - Body weight and serum sodium
    - About 60% body weight is body fluid
      - 40% ICF
      - 15% ECF
      - 5% IVF
  - For example:
    - Patient with 60 kg body weight, having Serum Na 120 mEq/L
    - About 60% of body weight—36 liters
    - Correction is done to 140 mEq/L
    - Deficit is 20 mEq/L
    - Total deficit is 36 × 20 = 720 mEq½ of the correction is done in 24 hours = 360 mEq.
  - Mode of administration of Na
    - With hypotension—parenteral
    - With normal BP—oral
  - Normal saline: 6 mL = 1 mEq of Na
  - 1.4% $NaHCO_3$: 6 mL = 1 mEq
  - 5% hypertonic saline: 1 mL = 1 mEq
    - 6 mL/kg, not >100 mL/hr
  - 3% saline: 1 liter = 513 mEq
  - 1 mEq = 2 mL of 3% saline
  - 1 g salt = 17 mEq of Na
  - 1 table spoon salt-5 g = 85 mEq
    In depletional hyponatremia, body will accept rapid and near correction, unlike in euhydrated hyponatremia.
- **Euhydrated hyponatremia—SIADH**
  - Principles of correction:
    - Slow correction
    - Subnormal correction to 125-130 mEq
    - Rate of infusion 1.5-2 mEq/L/Hr
    - Maximum correction-not >12 meq/L/24 hrs or up to 125 mEq (whichever is less)
    - 3% saline is used usually—1 liter = 513 mEq/L
    - 1 mEq = 2 mL.

  For example: Patient with 50 kg body weight and serum Na 115 mEq/L
    - Body fluid is 30 L
    - Correction is done to 125 mEq/L
    - Total deficit = 10 mEq/L (125-115) × 30 L = 300 mEq of infusion 1.5 mEq/L/hour = 30 × 1.5 = 45 mEq/hr = 90 mL of 3% saline/hr and 600 mL of 3% saline in 6.67 hours.
  - *Complication:* Rapid and full correction will lead on to osmotic demyelination of nervous system like pontine and nonpontine demyelination
    - 0.5 mEq/hr → 30 mL/hr → 8 drops/min
    - 1 mEq/hr → 60 mL/hr → 16 drops/min
- **Hyponatremia in over hydrated**
  - In CHF, cirrhosis and nephrotic syndrome
  - Principles of correction
    - Fluid restriction to 1L/24 hr
    - Promote diuresis by furosemide 0.5-1 mg/kg body weight
    - Replacement of Na and K
    - Treatment of primary disease.

Hypernatremia

Sodium > 150 mEq/L.

Correction of Hypernatremia

To calculate the replacement:

- [(Serum Sodium-140)/140] *30 in liters is the replacement needed. It should be given as 5% dextrose or plain water.
- Normal correction in 24 hour period.

If replacement volume is more than 3 liters, correct in 2 days time (24-48 hours).

CHAPTER 10

Examination of Hemopoietic System

SYMPTOMATOLOGY

- **Anemia**
  - Central cause—bone marrow failure, nutritional
  - Peripheral cause—hemolysis, hemorrhagic
  - Multifactorial—anemia of chronic disease.
- **Jaundice**—hemolysis
- **Bleeding**
  - Site
    - Cutaneous—petechiae, purpura, ecchymosis
    - Mucous membrane—oral mucosa, nasal mucosa and gum
    - Deep plane bleed—muscle, joint.
  - Systemic
    - Gastrointestinal tract—hematemesis, melena
    - Respiratory system—epistaxis, hemoptysis
    - Genitourinary—hematuria, bleeding per vaginum.
  - Platelet disorder—cutaneous and mucous membrane bleed
  - Coagulation disorder—deep plane bleed-hemarthrosis
- **Lymphadenopathy**
  - Localized—Hodgkin's lymphoma
  - Generalized
    - Lymphatic
    - Leukemia
    - Non-Hodgkin's lymphoma (NHL)
    - Miliary tuberculosis
- **Fever**
  - Hematological malignancy—leukemia, lymphoma
  - Infection—malaria, bartonellosis
  - Aplastic anemia with neutropenia
  - Immunocompromized hematological malignancy
  - Intravenous (IV) hemolysis.
- **Bone and joint pain**
  - Acute leukemia
    - Subperiosteal infiltration
    - Widening of marrow diploe
    - Articular and periarticular infiltration
    - Nutrient artery occlusion.
  - Myeloma—osteolysis
  - Osteoporosis.
- **Skin**
  - Pruritus—lymphoma, chronic lymphoblastic leukemia (CLL), chronic renal failure (CRF)
  - Warm urticaria—polycythemia vera (warm water bath-pruritus)
  - Bleeding
  - Pigmentation—megaloblastic anemia, lymphoma
- **Hair**
  - Premature graying—megaloblastic anemia
  - Alopecia—cyclophosphamide therapy
- **Leg ulcers**
  - Sickle cell anemia
  - Paraproteinemia
  - Thrombocytosis
  - Thrombotic thrombocytopenic purpura (TTP)
- **Edema**
  - Venous thrombosis
    - Thrombophilic state
    - Antiphospholipid (APL) syndrome
    - Paroxysmal nocturnal hemoglobinuria (PNH)
  - Anemia with congestive heart failure (CHF)
- **Gastrointestinal (GI) symptoms**
  - Bleeding—hematemesis, melena
  - Symptoms of malabsorption
  - Symptoms of GI malignancy
  - Symptoms of inflammatory bowel disease (IBD)
- **Cardiovascular symptoms**
  - palpitation, dyspnea—anemia
  - Angina—anemia, polycythemia
  - Anemia—infective endocarditis (IE)
- **Central nervous system (CNS) symptoms**
  - Paresthesia, ataxia—B_{12} neuropathy
  - Headache—increased intracranial pressure (ICP), neuroleukemia

- Focal neurological deficit—neuroleukemia, myeloma
- Bleeding diathesis
- **Genitourinary symptoms**
  - CRF—anemia
  - Polycystic kidney—polycythemia
- **Respiratory symptoms**
  - Chronic obstructive pulmonary disease (COPD)/Interstitial lung disease (ILD)—secondary polycythemia
  - Pulmonary TB—anemia
- **Endocrine symptoms**—hypothyroidism, hypopituitarism—anemia.

HISTORY TAKING

- Presenting symptoms
  - Anemia, jaundice, bleeding, fever, organomegaly, bone and joint pain
- History of presenting complaints
  - Detailing the symptom
- Past history
  - GI surgery
  - Excessive bleeding after surgical procedure
  - History of chronic systemic disease.
- Treatment history
  - Anticonvulsant
    - Diphenylhydantoin (DPH)
    - Folate-deficiency.
  - Bone marrow suppression
    - Antibiotics
    - Antimalignants
    - Immune suppressants
    - Antithyroid.
  - Hemolysis
    - G6PD deficiency
    - Primaquine
    - Dapsone.
  - GI bleed— nonsteroidal anti-inflammatory drugs (NSAIDs), aspirin
- Personal history
  - Vegetarian diet—B_{12} deficiency
  - Poor nutrition—deficiency anemia, poor hygiene—helminthic infestation.
- Social history
  - Racial origin—thalassemia, sickle cell anemia
- Family history
  - Hereditary hematological disorders
  - Hemophilia and Christmas disease—X-linked recessive
  - G6PD deficiency—X-linked recessive
  - Hemoglobinopathies—autosomal dominant
  - Von Willebrand's disease—autosomal dominant.

EXAMINATION OF HEMOPOIETIC SYSTEM

General

- Leg and buttock purpura—Henoch-Schonlein (HS) purpura (Fig. 10.1)
- Anemia (refer General Examination)
- Jaundice (refer General Examination)
- Bleeding—cutaneous—Petechiae (Fig. 10.2), purpura (Fig. 10.3), ecchymosis (Fig. 10.4).
- Palpable purpura—Henoch-Schonlein (HS)
- Purpura, paraproteinemia, vasculitis
- Mucous membrane—bleeding gum and oral mucosa
- Lymphadenopathy
  - Localized—Hodgkin's lymphoma
  - Generalized
    - Lymphatic leukemia
    - NHL
    - Miliary tuberculosis (TB)

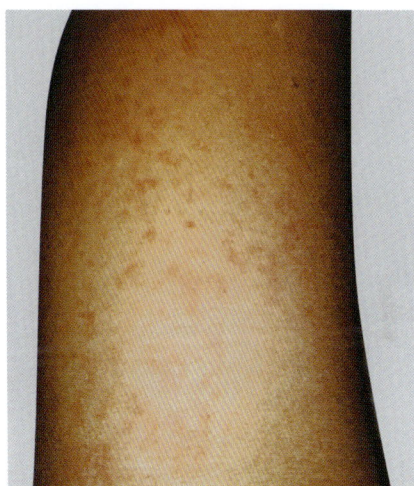

Fig. 10.1: Leg purpura in Henoch-Schonlein purpura.

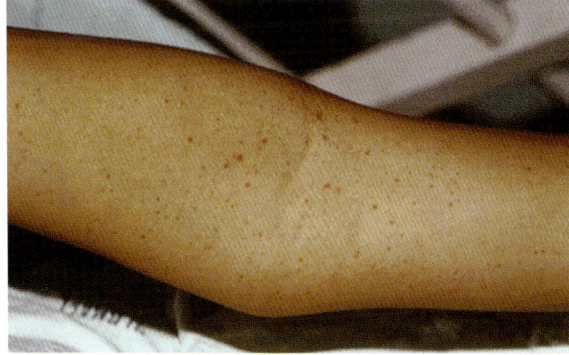

Fig. 10.2: Dengue fever-Positive 'Hess test' showing Petechiae developing distal to the site of an inflated sphygmomanometer cuff.

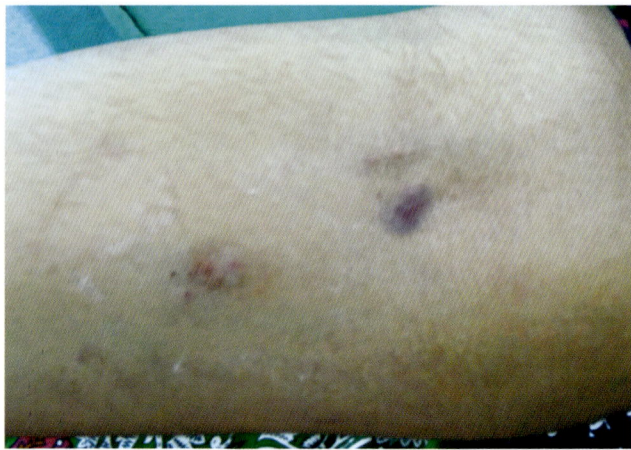

Fig. 10.3: Purpura forearm—Glanzmann's thrombasthenia.

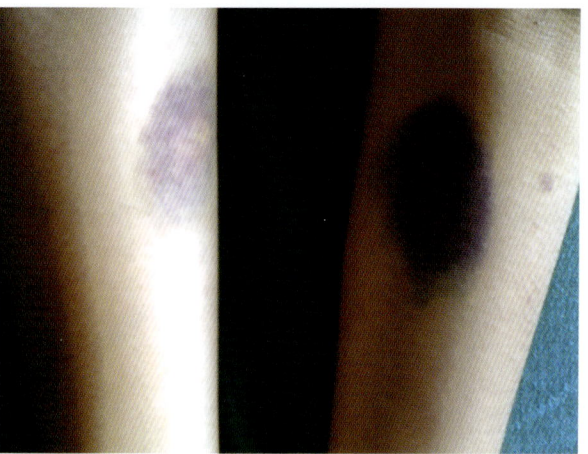

Fig. 10.4: Ecchymosis in a patient with bleeding diathesis.

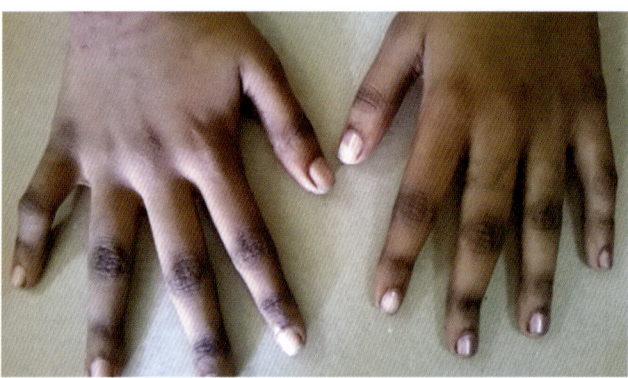

Fig. 10.5: Knuckle pigmentation—megaloblastic anemia.

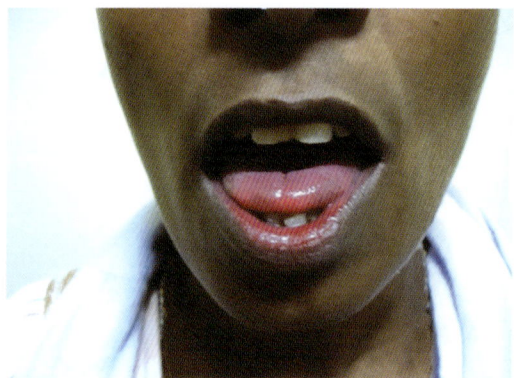

Fig. 10.6: Redness of the lips and tongue due to polycythemia.

- Nail
  - Koilonychia—Fe deficiency anemia
  - Clubbing and splinter hemorrhage—infective endocarditis
- Skin
  - Cutaneous bleed, pallor, jaundice, pruritus, warm urticaria
  - Pigmentation—megaloblastic anemia (Fig. 10.5), lymphoma
  - Plethora—polycythemia vera (Fig. 10.6)
  - Busulfan therapy.
- Cyanosis
  - Secondary polycythemia—COPD, ILD, cyanotic congenital heart disease
  - Primary polycythemia.
- Eye
  - Pallor, jaundice, cyanosis, conjunctival congestion → Polycythemia
  - Subconjunctival hemorrhage→bleeding diathesis and acute leukemia
  - Proptosis→chloroma—tumor of leukemic cells in acute myeloid leukemia (AML)
  - Optic fundi
    - Hemorrhage
      - Bleeding diathesis
      - Acute leukemia
      - Megaloblastic anemia
      - Infective endocarditis.
    - Engorged retinal vein
      - Hyperviscosity
      - Paraproteinemia
      - Polycythemia vera
    - Sausage shaped retinal vein
      - Waldenstrom's macroglobulinemia
    - Papill edema—hyperviscosity
- Digital gangrene
  - Sickle cell anemia
  - Polycythemia vera
  - Essential thrombocytosis.

- Bone tenderness—acute leukemia, multiple myeloma
- Arthritis—HS purpura, hemarthrosis and acute leukemia
- Fever—malaria, Bartonellosis, infective endocarditis, hematological malignancies
- Leg ulcers—sickle cell anemia, paraproteinemia, TTP, thrombocytosis.

Systemic Examination

Gastrointestinal Tract

- **Mouth**
  - Gum hypertrophy—acute monocytic leukemia
  - Bleeding gum–bleeding diathesis, acute leukemia
  - Ulcers—acute leukemia, aplastic anemia, immunosuppressants
  - Mucositis—methotrexate therapy
  - Glossitis—Fe deficiency anemia, B_{12} and B_2 deficiency
  - Oral and palatal mucosa—pallor, jaundice, purpura
  - Throat—Waldeyer's ring—enlarged in NHL
  - Dysphagia
  - Fe-deficiency anemia—Plummer-Vinson syndrome
  - Ca esophagus → anemia
  - Peptic esophagitis—bleeding → anemia.
- **Abdomen**
  - **Splenomegaly**
    - Mild
      - Chronic iron deficiency anemia
      - Megaloblastic anemia
      - Myeloma
      - Polycythemia vera
      - Infective endocarditis.
    - Moderate
      - Hemolytic anemia
      - Leukemia
      - Lymphoma
      - Osteopetrosis.
    - Massive
      - Chronic myeloid leukemia
      - Myelofibrosis
      - Chronic malaria
      - Kala-azar.
    - Absence of splenomegaly
      - Aplastic anemia
      - Sickle cell anemia
      - Idiopathic thrombocytopenic purpura (ITP).
- **Hepatomegaly**
  - Fatty infiltration in chronic anemia
  - Tender hepatomegaly—anemia and CHF
  - Extramedullary hemopoeisis
    - Hemolytic anemia
    - Myelofibrosis
    - Osteopetrosis
    - Leukemia and lymphoma
    - Hepatic fibrosis in methotrexate therapy.

- **Lymph node mass**
  - Lymphoma
  - Lymphatic leukemia
    - Testis—enlarged in ALL
    - Pancreatitis—L-asparaginase therapy
    - Rectal examination for—hemorrhoids, ulcer, malignancy.

Cardiovascular System

- Pulse—sinus tachycardia, high volume collapsing—anemia
- Jugular venous pressure (JVP)—increases due to increased blood volume in anemia, CHF in anemia
- Nonpulsatile jugular—superior mediastinal obstruction in mediastinal adenopathy—leukemia, lymphoma
- Cardiomegaly, hemic murmur—anemia
- Venous hum—anemia
- Myocarditis—Daunorubicin therapy
- Hypertension, anemia—CRF polycythemia—polycystic kidney disease
- Gaisbock's syndrome (polycythemia and hypertension)
- Venous and arterial thrombosis—polycythemia vera, thrombocytosis.

Respiratory System

- Pulmonary TB—anemia
- COPD, ILD—secondary polycythemia
- Hemoptysis—bleeding diathesis
- Pulmonary fibrosis—methotrexate therapy, busulfan.

Nervous System

- Peripheral neuropathy—B_{12} deficiency, vincristine therapy
- Subacute combined degeneration—B_{12} deficiency
- Reversible dementia—B_{12} deficiency
- Bilateral lower motor neuron (LMN) facial palsy—ALL
- Focal neurological deficit—bleeding diathesis, myeloma, neuroleukemia
- Signs of meningeal irritation—neuroleukemia
- Papilledema—hyperviscosity - Paraproteinemia
- Herpes zoster infection—immunocompromized—Leukemia, immunosuppressants.

Genitourinary System

- CRF—anemia and bleeding
- Polycystic kidney disease (PKD)—polycythemia
- HS purpura—hematuria, glomerulonephritis and CRF
- Glomerulonephritis, purpura-vasculitis-Wegener's granulomatosis, Churg-Strauss syndrome, microscopic polyangitis
- Hematuria—bleeding diathesis.

Locomotor System

- Rheumatoid arthritis—anemia
- HS purpura

- Bone pain, polyarthritis—acute leukemia
- Hemarthrosis, ankylosis of joint—hemophilia
- Secondary gout—myeloproliferative disorders.

COMMON DISORDERS OF HEMOPOIETIC SYSTEM

ANEMIA

Definition: Male—Hb <13 g%, PCV <42, RBC count <4.5 million/mm^3
Female—Hb <12 g%, PCV < 36, RBC count <4 million/mm^3.

Morphological Classification

- Microcytic (Fig. 10.7)—iron-deficiency anemia, thalassemia, sideroblastic anemia
- Normocytic—aplastic anemia, CRF, anemia of chronic disease, posthemorrhagic anemia.
- Macrocytic—
  - Megaloblastic—B$_{12}$ and folate deficiency
  - Nonmegaloblastic—hypothyroidism, chronic liver disease, posthemorrhagic anemia, posthemolytic anemia.

Etiological Classification

- Hypoproliferative
  - Hypoplastic anemia
  - Myelophthisic anemia
  - Dyshemopoetic –maturation disorder
    - Cytoplasmic defect
      - Iron deficiency
      - Thalassemia
      - Sideroblastic.
- Nuclear defect
  - B$_{12}$ and folate deficiency
- Hyperproliferative
  - Posthemorrhagic anemia
  - Hemolytic anemia.

Iron-Deficiency Anemia

It is characterized by microcytic hypochromic anemia with low plasma iron, ferritin and decreased saturation of transferrin (Table 10.1).

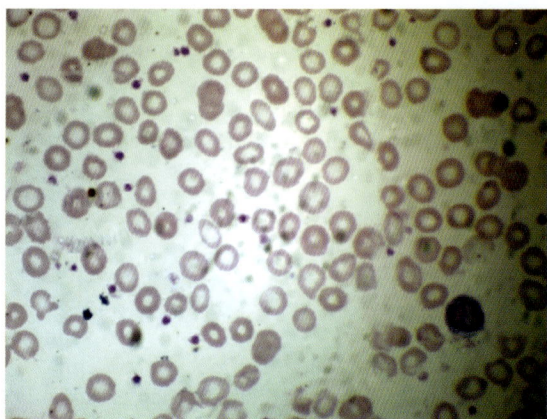

Fig. 10.7: Microcytic hypochromic anemia.

- Incidence—3% men, 20% women
- Ferrokinetics
  - Usual diet contains 10–20 mg of iron
  - Daily requirement—
    - Male—5–10 mg/day
    - Female—15 mg/day
    - Pregnancy 20 mg/day
- Children 0.5 mg/kg/day
- Absorption of iron—1 mg/day
- S. iron—75–150 mg%
- Whole blood 1 mL contains 0.4 mg
- Distribution of body iron
  - Total—4.5 g
  - Hemoglobin—2.5 g (70%)
    - Storage iron—1.5 g (20%)
  - Myoglobin—5%
  - Enzymes—5% (cytochrome, peroxidase, catalase)
  - Excretion—1 mg/day.

Etiology of Fe Deficiency Anemia

- Decreased uptake—malnutrition
- Decreased absorption—achlorhydria, upper GI surgery, celiac disease
- Increased blood loss—GI loss—ulcer, hemorrhoids, varices, neoplasm hookworm, polyp, diverticula and IBD menorrhagia
  - Bleeding diathesis
- Increased requirement—infants, adolescent and pregnancy.

Table 10.1: Characteristic features of iron deficiency anemia.

Stages	Normal	Negative Fe balance	Fe deficiency hemopoiesis	Microcytic-hypochromic anemia
Storage Fe (marrow)	Normal (1–3+)	Decreased (0–1+)	Decreased 0	Decreased 0
S. ferritin (mg/L)	50–200	<20	<15	<15
S. iron (mg/dL)	75–150	75–150	<50	<30
TIBC (mg/dL)	300–360	300–360	>380	>400
RBC	Normal	Normal	Normal	Microcytic hypochromic

Clinical Features

- Gradual onset of anemia, pallor, palpitation, dyspnea and dizziness
- Glossitis, angular stomatitis, koilonychia, dysphagia (Plummer-Vinson syndrome), pica, anorexia, splenomegaly in 10%, chlorosis–greenish hue complexion, atrophic rhinitis with foul nasal discharge (ozena)
- Features of diseases → Iron deficiency

Differential Diagnosis

Thalassemia, sideroblastic anemia, copper deficiency.

Investigations

- Hb low, RBC—hypochromic microcytic, anisocytosis, poikilocytosis
- Mean corpuscular hemoglobin (MCH), mean corpuscular volume (MCV), and mean corpuscular hemoglobin concentration (MCHC) are decreased
- S. iron and S. ferritin are decreased
- Bone marrow—erythroid hyperplasia and decreased stainable iron
- Investigations for diseases → iron deficiency
  - Motion occult blood
  - GI endoscopy
  - Chromium-labeled red blood cell (RBC)—to detect mild GI blood loss
  - Celiac disease
    - S. antigliadin, antiendomysium antibody
    - Duodenal biopsy.
- Stages of iron deficiency anemia
  - Stage of negative iron balance
  - Stage of iron deficiency hemopoiesis
  - Stage of microcytic hypochromic anemia.

Management

- Principles—correction of anemia
- Replacement of Fe stores
- Elimination of cause.

- **Foods containing iron**
  - >5 mg Fe/100 g of food
    - Liver, egg yolk, dried fruits, wheat germ
  - 1–5 mg Fe/100 g of food
    - Meat, fish, cereals, green leafy vegetables
  - < 1 mg Fe/100 g of food
    - Milk, nonleafy vegetables
- **Oral iron therapy**
  - Ferrous sulfate—300 mg—elemental iron 80 mg
  - Ferrous gluconate—300 mg—elemental iron 40 mg
  - Ferrous fumarate—200 mg—elemental iron 60 mg
  - Ferrous succinate—150 mg—elemental Fe 35 mg
  - 200 mg elemental Fe/day for 6–12 months
  - Rise in Hb 1 g/7–10 days.
- **Parenteral iron therapy**
  - Indications
    - Intolerance to oral iron
    - GI abnormality and malabsorption
    - Pregnancy.
  - Drugs
    - Iron dextran complex
    - Iron sorbitol complex
  - Dose—1.5 mg/kg IM/day
  - Complications of parenteral iron therapy: Fever, tissue necrosis, arthralgia Anaphylaxis, encephalopathy
- **Blood transfusion**—Anemia with CHF (packed cell)
- **Good response of iron therapy**—rise in reticulocyte count after 5 days of therapy
- **Failure of response**
  - Incorrect diagnosis, more blood loss
  - Marrow failure with decreased erythropoiesis.

Megaloblastic Anemia

- Anemia due to impaired DNA synthesis
- Cells affected are hemopoietic cells and GI epithelium and neurons.

Classification

- **Vitamin B_{12} deficiency:**
  - Decreased intake
    - Vegetarians
    - Malabsorption
  - Decreased intrinsic factor production
    - Pernicious anemia
    - Gastrectomy
    - Congenital absence—Juvenile pernicious anemia
  - Distal ileopathy
    - Tropical sprue
    - Regional ileitis—Crohn's, TB
    - Intestinal resection
    - Selective malabsorption of B_{12} (Imerslunds syndrome)
    - Back wash ileitis—ulcerative colitis.
  - Competition for vitamin B_{12} absorption
    - Fish tape worm
    - Blind loop syndrome (bacterial overgrowth)
    - Drugs: Neomycin, PAS, metformin.
- **Folic acid deficiency:**
  - Decreased intake
    - Alcoholic and infants
  - Increased requirement
    - Infancy, pregnancy, hemolytic anemia, malignancy
  - Malabsorption
    - Tropical sprue
    - Nontropical sprue
    - Drugs—phenytoin, barbiturate

- Impaired metabolism
    - Inhibiting dihydrofolate reductase
        - Methotrexate
        - Pyrimethamine
        - Triamterene
    - Alcohol
    - Deficiency of dihydrofolate reductase
- **Other causes**: Megaloblastic anemia unresponsive to B_{12} and folic acid
    - Drugs impairing DNA synthesis
        - Purine antagonist—6MP
        - Pyrimidine antagonist cytosine arabinoside 5 FU
    - Metabolic
        - Hereditary orotic aciduria (uridine 5 monophosphate synthetase deficiency)
        - Lesch-Nyhan syndrome (HGPRTase deficiency)
    - Megaloblastic anemia of unknown etiology
        - Congenital dyserythropoietic anemia.

Metabolism of B12 and Folic Acid

B_{12}
- Animal source only
- Daily requirement is 2.5 µg/day
- Absorption at terminal ileum
- Storage 2 mg in liver and 2 mg in other tissues.

Folic acid
- Source—fruits, vegetables
- Daily requirement—50 µg/day
- Absorption at proximal jejunum
- Storage—5–20 mg (half in liver).

Metabolic Pathways

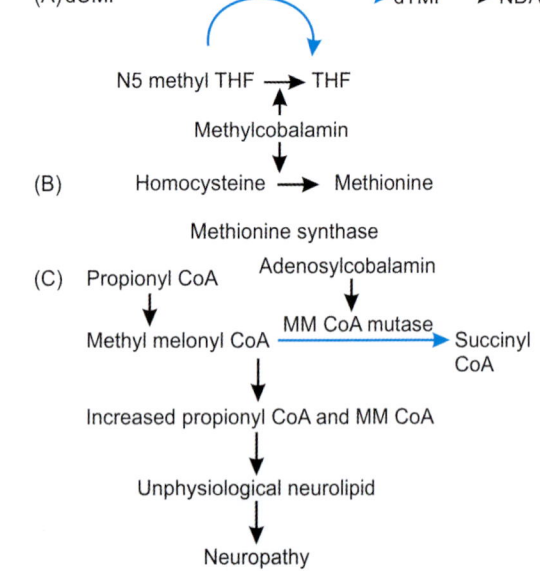

Abbreviations: dUMP: deoxyUridylate monophosphate; dTMP: deoxythymidylate monophosphate; CoA: coenzyme A

Clinical Features

Confined to hemopoietic system, nervous system and GIT.
- Anemia, thrombocytopenia, pancytopenia
- Mild hepatosplenomegaly
- Pigmentation of palm, sole and face—B_{12} deficiency
- Premature graying of hair—B_{12} deficiency
- Mild jaundice
- GIT—glossitis, beefy red tongue, diarrhea
- Pernicious anemia.
- Age: 60 years, not <30 years, intrinsic factor secretion reduced.
    - Autoimmune disease-antiparietal cell antibody—90%
    - Anti-intrinsic factor antibody 60%
    - Gastric atrophy and achlorhydria
    - Juvenile pernicious anemia—congenital intrinsic factor deficiency.

Investigations

- White blood cell (WBC): Leukopenia, hypersegmented neutrophil (macropolycyte) (Fig. 10.8)
- Red blood cell (RBC): Macrocytic, anisopoikilocytosis, macroovalocyte (Fig. 10.9)
- Platelet thrombocytopenia
- Decreased reticulocyte count, decreased Hb
- Bone marrow: Hypercellular, RBC precursors are large
- Megaloblastic erythropoiesis, nuclear cytoplasmic asynchrony.
- Serum lactate dehydrogenase (SLDH) isoenzyme ↑, S bilirubin ↑ (unconjugated)
- S B_{12}: Normal 200–900 pg/mL, <100 pg/mL → deficiency
- S. folate: 6–20 ng/mL; <4 ng/mL → deficiency
- RBC folate estimation
- Antibody to intrinsic factor and parietal cells
- Schilling test: To detect the cause of B→ deficiency: 1 mg (0.5 micro curie) of cobalt-labeled B_{12} orally, 2 hours later

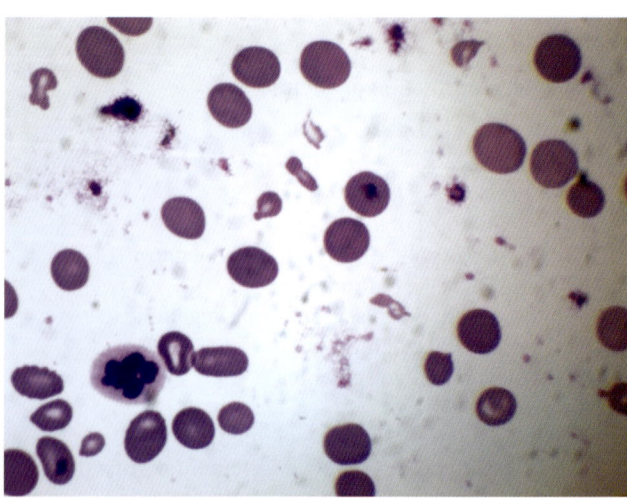

Fig. 10.8: Hypersegmented neutrophil.

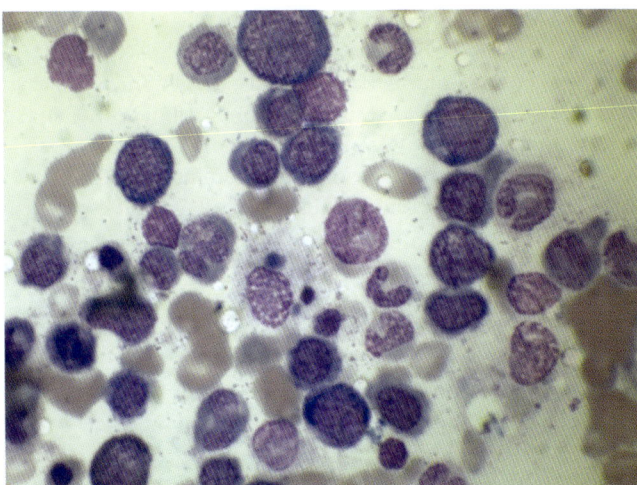

Fig. 10.9: Bone marrow showing megaloblastic erythropoiesis.

1,000 µg of B_{12} IM, urinary excretion of labeled B_{12} for next 24 hours is estimated. Normal is >15%, <8% if absorption is poor, this test can be repeated with IF and after a course of antibiotics to identify the defect.

Treatment

B_{12} deficiency
- Replacement therapy
  - 1000 mg IM twice weekly for 1 week
  - 1,000 mg IM weekly till normal blood count
- Maintenance therapy
  - 1,000 mg IM once in three months: for hematological manifestation
  - 1,000 mg IM once in a month for neurological manifestation.

  Response of treatment: Within 48 hours change in marrow morphology, reticulocyte count peak → 5–10th day Hb rise 1 g/week

Folate Deficiency
- Replacement therapy 5 mg/day for three weeks orally
- Maintenance therapy 5 mg/week.

Prevention
0.5 mg folic acid/day during pregnancy and for children.

Megaloblastic Anemia Unresponsive to B_{12} and Folate
- Enzyme dihydrofolate reductase deficiency
- Transcobalamine II deficiency
- Metabolic diseases:
  - Lesch-Nyhan syndrome
  - Hereditary orotic aciduria.
- Congenital dyserythropoietic anemia

- Manifestation of other hematological disorders
  - Megaloblastic crisis of hemolytic anemia
  - Acute myeloid leukemia –M6 (Di Guglielmo syndrome)
  - Myelodysplastic syndrome.
- Drugs
  - 6-mercaptopurine
  - 5-fluorouracil.

Aplastic Anemia

It is characterized by hypocellular bone marrow with pancytopenia.

Incidence: 1–2% of all anemia.

Etiology
- Primary: 75%
  - Idiopathic
  - Congenital (Fanconis' anemia).
- Secondary: 25%
  - Drugs and physical agents chloramphenicol, antimalignant drugs radiation, benzene
  - Hepatitis B virus (HBV), SLE, thymoma
  - Paroxysmal nocturnal hemoglobinuria
  - Immune mediated-cellular autoimmune process.

Clinical Features
- Insidious onset, progressive fatigue and anemia
- Bleeding diathesis, neutropenia and infection
- Lymphadenopathy and splenomegaly notably absent.

Investigations
- Blood count: Pancytopenia
- Peripheral smear: Normocytic-normochromic anemia
- Reticulocyte count: <1%
- Bone marrow: Dry tap
- Biopsy: Hypocellular bone marrow, marked depression of megakaryocytes myeloid cells and erythroid precursors.
- Severe aplastic anemia
  - Granulocyte <500/mm^3
  - Platelet<20,000/mm^3
  - Reticulocyte count <1%.

Differential Diagnosis of Pancytopenia Other than Aplastic Anemia
- Myelophthisic anemia
- Leukemia, lymphoma, myeloma myelofibrosis, miliary TB
- Hansen's disease (lepromatous).

Pancytopenia with Hypercellular Bone Marrow
- Hypersplenism, MDS, megaloblastic anemia
- Paroxysmal nocturnal hemoglobinuria
- Infections—kala-azar, TB, brucellosis.

Treatment

- Avoid offending drugs and chemicals
- General measures
  - Avoid IM injection, drugs like aspirin
- Prevent infection
- Supportive measures:
  - Packed cells in anemia
  - Platelet transfusion: Thrombocytopenia <20,000 or bleeding
  - Granulocyte transfusion
    - Granulocytopenia ± infection
  - Hemopoietic growth factor
    - Granulocyte-monocyte colony-stimulating factor (GM-CSF)
    - Granulocyte colony-stimulating factor (G – CSF)
- Marrow stimulants:
  - Lithium, methyl prednisolone, androgen
- Bone marrow transplant:
  - Allogeneic bone marrow—in young patient
- Treatment of underlying cause in secondary aplastic anemia
- Immunosuppressive therapy with cyclosporine and anti-thymocyte globulin in older patients.

Hemolytic Anemia

Two types of hemolysis are as follows:
1. Intravascular:
   - Exogenous toxin
   - Complement fixation
   - Trauma to RBC
2. Extravascular: By mononuclear macrophage system of spleen and liver.

Pathogenesis

Excessive destruction of RBC → increased catabolism of Hb → unconjugated hyperbilirubinemia and increased urobilinogen in urine.

Bone marrow stimulation → erythroid hyperplasia, normoblastosis, reticulocytosis.

Etiology

1. Inherited disorders
   - RBC membrane defect—spherocytosis, elliptocytosis, acanthocytosis
   - Intracorpuscular defect
     - Enzymopathy—G6PD deficiency, pyruvate kinase deficiency
     - Hemoglobinopathy.
   - Sickle cell anemia
   - Thalassemia
2. Acquired disorders
   - Immune hemolysis
     - Autoimmune hemolytic anemia (cold and warm Ab)
     - Mismatched transfusion
     - Hemolytic disease of newborn
   - Infection: Malaria, Bartonellosis, *Cl. welchii*
   - Drugs and toxins- Sulfa, dapsone, primaquine, snake venom
   - Microangiopathic: Hemolytic anemia
     - Hemolytic uremic syndrome
     - Thrombotic thrombocytopenic purpura.
   - Mechanical causes
     - Prosthetic valve
     - March hemoglobinuria.
   - Hypersplenism
   - Paroxysmal nocturnal hemoglobinuria: Acquired red cell membrane defect.

Clinical Features

Clinical triad—anemia, jaundice, splenomegaly.

Facies
- Parietal and frontal bossing
- Malar bone overgrowth
- Depressed nasal bridge
- Chip munk facies
- Cholelithiasis—pigment stone
- Chronic leg ulcers—sickle cell anemia
- Hyperpigmentation—hemosiderosis.

Crisis
- Aplastic crisis
- Megaloblastic crisis
- Hemolytic crisis
- Sequestration crisis.

Investigations

Biochemical triad—unconjugated hyperbilirubinemia, increased urobilinogen and reticulocytosis.
1. Evidence of increased hemolysis
   - Unconjugated hyperbilirubinemia
   - Increased urobilinogen, hemosiderin in urine
   - Increased serum haptoglobin
   - Increased serum LDH
2. Evidence of increased BM activity
   - Erythroid hyperplasia
   - Reticulocytosis
   - Normoblastosis
3. Tests for etiological diagnosis
   - Peripheral smear—spherocytosis, stomatocytosis
   - Fragility test—spherocytosis
   - Autohemolysis—spherocytosis
   - Sickling phenomenon—sickle cell anemia
   - Hemoglobin electrophoresis—hemoglobinopathy
   - Coombs' test—autoimmune hemolytic anemia
   - RBC enzyme study—G6PD deficiency
   - Ham test—acid hemolysin test—paroxysmal nocturnal hemoglobinuria (PNH).

Treatment

Depends on the cause
- Blood transfusion to keep Hb > 9g
- Washed RBC transfusion—PNH
- Folic acid 1 mg/day—hereditary spherocytosis, hemoglobinopathies
- Corticosteroid—autoimmune hemolytic anemia, PNH
- Splenectomy—hereditary spherocytosis, thalassemia, autoimmune hemolytic anemia
- Immunosuppressants—cold agglutinin disease, steroid and splenectomy failure in autoimmune hemolytic anemia
- Hydration with hypotonic alkaline solution—sickle cell anemia—decreased sickling in crisis
- Dextran IV—sickle cell anemia—decreased sickling in crisis
- Partial exchange transfusion—sickle cell anemia
- Bone marrow transplantation—sickle cell anemia, thalassemia
- Deferoxamine-iron overload in β thalassemia.

Hereditary Spherocytosis

- Most common congenital abnormality of RBC membrane
- Gene locus-chromosome 8 or 12
- Inheritance—autosomal dominant
  - Rarely recessive.

Pathogenesis

- Deficient membrane protein—ankyrin, spectrin
- Deficient membrane lipid increased permeability of sodium(Na).

Clinical Features

- Anemia, intermittent jaundice, splenomegaly
- Hemolytic facies, polydactyly, palate deformity.

Investigations

- Peripheral smear—microspherocyte >30% (Fig. 10.10)
- Osmotic fragility increased
  - Autohemolysis
  - Sterile incubation of RBC for 48 hours, hemolysis prevented by adding glucose in HS (normal <4% lysis, in HS >10-15% lysis)
  - HS excess entry of Na is prevented by ATP from glycolysis. If ATP decreases then hemolysis increased by adding glucose → increases ATP → decreases hemolysis
- Coombs' test negative
- Assay of red cell membrane spectrin content.

Complication

- Pigment gallstones and cholecystitis (Fig. 10.11)
- Crisis:
  - Hemolytic crisis—RES hyperplasia in infection
  - Aplastic crisis—infection by parvovirus, invade RBC precursors

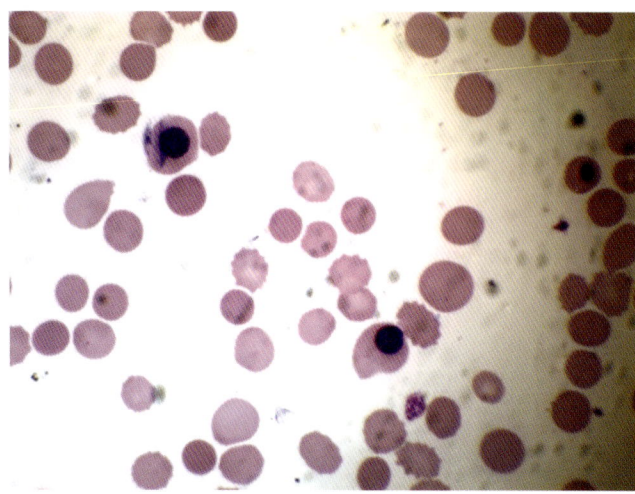

Fig. 10.10: Spherocyte.

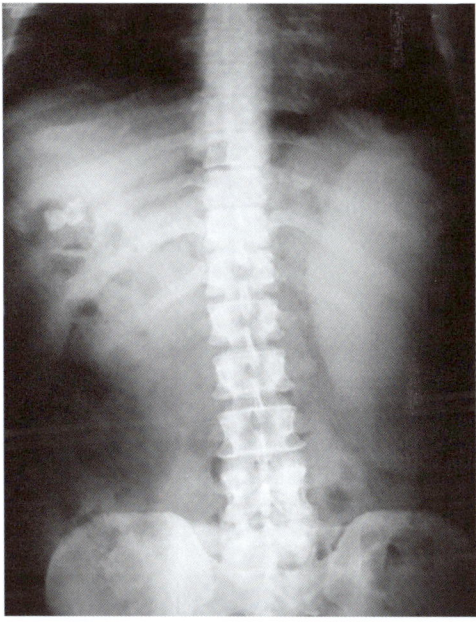

Fig. 10.11: X-ray abdomen showing splenomegaly with gallbladder stone in a patient with hereditary spherocytosis.

  - Megaloblastic crisis—folic acid deficiency with pregnancy.

Differential Diagnosis

Spherocytosis:
- Immune spherocyte, G6PD deficiency, ABO incompatibility
- Burns and uremia.

Diagnosis

Anemia, jaundice, splenomegaly, positive family history.
Spherocytosis, negative Coombs' test, autohemolysis prevented by glucose.

Treatment

- Folic acid prophylaxis: 1 mg/day
- Splenectomy:
  - Indications
    - Anemia with significant hemolysis—retic count >5%
    - Growth retardation
    - Recurrent crisis
    - Symptomatic cholecystitis
    - Death of other family members from same disease.
  - Age of surgery after 5–6 years
  - Complication
    - Postsplenectomy infection
    - Relapse—wrong diagnosis/splenic regrowth.

HEMORRHAGIC DISORDERS

Hemostatic Balance

- Promoters of thrombosis
  - Vessel wall damage
  - Platelet
  - Coagulation factors
- Inhibitors of thrombosis
  - Vessel wall
  - Protein C or protein S
  - Antithrombin III
  - Fibrinolytic system.

Hemostasis

- Extravascular factor: Tissue tension
- Support of vessel
- Vascular phase:
  - Vasoconstriction
  - Exposure of collagen fibers
  - Release of tissue factors
- Platelet phase:
  - Adhesion, release, aggregation
  - Platelet plug formation
- Coagulation phase - Intrinsic and extrinsic pathway
- Thrombus formation
- Stable hemostatic plug.

Classification

Defect of Blood Vessel

Vascular Purpura

- Congenital:
  - Hereditary hemorrhagic telangiectasia (Figs 10.12 and 10.13)
  - Hereditary capillary fragility
- Acquired:
  - Purpura simplex
  - Senile purpura
  - Infections—measles, typhus, infectious mononucleosis
  - Uremia, scurvy
  - HS purpura, vasculitis.

Disorders of platelet

- Quantitative
  - Thrombocytopenia (<1 lakh), e.g. immune thrombocytopenia
  - Thrombocytosis (>4 lakhs), e.g. essential thrombocytosis or essential thrombocythemia.
- Qualitative
  - Adhesion defect
    - von Willebrand's disease
    - Bernard-Soulier syndrome.
- Aggregation defect
  - Glanzmann's thrombasthenia
  - Uremia, drugs (aspirin).

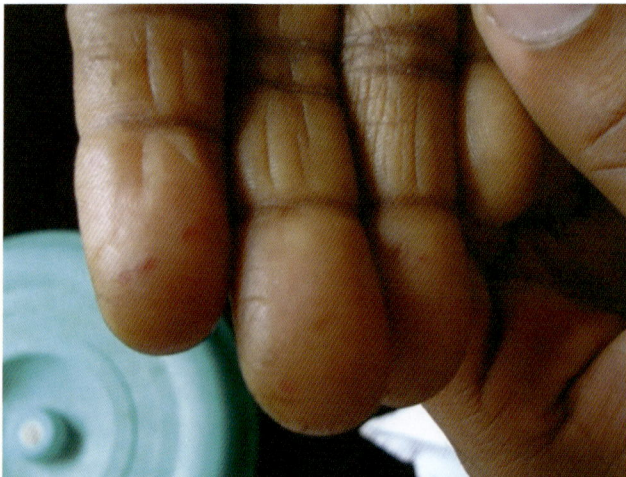

Fig. 10.12: Telangiectasia present over the fingertips in a patient with hereditary hemorrhagic telangiectasia.

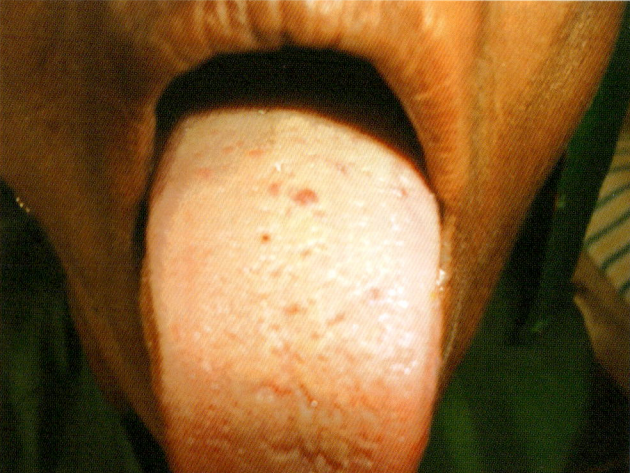

Fig. 10.13: Telangiectasia present over the tongue in a patient with hereditary hemorrhagic telangiectasia.

Coagulation Disorders

- Congenital:
  - Hemophilia—Christmas disease
  - Acquired:
    - Liver disease
    - Vitamin K deficiency
    - Oral anticoagulant.

Thrombocytopenia

About <1 lakh/mm^3.

Etiology

1. Decreased production:
   - Aplastic anemia
   - Myelophthisic anemia
   - Fanconis' anemia
   - Megaloblastic anemia
   - Heavy alcoholism
   - Hereditary-Wiskott-Aldrich syndrome
   - May—Hegglin anomaly.
2. Increased destruction:
   - Immune mediated:
     - Immune thrombocytopenic purpura (ITP)
     - Secondary thrombocytopenia
     - SLE, acquired immunodeficiency syndrome, lymphoma
     - Lymphatic leukemia
     - Post-transfusion thrombocytopenia
     - Isoimmune neonatal purpura
     - Drug-induced thrombocytopenia.
   - Nonimmune mediated:
     - Thrombotic thrombocytopenic purpura (TTP), disseminated intravascular coagulation
     - Hemolytic—uremic syndrome
     - Septicemia
     - Hemangioma
     - Prosthetic valves.
3. Sequestration: Splenic sequestration.

Idiopathic Thrombocytopenic Purpura

- Autoimmune thrombocytopenic purpura.
- Werlhof's disease.

Two types:
1. Acute ITP—more in children
2. Chronic ITP—following acute or insidious onset.

Pathogenesis

- Ab IgG + platelet → splenic macrophage destruction
- Splenic macrophage receptor for Fc portion of IgG
- Platelet coated with IgM (20%) removed by liver
- Platelet antibody
- IgG = 75%, IgM = 5%, IgG and IM = 20%
  Antibodies are produced by spleen and bone marrow.

Clinical Features

Acute ITP
- Children 2–6 years, preceding upper respiratory tract infection
- Antibody against viral antigens cross react with platelets
- Petechial hemorrhage, purpura, hemorrhagic bullae in oral cavity, epistaxis, GI and genitourinary bleed, fatal intracerebral bleed.

Chronic ITP
- Age 20–40 years
- Females >Males
- Insidious onset, mucocutaneous bleed
- Ecchymosis, epistaxis, menorrhagia
- Remission and relapses present.

Differential Diagnosis

Systemic lupus erythematosus (SLE), Evans syndrome, lymphoma, lymphatic leukemia.

Investigations

- Platelet count—thrombocytopenia
- Peripheral smear—megathrombocytes
- Bleeding time-prolonged, clothing time(LT)—normal, prothrombin time(PT)—normal, activated partial thromboplastin time(aPTT)—normal
- Hess's test is positive
- Clot retraction—defective (if platelet count <50,000/mm^3)
- Bone marrow—increased megakaryocytes without budding activity
- Demonstration of antiplatelet antibody.

Treatment

- Measures—observe without drugs
- Corticosteroids
- High dose immunoglobin
- Platelet transfusion (<20,000/mm^3)
- Plasmapheresis
- Splenectomy
- Immunosuppressants and danazole.

Acute ITP
- No treatment unless atraumatic bleeding
- Short-term prednisolone 1–2 mg/kg (4 weeks)
- Life-threatening bleed—platelet transfusion
- IV high dose immunoglobulin 1–2 g/kg (Ig blocks the Fc receptor of splenic macrophage)
- Poor response with corticosteroids for 6–12 months → splenectomy.

Chronic ITP
- Spontaneous recovery <10%
- Corticosteroids—thrombocytopenia <40,000/mm^3
  - Action:
    - ↓IgG production
    - ↓Platelet antibody interaction

- ↑ Platelet production
- ↓Destruction of antibody coated platelet).
  - Dose: 1 mg/kg, slow tapering to maintenance dose to keep platelet count > 40–60,000/cmm
- Splenectomy:
  - Unresponsive to steroid high dose maintenance
  - Relapse during pregnancy
  - Relapse 2 or more
  - Preparation: Pneumo vaccine 1–2 weeks prior to surgery, platelet transfusion and IV Ig if severe thrombocytopenia present.

Refractory ITP

- Unresponsive to corticosteroid and splenectomy
- Immunosuppressants
  - Cyclophosphamide 1–2 mg/kg/day
  - Azathioprine 1–4 mg/kg/day
  - Vincristine 1 mg/m^2
- If severe bleeding → IV Ig and platelet transfusion
- Danazol: 200–400 mg/day
- Other drugs—rituximab (anti CD 20), dapsone
- TPO receptor agonist
  - Romiplostim (subcutaneous)
  - Eltrom-bopag (oral).

Hemophilia-A

- Factor 8 deficiency, 1/10,000 males
- Genetic defect in X chromosome
- X-linked recessive transmission
- Female carriers—half of daughters carriers
- Half of sons suffer
- Hemophilic—daughters carriers
- Sons unaffected
- Severity:
  - <30%—bleeding manifests
  - >5%—mild post-traumatic bleed
  - <5%—mild spontaneous bleeding
  - 1–5%—moderate spontaneous bleeding
  - <1%—severe spontaneous bleeding.
- Majority of patients will have factor 8 <5%
- Factor 8 is produced by vascular endothelial cells, spleen and kidney.

Clinical Features

Are due to deep tissue bleeding:
- Bleeding into muscles, joints and body cavities
  - Arthropathy = Weight bearing joints
  - Hemarthrosis
  - Synovial hypertrophy
  - Cartilage destruction
  - Secondary osteoarthrosis
  - Ankylosis.
- Hematomas → pressure effect, muscle necrosis of calf and psoas → calcification → pseudotumor
- Psoas hematoma → femoral nerve palsy
- Calf muscle hematoma → ischemic necrosis → fibrosis → contracture
- GI and GU bleeding
- Fatal bleeding → CNS and oropharyngeal bleed.

Investigation

- Prothrombin time—normal
- Bleeding time—normal
- Clotting time—prolonged
- Platelet count—normal
- aPTT—prolonged, corrected with plasma factor 8
- Assay of factor 8.

Diagnosis

- Positive family history
- Joint and soft tissue bleeding
- Abnormal coagulogram as above.

Treatment

- Replacement of factor 8
- Cryoprecipitate
- Freeze dried antihemophilic globulin (AHG)
- **AHG by recombinant DNA technology**
  - Calculation of dose
    - Desired % rise in factor 8 × weight in kg divided by 2
  - Each unit of AHG will rise the plasma level by 2%/kg
  - Half-life of AHG is 8–12 hours
  - Soft tissue bleeding and hemarthrosis → one infusion to keep AHG 15–20%
  - Internal bleeding–infusion
    → 25–50% BID × 3 days
  - Intracerebral bleed–infusion
    → >50% BID × 2 weeks.

Hemophilic with inhibitors to AHG
- Two types of inhibitors
  - Type 1: High titer antibody with anamnestic response
  - Type 2: Low titer antibody
- For type 1 inhibitor → porcine factor 8 concentrate or prothrombin complex concentrate is given
- For type 2 inhibitor → higher doses of factor 8 is given Desmopressin acetate (1-deamino-8-D-arginine vasopressin) DPAVP is given in mild cases
- Epsilon-aminocaproic acid (EACA)—4–6 g QID × 3–4 days in mild cases.

Carrier Detection

- About 15% genetic mutation
- Daughter of hemophilic
- Mother of hemophilic son.

Antenatal Diagnosis

- Estimation of factor 8
- Chorionic villi sampling (11th week)

- Amniocentesis (16th week)
- Fetal blood (19th–20th week).

Complication

- Hemophilic arthropathy
- Inhibitors of AHG
- Hepatitis-B
- AIDS.

Prophylaxis

- Hemophilic should carry card with blood group
- Avoid IM injections
- Avoid antiplatelet drugs like aspirin
- Avoid trauma
- Proper dental care.

PLASMA CELL PROLIFERATIVE DISORDERS

Classification

1. Monoclonal gammopathy of undetermined significance (MGUS)
   - Ig < 3 g/dL, plasma cell <10%
2. Malignant monoclonal gammopathy
   - Multiple myeloma and its variants
   - Plasmacytoma
   - Plasma cell leukemia
   - Waldenstrom's macroglobulinemia
   - Heavy chain disease (α HCD, μ HCD, γ HCD)
   - Light chain disease
   - Primary amyloidosis.

Multiple Myeloma

Definition: Malignant proliferation of plasma cells derived from a single clone of B cells.

Classification

- IgG—55%
- IgA—21%
- IgD and IgE—2%
- Light chain (BJ myeloma)—22%.

Incidence: 4 new cases/lakh/year
- Male: female = 2:1
- Age > 60 years, 60–70 years
- < 2% before 40 years.

Pathogenesis

- Plasma cells → Ig of single heavy and light chain-monoclonal protein (M protein) or paraprotein, free light chain → urine—Bence-Jones (BJ) protein, dimer of light chain.
- M protein in urine is due to glomerular damage
- Proliferation of myeloma cells—(IL6 dependant) leads to—cytokines, IL1, osteoclast activating factor → bone resorption and osseous
   - Paraprotein → hyperviscosity, renal changes and amyloidosis
   - Bone marrow and extramedullary infiltration → anemia and thrombocytopenia
   - Reduction in normal Ig → infection.

Clinical Features

General, osseous and extraosseous.

General: Weight loss, malaise and fatigue.

Osseous:
- Bone pain, lytic lesion
- Pathological fracture, osteoporosis
- Hypercalcemia.

Extraosseous:
- Anemia (normocytic, normochromic) 80%
- Myelophthisic anemia, hemolytic
- Nephropathy—25% (myeloma nephrosis)
- Renal damage is due to:
   - Light chain—renal toxic effect
   - Hypercalcemia
   - Urate nephropathy
   - Amyloidosis
   - Infiltration by plasma cells
   - Pyelonephritis.
- Renal manifestation
   - Renal failure 25%
   - Proximal renal tubular acidosis
   - Nephrotic syndrome
   - Light chain deposit disease (light chain deposit in glomerulus)
- Neurological—due to:
   - Hyperviscosity
   - Cryoglobulinemia
   - Amyloid deposit
      - Carpal tunnel syndrome
      - Peripheral neuropathy.
   - Hypercalcemia
   - Spine destruction—myelopathy.

Infections: Due to decreased production and increased destruction of Ig decreased CD4 cells, decreased polymorphs.
- Pneumonia
- Pyelonephritis.

Hypercalcemia:
- Lethargy
- Weakness
- Depression
- Encephalopathy.

Hyperviscosity:
- Headache
- Loss of vision—retinopathy, sausage shaped retinal veins
- Normal serum viscosity is 1.8
- Symptoms seen if serum viscosity is 5–6
- Hyperviscosity and M protein
- IgM >4 g/dL
- IgG_3 >5 g/dL
- IgA >7 g/dL.

Bleeding:
- Due to paraprotein interfering with clotting factor
- Amyloid damage of endothelium
- Platelet dysfunction.

Diagnosis

Diagnostic triad:
1. Plasmacytosis >10%
2. Lytic bone lesions
3. Presence of serum/urine M protein.

Diagnostic criteria: Plasmacytosis>10% or plasmacytoma
+
One of the following:
1. M protein in serum >3 g/dL
2. M protein in urine
3. Lytic bone lesions.

Staging (Salmon and Durie)

Stage 1—$< 0.6 \times 10^{12}$ cells
All of the following:
- Hb >10 g/dL
- Serum calcium <12 mg%
- Normal X-ray/solitary lesion
- Low M component–IgG <5 g/dL
- IgA <3 g/dL
- Urine light chain <4 g/24 hours

Stage 2—$0.6\text{-}1.2 \times 10^{12}$ cells
Between stage 1 and stage 3.

Stage 3 $>1.2 \times (10)\ 12$ cells
One or more of the following:
- Hb <8.5 g/dL
- Serum calcium >12 mg dL
- Multiple lytic lesions of bone
- M.component—IgG>7 g/dL
- IgA >5 g/dL
- Urine light chain>12 g/24 hr.

Investigations

- Complete blood count, erythrocyte sedimentation rate (ESR) increases
- Urine—BJ protein and M protein in 24 hours

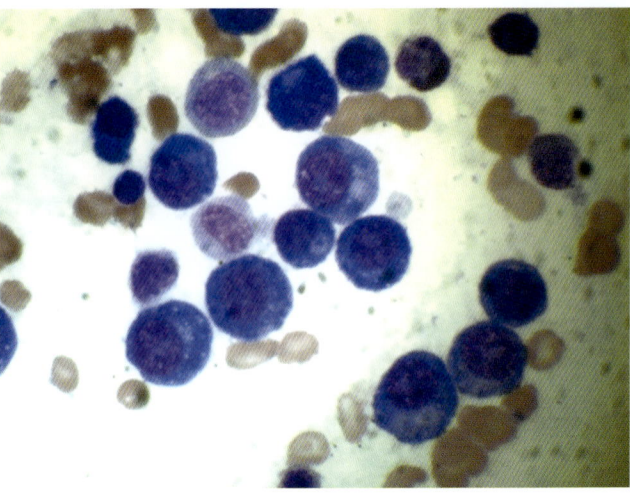

Fig. 10.14: Multiple myeloma—plasmacytosis.

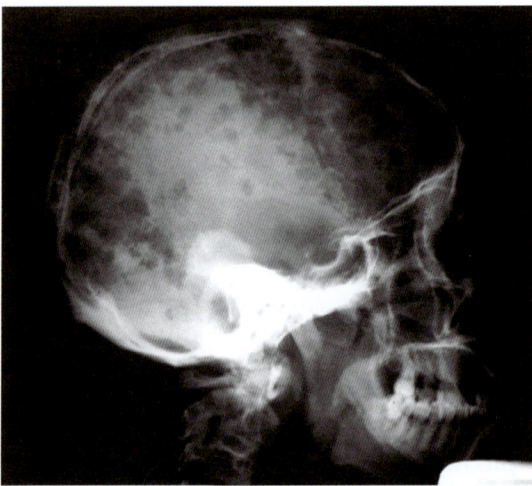

Fig. 10.15: X-ray skull lateral view showing multiple punched out lytic lesions—multiple myeloma.

- Hb decreases, normocytic normochromic anemia
- Bone marrow—plasma cells >10% (Fig. 10.14)
- X-ray bone—skull (Fig. 10.15), spine, pelvis-osteolytic lesion
- Isotope bone scan
- Serum calcium and alkaline phosphatase raised
- Renal function test
- Bleeding time coagulation screening
- Plasma viscosity
- Serum protein electrophoresis for M protein
- Immunoelectrophoresis
- β_2 microglobulin.

Variant forms of Multiple Myeloma

1. **Smoldering multiple myeloma**
   - M protein >3 g/dL
   - Plasma cells >10%
   - No anemia, no renal failure, no bony lesion

2. **Plasma cell leukemia**
   - Primary—60%
     - Lymphadenopathy
     - Hepatosplenomegaly
     - Anemia
     - No bony lesion
     - Peripheral smear-plasma cells >20%
   - Secondary—40%
     - Multiple myeloma → plasma cell leukemia
     - Bony lesion present.
3. **Nonsecretory myeloma**
   - No M protein in serum and urine
   - Paraprotein within the cell, detected by immunofluorescence
   - Renal lesions less
   - ESR—normal
4. **IgD myeloma:** Amyloidosis and extramedullary plasmacytoma are more.
5. **POEMS syndrome**
   - **P**olyneuropathy
   - **O**rganomegaly
   - **E**ndocrinopathy
   - **M** protein
   - **S**kin changes
   - Endocrinopathy—gynecomastia, testicular atrophy
   - Skin—hypertrichosis, hyperpigmentation
   - Polyneuropathy—CIDP type
   - Osteosclerotic lesions.
6. **Solitary plasma cytoma of bone**
   - Bone marrow—plasma cells <10%
   - No M protein in serum/urine
   - No other bony lesion.
7. **Extramedullary plasmacytoma**
   - Arising outside bone marrow
   - Usually in upper respiratory tract (80%).

Treatment

Indications
- Anemia, hypercalcemia, renal failure, lytic bone lesion
- Extramedullary plasma cytoma
- No specific treatment for MGUS and smoldering multiple myeloma.

Measures:
- Chemotherapy
  - Melphalan 8-10 mg/day + prednisolone 60 mg/day × 7 days once in six weeks, OR
  - Cyclophosphamide 200 mg/day or
  - Chlorambucil 8 mg/day ×1-2 years
  - Alkylating agent resistant cases—Vincristine, adriamycin and dexamethasone (VAD)
  - Thalidomide 100 mg daily + Prednisolne 60 mg/day for 7 days per month till remission **OR**
  - Lenalidomide 25 mg once daily for 21 days and 7 days off drug + Prednisolne 60 mg/day for 7 days per cycle till remission.

- Autologous stem cell transplantation
- Allogeneic bone marrow transplantation
- Radiotherapy for local lesions.

Treatment for Complications

- Hypercalcemia: Hydration, prednisolone and bisphosphonate
- Renal failure—treatment of the causes, plasmapheresis
- Infection—appropriate antimicrobial
- Bony lesion—radiotherapy, long-term bisphosphonate therapy
- Hyperviscosity—plasmapheresis.

Poor Prognostic Factors of Multiple Myeloma

- Hb <7 g/dL
- Hypercalcemia
- Hypoalbuminemia
- Renal failure
- Thrombocytopenia
- High β_2 microglobulin >4 mg/dL
  - Plasma cell leukemia.

HEMATOLOGICAL VALUES

White Blood Count

- Total leukocyte count—4000-11000/mm^3
- Leukocytosis—> 11000/cmm
- Leukopenia < 4000/mm^3.

Differential Leukocyte Count

- Neutrophil 50—70%
  - Absolute count 3000-6000/cmm
  - Neutrophilia >6500/mm^3
  - Neutropenia <1500/mm^3
- Eosinophil 1-4%
  - Absolute count 100-400/mm^3
  - Eosinophilia >500/mm^3
  - Eosinopenia <50/mm^3
- Basophil 0-1%: Absolute count 0-100/mm^3
- Lymphocyte 20-40%
  - Absolute count 1500-3500/mm^3
  - Lymphocytosis >4000/mm^3
  - Lymphocytopenia <1400/mm^3
- Monocyte 2-7%: Absolute count 200-600/mm^3

RBC Count

- Normal
  - Male: 4.4-6 million/mm^3
  - Female: 4.2-5.4 million/mm^3
- Anemia
  - Male: <4.5 million/mm^3
  - Female: <4 million/mm^3

- Polycythemia
    - Male: >6 million/mm^3
    - Female: >5.5 million/mm^3.

Reticulocyte Count

- 0.5–2%

Corrected reticulocyte count =

$$\text{Observed reticulocyte count} \times \frac{\text{Patient's PCV}}{\text{Normal PCV}}$$

Red Cell Indices

- MCH 27–32 pg
- MCV 76–94 fL
- MCHC 32–36 g/dL.

Normal Hemoglobin Values

By World Health Organization
- Children 6 months–6 years → 11 g/dL &>
- 6–14 years → 12 g/dL &>
- Adult male → 13 g/dL &>
- Adult female (nonpregnant) → 12 g/dL &>
- Adult female pregnant → 11 g/dL &>

Anemia:
- Male < 13 g/dL
- Female < 12 g/dL.

Polycythemia:
- Male > 18 g/dL
- Female > 16 g/dL.

Platelet Count

- Normal 1.5–4 lakhs/cmm
- Thrombocytopenia <1 lakh/mm^3
- Thrombocytosis > 4 lakhs/mm^3.

ESR

- Male: 0–10 mm/hr
- Female: 3–15 mm/hr.

PCV

- Male: 47 ± 7%, Female 42 ± 5%
- Anaemia: Male: < 42% , Female: < 36%
- Polycythemia: Male: > 55%, Female: > 47%.

Bone Marrow

Cellular Components

- Myeloid precursors — 57%
- Erythroid precursors — 25%
- Neutrophilic series — 53%
- Eosinophilic series — 3%
- Basophilic series — <0.1%
- Myeloblast — 0.9%
- Lymphocytes — 16%
- Monocytes — 3%
- Plasma cells — 1.3%
- Megakaryocytes — 0.1%
- Reticulum cells — 0.3%

Coagulation Parameters

- Bleeding time < 8 minutes
- Clotting time 5–10 minutes
- Prothrombin time 8–10.5 seconds
- aPTT - 26–37 seconds.

Blood Volume

- Male: 75 ± 10 mL/kg
- Female: 70 ± 10 mL/kg.

Index

Page numbers followed by f refer to figure and t refer to table.

A

Abdomen 194, 204, 289
 auscultation of 202
 causes, distension of 189
 clinical signs of 205
 distension of 189, 272
 examination of 194, 273
  acute 204
 inspection of 195
 measurements of 201
 palpation of 197
 percussion of 201
 pulsations of 196
 regions over 195f
 shape of 195
 upper 201
 veins over 196
Abdominal aorta 196
 arteritis 117
Abdominal aortic aneurysm 201, 203
Abdominal aortoarteritis 203
Abdominal examination 204
Abdominal group 18
Abdominal mass
 causes of 201
 palpation of 201
Abdominal migraine 188
Abdominal organs, surface marking of 195
Abdominal pain 187
 causes of
  acute 187
  chronic 188
 lateral 187
 lower 187
 mechanism 187
 medical disorders producing 188
 site of 187
 types of 187
 upper 187
Abdominal reflex, superficial 81
Abdominal wall
 masses, causes of anterior 201
 movement of 196
 veins of 197f

Abducent nerve 43, 52
Abscess 166
Absorption disorders 210
Acanthosis nigricans 14, 15, 194, 249
Accommodation reflex 38, 49
Achalasia cardia 183, 183f
Achilles bursitis 229
Achilles enthesitis 229
Achilles tendinitis 229
Achondroplasia 20
Acid
 eructation 180, 182
 hemolysin test 294
 peptic disease 188
  chronic 188
Acquired immunodeficiency syndrome 297
Acromegaly 254
 clinical features 255
 complications 255
 etiology 254
 incidence 254
 investigations 255
 management 256
Acute encephalopathy, differential diagnosis of 224
Acute glomerulonephritis, etiology of 275
Adalimumab 238
Addison's disease 14, 15, 19, 20, 182, 192, 194, 245, 246, 249, 264
Adefovir 217
Adenovirus 185
Adrenal crisis 265
 therapy of 266
Adrenal insufficiency
 acute 265
 causes 265
 chronic 265
 management of primary 265
 primary 265t
 secondary 265t
Adrenal neoplasm 264
Adriamycin 301
Adventitious sounds 163

Adversive seizure 50
Agnosia 36, 37
Agranulocytosis 194
Airway source, upper 153
Akathisia 90
Albumin-globulin ratio, reversal of 219
Alcohol, abstinence of 219
Alcoholic cirrhosis 218
Alcoholic hepatitis 216
Alcoholic liver disease 190, 206
Alcoholism 2
 neurological, manifestation of 205
Alfred de Musset's sign 135
Alimentary causes 180
Alimentary disorders, examinations in 205
Alimentary system 3, 189
 examination of 180, 191
 general examination in 190
Alkaptonuria 7f, 229f
Allergic asthma 242
Alopecia 17
Alpha-glucosidase inhibitors 252
Alport's syndrome 272, 276
Aluminum-containing antacids 186
Alveolar macrophage 152
Alveolar sac lined 151
Alzheimer's disease 34
Amebiasis cecum 201
Amebic liver abscess 206
Amenorrhea 248
 primary 248
 secondary 248
Amiodarone 167
Amnesia 34
Ampicillin 186
Amyloid arthropathy 232
Amyloidosis 206, 207
Anacrotic pulse 115, 116, 116f
Anakinra 238
Anal reflex 82
Analgesic nephropathy 232
Androgen deficiency 265
Android obesity 5

Anemia 4, 5, 6f, 9, 111, 155, 190, 286, 290
  chronic deficiency 207
  correction of 282
  etiological classification 290
  morphological classification 290
  sign of 6f
Anesthesia dolorosa 92
Angina, causes of 110
Angiodysplasia 187
Angular cheilitis 191
Angular stomatitis 191
Anisocoria 48
  causes of 48
Anisosphygmia 115
Ankle
  and foot 229
  clonus 85
  jerk 84, 84f
    absent 105
Ankyloglossia 193
Ankylosing spondylitis 20, 229, 231, 241, 244
  juvenile 241
Anomalies, congenital 2
Anomalous pulmonary venous
    connection 119
Anorexia 180, 246
  causes of 180
  nervosa 188
Anosmia 37
Antacids 186
Anterograde amnesia 34
Anthropometry 4
  types of 4
Antialdosterone 150
Antibody 216
Anticoagulant therapy 153, 205
Anticytokine treatment 238t
Antigen 216
Antineutrophil cytoplasmic antibody 213
Antinuclear antibody 234
Antiphospholipid antibody syndrome 234
Antiphospholipid syndrome 239, 272, 286
Antirheumatic drugs, disease modifying 237t
Antituberculous drugs 155
Anuria 269
Anuric renal failure 278
Anus, examination of 204
Aorta
  dissecting aneurysm of 188
  palpation of 200
Aortic arch arteritis 242
Aortic area 129
  second 129
Aortic component, accentuation of 124
Aortic ejection click 125
Aortic regurgitation 134
  causes of 134
  clinical features 134
  complications of 135
  etiology 134
  investigations 135
  management 136
  pathophysiology 134
Aortic root, aneurysm of 125
Aortic stenosis 133
  auscultatory signs of 133f
  clinical features 133
  complications 133
  etiology 133
  investigations 134
  management 134
  pathophysiology 133
  prognosis 134
Aortoiliac arteritis 117
Apathetic thyrotoxicosis 263
Apex of lung, percussion of 160f
Apex, position of 158
Aphasia
  clinical types of 35
  type of 36
  with repetition 35
  without repetition 35
Aphthous ulcer 192, 194, 211
Apical impulse 121, 157
Apical systolic murmur 128
Aplastic anemia 216, 293
  clinical features 293
  etiology 293
  investigations 293
Apneustic breathing 156
Appendix, gallbladder 188
Appetite 2, 246
  reduced 259
Apraxia 36
  of gait 88
Arachnodactyly 112f
Areflexia 250
Argyll Robertson pupil 49
Arnold-Chiari malformation 98
Arsenic poisoning 14
Arterial hypoxia 11
Arterial pulsation 119
Arterial waves, normal 113
Arthralgia 226
Arthritis 226, 232f, 240
  differential diagnosis of 232, 233
  in adult 232
    degenerative arthropathy 232
    endocrine 232
    hematological 232
    immune mediated 232
    infections 232
    postinfectious 232
  in children 232
Asbestos 155

Ascites 202
  causes of 208
  clinical clues to 209
  clinical evaluation of 207
  detection of 202
  etiology of 208
  fluid study 209
  investigations in 209
  mechanism of 218
  signs of 208
  symptoms of 207
  with bleeding manifestations 209
  with dyspnea 209
  with fever 209
  with hepatosplenomegaly 209
  with pain 209
  with pedal edema 209
  without bleeding manifestations 209
  without dyspnea 209
  without jaundice 209
  without pain 209
  without pedal edema 209
Ascitic fluid infection, types of 209
Aspergilloma 153
Asthenia 4
Asthma
  exercise induced 171
  extrinsic 170
  intrinsic 170
Ataxia telangiectasia 98
Ataxic breathing 156
Ataxic dysarthria 36
  types 36
Ataxic gait 87
Ataxic neuropathy 108
Ataxic nystagmus 50
Atherosclerosis 117
Athetosis 89
  etiology of 89
Atmospheric oxygen content, defect in 7
Atonic bladder 106
Atrial fibrillation 130
Atrial septal defect 138
  clinical evaluation of 138
  clinical features 138
  complications 138
  investigations 139
  management 139
  pathophysiology 138
  type of 138f
    lesion with 139
Atrial sound 124
Auditory agnosia 37
Auscultation 161, 123
  breath sounds 161
  method of 128
Austin flint murmur 128

Autoimmune
    chronic hepatitis 217
    hepatitis 216
    polyglandular syndromes 265
Automatic bladder 106
Autonomic nervous system
    division of 45f
    symptoms 31
Autonomic neuropathy 250
Autonomous bladder 106
Axillary area 159
Axillary group 18
Azathioprine 213, 282
Azoospermia, obstructive 169
Azotemia 181, 274
Azure lunula 12, 32, 190
Azygos vein, lobe of 151

B

Babinski's sign 82
Back pain 230
Band keratopathy 250, 272
Barium swallow 183f
Basal pneumonia 188, 205
Basedow's disease 260
Basilar artery 28, 103
Basophil 301
Bassen-Kornzweig syndrome 42, 98, 107
Beau's lines 12
Bedside test 64
Behcet's syndrome 194, 227, 231, 234, 273
Beighton score 231, 231t
Bell's palsy 63
    right side 63f
Bell's phenomenon 61
Bernard-Soulier syndrome 296
Berry aneurysm 83f
Bickerstaff encephalitis 53
Bifid apex beat 121
Biguanides 210
Bile duct, carcinoma 199
Bile salt 210
Biliary atresia 214
Biliary colic 187
Biliary disease 206, 217
Bilious vomitus 182
Binocular diplopia 46
Biochemical triad 294
Biot's breathing 22, 156
Bipyramidal signs 105
Bird Fancier's lung 155
Bisferiens pulse 115, 116, 116f
Bitemporal hemianopia 250
Biventricular failure 149
Bjerrum's screen 39
Bladder
    innervation of 106f
    neck 106

    percussion of 202
    symptoms 103
Bleeding 286
    diathesis 2, 153, 188, 205
    gum 180, 192
    causes 181
Bleomycin 155, 167
Blind loop syndrome 291
Blindness, bilateral 38
Blood
    flow through vessels, increased 128
    gas abnormality 173, 173t
    loss, assessment of 222
    pressure 21, 32, 113, 249, 260
        for adults, classification of 22
        procedure 21
    source of 184
    sugar test 253
    transfusion 291
    vessel, defect of 296
    volume 302
Blue nail 12
Body habits 4
Body habitus 20, 249
Body mass index 5
Bogarad's syndrome 63, 64
Bone 301
    and joint pain 286
    marrow 302
        cellular components 302
    tenderness 289
Bonnier's syndrome 65
Bouchard's node 228
Boutonniere deformity 235
Bovine cough 153
Bowel and bladder
    habits 2
    symptoms 31
Bowel sounds 202
    decreased 203, 205
    increased 203, 205
Bowel visible peristalsis, large 196
Bowel/bladder
    features 104
    symptoms 103
Brachial plexus lesion, lower 164
Bradycardia, relative 21
Bradypnea 155
Brain
    blood supply to 27
    lateral surface of 27f
    medial surface of 27f
    principal arteries of 28f
    venous drainage of 29
Brainstem 42
    damage, upper 22
    lesion 26, 65, 95, 102
    lesion, upper 95f

Brassy cough 153
Breast 249
    examination of 251
    symptoms referable to 247
Breath sounds
    intensity of 162
    types of 162f
Breathing, type of 99
Broca's aphasia 36
Broca's area 35
Bronchial adenoma 177f
Bronchial asthma 149, 164, 170
    clinical features 170
    clinical types 170
    diagnosis of 171
    drugs in 171
    etiological types 170
    factors precipitating 170
    investigations 171
    management 171
    pathophysiology 170
Bronchial breathing
    mechanism of 163f
    types of 162
Bronchiectasis 2, 153, 169, 205
    bad prognostic signs 169
    clinical features 169
    complications 169
    etiology 169
    morphological types 169
    pathological process 169
    sicca 169
Bronchitis 153
    chronic 172, 172t
Bronchodilator 155
    therapy 173t
Bronchogenic carcinoma 11, 155
Bronchomalacia 169
Bronchopulmonary anastomoses 128
Bronchopulmonary segments 151, 151t
Brown's syndrome 227, 235
Brown-Sequard lesion 96f
Brucellosis 234
Brudzinski sign 98
Buccal mucosa 194
Budd-Chiari syndrome 206, 207, 239
Budesonide 213
Bulbar myopathy 250
Bulbar palsy, progressive 69
Bulbocavernosus reflex 82
Bulimia nervosa 181
Bursitis 226
Busulfan 12, 167

C

Cachexia, causes of 5
Cachexia/wasting 190
Café-au-lait spot 32f

Calcified retroperitoneal tumor 188f
Calcium
    functions of 266
    homeostasis, disorders of 266
    metabolism 266
Calf muscle
    hypertrophy 258f
    hypothyroidism, hypertrophy of 72f
Calf syndrome 258
Campylobacter 185
Cannon sound 123
Capillary leak syndrome 9f
Caplan's syndrome 231, 235, 236
Capsular lesion, internal 102
Caput medusa 196, 218
Carcinoid syndrome 165, 246
Carcinoma 268
    ampulla of Vater 199
Cardiac asthma 164
Cardiac cachexia 130
Cardiac cause, ascites of 209
Cardiac cyanosis 7
Cardiac edema 8
Cardiac failure
    congestive 152
    precipitating causes for 149
Cardiac tamponade, causes of 146
Cardiopulmonary 281
    system 227
Cardiovascular disease, skin in 15
Cardiovascular disorders
    clinical features of 129
    history in 111
Cardiovascular factors 150
Cardiovascular symptoms 286
Cardiovascular system 3, 182, 205, 235,
        250, 251, 255, 258, 260, 289
    examination of 109
    general examination in 111
Cardiovocal paralysis 141
Carey Coombs murmur 128
Caries teeth 192
Caroli's disease 214
Carotenemia 6, 6f, 258f
Carotenoderma 6
Caroticocavernous fistula 52
Carotid artery, internal 28, 102
Carotid disease, internal 101
Carotid pulsation 120
Carpal tunnel syndrome 235, 299
Castell's method 202
Castleman Bland syndrome 145
Castleman's disease 19
Cataract 250
Catecholamine cardiomyopathy 250
Cauda equina 27
    lesion 96f
Causalgia 92
Cavernous breathing 162

Cavernous malformation 220
Cavernous portion 42
Cavitary lesion 168
    causes 168
    clinical features 168
    pathognomonic sign of 164
Cecum 198
Celiac axis 203
Celiac disease 194, 211
Cellulitis 13f
Central abdominal pain 187
Central cord lesion 96f
Central cyanosis 7, 142, 155, 190
Central nervous system 182, 267, 273, 281
    symptoms 286
Cerebellar artery
    anterior inferior 103
    posterior inferior 102
    superior 103
Cerebellar ataxia 87, 250
Cerebellar degeneration 164
Cerebellar disorder
    acute 97
    chronic 98
    etiology of 97
    recurrent 98
Cerebellar lesion 26, 88
    localization of 26
Cerebellar peduncle 26
Cerebellar signs 101
    examination of 96
Cerebellum 26
    disorder of 30
    functions 26
Cerebral artery
    anterior 29, 102
    middle 28, 102
    posterior 28, 29, 102
Cerebral coma 100
Cerebral cortex 26, 27
    blood supply of 27f
    input from 26
Cerebral lipidosis 90
Cerebral portion, branches of 28
Cerebral thrombosis 239
Cerebral vessels 144
Cerebrovascular accident 182
Cervical group 18
Cervical lymph nodes 251
Cervical lymphadenopathy 18f
Cervical portion 45f
Cervical spine 229
Chaddock's sign 82
Chalk white patches 192
Charcot's joint 252
Charcot-Marie-Tooth disease 20, 72f
Charcot-Wilbrand syndrome 40
Chediak-Higashi syndrome 17
Cheilitis 192

Chemodectoma 65
Chest
    and upper limbs 12f
    examination of 156
    expansion, measurement of 159
    lower anterior 158f
    movement of 157, 158
    pain 109, 154
        types of 154
    signs 176
    unilateral flattening of 157
    upper anterior 158f
    wall
        anterior 160f
        lateral 159, 160f
        palpation of 159
        posterior 159, 160f
    X-ray thymic mass 179f
Chewing tobacco 2
Cheyne-Stoke's breathing 22
Chiasmal lesion 39
    anterior 39
    middle 39
    posterior 39
Chickenpox 2
    vesicles of 12f
Chikungunya 232f
Childhood respiratory disease 2
Childhood thyrotoxicosis 262
Child-Pugh classification 220
Chip munk facies 19
Chlamydia 166, 167
    proctitis 212
Chloroquine 237
Cholestatic jaundice 213, 214
Chorea 69, 88
    clinical signs 89
    clinical triad of 89
    site of lesion 88
    variants of 89
Choreoathetosis 89
Choria gravis 89
Choroid tubercle 164
Christmas disease 287
Chronic arthritis, juvenile 241t
Chronic encephalopathy, differential
        diagnosis of 224
Chronic hepatitis, drug induced 216
Chronic kidney disease, stages of 281
Chronic liver disease, stigmas of 190
Chronic persistent asthma, treatment of 171
Churg-Strauss syndrome 231, 242, 289
Chylous ascites, milky fluid of 208f
Circle of willis 28f
Circumoral pigmentation 192
Cirrhosis
    compensated 219
    decompensated 219
    prognosis in 220

Cirrhosis liver 7, 190, 205-207, 208, 208f, 217, 218f
   advanced 202
   complications of 219
   investigations in 219
   prognosis of 220
Cirrhosis with
   ascites and pedal edema 220
   encephalopathy 220
Citelli's syndrome 52
Clawing of foot 229
Clenching jaws 57
Clonus 85
Clostridium 185
   difficile 185
Clubbing 11, 11f, 111, 155, 155f, 191f
   causes of 11
   grades of 11
   pathogenesis 11
   unilateral 12
Coagulation disorders 297
Coagulation parameters 302
Coal miner's 155
Coarctation of aorta 117, 143
   added anomalies 144
   clinical features 143
   complications 144
   etiology 143
   investigations 144
   management 144
   pathogenesis 143
Coarse crackles 163
Cochlear function, tests for 64
Cochlear lesion 65
Cochlear nerve 64
   lesion 65
Coenzyme A 292
Coin sound 164
Colchicine 210
Cold agglutinin 166
Cold intolerance 245, 259
Cold moist hand 19
Colicky pain 187, 202
Collagen vascular disease 107
   skin markers in 14
Collapse, types of 168
Collapsing pulse, demonstration of 116f
Color vision 41
   anomaly 41
Columnar epithelium 151
Coma 33
   deep 33
   etiology of 100
Communicable diseases 2
Community acquired pneumonia 165
Compressive myelopathy 104
   surgery for 105
Conduction deafness 65
   causes of 65

Condylomata accuminata 204
Conjuctival hemorrhage 147
Conjunctiva 6f
Conjunctival reflex 57, 81
Conn's syndrome 245, 249, 250, 254
Connective tissue disease, mixed 243
Consciousness, level of 33
Constipation 180, 186, 259
   causes 186
   features 186
Constrictive pericarditis, causes of 146
Constructional apraxia 37, 219
Continuous fever 20
Continuous murmur 127
   mechanism of 127
   with cyanosis 128
Conus medullaris 27
   lesion 96f
Convergent divergent nystagmus 50
Coomb's test 240, 294, 295
Copper kinetics 216
Cor pulmonale 169
Cord compression 96f
Corneal reflex 57, 81
Corneomandibular reflex 58
Corona radiata 102
Coronary artery disease 2
Corrigan's pulse 115
Cortical blindness 40
Cortical necrosis, acute 278
Cortical sensation 94
Corticonuclear fibers 23
Corticosteroid 268
   suppression test 268
Cough 110, 152
   dry cough 152
   phases of 152
   reflex arc 152
   types of 152
Courvoisier's law 199
Cover test 47
Cowpox 13f
Crack pot resonance 161
Crackles 163
Cranial fossa, posterior 42
Cranial nerve 104
   disorders of
     10th 66
     9th 66
   examination of 37
   lesion, symptoms of 5th 57
   palsy, causes of 6th 51
C-reactive protein 236
Crepitation 163, 164t
   types of 163
Cretinism 19
Cribrosa 41
Cricopharyngeal achalasia 167
Cricopharyngeal spasm 67

Crigler-Najjar type 213
Crocordile tears syndrome 63
Crohn's colitis 241
Crohn's disease 194, 201, 210-213
   small bowel 213
Cruveilhier-Baumgarten murmur 128, 203
Cuboidal epithelium 151
Cuirasse analgesia 96f
Cushing's disease 165, 264
Cushing's syndrome 15, 19, 20, 31, 34, 196, 245, 246, 248, 249, 250, 254, 263, 264
   clinical features 263
   etiology 263
   in baby 263f
   investigations 264
   juvenile 245
   management 264
   test for 264
Cutaneous lupus
   acute 240
   chronic 240
Cutaneous polyarteritis nodosa 242f
Cutaneous vasculitis 235
Cutis laxa 13f
Cyanosis 4, 7, 31, 110, 111, 193, 218, 288
   clinical types of 7
   differential 8
   early 7
   mixed 7
   with hypoxemia 7
   without hypoxemia 7
Cyanotic congenital heart disease 31
Cyclosporin A 282
Cyclosporine 213
Cystic bronchiectasis 169
Cystic fibrosis 169
Cystic masses in abdomen, causes of 201
Cytomegalovirus 215

D

Dapsone 16f
de Morsier's syndrome 37
Deep reflexes 82
Deep tendon reflex 82, 250
Defense mechanism, defect in 167
Deforming polyarthropathy, differential diagnosis of 233
Dehydration, signs of 11
Delayed puberty 248
   female 248
   male 248
Delirium 33
   tremens 33
Deltopectoral 18
Delusion 33
Dementia 34
   causes of 34
   primary causes 34
   secondary causes 34

Demyelinating disorders 52
Dengue fever 21f
   positive 287f
Dengue rash 16f
Dental ulcer 194
Deoxythymidylate monophosphate 292
Deoxyuridylate monophosphate 292
Depletional hyponatremia 285
Depressive illness 186, 250
Depressive psychosis 181
Dermatomyositis 15
Dermopathy 260f, 261
Dextrocardia 121f
Di Guglielmo syndrome 293
Diabetes mellitus 2, 232, 248, 249, 255
   insulins in 253
   skin changes in 15
   type 1 252, 253
   type 2 252, 253
Diabetic dermopathy 15
Diabetic hand syndrome 252
Diabetic ketoacidosis 181, 182, 188, 205, 246
Diabetic patient
   examination of 251
   treatment of 252
Diabetic pseudotabes 252
Diabetic rubeosis 15, 249
Dialated veins 219
Diarrhea 180, 185, 246
   causes of
     acute 185
     chronic 186
     large bowel 185
     small bowel 185
Diastolic murmur 127
   early 127f
Dicrotic pulse 116, 116f
Dietetic history 2
Dieulafoy's lesion 185
Diffuse apex 120
Diffusion defect 153
Digestive disorders 210
Digit span test 34
Dilated veins 196
   over abdomen 196
Dilated vessel conduct 125
Diminished movement, causes of 158
Diplopia
   analysis 46
   method of test for 46
   rules of 46
Dipping palpation 200
Disaccharidase deficiency 210
Disorder, site of 189
Displaced apex 120
Displaced apical impulse 121
Dissecting aneurysm 188, 205
Dissociated sensory loss 92

Distal ileopathy 210
Distal muscle wasting 70
Distant vision 38
Dobutamine 150
Doll's eye movement 55
Dome pulse 116
Domestic and marital relationship 2
Dominant hemisphere 102
Dopamine 150
Dorsum of hand 100f
Double outlet right ventricle 140
Down beating nystagmus 50
Downward gaze palsy 53
D-penicillamine 237
Dressing apraxia 37
Dropped head syndrome 68
Drowsiness 33
Drug abuse 2
Drug, groups of 252
Drug-induced rash 16f
Dry skin 259
Dryness 193
Duane's retractor phenomenon 52
Dubin-Johnson syndrome 213
Dupuytren's contracture 19, 190
Duroziez's murmur 135
Dwarfism 5f
   causes of 5
D-xylose test 211
Dysarthria 35, 36, 184
Dysconjugate gaze palsy 54
Dyslipidemia 2, 15, 249
Dysmetria 97
Dyspepsia 184
   alarming features in 184
   functional 184
Dysphagia 35, 180, 182, 183
   duration of 183
   groups of 183
   painful 184
   site of 183
   types of 182
Dysphonia 184
Dyspnea 4, 9, 99, 109, 111, 153, 154, 246, 259
   acute 10
   at rest 155
   change in 10
   clinical types 10
   exertional 10
   in respiratory disease 153
     clinical types of 153
   paroxysm of 10
   severe 10
   threshold 10
   tolerance of 10
Dystonia 89
   types 89
Dystrophia myotonica 19, 20, 58
Dystrophic gait 87

E

Ear 32
   lobe crease 15
Eaten Lambert syndrome 164
Ecadotril 150
Ectopic pregnancy 204
Ectopic thyroid tissue-induced
   thyrotoxicosis 263
Edema 4, 8, 9, 32, 110, 111, 190, 246, 249,
   271, 276, 286
   causes of 8
   clinical demonstration 8
   formation, factors responsible for 8
   generalized 8
   localized 8
   mechanism of 8
   pathogenesis of 8f
   procedure 8
   sites of 8
   treatment of 277
   types of 8
   unilateral 9f
Edinger-Westphal nucleus 38
Efferent lesion 49
Ehlers-Danlos syndrome 12, 13f, 134, 231
Eight and half syndrome 55
Eisenmenger syndrome 141, 142, 145f
   differential diagnosis of 142
Ejection systolic murmur 126, 126f
Ekbom syndrome 90
Elbow joints 228
Electrolyte disturbances 283
Elephantiasis 8f
Elfin facies 20
El-Tor vibrio 185
Emesis 181
Emotional state 33
Emotional stress 170
Emphysema 172, 172t
   types of 172
Empyema 11, 155
Encephalopathy 218
   acute 224
   chronic 224
Encysted effusion 176f
Encysted pleural effusion 176, 179f
Endocrine changes 255
Endocrine diseases, skin markers in 15
Endocrine disorders 3, 208, 248, 254
   symptoms of 245
Endocrine gland 248
Endocrine symptoms 287
Endocrine system 232
   disorders of 254
   examination of 245, 249
Endopeptidase inhibitors 150
Engorged veins 157f
Entamoeba histolytica 186

Enteric anaerobic 166
Enteric fever 2
Enteropathic arthropathy 241
Entrapment neuropathy 250, 258
Enuresis 271
Enzyme dihydrofolate 293
Eosinophil 301
Epiconus 27
Epigastrium 195
Epithelioma 192
Epsilon-aminocaproic acid 298
Epstein-Barr virus 215
Equilibratory coordination, testing 87
Erosive gastritis 184
Erythema multiforme 194
Esophageal disorder 182
Esophageal smooth muscles, disorders of 183
Esophagus 184
    carcinoma 188
    examination of 194
Establish Graves' disease 262
Etanercept 238
Euhydrated hyponatremia 285
Evans syndrome 297
Exanthematous fever and skin 16
Excessive appetite 180, 181
Exertional angina 133
Exertional dyspnea 246
    grading of 10
Extra-alimentary causes 182
Extra-articular manifestation 235
Extracardiac factors 150
Extracorporeal liver
    assist device 225
    perfusion 225
Extrahepatic cholestasis 214
Extraintestinal manifestations 212
Extramedullary hemopoiesis 206
Extramedullary lesion 95
Extramedullary plasmacytoma 301
Extraocular muscles 44t
Extrapyramidal system 26
    disorder, symptoms of 30
Extrapyramidal tracts 23
Eye 32, 164, 235, 249, 272, 288
    changes 227
    field, frontal 53
    movement
        abnormal 45, 50
        horizontal 45f
        normal range of 44
        vertical 44f
    reflex movement of 55
    skew deviation of 50
Eyeball, abducted 47f
Eyelid 100f
    disease of 47
    retraction of lower 48
    retraction of upper 48

F

Fabry's disease 276
Face
    and facial edema 275f
    and neck, partial lipodystrophy of 20f
    angioedema of 14f
    bizarre movement of 90
Facial muscles, abnormal movements to 63
Facial nerve 59, 59f, 63
    functions of 60
Facial palsy
    etiology of 62
    recurrent 63
    symptoms of 60
    types of 61
Fanconis' anemia 297
Fasciculation 90
Fasting blood sugar 265
Fatigue 110
Fatty liver 206
Felty's syndrome 235, 236
Female reproductive system, examination of 251
Femoral arteries, palpation of 200
Femoral hernia 203
Femoral nerve stretch test 230
Fenfluramine 181
Ferrous fumarate 291
Ferrous gluconate 291
Ferrous succinate 291
Ferrous sulfate 291
Festinant gait in parkinsonism 87
Fetor hepaticus 191
Fever 286
    and sweating 154
    in alimentary disorders 189
    in genitourinary disorder 272
    in heart disease 112
    types of 20
Fiber neuropathy
    large 108
    small 108
Fiber sensory neuropathy, large 108
Fibers in posterior column, lamination of 25
Fibrosing alveolitis 3, 216, 227, 236
Fibrosis of lung 167
    anatomical types 167
    clinical features 167
    differential diagnosis 168
    investigation 168
    management 168
    signs 167
Field of vision 38
Finger flexion reflex 83
Finger nose test 86
Finger to finger test 86
First heart sound 123
    clinical abnormality 123

Fisher's one and half syndrome 55
Fixed drug eruption 16f
Fixed monomorphic rhonchi 164
Flaccid dysarthria 36
Flank dullness 205
Flapping tremor 164, 191, 219
Flat chest 156
Flatulence 180, 184
Fleeting arthritis, differential diagnosis of 234
Floppy head syndrome 68
Flow murmur 135
Fluid and electrolyte imbalance 281
Fluid imbalance, correction of 282
Fluid overload states 149
Focal dystonia 89
Focal segmental glomerulosclerosis 274
Foetor hepaticus 219
Folate deficiency 293
Folic acid 210, 292
    deficiency 291
Follicular tonsillitis, acute 194
Food
    containing iron 291
    type of 183
Footdrop 230
Foramen ovale 138
Forcible apex beat 121
Forefoot 230
Foreign body 164
Fothergill's disease 59
Foville's syndrome 52, 62, 63
Frey's syndrome 59
Friction rub 203
Friedreich's ataxia 85, 93, 98, 105
Friedreich's sign 120
Fröhlich syndrome 245
Frontal lobe 27
    lesion 26, 33
Fronto-ponto-cerebellar tract 26
Fulminant hepatocellular failure 215, 223, 225
    nonparacetamol induced 225
    paracetamol induced 225
Fur on tongue 181

G

Gag reflex 66
Gaisbock's syndrome 289
Gait 87, 230
    abnormalities of 87, 230t
    bilateral, high stepping 87
    high stepping 87
    in hyperkinesias 87
    unilateral, high stepping 87
Galactorrhea 247, 255
Gallbladder 195
    carcinoma of 199
    mucocele of 199
    palpation of 199

Gardener's syndrome 15
Gastric antral vascular ectasia syndrome 185
Gastric ulcer 184, 231
Gastric varices 184
Gastric visible peristalsis 196
Gastroesophageal reflux disease 152
Gastrointestinal bleeding, upper 184, 222
    symptoms 180
Gastrointestinal loss 285
Gastrointestinal symptoms 246, 286
    lower 180, 185
Gastrointestinal tract 250, 251, 256, 258, 260, 289
Gattron's papules of dermatomyositis 243f
Gaucher's disease 206, 207
Gaze movement, cortical centers for 43
Gaze palsy 53
    downward 53
    lateral 53
    upward 53
    vertical 53
Gegenhalten phenomenon 73
Gemfibrozil 271
Geniculate body, lateral 39
Geniculocalcarine fibers 38
Genitalia, examination of external 203, 273
Genitourinary symptoms 287
Genitourinary system 227, 231, 255, 289
Geographical tongue 193
Giant cell arteritis 242
Gibbus deformity 98
Gibson's murmur 128
Gigantism 5
Gilbert's syndrome 213
Gilles de La Tourette syndrome 90
Gingival recession 192
Gingivitis 192
Glabellar reflex 86
Glabellar tap 61
Glanzmann's thrombasthenia 288f, 296
Glassy nail 12
Glibenclamide 252
Gliclazide 252
Glimepiride 252
Glipizide 252
Globus hystericus 67
Globus pharyngeus 180
Glomerular damage, control of 277
Glomerular disease 278
    primary 274
Glomerular hematuria 270
Glomerular proteinuria 270t
Glomerulonephritis 147
    rapidly progressive 274
Glomerulonephritis, acute 274, 275f, 278
    clinical features of 275
    complications of 275
    investigations 275
    management 275
    pathogenesis 274
    prognosis 275
Glomus jugulare 65
Glossopharyngeal nerve 65
Glossopharyngeal neuralgia 67
Glossopharyngeal reflex 66
Glove and stocking analgesia 96f
Glucocorticoid deficiency 265
Gluteal enthesopathy 228
Gluteal tendinitis 228
Glycogen storage disease 206, 207
Goiter 257f
Good Pasteur's syndrome 153
Goodpasture's syndrome 274, 278
Gordon's sign 82
Gottron's papule 19
Gouty arthritis 233f
Gradenigo's syndrome 52, 53, 59
Graham-Steel murmur 128
Gram-negative septicemia 219
Granulomatous aortitis 208, 235
Graphesthesia 94
Grasp reflex 86
Graves' disease 249, 260, 260f, 261
    acropachy in 261f
    differential diagnosis of 262
    etiology 260
Greater auricular nerve 56
Groin and external genitalia, inspection of 197
Groin lump, differential diagnosis of 203
Growth hormone 254
Growth retardation 272
Guillain-Barré syndrome 58, 104, 108
Gum 192
    features to 192
    hyperplasia 272
    hypertrophy 193, 289
Gustatory hyperhidrosis 245
Gut hormones 252
Gynecomastia 165, 219, 247
    in boy 248f
Gynoid obesity 5

H

Hair 17, 32, 249, 286
    causes 17
    examination of 17
    graying of 17
    loss of 218f, 219, 246
    over abdomen 196
    premature graying 17
Hairy leukoplakia 193, 193f
Half-half nail 12
Halitosis 165, 180
    causes 181
Hallervorden-Spatz disease 90
Hallucination 33
Ham test 294
Hand 4, 228
    deformities of 228
    disease 19
    in rheumatoid arthritis 234
Handedness 33
Hand-foot-mouth disease 13f, 192f
Hansen's disease 106, 107, 232, 234, 236
Harrison's sulcus 156
Hartnup disease 98, 210
Hashimoto's thyroiditis 251
Headache 30, 104, 246
    extracranial 30
    intracranial 30
    mechanism 30
Hearing
    decreased 259
    defective 250
Heart
    borders, percussion of 122
    defect in 7
    disease 111
        congenital 137
    failure
        acute 148
        chronic 148
        clinical evaluation of 148
        clinical features 149
        congestive 140, 141
        diastolic 148
        etiology of 148, 149
        left sided 149
        pathophysiology 148
        right sided 149
        systolic 148
        types of 148
    left border of 122
    sound 119f, 123
        accentuated 122
        fourth 124
        in cardiac cycle 125f
        intensity first 123
        second 123
        soft first 123
        third 124
        wide split of 2nd 124
Heartburn 180, 182
Heaving apical impulse 121
Heberden's node 19, 228
Heel knee test 86
Heel pain, causes of 229
Heerfordt syndrome 64
Heliotropic rash 243f
Helminthiasis 188
Hematemesis 184, 185
Hematochezia 180, 186
Hematological diseases, skin in 16
Hematological disorders 31, 205

Hematological values 301
Hematuria 269
　causes of 269
　differential diagnoses of 270
Hemianalgesia, total 95f
Hemianopia 39
Hemiballismus 89
Hemifacial atrophy 70f
Hemiplegia 75, 87
　causes of 102
　clinical evaluation of 100
　localization of 101
　recurrent 102
Hemiplegic gait 87
Hemispheric lesion 102
Hemithorax pulsation, right 120
Hemochromatosis 190, 192
Hemodialysis 282
Hemodynamic changes 148
Hemodynamic obstruction 129
Hemoglobin values, normal 302
Hemoglobinuria 270
Hemolytic anemia 6, 240, 294
　clinical features 294
　etiology 294
　investigations 294
　pathogenesis 294
　treatment 295
Hemolytic crisis 295
Hemolytic facies 19
Hemolytic jaundice 213
Hemolytic uremic syndrome 294
Hemophilia disease 287
Hemophilia-A 298
　clinical features 298
　complication 299
　diagnosis 298
　investigation 298
　treatment 298
Hemopoietic system
　disorders of 290
　examination of 286, 287
Hemoptysis 110, 153, 185
　causes for 153
Hemorrhagic ascites, causes of 208
Hemorrhagic disorders 296
Hemorrhagic pericardial effusion, causes of 146
Hemostasis 296
Hemostatic balance 296
Henoch-Schonlein purpura 188, 216, 274, 287, 287f
Hepatic amebiasis 206
Hepatic bruit 203
Hepatic calcification, causes of 207
Hepatic complications 215
Hepatic dullness, obliteration of 205
Hepatic edema 9

Hepatic encephalopathy 223
　acute 223
　chronic 223
　clinical features 223
　diagnosis of 224
　differential diagnosis of 224
　etiology 223
　grading of 224
　mechanism of 224f
　precipitating factors for 219
　subclinical 223
　types of 223
Hepatic fibrosis, congenital 220
Hepatic rub, causes of 203
Hepatitis
　A virus 215
　acute 206
　B virus 215
　C virus 215
　chronic 215, 216
　　active 216, 236
　　etiology 216
　　investigations 216
　　pathological types 216
　D virus 215
　E virus 215
　G virus 215
　management of chronic 216
　viruses 217
Hepatobiliary disease, symptoms of 180
Hepatocellular carcinoma 219
Hepatocellular disease, acute 180
Hepatocellular failure 181
　chronic 225
　complications of fulminant 224
　investigations 224
　management 224
Hepatocellular jaundice 6, 213, 214
Hepatojugular reflex 118
Hepatomegaly, differential diagnosis of 206
　irregular 206
　massive 206
　mild 206
　moderate 206
　pathogenesis of 206
Hepatorenal syndrome 219
Hepatosplenomegaly
　differential diagnosis of 207
　with anemia, causes of 207
　with ascites, causes of 207
　with fever, causes of 207
　with jaundice, causes of 207
　with leeding tendency, causes of 207
　with lymphadenopathy, causes of 207
Hereditary angioedema 188
Hereditary ataxia 98
Hereditary hemorrhagic telangiectasia 15, 184, 296f

Hereditary spherocytosis 295
　clinical features 295
　complication 295
　diagnosis 295
　differential diagnosis 295
　investigations 295
　pathogenesis 295
　treatment 296
Hereditary-Wiskott-Aldrich syndrome 297
Heredofamilial disease 276
Hernias 203
Herpes simplex
　labialis 192
　virus 215
Herpes zoster 188, 205
Herpetic gingivostomatitis 193f
　acute 193
Hess test 287f
Heubner's artery 29
Hilar adenopathy, bilateral 178f
Hill's sign 22, 135
Hindfoot 230
Hip
　abduction, abnormality of 230
　arthropathy 230
　joint 228
　measurement 5
Hippocratic facies 19, 204
Hippus 48
　causes 48
Hirschsprung's disease 186
Hirsutism 17, 245
Hoarseness 259
　of voice 154, 164, 184, 246, 250
Hodgkin's lymphoma 21, 286
Hoffman syndrome 258
Hoffmann's sign 85
Hoffmann's syndrome 247, 250
Holmes-Adie's syndrome 49
Homocystinuria 5
Hormone deficiency, isolated 256
Horn cell, anterior 104
Horner's syndrome 19, 43, 47-49, 49f, 101, 102, 164
　bilateral 48
　complete 43
　incomplete 43
Hospital-acquired pneumonia 165
Huebner's artery 29
Human leukocyte antigen, basis of 282
Huntington's chorea 34
Hydration 4, 11
Hydropneumothorax 175
　left side 175f
Hydrostatic pressure 8
Hydrothorax, causes of 175
Hyperacute hepatocellular failure 223
Hyperbilirubinemia, isolated 214

Hypercalcemia 188, 299
  differential diagnosis of 267
  management of 268
Hypercalciuria 267
Hypercellular bone marrow 293
Hyperkalemia 284
  clinical features 284
  etiology 284
  pathogenesis 284
  principles of management 284
Hyperkinetic dysarthria 36
Hyperkinetic portal hypertension 220
Hyperkinetic pulmonary
  blood flow 140
  hypertension 144
Hypernatremia 285
  correction of 285
Hyperparathyroidism 267
  causes 267
Hyperplasia 268
Hyperpyrexia 20, 21
Hyper-reflexia, signs of 85
Hypertelorism 112f
Hypertension 2, 144, 145
  accelerated 22
  cause for 254
  control of 275
  dyslipidemia 3
  malignant 22
  pregnancy-induced 272
Hypertensive congestive heart failure 276
Hypertensive emergency 22
Hypertensive patient
  examination of 253
  monitoring of 254
Hyperthyroidism 249
  types of 261
Hypertonia 73
Hypertrichosis 17
Hypertrophic osteoarthropathy 155, 232
Hypoadrenalism 264
  clinical features 265
  etiology 264
  investigations 265
Hypoalbuminemia 9, 208, 218, 276
  correction of 277
Hypocalcemia, differential diagnosis of 266
Hypogastric ganglion 106
Hypogastric plexus
  inferior 106
  superior 106
Hypogastrium 195
Hypoglossal nerve 68
  arises 68
Hypoglossal palsy, symptoms of 68
Hypoglycemia 247
Hypokalemia 250, 283
  causes 283
  clinical features 283

diagnosis 283
  treatment of 283
Hypokinetic dysarthria 36
Hyponatremia 258, 285
  clinical features 285
  clinical types 285
  correction of 285
  etiology 285
  in over hydrated 285
  mechanism 285
Hyponatremic disorders 284
Hypoparathyroidism 266
  causes of 266
Hypopigmented lesions 14
Hypopituitarism 256
  etiology 256
  investigations 257
  management 257
Hyporeflexia, causes of 85
Hyposmia 37
Hypothalamic disorder 181
  primary 245
Hypothalamic tumors 254
Hypothalamo-pituitary tumors 31
Hypothermia 20, 21
Hypothyroid cases 259
Hypothyroidism 19, 31, 33, 250, 257, 258f
  clinical features 257
  differential diagnosis of 259
  etiology 257
  goitrous 257
  juvenile 258
  non-goitrous 257
  presentation of primary 258
  primary 257, 260t
  secondary 260t
  subclinical 257
  symptoms of 259
Hypotonia 72
  causes 73
Hypovolemia 114
Hypoxemia 7
  without cyanosis 7
Hysterical gait 88

I

Ideational apraxia 37
Ideomotor apraxia 36
Idiopathic cyclical edema 9
Idiopathic pulmonary hemosiderosis 153
Idiopathic thrombocytopenic purpura 297
  acute 297
  chronic 297
  clinical features 297
  differential diagnosis 297
  investigations 297
  pathogenesis 297
  refractory 298
  treatment 297

Ileocecal tuberculosis 213
Iliac fossa
  left 195, 201
  right 195, 201
Iliopectineal bursitis 229
Illness, course of 2
Illusion 33
Imerslunds syndrome 291
Immune thrombocytopenic purpura 192, 297
Immunologic phenomena 147
Impalpable apex 158
  beat 121
Impotence 248
Individual muscles, testing 45
Infantile hypothyroidism 258
Infection
  myonecrosis 194
  source of 166
Infective endocarditis 11, 146, 147, 205, 236
  clinical features 147
  etiological factors 147
  investigations 147
  management 148
  markers of 111
  pathology 146
Infiltrative lesions 220
Inflammatory bowel disease 185, 205, 211, 212, 227
  clinical features 211
  differential diagnosis of 212
  etiology 211
  pathology 211
Inflammatory disease 256
Inflammatory pain 226
Infliximab 238
Inguinal group 18
Inguinal hernia 203
  direct 203
  indirect 203
Inhaled allergens 170
Inspiratory dyspnea 246
Insulin 253
  aspart 253
  degludec 253
  detemir 253
  glargine 253
  glulisine 253
  preparations, action of 253
Intercostal neuralgia 164
Intercostal pulsation 120
Interlobar effusion 130
Intermittent colic 187
Intermittent fever, types of 20
Intermittent porphyria 188
Internal capsule 23
  blood supply of 29
Internal malignancy 188, 205
  skin markers in 15

Internal mammary artery 128
Internuclear ophthalmoplegia 54
   inferior 54
   superior 54
Interpupillary distance, increase in 112f
Interstitial lung disease 11, 155
Interstitial nephritis, acute 278
Interstitial nucleus of Cajal 43
Interventricular septum, development of 139f
Intestinal manifestation 211, 212
Intestinal obstruction 202
Intestinal tuberculosis 210
Intestinal ulcer 231
Intestinal visible peristalsis, small 196
Intracranial hemorrhage 147
Intracranial pressure, increased 255
Intrahepatic cholestasis 214
Intramedullary lesion 95, 96f
Intraorbital portion 43
Intrapartum, history of 3
Intrarenal obstruction 278
Involuntary movements 88
Iodine-induced thyrotoxicosis 263
Ipratropium bromide 171
Iritis 190
Iron 210
   kinetic study 219
   therapy, good response of 291
Iron-deficiency anemia 181, 290, 290t
   clinical features 291
   investigations 291
   management 291
Ischemic optic neuritis, anterior 38
Ischiogluteal bursitis 229

J

Jack in box tongue 89
Jacobson's neuralgia 67
Janeway lesion 111, 147
Jargon aphasia 36
Jaundice 4, 6, 7f, 32, 190, 190f, 218f, 286
   biochemical types of 214
   clinical evaluation of 213
   history taking in 214
   mechanism 6
   obstructive 6
   pathogenesis of 213
   patient, examination of 214
   types of 213, 215
Jaw jerk 57, 83
Jaw, opening of 57
Jendrassik maneuver 83
Jerky pulse, high volume 116
Jod basedow phenomenon 263
Joint
   hyperextensibility of 231f
   hypermobility of 231

involvement
   pattern of 226, 234
   precipitating factors for 226
metacarpophalangeal 200, 230
metatarsophalangeal 233f
tenderness, assessment of 227
Jones criteria 241
Jugular venous pressure 113, 117, 118f
   decreased 118
   measurement of 117, 118f
Jugular venous pulsation 117, 119, 119f, 142
   clinical abnormality of 119
   physiology of 119
Junctional rhythm 130

K

Kala-azar 206, 207, 236
Kallmann's syndrome 37
Kartagener's syndrome 169
Kawasaki disease 242
Kayser-Fleischer ring 190
Keratoconjunctivitis sicca 235
Keratoderma blenorrhagica 227
Kernig's sign 98
Ketotifen 171
Kidney 195, 252
   disease
      acute 274
      chronic 274
   examination of 269, 272
   injury, acute 274
   palpation of 200
   percussion of 202
Kikuchi's disease 19
Kinesia paradoxa 87
Klebsiella 166, 167
   pneumoniae 166
Klinefelter's syndrome 5, 20, 245, 247
Klippel feil syndrome 98
Knee 230
   jerk 84, 84f
      hung up 84
   joint 229
Knuckle deformity 98
Knuckle pigmentation 288f
Koilonychia 4, 12
Koplik's spots 194
Korotkoff's sounds 22, 115
Korsakoff's psychosis 37
Kronig's isthmus 159
Kugelberg-Welander syndrome 70
Kussmaul's breathing 22, 156
Kussmaul's pulse 114
Kussmaul's sign 120

L

Labyrinthine 182
   lesion 65
Lamina cribrosa 41

Laryngeal nerve
   palsy, recurrent 67
   superior 67
Laryngeal spasm 67
Laryngeal stridor 154
Lassegue's sign 230
Laurence-Moon-Biedl syndrome 42
Lawrence-Moon-Bardet-Biedel
   syndrome 112f
Lead poisoning 188
Leflunomide 237
Left diaphragm, eventration of 178f
Left eye, partial ptosis of 49f
Left iliac fossa, colon in 198
Left nostril, rhinosporidiosis of 156f
Leg 230
   muscle, wasting of 72f
   purpura 287f
   raising test, straight 230
   ulcers 286
Legionella 166, 167
   pneumoniae 166
Lenalidomide 301
Leonine facies 19
Leptospirosis 3, 214, 216
Lermoyez's syndrome 65
Lesch-Nyhan syndrome 292, 293
Lesion
   at cavernous sinus 58
   at gasserian ganglion 58
   at superior orbital fissure 58
   extramedullary 107t
   extrinsic 183
   for hemiplegia 101f
   in apraxia 37
   in visual pathway 39
   intramedullary 107t
   intrinsic 183
   of cauda equina 107t
   of conus medullaris 107t
   over eye, pigmented 7f
Lesser-Trelat sign 15
Lethargy 259
Leuconychia 12, 219
Leukemia, acute 286
Leukocyte count, differential 301
Leukopenia 240
Leukoplakia 193
Levator palpebrae superioris, testing 47
Lhermitte's syndrome 54
Libman-Sack's endocarditis 239
Life threatening
   infection 16
   signs 170
Ligament of trietz 184
Light reflex 49
   direct 49
   indirect 49
   pathway 38

Limb
  lower 71
  upper 71
Lindsay nail 12
Lingua nigra 193
Lip 191
  angioedema of 14f
  ulcer of 192
Lipid profile 253
Lipoma 201
Lipoprotein deficiency 98
Livedo reticularis 239
Liver 100, 195
  biopsy 219
  consistency of 207
  disease 7, 31, 212, 223
    chronic 14, 188
    decompensated 190
    signs of chronic 191f
  dullness 201
  function test 236
  lower border 195
  malignancy of 206, 207
  palpation of 198, 198f
  percussion of 201
  span 201
  support, artificial 225
  upper border 195
Lobe fibrosis, upper 167
Lobes, surface marking of 152
Lobular hepatitis, chronic 216
Locomotor symptoms 226
Locomotor system 112, 289
  examination 227
Louis Bar syndrome 98
Lower gastrointestinal bleeding, causes of 186
Lower limb
  left 9f
  muscles of 80f
  testing tone in 72
Lower motor neuron 24, 54
  facial palsy 62t
    bilateral 62, 63
    unilateral 61, 62
  lesion 24
Lower quadrant homonymous defect 39
Lower respiratory tract infection, acute 152
Lumbar region
  left 195
  right 195
Lundh test 211
Lung
  abscess 153
    causes 167
    clinical features 167
    investigations 167
    management 167
    predisposing factors 167

active collapse of 168
collapse of 168
  causes of 169
  investigations 169
  management 169
defect in 7
disease 234
malignancy, bronchial asthma 152
nodular lesion of 178f
sequestration of 151
syndrome, small 239
Lupus nephropathy, WHO classification of 239
Lutz internuclear ophthalmoplegia 54
Lyme arthritis 234
Lymph node 190
  enlargement 4, 155, 249
    causes of 18
  examination of 17
  mass 289
Lymphadenopathy 18, 32, 286
  localized 19
Lymphocyte 301
Lymphoma 211
Lyspro insulin 253

M

Maccallum patch 130
Macroglassia 258f
Macronodular cirrhosis 206
Macula 41
  lutea fovea 41
Macular rash 21f
Malabsorbed substance 210
Malabsorption 267
  diarrhea 185
Malabsorption syndrome 188, 190, 210
  clinical features 210
  etiology 210
  investigations 210
  pathogenesis 210
Malaria 20
  chronic 206
Male reproductive system, examination of 251
Mallory-Weiss syndrome 184
Mandibular division 56
Maniacal chorea 89
Mantoux test 177
Marcus Gunn pupil 49
Marcus-Gunn phenomenon, reverse 63
Marfan's index 5
Marfan's syndrome 5, 19, 20, 112f, 131, 134, 135, 137, 144, 174, 231
Marin-Amat syndrome 63, 64
Massive pericardial effusion 161
Massive pulmonary embolism 153
Massive splenomegaly 161, 206
Mastication, muscles of 57f

Maxillary division 56
May-Hegglin anomaly 297
McCune-Albright's syndrome 248
Measles 2
Mechanical dysphagia, causes of 183
Mechanical ventilation, indication of 172, 173
Medial rectus palsy, right 42f
Median rhomboid glossitis 193
Mediastinal group 18
Mediastinal mass, anterior 178f
Mediastinal pleura 152
Medulla 23
Medullary lesion, lateral 95f
Medullary syndrome, lateral 95, 102
Mee's lines 12
Megaloblastic anemia 14, 19, 31, 288f, 291, 293
  classification 291
  treatment 293
Megaloblastic crisis 295
Meige's syndrome 64
Meissner's corpuscles 24
Melanoma, malignant 16f
Melena 180, 186
Melkersson syndrome 64
Membranoprolifeative glomerulonephritis 275
Membranous nephropathy 274
Memory 33
  disorder of 34
Meniere's disease 65
Meningeal irritation, signs of 98
Menorrhagia-blood loss 3
Menstrual history 3, 248
Mental neuropathy, isolated 58
Merkel's disc 24
Mesalazine 213
Mesenteric artery
  superior 203
  thrombosis 188
Mesenteric occlusion 188
Metabolic acidosis, correction of 282
Metabolic coma 100
Metabolic disease 2, 98
Metabolic disorders 53, 205
Metabolic pathways 292
Metastatic nodule 157
Methemoglobinemia 7
Methotrexate 167, 213, 237
Methylxanthines 171
Meyer's loop 38
Microalbuminuria 253, 270
Microaneurysm 41
Microcytic hypochromic anemia 290f
Micturition
  disorders of 271
  reflex 106, 106f
  symptoms of 271

Midabdomen 204
Midbrain 23
Midclavicular line 201
Mid-diastolic murmur 125, 127, 128
Midfoot 230
Migraine 30, 33
   complicated 30
Migratory thrombophlebitis 15
Miliaria 21
Milking sign 89
Millard-Gubler syndrome 52, 62, 63
Miller-Fisher syndrome 51
Milrinone 150
Milroy's edema 9
Mimic facial palsy 62
Mineralocorticoid deficiency 265
Miosis 48
   causes 48
Mitral facies 129
Mitral opening 125
Mitral regurgitation 131
   auscultatory signs of 132f
   clinical features 131
   complications 132
   etiology 131
   investigations 132
   management 132
   pathophysiology 131
Mitral stenosis 129, 135, 153
   complications of 130
   etiology 129
   hemodynamic 129
   pathophysiology 129
   severity of 130
Mitral valve
   calcification of 130
   prolapse 131, 132
      clinical features 132
      complications 133
      management 133
      pathogenesis 132
Mitral valvular disease 133
Mobility, absence of 251
Moebius disease 52
Moebius syndrome 52, 64
Moistness 193
Mollaret's triangle 67
Monckeberg's medial calcific sclerosis 117
Mongolism 259
Monilial stomatitis 194
Monoarthritis 226
   acute 232
   chronic 232
   differential diagnosis of 233
Mononeuritis 25
   cranialis 25
   multiplex 25
Mononeuropathy 25
Mono-ocular diplopia 46

Monoplegia 75
Morquio syndrome 98
Motility disorder 185, 251
Motor aphasia 36
Motor component 58
Motor cortex 23
Motor dysphagia, causes of 183, 184
Motor function 57
Motor neuron disease 184
Motor nucleus 56, 65, 66
Motor paralytic bladder 106
Motor root 56
Motor supply 56
Motor symptoms 103
Motor system 23, 101, 104
   disorder, symptoms of 30
   examination of 69
Mouth 32, 289
   and throat, examination of 191
   bizarre movement of 90
   ulcers 192f
Mucoid sputum 153
Mucopolysaccharidosis 5f, 19, 20, 134
Mucosa 211
Mucosal ulcer 227, 272
Mucous gland, retention cyst of 192
Mucous membrane lesions 227
Mucoviscidosis 205
Muller's muscle 43
Multiple black macules 12f
Multiple extrasystole 114
Multiple hydatid cyst 177f
Multiple myeloma 299, 300f, 301
   classification 299
   clinical features 299
   diagnosis 300
   investigations 300
   pathogenesis 299
   variant forms of 300
Multiple punched out lytic lesions 300f
Multiple sclerosis 33
Multiple umbilicated papules 16f
Multisystem diseases with arthritis 234
Mumps 2
   virus 215
Murmur 123, 125
   depending on site, differential diagnosis of 128
   description of 125
Murphy's sign 199
Muscle
   action of 56
   bulk of 69
   cramps 247
   disease 104
   hypertrophy of 72, 247, 250
   individual 44f
   inferior
      oblique 46
      rectus 46

   lateral rectus 46
   medial rectus 46
   observe wasting of 57
   power, grading of 73
   stretch reflex 82
      disorders of 85
      grading of 83
      hyperactivity of 85
      of lower limb 84
      of upper limb 83
   superior
      oblique 46
      rectus 46
   tone of 72
   wasting of 70, 71, 219
   weakness 74, 247, 250
      clinical signs of 46t
Muscular pains 259
Musculoskeletal system, examination of 226
Myasthenia gravis 58, 184
Myasthenic facies 19
Myasthenic syndrome 164
Myasthenic weakness 75
Mycophenolate mofetil 282
Mycoplasma pneumoniae 166
Mycotic aneurysm 147
Mydriasis 48
   causes 48
Myelodysplastic syndrome 293
Myelofibrosis 206
Myeloid leukemia, chronic 206
Myeloma 236
Myelopathy 108
Myelophthisic anemia 297
Myerson's sign 61
Myocardial infarction 188
Myocardial remodeling 148
Myoclonus 218
   abrupt 90
Myocyte loss 148
Myoedema 73
   causes 73
Myoglobin, presence of 271
Myoglobinuria 271
Myokimia 90
   etiology 90
Myopathic weakness 75
Myopathy 226
Myositis 226
Myotatic irritability 73
Myotonia 73
   causes 73
Myotonic disorders 19
Myotonic dystrophy 184
Myotonic reflex 85
Myxedema 15, 20, 249
   madness 258
Myxoma 127

N

Nail 190, 272, 288
   changes 227
   clubbing 4
   discoloration of 12
   examination of 11
   growth 12
   pitting of 12
Nailbed infarct 12
Nailfold telangiectasis 12
Nasal spine, posterior 151
Nasal ulcers 240
Nasobronchial allergy 3
Near vision 38
Neck 249
   rigidity 98
      causes of 98
   short 5f
Necrobiosis diabeticorum 15
Necrobiosis lipoidica diabeticorum 249
Necrolytic migratory erythema, acute 15
Nedocromil sodium 171
Nelson's syndrome 14, 246, 264
Neomycin 210
Neonatal thyrotoxicosis 262
Neoplasms 206
Nephritic syndrome, acute 273
Nephritis 231
Nephrolithiasis 274
Nephropathy, minimal change 274
Nephrotic syndrome 208, 235, 259, 274, 276, 299
   clinical features 277
   complications 277
   congenital 276
   etiology 276
   investigations 277
   management 277
   pathogenesis 276
Nerve
   accessory 67
   biopsy 242
   causes of thickening 99
   deafness 65
      causes of 65
   fascicle 43
   fiber
      classification of 108
      infarct, superficial 239
   functions of 5th 56
   lesion
      clinical signs of 3rd 45
      clinical signs of 4th 45
      clinical signs of 6th 46
   palsy
      causes of 3rd 51
      left 3rd 47f

Nervous system 3, 164, 205, 231, 235, 250, 252, 255, 258, 289
   disorder 29, 31
      general examination in 31
   examination 23, 32, 99, 101, 104
   symptoms 246
Nervus intermedius 60
Neural dysfunction 248
Neuralgia 67
Neuroanatomy 37, 38, 43
Neurocutaneous diseases 15
Neurocutaneous syndrome 32
Neurodegenerative disease 2
Neuroendocrine 31
Neurogenic bladder 105
   symptoms of 106
   types of 106
Neurohumoral stimuli 11
Neurologic involvement 240
Neurological signs 100
Neuromuscular and muscle lesion 85
Neuromuscular junction cause 104
Neurovascular syndromes 102
Neutrocytic ascites, culture negative 209
Neutrophil 301
Nicotine staining of finger 155, 157f
Night pain 226
Nocturia 247
Nocturnal asthma 171
Nocturnal cough 153
Nodular lesion 16f
Nominal aphasia 36
Nonarticular rheumatic features 235
Noncirrhotic portal fibrosis 220
Noncompressive myelopathy 104
Nondominant hemisphere 102
Nonejection click 125
Nonequilibratory coordination, testing 86
Nonglomerular hematuria 270
Nonhemolytic jaundice, congenital 214
Nonhepatic complications 216
Noninvasive ventilation, indications for 173
Nonoliguric renal failure 278
Nonparalytic squint 47
Nonpitting edema 8f
Nonpulsatile engorged jugular vein 118f
Nonscarring alopecia 240
Nonsecretory myeloma 301
Nonselective proteinuria 270
Non-sulfonylurea insulin 252
Nonulcer dyspepsia 184
Nonvariceal bleed, management of 222
Nonviral hepatitis 214
Normosthenia 4
Nourishment 5
Nuclear column, unpaired 42

Nuclear lesion 43
   at pons 58
Nutritional anemia, chronic 207
Nystagmus 49
   testing 50

O

Obesity
   grades of 5
   types of 5
Oblique myokymia, superior 51
Oblique tendon, superior 227
Obliterative pulmonary 144
Obstetric history 3
Obstruction, causes of 127
Obstructionat porta hepatis 220
Obstructive pulmonary disease, chronic 145, 152, 172, 205, 287
   clinical features 172
   complications 173
   etiopathogenesis of 172
   investigations 173
   management 173
   pathological changes 172
   signs 172
   therapy 173t
Occipital gaze center 43
Occipital lobe 27
   lesion 33
Occupational history 3
Occupational respiratory disease 3
Ocular apraxia 51
Ocular bobbing 50
Ocular dysmetria 50
Ocular flutter 51
Ocular motor
   nerves 42
   system, symptoms of 44
Ocular movement
   physiology of 44
   slow 51
   testing 44
   types of 44
Ocular muscle 44
Ocular myoclonus 50
Ocular signs 261
Ocular symptoms 247
Oculocephalic reflex 55
Oculofacial diplegia 52
Oculogyric crisis 50
Oculomotor nerve 42
Oculopharyngeal myopathy 184
Odor 182
Odynophagia 184
Olecranon bursitis 228
Olfactory nerve 37
   clinical disorders of 37

Oligoarthritis
    differential diagnosis of 233
    disease 226
Oliguria 269
    in acute renal failure, mechanism of 279
Omonymous hemianopia 39
Onychomyosis 12
Ophthalmic area 56
Ophthalmic division 56
Ophthalmoplegia 104, 250
    clinical approach to 51
    duration of 53
    etiology of 52
    external 51
    internal 51
    painful 53
    total 51
Oppenheim's sign 82
Opsoclonus 51
Optic atrophy 42
    causes 42
    primary 42
    secondary 42
Optic disc 41
Optic fundus examination 41
Optic nerve 38, 104, 250
Optic neuritis 39, 42, 164
Optic pathways 38f
Optic radiation 38, 39
Optic tract 39
Optica-Devic's disease 104
Optokinetic nystagmus 50
Oral antidiabetic drugs 253
Oral iron therapy 291
Oral lichen planus 194
Oral ulcers 240
Orbicularis oculi 61
Orbicularis oris 61
    reflex 61
Orbital fissure, superior 43
Organic causes 184
Organic disease 33
Orofaciolingual dyskinesia 69, 90
Oropharyngeal disorder 182
Oropharyngeal ulcer 231
Oropharynx 151
    swelling of 194
Orthopnea 10
    mechanism 10
Ortner's syndrome 130
Osalazine 213
Oscillating intracardiac mass 147
Oscillopsia 51
Osler's node 15, 19, 111, 147
Osler's sign 7f
Osmotic diarrhea 185
Osmotic pressure 8
Ovarian cyst 202
    large 202

Ovarian tumor 201
Overnight joint swelling 234
Overt albuminuria 270

P

Pain 226
    character of 204
    deep 93
    types of 94
Palatal paralysis 66
Palm of hand, vesicular lesion on 13f
Palmar crease, pallor of 19
Palmar erythema 190, 218, 219, 227
Palmar tylosis 15
Palmomental reflex 61, 86
Palmoplantar keratoderma 15
Palpable gallbladder, causes of 199
Palpable kidney, causes of 200
Palpable left kidney 200
Palpable liver 206
Palpable mass in rectum, causes of 204
Palpable peripheral nerves 99
Palpable rhonchi 159
Palpable shock 122
Palpating respiratory movement 158f
Palpitation 109
    mechanism 109
Palsy
    bilateral 67
    unilateral 67
    upward gaze 53
Pancoast's tumor 164
Pancreas, carcinoma head of 199
Pancreatic disease, symptoms of 180
Pancreatitis 231
Pancytopenia 293
    differential diagnosis of 293
Pandiastolic murmur 127
Pansystolic murmur 126
Paper money skin 190
Papillary muscle dysfunction 132
Papilledema 41
Paracentesis abdominis 219
Paradoxical triceps reflex 83
Paragonimus westermani 153
Paralysis
    neural pattern of 78
    of insane 33
Paralytic chorea 89
Paralytic dysphagia 183
Paralytic squint 47
Paraneoplastic syndrome 98
Paraplegia
    acute 104
    chronic 104
    etiology of 104
    in extension 105
    in flexion 105
    recurrent 104

Parasternal heave, left 121
Parasympathetic nucleus 65
Parathormone 266
    actions of 266
Paratonia 73
Parenchymal fibrosis, etiology of 167
Parenchymal liver disease, acute 214
Parenchymal source 153
Parenteral iron therapy 291
Paresthesia 259
Parietal lobe 27, 96
    function 94
Parietal pleura 152
Parkinson's syndrome 49
Parotid enlargement 219
Paroxysmal cough 153
Paroxysmal nocturnal dyspnea 10
    mechanism 10
Parry-Romberg syndrome 70f
Past illness, history of 2
Patella syndrome 276
Patellar clonus 85
Patent ductus arteriosus 140
    associated anomalies 141
    clinical features 140
    complications 141
    etiology 140
    investigations 141
    management 141
    severity of 141
Pauciarticular disease 226
Pectoral girdle muscles, wasting of 72f
Pectus carinatum 156
Pectus excavatum 156
Pedal edema 9, 155
Pegion chest 156
Pel-Ebstein's fever 21
Pellagra 15
Pelvis 201
Pemberton's sign 250
Pendular knee jerk 84
Pendular nystagmus 49
Pentalogy of Fallot 143
Percussion notes, types of 161
Perfusion defect 153
Periarthritis shoulder 252
Periarticular lesions 228
Pericardial disease 145, 207
    causes of 146
    clinical features 146
    clinical types 145
    depends on duration 145
    investigations 146
    management 146
Pericardial effusion 145f
Pericardial fluid, aspiration of 146
Pericardial rub 122, 123, 128
Pericardium, inflammation of 146
Perihilar flare 130

Periodic lingual numbness 58
Periorbital edema 9f
Peripartum cardiomyopathy 3
Peripheral cyanosis 7, 19
    etiopathogenesis 7
    types 7
Peripheral extensor plantar response 82
Peripheral lesion 25, 50
Peripheral nerve 84, 94, 99
    causes of 99
    innervation 91f, 92f
    involvement 108
    lesions, common 97f
    thickened 108
Peripheral nervous system 106
Peripheral neuropathy 25, 106, 108, 164, 216
    hysteria 96f
    with cerebellar involvement 108
    with cranial nerve involvement 108
Peripheral pulsation 117
    absence of 117
Peripheral vascular disease 117
Peritoneal dialysis 282
Peritoneal disease 208
Peritonitis 204
Pernicious anemia 205
Peroneal muscular atrophy 72f
Persistent asthma, chronic 170
Persistent hepatitis, chronic 216
Persistent pain 226
Peutz-Jeghers syndrome 192, 194
Phantom limb 92
Phantom sensation 92
Pharyngeal muscle 66
Phasic nystagmus 50
    causes of 50
Phenindione 210
Phenothiazine 12
Pheochromocytoma 245, 250
Phlycten 164
Phosphodiesterase inhibitors 150
Phrenic nerve palsy 164
Physical examination 4
    apparent age 4
    appearance of patient 4
    build and nourishment 4
    consciousness 4
    cooperation 4
Pica 181
    causes 181
Pick's disease 34
Pierre-Robin syndrome 144
Pigmented lesions in mouth, differential diagnosis of 192
Pimobendan 150
Pistol shot sound 135
Pitted scar 13f
Pituitary adenoma 264
Pituitary hormones, deficiency of 260

Pituitary thyrotrophs 262
Pityriasis rotunda 15
Plantar fasciitis 229
Plantar reflex 81
    extensor response 81f
    flexor response 81f
Plasma cell
    leukemia 301
    proliferative disorders 299
        classification 299
Plasmacytosis 300f
Platelet
    count 302
    disorders of 296
Pleura 152
Pleural biopsy 177
Pleural effusion 169, 175, 250
    causes of
        left sided 175
        right sided 175
    clinical features 175, 177
    complications 177
    etiology 175
    investigations 176
Pleural fluid
    aspiration, indication for 176
    biochemistry of 176
    cytology of 176
    dynamic 152, 152t
Pleural rub 164, 164t
Pleuritic pain 154
    causes of 154
Pleuropericardial rub 164
Plummer's nail 12
Plummer-Vinson syndrome 194, 289, 291
Pneumaturia 271
Pneumonia 165
    antibiotic therapy in 167t
    causes of unresolved 166
    stages of 166
Pneumothorax 174
    clinical features 174
    etiology 174
    investigations 174
    management 175
    types of 174
POEMS syndrome 301
Polyangiitis, microscopic 242
Polyarteritis nodosa 107, 242
Polyarthritis 226, 232
    acute 232
    and infection 234
    chronic 233
    differential diagnosis of 233
Polycystic kidney 144
    disease 272, 289
Polycystic ovarian disease 245

Polycythemia 4, 6, 111, 155
    redness of
        lips to 288f
        tongue to 288f
    vera 288
Polydipsia 245
Polyglandular deficiency syndrome 266
Polymyositis 184
Polyneuritis cranialis 25
Polyneuropathy 25
Polyuria 245, 247
Poncet's disease 234
Pons 23
Pontine lateral gaze center 43
Poor memory 259
Portal hypertension 196, 218, 220
    clinical features of 221
    complications 221
    etiology of 220, 221f
    in cirrhosis, mechanism of 219
    investigations 222
    management of 222
Portal vein
    atresia 220
    blood 220
    thrombosis 220
        causes of 220
Portosystemic anastomosis 196, 220
Portosystemic mylopathy 219
Positional nystagmus 50
Positive rheumatoid factor, disease with 236
Postglucose suppression 255
Postrenal causes 279
Postsubclavian CoA 117
Post-tussive crepitation 164
Post-tussive suction 164
Postural cough 153
Posture 4
Potassium homeostasis, disorders of 283
Pott's disease 98
Power of muscle 73
Precocious puberty 248
    female 248
    male 248
Precordial signs 135
Precordium
    examination of 113, 120
    inspection of 120
    palpation of 120
    shape of 120
Prednisolne 301
Pregnancy, toxemia of 272
Premenstrual tension and edema 3
Present illness, history of 1
Pressure pain 93
Presystolic accentuation
    absence of 130
    mechanism of 130
Presystolic murmur 127, 127f

Pretibial myxedema 260f
Primary syphilis, chancre of 192
Progressive exertional dyspnea 129
Progressive systemic sclerosis 205, 244
Proliferative glomerulonephritis 274
    pathology of 274
Pronator sign 89
Proportionate dwarfism 256f
Proteinuria 270
    clinically 270
    quantitative assessment of 270
Proximal muscle wasting 70
Proximal myopathy 250
Pruritus 15
Pseudoathetosis 89
Pseudo-Babinski's sign 82
Pseudobulbar palsy 33, 69, 184
Pseudo-Cushing's syndrome 232
Pseudoextensor response 82
Pseudo-Gradenigo's syndrome 52
Pseudohypoparathyroidism 20, 267
Pseudointernuclear ophthalmoplegia 55
Pseudomonas 166
Pseudopancreatic cyst 201
Pseudostratified ciliated columnar 151
Psittacosis 155
Psoas abscess 201
Psoriasis 14f
Psoriatic arthritis 229
Ptosis 47
    bilateral 48, 48f
        causes 48
    myogenic 47
    neurogenic 47
    neuromuscular 47
    of left eye, complete 47f
Ptyalism 180, 181
Puddle's sign 201, 202
Puffiness of face 155
Puffy eyelid 249
Pulmonary arterial hypertension 130, 239
Pulmonary arteriovenous
    fistula 218
    malformation 153
Pulmonary artery
    dilated 124
    hypertension 145f
    pulsation 122
Pulmonary atresia 128
Pulmonary component, accentuation of 124
Pulmonary cyanosis 7
Pulmonary edema 130, 132
Pulmonary endometriosis 153
Pulmonary hypertension 124, 144
    causes of 144
    clinical features of 145
    investigations 145
    passive 144
Pulmonary oligemia 137

Pulmonary plethora 137
Pulmonary regurgitation 137
    clinical features 137
    etiology 137
    investigations 137
    management 137
Pulmonary sequestration 169
Pulmonary stenosis 136
    clinical features 136
    complications 137
    etiology 136
    investigations 137
    management 137
Pulmonary tuberculosis 11, 155
Pulmonary valvular disease 136, 153
Pulmonary vascular source 153
Pulmonary venous hypertension 130
Pulsation over interscapular space 120
Pulse 21, 32, 113, 249
    character of 115
    collapsing 115, 115f
    irregular 249
    normal characters of 115f
    paradoxus, reverse 115
    pressure 114
    volume of 114
Pulsus alternans 114
Pulsus paradoxus 114
Pupil 48
    and light reflex 48
    examination 48
Pure motor paraplegia 104
Purpura forearm 288f
Pursuit movement, disorders of 55
Pyelonephritis, acute bilateral 278
Pyemic liver abscess 206
Pyloric stenosis 201
Pyoderma gangrenosum 211-213, 227
Pyogenic granuloma 192
Pyorrhea alveolaris 192
Pyramidal sign, without 71
Pyramidal system 23
Pyramidal tract 23f
Pyrosis 180, 182
Pyuria 270

R

Radial artery 117
Radial pulse, palpation of 113f
Raeder's paratrigeminal syndrome 58, 59
Ramsay-Hunt syndrome 64
Rapamycin 282
Raymond's syndrome 52
Raynaud's disease 230
Raynaud's phenomenon 243
RBC count 301
Reactive arthritis 234
Reactive arthropathy 241, 244

Reactive pulmonary 145
Reader's paratrigeminal syndrome 49
Rebound tenderness 198
Recent memory 34
Rectum, examination of 204
Rectus abdominis 198
Red cell indices 302
Referred pain 187
Reflex
    function 57, 61
    iridoplegia 49
    movement 66
    reinforcement of 83
    superficial 81
Refractory heart failure 150
Refsum's disease 98
Refsum's syndrome 42
Reiter's arthropathy 241
Reiter's disease 194, 229
Reiter's syndrome 227, 273
Relapsing fever 21
Remittent fever 20
Remote memory 34
Renal artery stenosis 203
Renal biopsy, indications of 276
Renal colic 187
Renal disease 31, 254, 271, 273
Renal disorders, history taking in 272
Renal edema 8
Renal failure
    course of acute 279
    hypercatabolic 279
Renal failure, acute 274, 278
    clinical features 279
    complications 280
    etiology 278
    investigations 279
    management 279
    pathogenesis 278
    pathology 279
    prevention 280
    prognosis 280
    types 278
Renal failure, chronic 227, 259, 267, 274, 280
    clinical features of 280
    etiology of 280
    investigation 281
    management 281
    pathogenesis 280
Renal function test 236, 253
Renal involvement 240
Renal loss 285
Renal manifestation 299
Renal osteodystrophy 231
Renal replacement therapy 282
Renal rickets 231
Renal symptoms 247
Renal system 165

Renal transplantation 282
Renal tubular
　defect 274
　obstruction 278
Renal vasculitis 232
Reproductive symptoms 248
Respiration
　rate of 155
　rhythm of 156
　type of 156
　variation with 126
Respiratory airways 151
Respiratory causes 154
Respiratory disease 154, 158
　clinical features of 165
　drugs for 155
　history taking in 154
　signs in 165t
Respiratory disorders, systems in 164
Respiratory distress syndrome, acute 224
Respiratory failure 31, 173
　causes of 174t
　chronic 173
　management 173
　types of 173, 173t
Respiratory infection, upper 167
Respiratory obstruction, upper 153
Respiratory rate 22
Respiratory symptoms 31, 246, 287
Respiratory system 3, 11, 21, 100, 205, 231, 235, 250, 251, 255, 273, 289
　examination of 151, 155
　general examination in 155
Rest pain 226
Restless leg syndrome 90
Reticulocyte count 302
Retina, rest of 41
Retinal disease 42
Retinitis pigmentosa 41, 42
　causes 42
Retrograde amnesia 34
Retroperitoneal lymphadenopathy 201
Retropharyngeal abscess 194
Retrosternal goiter 246
Retrosternal pain 154
　upper 154
Reversible renal factors, treatment of 282
Rhagades 192
Rheumatic fever 2, 234, 241
　markers of 111
Rheumatic heart disease 149
Rheumatic valvulitis 129
Rheumatoid arthritis 19, 227, 228, 230, 231, 233, 234, 241
　etiology 234
　immunopathology 234
　juvenile 236, 241
Rheumatoid disease, malignant 236

Rheumatoid factor 147, 234
Rheumatological disorders 205, 230t, 234, 241
Rheumatology 226
Rhonchi 163
　causes of 164
Rhonchial fremitus 159
Rhythm of respiration, changes in 22
Rib, tuberculosis of 179f
Rickets 20, 267
Riedel's lobe of liver 199
Riedel's thyroiditis 251
Rifampicin 214, 216
Right hip, flexion of 204
Rinne test 65
Rituximab 238
Rosai-Dorfman syndrome 19
Rotatory nystagmus 50
Roth's spots 147
Rotor's syndrome 213
Rovsing's sign 198
Ruffini's corpuscle 24
Rupture aneurysm 204
Rusty sputum 153

S

Saccadic movement 44
　disorders of 55
Sacroiliac joint 230
Saddle analgesia 96f
Saddle anesthesia 95
Salam's sign 252
Salbutamol 171
Salivary gland, diseases of 181
Salmonella 185, 212
Sandiego criteria 244
Sanfrancisco criteria 244
Sarcoidosis 220
Scar 157, 196
Scarlet fever 193
Schaeffer's sign 82
Schistosomiasis 220
Schober's test 230
Schwabach test 65
Scissor gait 87
Sclera, yellowish discoloration of 7f
Scleredema diabeticorum 15
Scleroderma, pitted scar of 243f
Sclerosing glomerulonephritis, chronic 274
Sclerosing tenosynovitis 227
Scrotal swelling 203
　differential diagnosis of 203
Sea blue hystiocytosis syndrome 53
Seagull murmur 132
Sebaceous cyst 201
Secretory diarrhea 185
See saw nystagmus 50

Segmental dystonia 89
Segmental nerve innervation 92f
Semantic aphasia 36
Sensorium, altered 247, 252, 257
Sensory
　aphasia 36
　ataxia 87
　component 58, 65
　cortex 24, 96
　division 56
　features 104
　fibers 65, 66
　function 57, 61
　inattention 92, 94
　nuclei 56
　paralytic bladder 106
　seizure 96
　symptoms 103
Sensory loss 97f
　global 108
　type of 96
Sensory pathways 25f
　applied anatomy of 24
Sensory system 24, 91, 101, 104
　anosognosia 92
　astereognosis 92
　disorder, symptoms of 30
　dysesthesia 91
　etiology 106
　examination of 90
　graphanesthesia 92
　graphesthesia 92
　hyperpathia 92
　lesion of 94
　pallanesthesia 92
　pallesthesia 92
　paresthesia 91
　stereoanesthesia 92
　stereognosis 92
　terms related to 91
　topanesthesia 91
　topesthesia 91
Septic pulmonary infarcts 147
Septum secondum 138
Seronegative spondyloarthropathy 241
Serositis 226, 240
Serous sputum 153
Serum
　bilirubin 216
　calcium 267
　cortisol level 265
　electrolyte 265
　growth hormone estimation 255
Sessile papilloma 194
Sex hair in female, development of 245
Sexual function 86
Sexually acquired reactive arthropathy 241
Sexually transmitted diseases 2

Sheehan's syndrome 3, 248
Shifting dullness 161
Shigella 185
Shiny nails in cirrhosis 191f
Shock 19
Shoulder
    joint 228
    position of 157
Shrunken liver 202
Sicca syndrome 239
Sickle cell
    anemia 288
    disease 188, 205
Silica dust 155
Silver Streni Corda syndrome 218
Sinus 29
    aplasia 169
    bradycardia 113
    histiocytosis 19
    paired 29
    tachycardia 113, 249
    unpaired 29
Sinusoidal 220
Sitophobia 180, 181
Situs inversus 121f, 169
Sjogren's syndrome 104, 107, 108, 181, 227,
    234, 235, 236, 240, 244
    primary 234
    secondary 235
Skeletal changes 255
Skeletal muscles, hypertrophy of 258
Skin 12, 21, 32, 235, 286, 288
    and hair 4
    bullous lesion of 13f
    color of 14
    flushing of 14, 15
    infection 15
    lesions 15
        primary 12
        secondary 12
    over abdomen 196
    over chest 157
Skull and spine examination 98
Sleep 2
Sleep apnea
    obstructive 259
    syndrome 250
Small intestine 186
    biopsy of 211
Small muscles of hand, wasting of 71f
Smallpox, healed 13f
Smoking, habit of 2
Smoldering multiple myeloma 300
Snake bite 9f
Sneddon's syndrome 239
Snellen's chart 38
Snout reflex 61, 86
Socioeconomic status 3

Sodium
    distribution of 284
    physiology of 284
Solitary adenoma 268
Solitary plasma cytoma 301
Somatic abnormalities 111
Somatic motor fibers 105
Somatization disorder 188
Spastic ataxic gait 87
Spastic dysarthria 36
Spastic gait 87
Speech 34
    abnormality of 35
    areas, anatomy of 35
    comprehension of 35
    fluency of 35
    function, examination of 35
Spherocyte 295f
Sphincter, external 106
Spider naevi 190, 218, 219
Spinal accessory 67
    nerve 67
        clinical disorders of 67
    palsy, symptoms of 67
Spinal artery occlusion, anterior 95
Spinal cord 26, 94
    ascending pathways 26
    blood supply of 29
    descending pathways 27
    diseases of 103, 186
    hemisection of 94
    lesion 85, 102
    pathways of 25f
    transection of 94
    venous drainage of 29
Spinal hemiplegia 102
Spinal segment 27, 84
Spinal tract, nucleus of 58
Spine 98, 229-231
    deformities 229
    involvement, symptoms of 103
    movement of 229
    normal curvature 229
Spinothalamic tract 24, 25
    central lesion of 25
    function 93
Spinoumbilical measurement 201
Spleen 195
    huge 200
    palpation of 199, 199f
    percussion of 202
Splenic rub, causes of 203
Splenomegaly 200, 207
    differential diagnosis of 205
    moderate 206
Splinter hemorrhage 12, 111
Spontaneous bacterial peritonitis 209, 218
    management of 209

Spotty necrosis 216
Spurious hematemesis 184
Sputum 153
Squint, analysis of 46
Staphylococcal skin lesion 13f
Staphylococcus 167
    aureus 147, 166, 185
Steele-Richardson syndrome 34
Sterile pyuria 270
Sternal border, left 128
Sternoclavicular pulsation 120
Sternocleidomastoid muscle, wasting of 68f
Still's disease 227
Stomach 184
    carcinoma 184
Stool, abnormal 180, 187
Strabismus 46
Strawberry tongue 193
Stress incontinence 271
Stridor 154, 246
Strongly positive mantoux test 177f
Stuporous 33
Sturge-Weber syndrome 15, 59
Subarachnoid space 42
Sub-cortical lesion 102
Subcutaneous edema 232f
Subcutaneous emphysema 159
Subcutaneous nodules 227, 233
Subfulminant hepatocellular failure 223
Subhyaloid hemorrhage 41
Sublingual varicosities 193
Subparietal lobe lesion 39
Subungual fibroma 12
Succussion splash 164, 203
Sulfhemoglobinemia 7
Sulphasalazine 237
Supinator jerk 83f
Suppurative lung disease 2, 11, 152, 155
Suppurative pneumonia 167
Supraclavicular area 159
Supranuclear lesion 58
Supranuclear ophthalmoplegia 53
Supraspinatus muscles, wasting of 71f
Suprasternal pulsation 120
    causes 120
Swallowing
    physiology of 182
    reflex 86
Swan neck deformity 235
Sweating, decreased 259
Swelling 226
Symmetrical deforming polyarthritis,
    differential diagnosis of 233
Symphysis pubis 195
Symptomatic migraine 30
Symptomatology 29, 152, 180, 245
Syncopal attack 110
Synovial fluid analysis 236
Synovitis 226

Syphilis 194, 234
Syringomyelia 59, 96f
Systemic disease 19
    sign of 12
    with alopecia 17
    with pruritus 15
Systemic examination 273, 289
Systemic hypertension 274
Systemic lupus erythematosus 238, 297
    clinical features 238
    etiology 238
Systolic hypertension, isolated 22
Systolic murmur 126, 128
    early 126
    late 126
Systolodiastolic murmur 128

T

Tabes dorsalis 188
Tabetic facies 19
Tachycardia, relative 21
Tachypnea 155
Tactile agnosia 37
Tactile localization 94
Takayasu's disease 117, 242, 243
Tall stature 20, 245
    causes for 5
Tangier's disease 98
Tapping apex beat 121
Tarsal tunnel syndrome 238
Teeth 192
    color of 192
    shape of 192
Telangiectasia 192, 219, 296f
Temporal lobe 27
    epilepsy 33
Temporomandibular joint 228
Tenacious sputum 153
Tender hepatomegaly, causes of 206
Tenderness 199
Tendinitis 226, 228
    adductor 228, 229
Tenofovir 217
Tenosynovitis 226
Teratoma 178f
Terbutaline 171
Terry's nail 12
Testes, tumors of 204
Testicular disease 248
Testing sensory system, purpose of 92
Tetanus 19
Tetany 247
Tetralogy of Fallot 140, 142
    associated anomalies 142
    clinical features 142
    components of 142
    embryology 142
    hemodynamics 142

Thalamoparietal projection 24
Thalamoparietal radiation 95
Thiazolidinedione 252
Thoracic kyphoscoliosis 156
Thoracolumbar spine 229
Thrombocytopenia 240, 297
    etiology 297
Thrombosed external piles 204
Thrombosis, promoters of 296
Thrombus 127
Thyroid 4, 32, 112
    carcinoma 251
    disease 254
    function test 259
    gland 17
        examination of 250
        symptoms of 247
    swelling 257f
Thyroiditis 216, 263
    chronic 257
Thyromegaly, causes for 17
Thyrotoxicosis 20, 31, 250, 260, 262, 263
    bone 261
    etiology 260
    factitia 263
    general 260
    hemopoietic 261
    in pregnancy 262
    metabolic 261
    nail 260
    nervous 261
    psychiatric 261
    reproductive 261
    skin 260
Thyroxine 266
Tics 90
Tidal percussion 161
Titubant ataxia 87
Tolosa-Hunt syndrome 51
Tone, examination of 72
Tongue 193
    abnormal movements of 69
    balded 193
    bizarre movement of 90
    coating of 193
    dry brown 193
    fissuring of 193
    numbness 58
    pigmentation of 194
    precancerous lesions of 194
    sides of 193
    size of 193
    ulcer of 193
    underneath of 193
Tonsillar region 194
Torsion dystonia 89

Torsion testes 188
Touch sensation, pathway of 24
Toxic hepatitis 206, 216
Toxins 214, 276
Toxoplasmosi 214
Trachea
    palpating position of 157f
    position of 120, 156, 157
Tracheal shift, causes of 156
Tracheal stridor 154
Tracheobronchial source 153
Transcortical motor aphasia 36
Transcortical sensory aphasia 36
Transmitted murmur 126
Traube's double tone 135
Traube's space 161
    obliteration of 161
    upward shift of 161
Tremor 88, 247
    etiology of 88
Trendelenburg test 228
Triceps jerk 84f
Tricuspid area 129
Tricuspid regurgitation 119, 136
    clinical features 136
    etiology 136
    investigations 136
    management 136
Tricuspid stenosis 136
    causes 136
    clinical features 136
    investigations 136
    management 136
Tricuspid valvular disease 136
Trigeminal nerve 56
    disorders of 59
    distribution of 56f
    lesion of 58
    neuroanatomy 56
    palsy, etiology of 58
Trilogy of Fallot 143
Trochanteric bursitis 228
Trochlear nerve 43
    palsy, causes of 51
Troisier's sign 18, 190
Trophoblastic tumor 262
Tropical pulmonary eosinophilia 164
Tropical sprue 211
Trousseau's sign 22
Truncal obesity 5
Tuberculosis 2, 153, 211, 234
    pleural effusion, management of 177
Tuberculous cavity, left side 178f
Tuberculous pleural effusion 177
Tuberous sclerosis 15, 174
Tubular breathing 162

Tubular necrosis, acute 278
Tubular proteinuria 270t
Tubular vision 40
    causes 40
Tuft cyanosis 7
Tunica vaginalis, hydrocele of 203
Tuning fork 65
Turner's syndrome 19, 20, 144, 245, 248, 249

U

Ulcer 194
    frenulum 193
Ulcerative colitis 194, 211, 213, 241
    differential features of 212
    drug treatment of 213
    severity of 212
Umbilical region 195
Uncommon organism 166
Unconscious patient, examination of 99
Upper limb
    left 9f
    muscles of 78f
    testing tone in 72
Upper lobe
    collapse right 169f
    fibrosis, right 168f, 178f
Upper motor neuron 23
    bilateral 58
    facial palsy
        bilateral 62
        unilateral 62
    lesion 24
        acute phase of 24
Upper quadrant homonymous defect 39
Upper respiratory tract
    examination of 156
    infection, acute 152
Uremia 274
    prerenal 278t
    renal 278t
Uremic complications, treatment of 282
Uremic symptoms 271
Urethra, posterior 106
Urethritis 232
Urinary abnormalities, asymptomatic 274
Urinary bladder 195
    palpation of 200
Urinary composition, alteration in 269
Urinary deposit 278
Urinary sodium 278
Urinary system 252
    examination of 269, 272
Urinary tract
    infection 252, 274
    obstruction 274

Urine
    alteration in amount of 269
    incontinence of 271
    microscopy, normal 273
    normal 273
        chemical composition 273
    specific gravity 278
Urogenital tract disorders, pain in 271
Uterus 201

V

Vagus nerve 65, 66
Valsalva, ruptured sinus of 119
Valve cusp, deformity of 131
Valvular aortic stenosis 125
Valvular heart disease 2, 129, 239
Valvulitis-Rheumatic-Carey coombs
    murmur 127
Variceal bleed, management of 222
Vascular bruit 203
Vascular disorders 52
Vascular headache 30
Vascular phenomena 147
Vasculitic disorders 242t
Vasculitis 231
Vasoconstrictive pulmonary 145
Vegetations 127
Veins 29
    deep 29
    superficial 29
Vena cava obstruction
    inferior 196
    superior 196
Venous congestion of intestine, chronic 210
Venous flow, direction of 196
Venous pulsation 119
Ventilatory defect 153
Ventricular failure
    acute left 153
    left 114
Ventricular filling sound 124
Ventricular hypertrophy, left 141
Ventricular septal defect 139
    anatomical severity of 139
    associated anomalies 140
    complications 140
    investigations 140
    management 140
    pathophysiology 139
    types of 139
Vertebra 27
Vertebral artery 28
    deficiency 95f
Vertebral body level spinal segment 27
Vertebrobasilar system 28, 102

Vertiginous ataxia 87
Vessel vasculitis
    large 242
    medium 242
    small 242
Vessel, narrowing of 127
Vestibular disorders, causes of 65
Vestibular function, tests for 65
Vestibular lesion 50
Vestibular nerve 64
    lesion 65
Vestibulocochlear nerve 64
Vestibulo-ocular reflex 55
Vincristine 301
Viral
    hepatitis 214, 215
    markers 216
Virchow's intermittent biliary fever 187
Virchow's node 18
Viridians streptococci 147
Viscera, vasculitis of 205
Visceral leakage 208
Visceral pleura 152
Visceral reflexes 86
Viscus, perforation of 202
Visible peristalsis 196
Vision
    acuity of 38
    central field of 39
Visual acuity, loss of 38
Visual agnosia 37
Visual pathway 40f
Visual reflexes 38f
Vital signs 4, 20
    temperature 20
Vitamin
    A 210
    B_{12} 210
        deficiency 287, 289, 291, 293
        metabolism of 292
    C 210
    D 210, 266
        deficiency 266
        intoxication 267
    deficiency 34
    K 210
Vitiligo 14, 14f, 246, 265
    of fingers 246f
Vocal cord abnormality 66
Vocal fremitus 158
Vocal resonance 162
Vogt-Koyanagi syndrome 17
Vogt-Koyanagi-Harada syndrome 32
Voice, change in 259
Vomiting 181, 246
    causes of 182
    mechanism of 182
    phases of 182

Vomitus, examination of 182
von Hippel-Lindau syndrome 98
von Recklinghausen's disease 15
von Willebrand's disease 296

W

Waardenburg syndrome 17
Waddling gait 87
Waist-hip ratio 5
Waldeyer's ring 289
Wallenberg's syndrome 59, 66, 95, 102
Wartenberg sign 85
Wasting, types of 70
Water brash 180, 181
Water Hammer pulse 115
Waterhouse-Friderichsen syndrome 264
Watermelon stomach 185
Weakness, pattern of 75
Weber's syndrome 63, 102
Weber's test 65
Webino syndrome 55
Wegener's granulomatosis 153, 231, 242
Wegener's vasculitis 234
Weill-Marchesani syndrome 19
Wemino syndrome 55
Werner's syndrome 17
Wernicke's aphasia 36
Wernicke's area 35
Wernicke's encephalopathy 205
Wernicke-Korsakoff syndrome 34
Wheeze 154
Whipple's disease 205, 208, 210, 211
Whispering pectoriloquy 164
Whispering test 64
White blood count 301
White coat hypertension 22
White nail 12
Wilbrand's knee 38, 39
William's syndrome 20, 144, 190, 216, 218
Wilson's disease 32, 88, 90, 98
Wolfram's syndrome 252
Woltman's sign 85, 250
Wrist 228
    clonus 85
    sign 112f

X

X descend 119
Xanthelasma 100f, 190
Xanthoma 100f, 249
Xerostomia 180, 181
Xiphisternum 195

Y

Y descend 119
Yellow fever virus 215
Yellow nail 169
    syndrome 12, 169
Young syndrome 169

Z

Zidovudine 12
Zinc 210
Zollinger-Ellison syndrome 246